Respiratory Therapist Exam Review Guide

Edited by

CRAIG L. SCANLAN, EdD, RRT, FAARC
Professor, Department of Interdisciplinary Studies
School of Health Related Professions
University of Medicine and Dentistry of New Jersey
Newark, NJ

ALBERT J. HEUER, PhD, MBA, RRT, RPFT
Associate Professor, Program Director
Respiratory Care–North
School of Health Related Professions
University of Medicine and Dentistry of New Jersey
Newark, NJ

LOUIS M. SINOPOLI, EdD, RRT, AE-C
Professor and Director
Respiratory Care Program
Health Sciences and Athletics Division
El Camino College
Torrance, CA

JONES AND BARTLETT PUBLISHERS
Sudbury, Massachusetts
BOSTON   TORONTO   LONDON   SINGAPORE

World Headquarters

Jones and Bartlett Publishers
40 Tall Pine Drive
Sudbury, MA 01776
978-443-5000
info@jbpub.com
www.jbpub.com

Jones and Bartlett Publishers
Canada
6339 Ormindale Way
Mississauga, Ontario L5V 1J2
Canada

Jones and Bartlett Publishers
International
Barb House, Barb Mews
London W6 7PA
United Kingdom

Jones and Bartlett's books and products are available through most bookstores and online booksellers. To contact Jones and Bartlett Publishers directly, call 800-832-0034, fax 978-443-8000, or visit our website, www.jbpub.com.

Substantial discounts on bulk quantities of Jones and Bartlett's publications are available to corporations, professional associations, and other qualified organizations. For details and specific discount information, contact the special sales department at Jones and Bartlett via the above contact information or send an email to specialsales@jbpub.com.

The authors, editor, and publisher have made every effort to provide accurate information. However, they are not responsible for errors, omissions, or for any outcomes related to the use of the contents of this book and take no responsibility for the use of the products and procedures described. Treatments and side effects described in this book may not be applicable to all people; likewise, some people may require a dose or experience a side effect that is not described herein. Drugs and medical devices are discussed that may have limited availability controlled by the Food and Drug Administration (FDA) for use only in a research study or clinical trial. Research, clinical practice, and government regulations often change the accepted standard in this field. When consideration is being given to use of any drug in the clinical setting, the health care provider or reader is responsible for determining FDA status of the drug, reading the package insert, and reviewing prescribing information for the most up-to-date recommendations on dose, precautions, and contraindications, and determining the appropriate usage for the product. This is especially important in the case of drugs that are new or seldom used.

Production Credits

Publisher: David Cella
Associate Editor: Maro Gartside
Production Manager: Julie Champagne Bolduc
Production Assistant: Jessica Steele Newfell
Senior Marketing Manager: Sophie Fleck
Manufacturing and Inventory Control Supervisor: Amy Bacus
Composition: Publishers' Design and Production Services
Cover Design: Kristin E. Parker
Cover and Chapter-Opening Images: © Photodisc
Printing and Binding: Courier Stoughton
Cover Printing: Courier Stoughton

Library of Congress Cataloging-in-Publication Data

Certified respiratory therapist exam review guide / [edited by] Craig L. Scanlan, Albert J. Heuer, Louis M. Sinopoli.
    p. ; cm.
  Includes bibliographical references and index.
  ISBN 978-0-7637-5511-9 (pbk. : alk. paper)
  1. Respiratory therapy—Examinations—Study guides. I. Scanlan, Craig L., 1947– II. Heuer, Albert J. III. Sinopoli, Louis M.
  [DNLM: 1. Respiratory Therapy—methods—Examination Questions. WB 18.2 S283c 2010]
  RC735.I5C464 2010
  615.8'36076—dc22

2009008731

6048

Printed in the United States of America
13 12 11 10 09   10 9 8 7 6 5 4 3 2

To my family and my past, current, and future students, from whom I continue to draw enthusiasm and inspiration.

— CLS

To my wife, Laurel, as well as my fellow educators and respiratory therapists, who encouraged me to pursue this text and inspired me towards its completion.

— AJH

To my family, friends, and the profession, as they are the motivation for all I do, and I thank them for that every day.

— LMS

Contents

Contents

Contents

Contents

Preface

As the editors were preparing this text, colleagues often would ask us if another respiratory therapy exam review book was really needed. Our reply was "not another book, but a different one." With our combined experience of over 100 years in preparing students and graduates for the NBRC exams, we have come to realize that "book knowledge" alone does not assure a passing score. Over time, we have observed that the candidates most likely to do well on these tests are those who know exactly what and how to study, and who are confident in their test-taking abilities. Our goal is to share with all respiratory therapy students and graduates this basic formula: to provide you with the same test knowledge, skills, and strategies that successful candidates use to score highly on the CRT exam.

What makes this book fundamentally different is its approach. First, unlike many other review books, this one focuses your attention exclusively on the CRT exam content. Each topical chapter corresponds *exactly* to a specific content area covered on the current exam. This approach lets you concentrate on the specific knowledge and skills tested in each area, at the levels set by the NBRC for that specific content. Moreover, to distill this content down to what you absolutely need to know, we have formatted much of the book content using simple outlines and tables with a minimum of long-winded narrative.

Second, we provide you with a tried-and-true plan for success. Our plan is based on the decades of experience we have in successfully helping thousands of candidates pass the CRT exam. The basic strategy involves a minimum of 6–8 weeks of preparation, whereby you proceed systematically through each chapter of the text, using both a pre- and post-test to assess your knowledge and confirm its mastery. The plan culminates with you taking and passing a mock CRT-like exam (the chapter post-tests and mock exam are provided on the CD).

Third, we provide key test-taking guidance, designed specifically to allay anxiety, build confidence, and boost your CRT exam scores. Besides providing a full chapter on test-taking techniques, every topical chapter in the text includes critical lists of both common testing errors and the correct approaches you should always take in selected clinical problems or scenarios. Also, you can build additional confidence by repeating the practice tests that draw on our 800+ question item pool.

We also provide special guidance for those who heretofore have been unsuccessful in achieving their goal of becoming a Certified Respiratory Therapist. First, in every topical chapter we identify the latest content that the NBRC recently added to its 2009 CRT exam matrix. Given that there are over 40 new topical areas on the exam, no one should consider retaking this test without full knowledge of these important changes. Second, because our content parallels the CRT exam, you can easily focus you preparation for retesting on just those specific topics where you previously did poorly

Lastly, for those needing additional assistance beyond what the book provides, we provide access to some important supplemental resources. In addition to the testing software on the CD, you will find a wealth of exam-related World Wide Web resources. The editors and authors have sought out, evaluated, and selected the very best respiratory care resources on the Internet and organized them for you based on the NBRC matrix. In this manner, if you need to review a specific content area, you can simply select the relevant chapter/NBRC content area and link to the selected Web subject matter. For those needing additional personal support, including access to unlimited practice testing based on a 3,000+ item pool of NBRC-like questions (all automatically scored and provided with answer explanations), we recommend that you consider the Online CRT Examination Review course described in Appendix C. As an added benefit, purchasers of this book are eligible for a discounted enrollment fee for this comprehensive Web-based course.

Preparing for and passing the CRT exam is a major task. To achieve any major task, you need the right plan and the right materials. This book provides you with both. Follow our plan, use the tools we provide and the strategies we recommend, and you can achieve this important goal!

— *CLS, AJH, & LMS*

Contributors

Salomay R. Corbaley, MBA, RRT, NPS, AE-C
Professor
Respiratory Care Program
El Camino College
Torrance, CA

Sandra McCleaster, MA, RRT, NPS
Adjunct Faculty
Bergen Community College
Paramus, NJ

Roy Mekaru, BS, MHA, RRT, NPS
Director of Clinical Education
El Camino College
Torrance, CA

Narciso E. Rodriguez, BS, RRT, RPFT, NPS, AE-C
Assistant Professor, Department of Primary Care
School of Health Related Professions
University of Medicine and Dentistry of New Jersey
Newark, NJ

John A. Rutkowski, MBA, MPA, RRT, FACHE
Assistant Professor, Department of Primary Care
School of Health Related Professions
University of Medicine and Dentistry of New Jersey
Newark, NJ

Brian X. Weaver, MS, RRT, RPFT, NPS
Director of Respiratory Therapy
The University Hospital
University of Medicine and Dentistry of New Jersey
Newark, NJ

Robert L. Wilkins, PhD, RRT, FAARC
Clinical Professor, Department of Respiratory Care
University of Texas Health Science Center
San Antonio, TX

Kenneth A. Wyka, MS, RRT, FAARC
Cardiopulmonary Clinical Specialist
Anthem Health Services
Albany, NY

Preparing for and Passing the NBRC CRT Exam

Using This Book and CD: Your Roadmap to Success

Craig L. Scanlan

INTRODUCTION

To become a Certified Respiratory Therapist and to obtain a license to practice, you must pass the National Board for Respiratory Care (NBRC) Certification Examination for Entry-Level Respiratory Therapists (CRT exam). Preparing for and passing the CRT exam is no small task. Each year, despite intensive schooling and test-taking experience, a substantial portion of graduates fail this exam or require multiple and expensive retakes to pass it. Because in most states passing the CRT exam is a legal prerequisite to working in the field, you simply cannot afford to do poorly on this test.

To accomplish any major task, you need the right plan and the right materials. This book provides you with both. Our plan is based on our decades of experience helping thousands of candidates pass the CRT exam. Underlying our plan is a set of tried-and-true tools and materials adapted from a highly regarded online CRT examination review course that has helped hundreds of candidates achieve their goal of becoming a Certified Respiratory Therapist. Follow our plan and use the tools we provide and the strategy we recommend, and you too can achieve this important goal!

THE PLAN

A good plan has clear focus and structure. *Unlike many other review books, this one focuses exclusively on the CRT exam.* Some review texts mix preparation for both the CRT and Registered Respiratory Therapist (RRT) exams. Others attempt to review essentially all the topics covered in a typical respiratory therapy program curriculum. *To make the most of your preparation time, you need to focus solely on what is covered on the CRT exam.* You don't need to review everything you learned in school, nor do you need to confuse yourself by studying the different knowledge and skills required for the RRT exam.

Our exclusive focus on the CRT exam is reflected in the structure of this book. Each chapter corresponds *exactly* to a specific content area covered on the current CRT exam. Moreover, we present the topics in the same order as published by the NBRC in its CRT examination matrix (see Appendix A). This approach lets you concentrate on the exact knowledge and skills tested in each area at the levels set by the NBRC for that specific content. Organizing the book by NBRC content areas also helps you if you are preparing to retake the CRT exam. If you fall into this category, you likely scored below expectations in some content areas but did well in others. The best way to ensure success when retaking the exam is to focus your efforts on those content areas where you previously did poorly. Fortunately, this book makes that task easy. Simply review your NBRC score report to identify the content areas where you scored lowest, then focus your work on the corresponding text chapters.

THE TOOLS AND MATERIALS
Book Overview

This book and its supplemental resources provide you with all the tools and materials you need to pass the CRT exam. In addition to this overview chapter, Chapter 2 (Test-Taking Tips and Techniques) provides essential guidance to help you prepare for the exam. The next 17 chapters focus on the specific knowledge and skills needed in each of the current 17 CRT exam content areas. Finally, there is an additional chapter on performing relevant calculations (Chapter 20). Furthermore, the accompanying CD provides post-tests for each of the content area chapters, a mock CRT exam, links to carefully selected Web resources, and other materials useful in preparing for the CRT exam.

Chapter Structure and Content

Each of the 17 content-area chapters has a consistent structure designed to help make your exam preparation as efficient as possible.

Introduction, Objectives, What to Expect, and What's New

Each chapter begins with a short introduction, a set of explicit objectives, and a brief description of the category. The introduction emphasizes the relative importance of that content area and the recommended preparation time. The objectives correspond to the specific knowledge you need to master that section of the exam. The category description specifies the number and type of questions you can expect in this content area on the current NBRC exam. In addition, especially for those who took the exam prior to July 2009, we provide a section called *What's New for 2009*. This section specifies all new topics that the NBRC added to its CRT exam matrix for test administrations beginning in July 2009.

You will immediately note that the chapters in this text vary greatly in length. This variation is by design, based on the defined scope and weight of each NBRC content area. For example, Chapter 6 (Manipulate Equipment by Order or Protocol) is among the longest in the book because this category constitutes nearly 20% of the CRT exam content. In contrast, Chapter 18 (Assisting the Physician with Special Procedures) is among the shortest chapters because the current CRT exam contains only two questions in this category. It is based on these differences that the editors and contributing authors recommend more or less exam preparation time for each chapter.

Pre-Test Questions with Answers and Explanations

All chapters begin with a short practice test of the relevant objectives and content and end with the correct answers and explanations for each practice test question. Similar to chapter length, the number of questions on each pre-test varies with the relative emphasis given that content area on the CRT exam. In total, the 17 chapter pre-tests provide over 275 practice questions, answers, and explanations to help you prepare for the CRT exam.

A word of warning: We have found that many exam candidates try to memorize as many practice questions and answers as possible in hopes that doing so will help them pass the CRT exam. *This is a huge mistake and a waste of your time.* The likelihood of seeing the exact same questions from any review source (including this text) on the actual CRT exam is miniscule. Instead, we recommend that you use each chapter's pre-test to assess your existing knowledge of each content area. This information will help you (1) identify content areas needing priority and (2) adjust the amount of time you spend on each chapter.

In terms of prioritizing what to study, *use the practice questions to help you differentiate between the concepts you have mastered and those you still need to work on*. For example, if you notice that you consistently get practice questions on ventilator peak and plateau pressures wrong (or always have to guess at them), you have identified a shortcoming in your understanding of the mechanics of ventilation. You then would ideally seek out and review the relevant content, including (in this example) the meaning and measurement of total impedance, airway resistance, and compliance.

In general, the first source to review for any pre-test question you get wrong is the explanation of the correct answer provided at the end of the chapter. To ensure content mastery, you should always thoroughly review these explanations so that you understand *why* the correct answer is the right choice. If you are still unclear about a concept after reviewing a question's explanation, you should seek out the more detailed information provided in the chapter or on the CD.

Finally, based on how many concepts you identify by pre-testing as still needing your attention, you should adjust the total amount of time you plan to spend on each chapter according to your individual needs.

What You Need to Know: Essential Content

The *Essential Content* section is the "meat" of each chapter, containing the vital information you need to succeed on the CRT exam. Every effort has been made to distill this essential content down to the key *need-to-know* information most likely to appear on the exam. To do so, we have purposefully chosen a format that emphasizes outlines and tables with a minimum of long-winded narrative.

In addition, we have carefully organized chapter content to coincide directly with the objectives, making it easy for you to find any of the specific information covered in the NBRC CRT exam matrix. For example, if you need to review manipulating resuscitation devices (current NBRC matrix content area II-A-5), you will find a section by that name in Chapter 6.

Common Errors to Avoid

One of the unique aspects of this text is its use of prior candidates' common testing mistakes. We have identified these common errors by analyzing a large pool of question statistics from those who have previously taken an online CRT examination review course. These statistics allowed us to identify the most common mistakes on questions in each of the CRT exam's 17 content areas. The *Common Errors to Avoid* section of each chapter provides a short summary of these common areas of misunderstanding. You can improve your score on the CRT exam by avoiding these mistakes.

Sure Bets

Although you probably have been taught to be on guard for absolutes in questions (e.g., "always"), there are a few relative certainties that apply to responding to questions in each content area of the CRT exam. We have taken the time to highlight these *Sure Bets* at the end of each chapter. As with avoiding common mistakes, knowing in advance what is always the right approach to a clinical problem or scenario can add extra points to your CRT exam score!

Supplementary CD

The supplementary CD extends the resources provided in the book to include a post-test for each of the content area chapters, a mock CRT exam, links to carefully selected Web resources, and other materials useful in preparing for the CRT exam.

Post-Tests

A post-test for each chapter is available on the accompanying CD. Instructions for taking these post-tests are provided in Appendix B. In combination, these 17 post-tests provide hundreds of additional practice questions to help confirm your mastery of each chapter's objectives. We recommend that you take the applicable post-test after completing each chapter and before moving on to review any other content areas. Based on our experience, a score less than 75% correct on any post-test indicates that you need to spend additional time on that chapter's content and/or review the supplementary resources on the CD applicable to that chapter.

Mock Exam

The CD also provides a customizable mock CRT exam that draws questions from the entire item pool. We recommend that you take this mock exam only after completing all 17 of the book's content chapters, including passing each of the accompanying post-tests.

Web Resources

The supplementary CD offers you direct access to the wealth of resources available on the World Wide Web. The editors and authors have sought out, evaluated, and selected the very best respiratory care resources on the Internet and organized them for you based on the NBRC matrix. If you need additional review in any specific content area, you simply need to start up the CD, select the relevant chapter/NBRC content area, and click on the selected Web subject matter.

Other Materials

More details on the CD contents, including additional valuable resources compiled after book production, are described in Appendix B.

THE STRATEGY

Figure 1-1 outlines the strategy we recommend you follow to prepare for and pass the CRT exam. *You should devote at least 6 to 8 weeks to this process.* One of the most common reasons candidates do not pass the CRT exam is hasty or last-minute preparation. Do yourself a favor and follow a deliberate and unhurried process. Remember, it was the turtle who won the race, not the hare!

Some of you will implement this strategy on your own, while others may be guided in their preparation while still in a respiratory therapy program. In either case, it's important to proceed systematically through each chapter and not move forward until you are satisfied that you have mastered the relevant content.

For Those Who Have Previously Taken the CRT Exam

If you have previously taken the CRT exam, you are using this book because you did not achieve a passing score. Although you likely are unhappy with this outcome, this event actually gives you a significant advantage over those who have never taken this exam. First, you are experienced with the testing procedures, so you know what to expect. Second, your score report tells you *exactly* where on the exam you did well and where you did poorly. We recommend that you compute the percentage of correct questions for each of the 17 subscores on your NBRC score report. For example, based on the following section of an NBRC score report:

II. Equipment Manipulation, Infection Control, and Quality Control

	Subscore
A. Manipulate Equipment by Order or Protocol	11/22

you would compute the percentage correct for the Manipulate Equipment by Order or Protocol subsection of the CRT exam as $11/22 = 0.50 \times 100 = 50\%$.

After computing the percentage correct for each subsection, we recommend that you flag every subsection on which you got less than 75% of the questions correct. You should then focus your primary attention on these flagged subsections and their corresponding book chapters in preparing to retake the CRT exam. You should still review the book chapters corresponding to NBRC subsections where you scored above 75%, *but only after attending to your high-priority needs*.

Chapter Review Process

For this strategy to succeed, it is essential that you proceed systematically through each content area chapter. This normally involves the following steps:

1. Take and score the chapter pre-test
2. Review the pre-test to determine your shortcomings
3. Prioritize chapter content based on identified shortcomings
4. Review the applicable chapter content
5. Take and pass the chapter post-test (on CD)
6. Repeat steps 1 to 5 for each chapter

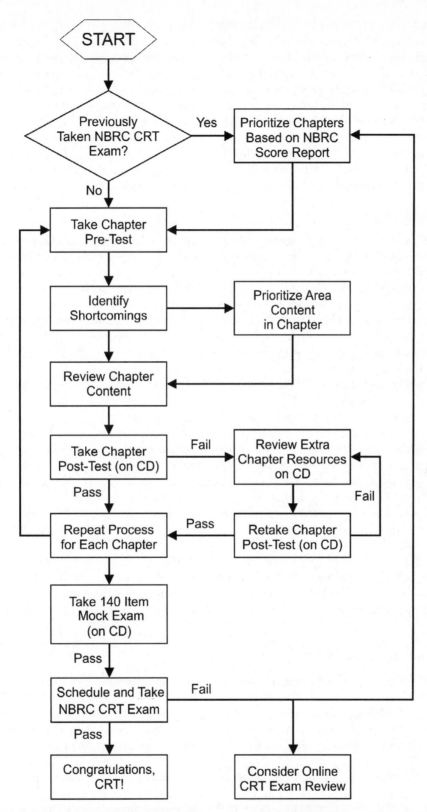

Figure 1-1 Recommended Strategy for Passing the CRT Exam. Spend at least the 6 to 8 weeks proceeding the exam date systematically reviewing the text (about 2 to 3 chapters per week). Upon completing all NBRC content-area chapters and fully examining Chapter 2 (Test-Taking Tips and Techniques), take the mock CRT exam on the CD. Only after successfully completing the mock exam should you schedule and take the NBRC CRT exam.

In regard to step 5 (taking and passing chapter post-tests), we recommend that you set a goal of achieving at *least 75% correct* on each chapter post-test. In addition, your post-test scores generally should be higher than your pre-test scores. The greater this difference, the more you have learned!

What if you fail a chapter post-test? Because chapter post-tests provide explanations for all answers, your first job should be to review these explanations thoroughly so that you understand *why* the correct answer is the right choice. We then recommend that you take full advantage of the CD and review the additional resources provided for the chapter in question. After reviewing both the post-test answers and the extra resources on the CD, *retake the applicable chapter post-test until you achieve at least 85% correct*. We suggest this higher "pass" score for post-test retakes due to the presence of some repeat questions. Lastly, we recommend that you not move forward with any new chapter until you are satisfied that you have mastered each preceding one.

Take the Mock Exam

The mock CRT exam is intended to simulate taking the real CRT exam. Like the chapter pre- and post-tests, our mock exam also gives you feedback on each and every question, including the correct answers and their explanations.

With this feedback, our mock exam becomes a critical learning tool in your path to success on the CRT exam. First, your overall score on this exam tells you how well you have learned and retained the content covered in the book and on the CRT exam. Second, careful review of the test item explanations should help further your understanding of the important concepts likely to be tested on the CRT exam. Last, review of the test item explanations on the mock exam also can help you identify any remaining areas of weakness that you need to address before scheduling your CRT exam date. Because the mock exam serves as a bridge between the book and the CRT exam, we recommend that you take it only after completing all 17 of the book's content chapters, including passing each of their post-tests. We also recommend that you complete our mock exam at least 2 weeks before you are scheduled to take the CRT exam. This way you will have time to review any persistent areas of misunderstanding you have identified as well as avoid the anxiety that last-minute cramming always causes. Instructions on how to take the mock CRT exam are provided in Appendix B.

Should you set a time limit for taking the mock exam? We definitely recommend timing your test. *Because the CRT exam requires that you answer 20 extra nongraded questions (160 total) in 3 hours, you will need to pace yourself to complete about 1 question per minute.* If you take significantly longer to answer each question, you will need to work on your pacing before taking the actual NBRC CRT exam.

What if you do not score well on our mock exam? If you carefully follow the strategy we outline here, it is highly unlikely that you will do poorly on our exam. In the unusual case that you score below 75% on this exam, it's "back to the books." In this case, careful review of the test items you get wrong on our mock exam should help you identify the content areas and book chapters that need review.

Schedule and Take the CRT Exam

After successfully completing all book chapters, their post-tests, and the mock CRT exam, it is time to schedule and take the real thing. If you have not already done so, we strongly recommend that you use some of the time you have set aside before sitting for the NBRC CRT exam to review Chapter 2 (Testing Tips and Techniques). Also, consider using a portion of your set-aside time to take a practice trip to and from your designated NBRC testing center, ideally during the same time period your exam is scheduled. This run through can help you gauge the travel time involved (including the likely traffic) and iron out little details like parking arrangements and where to get a light meal or cup of coffee before the exam.

What if you do not pass the CRT exam? There are several DOs and DON'Ts associated with a failed attempt on the exam. First, the DON'Ts:

- Don't get disheartened
- Don't give up
- Don't immediately reschedule a retake

Instead, take a proactive approach. DO the following:

- Do carefully analyze your NBRC score report
- Do use your score report to prioritize content areas needing further study
- Do revisit the key content area resources we provide in the book and on the CD
- Do give yourself adequate time to implement your new study plan (a minimum of 3 to 4 weeks)

Lastly, if you want or need access to *unlimited* practice testing based on a 2,800+ item pool of NBRC-like questions (all automatically scored and provided with answer explanations), we recommend that you consider the online CRT examination review course described in Appendix C. Purchasers of this book are eligible for a discounted enrollment fee for this course.

Test-Taking Tips and Techniques

Craig L. Scanlan

INTRODUCTION

To perform well on the CRT exam, you first must know the subject matter covered. However, to pass this exam, you also need good test-taking skills. **Figure 2-1** offers our simple two-part "formula" for success on the CRT exam.

Inspection of this formula reveals why many knowledgeable candidates fail the CRT exam. Typically, such individuals do poorly on the exam because they lack the *test-taking skills* needed to translate their mastery of the subject matter into consistently correct answers. The common refrain "I'm no good at taking tests" is a symptom of this problem. Fortunately, this condition is treatable. With good guidance and practice, everyone can develop good test-taking skills. The purpose of this chapter is to help you become a better test-taker. By doing so, you will improve your odds of passing the NBRC CRT exam.

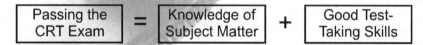

Figure 2-1 Formula for Success on the NBRC CRT Exam.

HOW TO FAIL THE CRT EXAM

It may seem a bit strange to begin with instructions on how to fail your test. However, knowing why people fail the CRT exam can actually help you avoid failure. Of course, the most common reason why candidates perform poorly on the CRT exam is lack of content knowledge. Other causes of failure include the following:

- Taking the test "cold" or unprepared
- Memorizing as many practice questions and answers as possible
- Reviewing everything you ever learned in school
- Cramming the night before the exam
- Letting anxiety get the best of you
- Not finishing the test

It always amazes us how some candidates insist on taking the CRT exam without the proper preparation. Of course, some of these folks do so because they planned poorly and simply ran out of time. Others take the test cold because they are overly confident in their abilities. Last and most foolish are those who take the exam without preparation just to "see how they will do." By not preparing for the exam, you risk both time and money should you fail and need to retake the exam. Although we do advocate "gambling" on specific test questions, taking the CRT exam without any preparation is a very bad bet that you are more than likely to lose. As indicated in our formula for success, you cannot pass the exam without good knowledge of the content covered on the exam. And good knowledge of the subject matter comes only with good preparation.

Another common cause of failure is the misguided strategy of memorizing hundreds of practice questions and answers. As mentioned in Chapter 1, this is a waste of your time. Instead, you should use practice questions and answers to help identify concepts that you know and those that you still need to work on.

We also know of candidates who prepare by surrounding themselves with the dozens of books and hundreds of pages of notes that they acquired while in school. Many of these folks simply do not know where to begin, and sooner or later most will feel overwhelmed by the sheer volume of these materials. Such a strategy typically begets both anxiety and confusion, which are among the most common causes of poor exam performance. To avoid the problems associated with this strategy, you first need to remember that the CRT exam does *not* test for isolated facts or the "book knowledge" covered in specific courses you took in school. Instead, *this exam assesses your job-related knowledge and skills*. So instead of reviewing everything you learned in school, your time is better spent focusing on the specific content of the exam as defined by the NBRC. That is exactly what the remaining chapters in this text do.

Cramming is perhaps the most common reason why candidates fail the CRT exam. Lacking a good study plan and being pressed for time due to job and/or family commitments, some individuals typically put off their preparation until the week *or even the night* before their scheduled test date. Besides producing even worse anxiety than trying to review everything ever learned, cramming typically results in a loss of sleep in the days leading up to the test. "Dazed and confused" best describes such candidates when they show up to take the test—and disappointed when they get their score report.

Anxiety is a common cause of poor CRT exam performance. More precisely, *overanxiety* can lead to failure. Some anxiety prior to taking a test is not only natural but can have positive benefits. Like getting "pumped up" in anticipation of a sports contest, the stress associated with taking a test can help motivate you to excel. Channeling the extra energy associated with test apprehension in a positive way can improve your exam performance.

Last, the surest way to fail the CRT exam is not to finish it. Unlike some exams in which the score is based on the number of questions you complete, the NBRC computes your CRT exam score based on the number of questions you answer correctly. Every question you skip or fail to answer is counted against you. When every question counts, you simply cannot afford to throw away points by omitting answers. To finish the CRT exam in the time allotted (3 hours), you will need to develop good pacing strategies, as described later in this chapter.

GENERAL PREPARATION TIPS

Be Prepared!

Good preparation is the key to success on the CRT exam. Good preparation involves knowing:

- WHAT to study
- WHERE to study
- WHEN to study
- HOW to study

What to Study

Know Your Enemy: The CRT Examination

A common strategy among generals planning a battle is to *know your enemy*. Thinking of the CRT exam as an adversary that you can and will conquer can help you prepare for your coming "battle" with this test. In this case, *knowing the enemy means understanding both the structure and the content of the CRT exam and applying this knowledge to your study plan*.

The structure and content of the CRT exam are well defined in the NBRC CRT examination matrix, published in the current version of the *Candidate Handbook and Application*. The current CRT

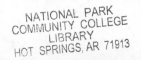

exam consists of 140 graded questions and 20 ungraded items being pretested for future use. The 140 graded questions fall under one of three major content sections: (I) Patient Data Evaluation and Recommendations, (II) Equipment Manipulation, Infection Control, and Quality Control, and (III) Initiation and Modification of Therapeutic Procedures. **Table 2-1** summarizes the current NBRC CRT examination matrix. The full matrix for the current CRT exam, including detailed content in each of these major areas, is reproduced in Appendix A.

Table 2-1 Summary of the Current NBRC CRT Examination Matrix (2009 Version)

Content Area	Number of Questions by Cognitive Level			
	Recall	Application	Analysis	Totals
I. PATIENT DATA EVALUATION AND RECOMMENDATIONS	11	14	1	26
A. Review Data in the Patient Record	4	0	0	4
B. Collect and Evaluate Additional Pertinent Clinical Information	6	11	1	18
C. Recommend Procedures to Obtain Additional Data	1	3	0	4
II. EQUIPMENT MANIPULATION, INFECTION CONTROL, AND QUALITY CONTROL	5	15	9	29
A. Manipulate Equipment by Order or Protocol	4	10	8	22
B. Ensure Infection Control	0	2	1	3
C. Perform Quality Control Procedures	1	3	0	4
III. INITIATION AND MODIFICATION OF THERAPEUTIC PROCEDURES	19	45	21	85
A. Maintain Records and Communicate Information	2	3	0	5
B. Maintain a Patent Airway Including the Care of Artificial Airways	2	2	3	7
C. Remove Bronchopulmonary Secretions	1	3	0	4
D. Achieve Adequate Respiratory Support	2	5	1	8
E. Evaluate and Monitor Patient's Objective and Subjective Responses to Respiratory Care	3	7	5	15
F. Independently Modify Therapeutic Procedures Based on the Patient's Response	2	9	7	18
G. Recommend Modifications in the Respiratory Care Plan Based on the Patient's Response	3	10	4	17
H. Determine the Appropriateness of the Prescribed Respiratory Care Plan and Recommend Modifications When Indicated by Data	1	3	0	4
I. Initiate, Conduct, or Modify Respiratory Care Techniques in an Emergency Setting	1	1	1	3
J. Act as an Assistant to the Physician Performing Special Procedures	1	1	0	2
K. Initiate and Conduct Pulmonary Rehabilitation and Home Care	1	1	0	2
TOTALS	35	74	31	140

In terms of major content levels, questions on Sections I (patient data evaluation) and II (equipment, infection control, and quality control) each constitute about 20% of the exam. The bulk of the current CRT exam (60%) focuses on questions in Section III (therapeutic procedures).

All questions on NBRC exams are also categorized by cognitive level. The cognitive level of a question is based on the mental process involved in answering it and generally is associated with its complexity or difficulty. As outlined in **Table 2-2**, the NBRC defines three cognitive levels of its exam questions. The *Recall, Application,* and *Analysis* columns in Table 2-1 specify the distribution of questions in each content area by their cognitive level. As indicated in the *Totals*, about half the test items are at the application level with about one-quarter each requiring recall or analysis.

Here are some examples of questions at each of these three levels covering the same content area, with the correct answers underlined (Subcategory III-E: Evaluate and Monitor Patient's Objective and Subjective Responses to Respiratory Care):

Recall Example

2-1. An otherwise healthy 25-year-old male patient who took an overdose of sedatives is being supported on a ventilator. Which of the following measures of total static compliance (lungs + thorax) would you expect in this patient?

    A. <u>100 mL/cm H_2O</u>
    B. 10 mL/cm H_2O
    C. 1 mL/cm H_2O
    D. 0.1 mL/cm H_2O

Comments: To evaluate and monitor a patient, you need to know what is normal and what is abnormal. This item tests your ability to recall normal static compliance. It also separately assesses your ability to differentiate the common bedside units used for this measure (mL/cm H_2O) from that typically employed in a pulmonary lab (L/cm H_2O).

Application Example

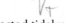

2-2. An adult patient receiving volume-oriented assist/control ventilation has a corrected tidal volume of 700 mL, a peak pressure of 50 cm H_2O, and a plateau pressure of 40 cm H_2O and is receiving 5 cm H_2O positive end-expiratory pressure (PEEP). What is this patient's static compliance?

    A. 200 mL/cm H_2O
    B. <u>20 mL/cm H_2O</u>
    C. 2 mL/cm H_2O
    D. 0.2 mL/cm H_2O

Comments: This item tests your ability to apply a formula to a clinical situation (most formula-type questions are at the application level). To answer it correctly, you need to "plug" the correct data into the formula for computing static compliance—i.e., C (mL/cm H_2O) = delivered volume ÷ (plateau pressure − PEEP).

Table 2-2 NBRC Exam Question Cognitive Levels

Level	NBRC Definition
Recall	The ability to recall or recognize specific information
Application	The ability to comprehend or apply knowledge to new or changing situations
Analysis	The ability to analyze information, to put information together to arrive at solutions, and/or to evaluate the usefulness of the solutions

Analysis Example

2-3. A patient in the intensive care unit with congestive heart failure receiving assist/control ventilation with a set volume of 650 mL exhibits the following data on three consecutive patient-ventilator checks:

Time	Peak Pressure	Plateau Pressure	PEEP
9:00 AM	40	25	8
10:00 AM	50	35	8
11:00 AM	60	45	8

The patient also exhibits diffuse crackles at the bases and some wheezing. Which of the following would you recommend for this patient?

    A. A diuretic
    B. A bronchodilator
    C. A mucolytic
    D. A steroid

Comments: This item assesses your ability to analyze monitoring data and apply this information to recommend a treatment approach for this patient. First, you must analyze the data, which should reveal that the patient is suffering from a progressive decrease in compliance (rising plateau – PEEP pressure difference). Second, you need to recognize that in patients with congestive heart failure, the most common cause for a progressive decrease in compliance is the development of pulmonary edema. Last, you need to apply these data and your knowledge of pathophysiology and pharmacology to recommend the correct course of action, in this case the administration of a diuretic like Lasix.

What conclusions can you glean from these examples? Key pointers that inspection of the NBRC CRT exam matrix reveals include the following:

- Only about one-quarter of the exam questions are based on recall—*you cannot pass this exam by simply memorizing facts!*
- About one-half of the questions on the exam require you to apply your knowledge in a variety of clinical situations; to do well in this area, it can help to visualize and relate your experiences at the bedside as you prepare for your test.
- Most of the exam focuses on therapeutic procedures—you should spend the majority of your preparation in this area!
- Over half of the current exam (75 items) focuses on *just four* of the 17 content areas, to which you should give high priority:
  - Collect and Evaluate Additional Pertinent Clinical Information (18 items)
  - Manipulate Equipment by Order or Protocol (22 items)
  - Independently Modify Therapeutic Procedures (18 items)
  - Recommend Modifications in the Respiratory Care Plan (17 items)
- Most analysis-type questions pertain to equipment and therapeutic procedures, making these areas the most critical overall in terms of both content and level of difficulty.

The "NBRC Hospital"

What you study also should take into account what we refer to as the NBRC hospital. What is the NBRC hospital? *It is not a place but a state of mind.* You "enter" the NBRC hospital whenever you take an NBRC or an NBRC-like exam. This hospital may or may not function the same as the clinical sites you rotated through as a student or the facility where you currently work. Instead, it represents an idealized institution. What do we mean by *idealized*? We mean that the NBRC hospital's "respiratory care department" always relies on generally accepted knowledge in the field, based in part on the various practice guidelines and standards described below. In addition, the NBRC hospital respiratory care department's "procedure manual" is based on broad national agreement among clinicians and educators as to what common clinical skills the *average* graduate performs when first employed. For these reasons, when entering the NBRC hospital, you may be expected to know and do different things from those you do or were trained to do.

For example, in your facility there may be a separate electrocardiogram (ECG) department responsible for taking 12-lead ECGs and maintaining the related equipment. And maybe nurses, physician assistants, or residents are the ones responsible for obtaining 12-lead ECGs in your special care units or the emergency department. But, in the NBRC hospital, you are expected to be able to both use an ECG machine to obtain a good 12-lead tracing and also troubleshoot the device should it not be properly functioning.

Another potential difference operating in the NBRC hospital is the level of independent judgment you are expected to exercise. In many hospitals, new graduates are very limited in what they can do without either supervisor or physician approval. However, a quick review of the CRT examination matrix reveals that the single most important subsection in the therapeutic procedures category is to modify these procedures *independently* based on the patient's response. And this expectation goes well beyond making adjustment to simple "floor therapy" to include using your judgment to alter many key mechanical ventilation parameters, such as the oxygen concentration (FIO_2) or PEEP level. In these cases, the NBRC hospital typically gives you free choice, without being constrained by having to get physician approval. Only if the scenario in question specifies checking with the physician as an option should you consider not exercising your independent judgment.

So how do you prepare to "work" in the NBRC hospital? We recommend the following:

- First, *treat the CRT exam matrix as your departmental procedure manual* focusing in particular on those things you either don't do or don't do frequently in your facility.
- Second, use the questions we include here to help you identify how the practices at the NBRC hospital differ from what you have learned in your training or experience.
- Lastly, when given the opportunity on the CRT exam, do not be afraid to exercise your independent judgment and modify a procedure when changes in the patient's status warrant it.

Study Resources

In terms of the needed knowledge in each content area of the CRT exam, we recommend you focus on what we provide here in Chapters 3–20, using the study plan outlined in Chapter 1. In addition, the NBRC recommends that you obtain or review the most current versions of the following publications in preparation for the CRT exam:

American Association for Respiratory Care (AARC)
- Evidence-Based Guidelines
- Expert Panel Guidelines

  Available online at http://www.rcjournal.com/cpgs

American Heart Association (AHA)
- 2005 American Heart Association Guidelines for Cardiopulmonary Resuscitation and Emergency Cardiovascular Care
  Available online at http://circ.ahajournals.org/content/vol112/24_suppl
- The following training texts:
  - 2008 Handbook of Emergency Cardiovascular Care for Healthcare Providers
  - Advanced Cardiovascular Life Support Provider Manual
  - Pediatric Advanced Life Support (PALS) Provider Manual and Course Guide

  Available online at http://aha.channing-bete.com

American Thoracic Society/European Respiratory Society
- Brusasco, V., Crapo, R., & Viegi, G. (Eds). (2005). Standardisation of spirometry. *European Respiratory Journal, 26,* 319–338.

  Available online at: http://erj.ersjournals.com/cgi/reprint/26/2/319.pdf

Clinical Laboratory Standards Institute
- Blood Gas and pH Analysis and Related Measurements (C46-A)
- Reference and Selected Procedures for the Quantitative Determination of Hemoglobin in Blood (H15-A3)
- Procedures for the Collection of Arterial Blood Specimens (H11-A4)
- Pulse Oximetry (HS3-A)

Not available online; check with your arterial blood gas or clinical lab

You should also have access to a good, comprehensive reference text on respiratory care. To that end, we highly recommend the current edition of *Egan's Fundamentals of Respiratory Care*. To help you find applicable CRT exam-related content, the publisher of the current version of *Egan's* provides an excellent cross-reference between the NBRC matrix and the current edition's content, available to registered users online at http://evolve.elsevier.com.

Where and When to Study

Obviously, where you study depends on your personal circumstances. That being said, it's always best to set aside a familiar and quiet place to do your exam preparation. Often, how quiet your chosen study location is depends on the time of day or night you intend to use it, so plan accordingly. We also recommend that you establish and *strictly follow* a set study schedule, for example, Wednesday and Friday evenings from 8:00 PM to 11:00 PM. In our experience, you must treat your planned study time like a required class or important appointment (with yourself!) to stick to your plan.

How to Study

We provide our principal guidance on how to study in Chapter 1, which describes the use of this text as the primary basis for your CRT exam preparation. Other general advice we provide to our students includes the following.

Prepare Yourself Mentally and Physically

Your brain is part of your body. To stay focused as you study and prepare for the CRT exam, you need to be in top mental *and* physical condition. Be sure to get enough sleep, eat healthy, and get regular exercise. In combination these activities boost your energy levels and keep you sharp.

Be Organized

As we previously discussed, being disorganized leads to confusion and anxiety. Taking the time needed to organize your resources and plot your "battle plan" may at first seem unproductive. However, putting things in order at the beginning of your study plan always pays off big in terms of time saved in the process. In addition, being organized also helps you reduce your anxiety levels as you prepare for the CRT exam.

Once you have set aside a good time and place to study and have all your needed resources in hand, we recommend you follow the systematic plan we outline in Chapter 1 (see Figure 1-1) or a version of this plan adapted to your personal needs and circumstances.

In addition, to help you focus on what content to prioritize, we also recommend that you maintain a problem list, what we call a "lousy log." You should maintain and update this log after each study session and include any problem areas that you discover as you progress through the book and supplementary materials. In most cases, these problem areas represent specific concepts that you have yet to fully master and/or CRT exam sections in which your pre- or post-test performance remains "lousy." In general, your lousy log should initially grow as you identify areas needing attention, then shrink as you master the relevant concepts or content. Of course one goal of your study plan should be that your lousy log be blank before you take the CRT exam.

Get Psyched

As we mentioned previously, anxiety can affect your test performance in negative or positive ways. To ensure that your anxiety helps improve your test performance, you need to "get psyched." *Getting psyched means creating and maintaining a positive attitude toward your test preparation and testing experience.*

Maybe you are not that affected by test anxiety and have already learned to channel your apprehension into a positive force to help you do well on exams. If so, you are in a distinct minority. Most of our students tend to let anxiety get the best of them when preparing for or taking tests, especially high-stakes tests like course finals or NBRC exams.

How do you know if you are negatively affected by test anxiety? How about taking a quiz to find out! The accompanying box provides a 12-question self-assessment developed by the Penn State University Learning Centers to help you determine if you are letting anxiety get the best of you. If several of these statements are true for you, you likely suffer from test anxiety.

Test Anxiety Self-Assessment

T	F	I have trouble sleeping at night and spend those last few minutes before sleep worrying about upcoming exams or projects.
T	F	The day of an exam, I experience drastic appetite changes and either overeat or skip breakfast and lunch.
T	F	While studying for or taking an exam, I often feel a sense of hopelessness or dread.
T	F	While studying or taking an exam, I have problems concentrating and I sometimes feel bored or tired.
T	F	I often yawn during an exam or while studying.
T	F	During an exam, I often feel confused or panicky.
T	F	During an exam, I experience sweaty palms, mental blocks.
T	F	While taking an exam, I sometimes experience headaches, vomiting, or fainting.
T	F	After the exam, I pretend the exam meant nothing to me and discard the result as meaningless.
T	F	When I am finished with an exam, I sometimes feel guilt and blame myself for not studying enough.
T	F	I sometimes get angry or depressed after an exam.
T	F	As a general rule, I view test taking as a stressful situation and dread it.

Adapted from: Penn State University Learning Centers. (2001). *Test taking and anxiety.* Retrieved August 28, 2008, from http://www.ulc.psu.edu/studyskills/test_taking.html

---

If you are an anxious test-taker, that anxiety tends to spill over into your test preparation. A good way to avoid anxiety is to maintain a positive attitude during exam preparation. To do so, we recommend that you reward yourself for studying. This gives you something to look forward to after each prep session and can help give you a regular sense of accomplishment. Some good ways to reward yourself when preparing for a major test include the following:

- When studying, be sure to have a few favorite snacks on hand; these not only can serve as a reward for doing well on small tasks—such as passing a post-test—but also can help maintain your blood sugar level, which is needed for focus and concentration.
- Schedule and complete your test prep sessions *before* enjoyable events, such as a good meal or favorite activity.
- Set a specific time schedule for studying; in this manner you can remind yourself as the end of the session nears (e.g., "just one more hour to go").
- Consider going out for dinner or a movie after completing major milestones in your study plan, such as finishing a set of chapters covering one of the NBRC major content areas.

Even with a positive rewards system, you will likely experience some periods of high anxiety when preparing for or taking your CRT exam. Anxiety often increases as your test date gets closer and closer. **Table 2-3** outlines some good ways to help you allay anxiety when it occurs.

Table 2-3 Ways to Decrease Anxiety

Method	Description
Stop and clear the clouds	If you feel yourself beginning to get overly anxious, force yourself to stop what you're doing and clear your mind for a minute or two before continuing. The time spent "clearing the clouds" generally will be less than that you lose due to stress-associated confusion.
Think good thoughts (daydream)	If you feel overwhelmed by the material, let your mind wander briefly. Thinking good thoughts can help you relax. Once you have released your tension, return to the task at hand.
Visualize success	High achievers always visualize success, not failure. Consistent with this approach, try to picture what it will feel like to pass the CRT exam. Think about getting your permanent state license to practice, getting or advancing in the job you want, becoming registry-eligible, etc. You might even try putting a "CRT certificate" on the wall in your study area with your name on it. Visualizing all these positive outcomes will help you get psyched to achieve them.
Focus, focus, focus	Trying to accomplish multiple tasks at the same time increases stress. When doing your exam prep, always focus on the task at hand, avoid or eliminate any distractions, and do not let outside influences occupy your thoughts. This approach not only reduces stress but also helps you make the most efficient use of your time.
Praise yourself	For every correct answer, every good score on a practice test, every chapter or review session completed, or every item crossed off your "lousy log," give yourself some deserved praise. If you do encounter difficulty with a concept or question, rather than getting "stuck on stupid," put the item in your lousy log and return to it after making progress elsewhere. Praise helps promote a positive attitude, and a positive attitude leads to success.
Avoid the "Nervous Nellies"	Many candidates organize peer study groups to help prepare for NBRC exams. If you are still in school, your class may be preparing for the CRT and RRT exams together. If you find study groups useful in preparing for a test, by all means join or create one. However, try to avoid working with peers whose anxiety overflows and increases your stress levels.

Adapted from: Penn State University Learning Centers. (2001). *Test taking and anxiety.* Retrieved August 28, 2008, from http://www.ulc.psu.edu/studyskills/test_taking.html

Crunch Time

The days immediately before your exam often are the most stressful. The key is to stick with your study plan, maintain your positive attitude, and continue to practice good health habits, including getting sufficient sleep, eating healthy, and exercising.

If you follow your study plan, you should feel confident and well prepared as exam day approaches. Do *not* try to do much additional review the day before the exam. Instead, plan to spend time doing something enjoyable and stress free. The night before the test, be sure to get a full night's rest. The day of the exam, eat a healthy but light meal before the test, and schedule your time so that you are not rushed getting to your testing center.

BECOME A WISE GUY (OR GAL): DEVELOPING TEST-WISENESS

Students and NBRC examination candidates who consistently do well on tests have two things going for them. First, *they know the content and are confident in that knowledge.* But these high performers also have a "secret weapon" in their back pocket. This weapon is the ability to apply knowledge of test design and specific reasoning skills to improve their exam scores. We call this ability *test-wiseness.*

Table 2-4 Hypothetical Impact of Test-Wiseness on Exam Performance

Candidate Response and Performance	Test-Unaware Candidate		Test-Wise Candidate	
	Questions Answered	*Questions Correct*	*Questions Answered*	*Questions Correct*
"Knows cold"	70	70	70	70
Guesses at	70	18	70	35
Raw score		88		105
Percentage		63%		75%
Result		FAIL		PASS!

How does test-wiseness work? **Table 2-4** demonstrates the difference between a test-unaware and a test-wise candidate on a hypothetical NBRC CRT exam. Both are comfortable enough with the content to "know cold" or be absolutely sure about their answers to half the questions on the exam (70 items). Both have to guess at the remaining 70 questions. Unfortunately, the test-unaware candidate does no better than chance on these questions, getting about one in four correct, resulting in a failing score of 88/140, or 63%. In contrast, the test-wise candidate applies knowledge of test design and question reasoning skills to get half of these questions correct, resulting in an overall score of 105/140, or 75%, sufficient to pass the exam.

Fortunately, test-wiseness is a skill that anyone can learn. It entails both techniques related to multiple-choice questions in general and specific rules of thumb applicable to NBRC-like questions. By developing this skill, you not only will improve your exam scores but will also increase your command over testing situations in general. The added benefits are increased confidence and decreased anxiety when taking tests.

General Tips for Multiple-Choice Items

Dissecting Questions: The Anatomy of Multiple-Choice Items

The NBRC CRT exam consists entirely of multiple-choice questions. Most of these are the simple "one best answer" type, but a small percentage use the multiple-true format, also known as complex multiple-choice items.

The first skill in becoming test-wise is to understand the various parts of these questions and to use that knowledge to improve your odds of identifying the correct answer. **Table 2-5** summarizes the key elements common to most NBRC CRT exam questions, and **Figure 2-2** provides a "dissected" example.

Table 2-5 Elements Common to NBRC CRT Multiple-Choice Questions

Question Element	Description
Scenario	Brief description of the clinical situation
Stem	The statement that asks the question or specifies the problem
Options	Possible answers to the question or solutions to the problem
Keyed response	The option that answers the question correctly (the *correct* answer)
Distractors	The remaining incorrect options (*wrong* answers)

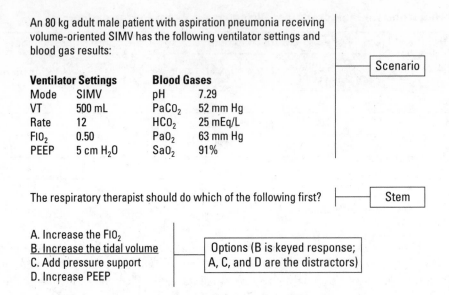

An 80 kg adult male patient with aspiration pneumonia receiving volume-oriented SIMV has the following ventilator settings and blood gas results:

Scenario

Ventilator Settings		Blood Gases	
Mode	SIMV	pH	7.29
VT	500 mL	$PaCO_2$	52 mm Hg
Rate	12	HCO_2	25 mEq/L
FIO_2	0.50	PaO_2	63 mm Hg
PEEP	5 cm H_2O	SaO_2	91%

The respiratory therapist should do which of the following first? — Stem

A. Increase the FIO_2
B. Increase the tidal volume
C. Add pressure support
D. Increase PEEP

Options (B is keyed response; A, C, and D are the distractors)

Figure 2-2 The Key Elements in a Typical NBRC-Like Question. In this example, the scenario and stem are separate. The scenario and stem may be combined in many cases.

Scenario

Typically, a question scenario briefly describes a clinical situation that you need to assess. We recommend that you thoroughly review the scenario before even looking at the stem or question options (note that sometimes the scenario and stem are combined and must be reviewed together). When assessing the scenario, look for the following critical information:

- The location or setting (e.g., ICU, outpatient clinic, patient's home)
- The available resources (e.g., equipment that is being used or is at hand)
- The patient's general characteristics (e.g., age, size, disease process, mental status)
- Any relevant objective data (e.g., from ABGs, PFTs)
- Any relevant subjective information (e.g., signs and symptoms)

Assume all the information in the scenario is there for a reason. As you assess the scenario, note in particular the patient's characteristics and any and all *abnormal* data or information, especially laboratory results. As an example, based on your assessment of the scenario in Figure 2-2, you should extract the following critical information:

1. The patient:
   a. Is an adult male weighing 80 kg (about 200 lbs)
   b. Has aspiration pneumonia (often a cause of hypoxemia)
2. The equipment is a ventilator capable of volume-oriented SIMV
3. In terms of the objective data:
   a. The set tidal volume may be a bit low for an 80-kg patient
   b. The FIO_2 is near the high end of its safe level
   c. The blood gas is abnormal:
      i. The primary/most severe problem is acute respiratory acidosis
      ii. The PaO_2 is low but adequate (SaO_2 > 90%)

Stem

The stem asks the question or directs your action. In Figure 2-2, the stem is asking what action the respiratory therapist should take. As with the scenario, you always must read the stem carefully. The stem often contains key words or phrases that may help you choose the correct answer. **Table 2-6** describes common key words or phrases that you should look for in question stems and what to do when you encounter them.

Table 2-6 Key Words or Phrases Found in Question Stems

Type of Clue	What to Look For	What to Do
Priority	Words such as *first, initially, best, priority, safest, most,* and *least*	Put a value on each available option and then place them in rank order
Sequence	Words such as *before, after,* and *next*	Apply procedural knowledge or logic to place the options in proper sequence
Negative polarity	Words such as *not, except, contraindicated, unacceptable,* and *avoid*	Switch from being concerned with what is correct or true to what is false; consider each option a T/F question and select the one that is *false*
Absolutes	Key words such as *always* and *never*	Find the only option that would be correct *in every case every time*
Verbal associations	Word or phrase in the stem that is identical or similar to a word in the correct answer	Select the option that includes wording similar to that found in the stem

In our sample question in Figure 2-2, the stem contains the key word *first*. This is a priority clue that directs you to choose the action *most immediately* needed. Based on our analysis of the blood gas data, we identified the primary/most severe problem as being acute respiratory acidosis. The keyed response or right answer should therefore be one that best corrects this problem, in this case option B, *Increase the tidal volume.*

In addition to the general clues described in Table 2-6, be on the lookout for other key words or phrases. For example, compare the wording of the following two question stems related to endotracheal tube positioning:

Stem Wording A

Which of the following assessment procedures would help determine proper positioning of an endotracheal tube in a patient's trachea?

Stem Wording B

Which of the following assessment procedures would confirm proper positioning of an endotracheal tube in a patient's trachea?

Note that the two stems are identical except for the verb. Question stem A specifies "help determine," while B specifies "confirm." This tiny variation in wording makes a huge difference in the likely best answer for these two questions. Whereas there are many potentially good answers for A (e.g., breath sounds, capnography, tube insertion length, esophageal detection device, chest X-ray, etc.), there is only one consistently correct response for B (i.e., a chest X-ray).

Although you should always be on the lookout for key words or phrases in CRT test items, we also recommend that you avoid reading anything into your exam questions. When you read too much into a test item, you usually end up answering a question differently than intended by the exam writers. Read all questions as is. Don't be led astray by either overanalyzing or oversimplifying any question. Last, avoid drawing any assumptions beyond those supported by the facts at hand. *The simplest interpretation is generally the correct one.*

You also might want to consider a useful strategy that many good test-takers employ. Good test-takers frequently paraphrase the question in their own words and then anticipate the answer—*before looking at the options available.* In the days of pencil-and-paper testing, this meant actually covering up each question's options with scratch paper or one's hand. This can help minimize any confusion that a question's options may cause, especially the distractors. In general, this technique works best when you can quickly and confidently identify the answer in your head.

Options

Options are the possible answers to a question. The good news is that every NBRC CRT exam item has only four options, labeled A through D. Also good news for well-prepared candidates is that a substantial portion of these questions will be straightforward and relatively easy to answer. Indeed, if you understand and can apply the information being tested, you will often recognize the correct answer immediately.

The bad news is that not even the smartest candidate knows all the correct answers. Indeed, we believe that on average most candidates will be forced to guess on between one-third to one-half of the questions on the exam. If the best you can do on these questions is to guess randomly at their answers, you'll only get about 25% of them correct. To do better you'll need to apply our recommended option selection strategies.

Option Selection Strategies

To do well on the CRT exam, you need to thoughtfully examine each question's options. *When you are sure of the correct response, select it and move on.* In contrast, if the correct response is not immediately apparent to you, you will need to apply specific skills to analyze the available options before selecting an answer.

First, do not panic when you encounter questions that appear difficult or unfamiliar to you. All CRT exam candidates will encounter dozens of such questions when they take this test. Instead of getting flustered, get resourceful. Whenever you encounter a difficult question, you need to rise to the challenge and use the strategies we provide here to select the most logical answer.

Useful general option selection strategies include the following:

- Always look for the best option, not just a correct one (two or more options may be correct, but one likely is the "most" correct in *the particular circumstances or with the specific patient described*).
- When you are unsure of the correct option, switch from finding the right answer to finding the wrong answer(s).
- Eliminate options you know to be incorrect; each time you can eliminate a true distractor, you dramatically increase your chances of answering the question correctly.
- When in doubt, give each option a "true–false" test as compared with the stem (the true statement is usually the most plausible answer).
- Be wary of options that are totally unfamiliar to you; more often than not unfamiliar options are distractors.
- If you encounter a "double negative" in a stem and option, remember that it creates the equivalent positive statement.
- Avoid impulsively selecting an option simply because it provides correct information as an option can provide correct information but still be the wrong choice because it does not answer the question asked.

If these selection strategies do not help, you'll need to apply more specific reasoning skills to identify the correct answer. These skills involve identification of absolutes and qualifiers, dealing with equally plausible options, weighing two options that are opposite to each other, addressing duplicate facts appearing in options, finding the most general or global option, and dealing with a range of option values. In addition, if the question involves using basic math skills, a few key strategies can help you succeed whenever you need to perform computations.

Absolutes (Specific Determiners)

As with question stems, some options may include absolutes or specific determiners. You know an option includes a specific determiner when you find words such as *always, never, all, every, none,* and *only.* These key words indicate that the option has no exceptions. Question 2-4 provides an illustrative example.

2-4. Which of the following is true regarding patients in the early stages of an asthmatic attack?

    A. They all exhibit respiratory alkalosis.
    B. They always have moderate hypoxemia.
    C. They have decreased expiratory flows.
    D. They never respond to beta adrenergics.

In this hypothetical example, options A, B, and D all contain specific determiners or absolutes. More often than not, options that use absolutes are false. Generally, you should avoid choosing any option that *must* be true or false every time, in every case or without exception. In this case, applying this strategy helps you easily zero in on the correct answer (C), the only one not containing an absolute.

Note that because specific determiners are easy to identify, the NBRC minimizes their use on its exams. So do not expect to encounter these frequently. Also note that some absolutes, especially those founded in rules or standards, may be a correct option. For example, most would agree that the statement "You always must properly identify the patient before treatment" holds without exception in general patient care situations. For this reason, if the scenario and stem are addressing policies, procedures, rules, or standards, you may need to allow for absolutes. *In contrast, if the question involves a patient in unique clinical circumstances, few if any absolutes pertain.*

Qualifiers

A qualifier is the opposite of a specific determiner. Qualifiers represent a conditional or "hedge" word or phrase such as *usually, probably, often, generally, may, frequently,* and *seldom.* Qualifiers may appear either in the question stem or in one or more options. Question 2-5 is a good example of the use of qualifiers.

2-5. A patient's advanced directive:

    A. Is usually obtained at the time of admission
    B. Can be found in the doctor's progress notes
    C. Represents a guideline, not a legal requirement
    D. Cannot be altered after it is written and signed

Options that contain qualifiers usually represent good choices. In this example, only option A contains a qualifier and is in fact the correct option. As with absolutes, note that the NBRC minimizes the use of qualifiers in its exam questions, especially in question options. Nonetheless, you need to be on the lookout for these key words and apply the appropriate strategy when needed.

Equally Plausible Options

Often, NBRC questions contain two options that are very similar or equivalent to each other, as apparent in question 2-6.

2-6. An intubated patient is receiving volume control ventilation. The patient's condition has not changed, but you observe higher peak inspiratory pressures than before. Which of the following is the most likely cause of this problem?

    A. There is a leak in the patient-ventilator system.
    B. The endotracheal tube cuff is deflated or burst.
    C. The endotracheal tube is partially obstructed.
    D. The endotracheal tube is displaced into the pharynx.

Note that options A and B are equivalent because a deflated or burst endotracheal (ET) tube cuff represents a leak in the patient-ventilator system. Usually when two items are very similar or equivalent to each other, they are distractors and should be eliminated from consideration. Then make your choice from among the remaining two options (in this case option C is the correct choice). By doing so, you immediately improve your odds of correctly answering this question from 25% to 50%. As noted previously, this is exactly what test-wise candidates do.

What if three of the options are very similar to each other? In this case, apply the "Odd Man Out" strategy, as applicable in answering question 2-7.

2-7. Over a 3-hour period, you note that a patient's plateau pressure has remained stable, but her peak pressure has been steadily increasing. Which of the following is the best explanation for this observation?

    A. <u>The patient's airway resistance has increased.</u>
    B. The patient is developing atelectasis.
    C. The patient's compliance has decreased.
    D. The patient is developing pulmonary edema.

In this example, options B, C, and D are similar in that they all correspond to a decrease in the patient's compliance. When this occurs, turn your attention to the different or "Odd Man Out" option, which is most likely the correct one (option A in this example).

Opposite Options

Another very common way NBRC item writers create distractors is to include a pair of direct opposites among the options, what we call "mirror-image options." Question 2-8 is an NBRC-like item with mirror-image options:

2-8. You are assisting with the oral intubation of an adult patient. After the ET tube has been placed, you note that breath sounds are decreased on the left compared with the right lung. What is the most likely cause of this?

    A. <u>The tip of the tube is in the right mainstem bronchus.</u>
    B. The cuff of the endotracheal tube has been overinflated.
    C. The endotracheal tube has been inserted into the esophagus.
    D. The tip of the tube is in the left mainstem bronchus.

In general, when you encounter two options that are opposites, chances are the correct choice is one of the two. In this example, options A and D are literally mirror images of each other, and one of them is likely the correct answer. Referral back to the scenario (breath sounds decreased on the left compared to the right) should help you decide which of these two responses is correct (A).

It is important to note that there are exceptions to this strategy. Although you will encounter them less frequently, some questions may include mirror-image options as distractors, meaning that *both* are incorrect choices. In these cases, the item writer is using option opposites to divert your attention from the correct answer, as in question 2-9.

2-9. A patient receiving long-term positive-pressure ventilatory support exhibits a progressive weight gain and a reduction in the hematocrit. Which of the following is the most likely cause of this problem?

    A. Leukocytosis
    B. Chronic hypoxemia
    C. <u>Water retention</u>
    D. Leukocytopenia

In this example, leukocytosis and leukocytopenia are polar opposites. Is one of them the correct choice, or are they both distractors? To make this decision often requires referring back to the scenario or stem (which are combined in this question). Logically, both leukocytosis and leukocytopenia are more often the result of abnormal processes (such as infection) and less often the *cause* (a key word in the stem). So here these two options are more likely both being used as distractors and should be eliminated. Now, by selecting from the two remaining two options, your odds of correctly answering this question have improved to 50-50. If you also remember that chronic hypoxemia tends to increase and not decrease the hematocrit, you can now be almost certain of selecting the correct option (C).

Duplicate Facts in Options

Item writers often create options that include two or more similar or identical statements among the choices. Question 2-10 is a good example of this question design.

2-10. In reviewing the PFT results of a 67-year-old smoker with an admitting diagnosis of emphysema and chronic bronchitis, you would expect which of the following general findings?

    A. Increased airway resistance and decreased lung compliance
    B. <u>Increased airway resistance and increased lung compliance</u>
    C. Decreased airway resistance and decreased lung compliance
    D. Decreased airway resistance and increased lung compliance

Note that this question's options contain two contrasting sets of statements: increased/decreased resistance and increased/decreased compliance. When you encounter this type of question and are unsure of the answer, you should try to identify any statement that you know is *either* true or false. Once you do so, you usually can eliminate at least two options as being distractors. In our example above, if you know that patients with emphysema and chronic bronchitis typically have high airway resistance, then you can immediately eliminate options C and D. Alternatively, if you know that patients with emphysema do *not* have decreased lung compliance, then you can eliminate options A and C. Either way, you have doubled the likelihood of selecting the correct answer (B).

Global Options

Question options often include a mix of general and specific statements, as in question 2-11.

2-11. In instructing a patient how to breathe during a small-volume nebulizer drug treatment, the respiratory therapist coaches the patient to hold his breath at the end of each inspiration. The purpose of this maneuver is to improve:

    A. <u>Drug delivery</u>
    B. Particle stability
    C. Aerosol penetration
    D. Inertial impaction

In this example, option A is the most general or global alternative, while options B through D are much more specific. Candidates who are test-wise know that global statements are more likely to be the correct option than choices that are very specific or limited in focus. This is because the most global option usually includes the most information. In this question, particle stability, aerosol penetration, and inertial impaction are all factors that *fall under the broader concept of enhanced drug delivery*, making option A the best choice here.

Options Constituting a Range

Some test questions, especially those focusing on recall, provide options representing a range of values, typically from early to late, or from big to small. Question 2-12 is a good example.

2-12. You obtain an SpO_2 measurement on a patient of 80%. Assuming this is an accurate measure of hemoglobin saturation, what is the patient's approximate PaO_2?

    A. 40 torr
    B. <u>50 torr</u>
    C. 60 torr
    D. 70 torr

When item writers create questions like this one, they often try to hide or mask the correct choice by placing it within a set of higher and lower values. In these cases, you should consider eliminating the highest and lowest values, choosing an option in the middle. Following this logic for this question would result in eliminating options A and D, giving you a 50-50 shot at the correct answer to this question (B). Of course this strategy should be applied only when you do not know the answer. Those familiar with the "40-50-60/70-80-90" rule of thumb might recognize its application to this question and immediately know that 80% saturation roughly corresponds to a PaO_2 of 50 torr.

Math Problems

Typically, the NBRC CRT exam will include a small number of questions that require a simple calculation in order to obtain the correct answer. To help you prepare for these questions, Chapter 20 reviews common cardiopulmonary calculations likely to appear on the CRT exam. Here we provide more general guidance in regard to selecting options when presented with questions involving math.

Because many candidates lack confidence in their math skills, they tend to panic when confronted with a question that requires a computation. This response generally is unwarranted because the math skills required on the CRT exam are rather basic and typically involve no more than one or two computational steps. So there is really no reason to get anxious over these questions.

To improve your confidence in approaching math questions and help you consistently select the correct answers, we recommend the following:

- Always set up the problem before you begin to solve it; use the scratch paper provided at the testing center to write out the applicable formula, *being sure to set it up properly to solve for the value being requested.*
- After setting up the formula, try *estimating* the answer without calculating it; prior estimation can help you avoid making formula or computational errors.
- After doing the computation, do it a second time to confirm that you get the same answer.
- Don't immediately select an answer that matches your calculation; most math question distractors are based on common formula or computation errors. Instead, reread the problem, recheck your formula, and if necessary redo your math.
- If you are completely stumped, "choose from the means and not the extremes." If you do not know the applicable formula or cannot come up with a good estimate, toss out the high and low numbers and select one near the middle.

Question 2-13 illustrates using math problem strategies to arrive at the correct answer.

2-13. A portable spirometer requires that you enter the patient's height in centimeters in order to derive normal values. The patient tells you that she is 5 feet 6 inches tall. What value would you enter into the device?

    A. 26 cm
    B. 66 cm
    C. <u>168 cm</u>
    D. 186 cm

First, you should set up the problem. This represents a straight unit conversion, from English to metric units (inches to centimeters). All such problems are based on a simple formula that requires knowledge of the applicable conversion factor:

measurement (X units) × conversion factor = measurement (Y units)

In this case the X units are inches, the Y units are centimeters, and the conversion factor is 2.54 cm/inch. So the proper setup of the formula for this problem is:

measurement (inches) × 2.54 cm/in = measurement (cm)

Slightly complicating this problem is your need to convert 5 feet 6 inches to inches. Since there are 12 inches to a foot, the patient is $(5 \times 12) + 6$, or 66 inches tall. Note that the numeric value 66 appears among the distractors. Including a value derived in an intermediate step as a distractor is a common ploy used by item writers. You can avoid succumbing to this ploy by completing all computations before comparing your answer to those provided.

Now that you are sure you have set the correct formula to answer the question, estimate the answer before you compute it. The answer should be about 2½ times greater than the patient's height in inches, 66 inches. Twice 66 is *about* 130 and ½ 66 is *about* 33, so the answer should be *about* 130 + 33 or 163 cm. Based on estimation alone, answer C, 168 cm, looks very good. Based on estimation, you also can eliminate option A because it is *less than* the patient's height in inches. Based on the setup of your formula, that would be impossible. Indeed, option A (26 cm) is lurking there to catch those who set up the formula improperly or use the wrong conversion factor. You would get 26 cm as the answer if you mistakenly *divided* the patient's height in inches by 2.54 instead of multiplying by this factor.

Last, after doing the initial computation, do not immediately select the answer. Instead, re-compute the answer after rereading the question and rechecking the setup of your formula.

What if you don't know the exact formula or factor to use? Hopefully your estimated answer will allow you to eliminate at least some of the distractors and improve your odds of answering the question correctly. And if elimination does not help, apply our last-ditch "choose from the means and not the extremes" strategy.

Specific Tips for Common NBRC-Type Items

Applying general option selection strategies will go a long way toward improving your NBRC CRT exam score. To boost your score even more, we have developed several item response guidelines that apply specifically to common NBRC question formats. By learning to apply these guidelines when you encounter these question formats, you will increase your likelihood of passing the exam!

The Triple S Rule

The "Triple S" rule is the most basic of all principles we recommend you apply to answering NBRC-type questions. Put simply, if a patient gets worse when you are giving therapy, *Stop, Stabilize,* and *Stay.* Stop what you are doing, try to stabilize the patient, and stay until help arrives. Question 2-14 is a good example of the Triple S rule.

2-14. During postural drainage of the left lower lobe, a patient complains of acute chest pain. Which of the following should you do?

- **A.** Give the patient supplemental oxygen
- **B.** Continue the treatment with the bed flat
- **C.** Ask the nurse to administer pain medication
- **D.** <u>Discontinue the treatment and monitor the patient</u>

A corollary to the Triple S rule is to *never start* therapy if the patient is exhibiting abnormal signs or symptoms that could be worsened by your action. Instead, as illustrated in Question 2-15, you should always contact the physician.

2-15. A 45-year-old patient with asthma is prescribed 0.3 mL of albuterol (Proventil) in 3 mL normal saline via small-volume nebulizer. Before initiating therapy, you note from chart review that the patient is severely hypertensive and has been experiencing episodes of superventricular tachycardia. You should do which of the following?

- **A.** Administer the treatment as ordered
- **B.** <u>Postpone the treatment and notify the physician</u>
- **C.** Dilute the albuterol with extra normal saline
- **D.** Decrease the amount of albuterol administered

Act First, Ask Questions Later

With all of the emphasis teachers place on assessing patients, students often forget that there are times you should act first, then gather information. The best examples are always emergency situations, where any delay for information gathering may cause harm to the patient. Question 2-16 provides a good example of this principle.

2-16. A patient is admitted to the emergency department comatose with suspected smoke inhalation. After confirming airway patency, which of the following should you do *first*?

    A. Measure the SpO_2
    <u>**B.** Initiate 100% oxygen</u>
    C. Obtain an arterial blood gas
    D. Request a STAT chest X-ray

In this scenario, getting more information is important, but the first priority is to ensure adequate oxygenation. Given that the patient is suspected of having a smoke inhalation injury, 100% O_2 should be administered STAT, without waiting for more information.

    Question 2-17 also illustrates this principle, which emphasizes that your patient's safety and welfare must always be your first priority.

2-17. You are called to the bedside of a patient by her ICU nurse to check the attached volume ventilator. You note that both the low-volume and high-pressure limit alarms are sounding on each breath. Your first action should be to:

    <u>**A.** Disconnect patient and manually ventilate with 100% O_2</u>
    B. Call the attending physician for further patient information
    C. Check the patient's chart for the original ventilator orders
    D. Ask the nurse about how recently the patient was suctioned

    In this example, the patient is in danger, as evident by the ventilator alarms. Although options B, C, and D might help you understand the cause of the problem, they waste valuable time and ignore the immediate needs of the patient. Since your priority always must be the patient's safety and welfare, option A is the best answer for this question.

If It Ain't Broke, Don't Fix It!

Another of our "top ten" principles is to *leave well enough alone*—i.e., if it ain't broke, don't fix it! Typically this will show up on an NBRC exam as a situation in which patient data indicate normal parameters, but you are given the option to change things. DON'T. Question 2-18 illustrates application of this item response guideline.

2-18. A 60-kg (132-lb) COPD patient is receiving SIMV with a V_T of 500 mL at a rate of 9/min with an FIO_2 of 0.35. Blood gases are as follows: pH = 7.36; PCO_2 = 61 torr; HCO_3 = 36 mEq/L; PaO_2 = 64 torr. Which of the following changes would you recommend at this time?

    A. Increase the IMV rate
    B. Increase the FIO_2
    <u>**C.** Maintain settings</u>
    D. Increase the V_T

Back Off Bad!

Exam candidates love to complain about NBRC questions with "two right answers." Of course, according to the NBRC, there is only one best answer for each question. One perfect example of this type of question is the "double effect" scenario. Typically, a patient who is receiving multiple therapies at the same time either worsens or improves. At least two different changes could help the situation—which do you choose? Question 2-19 is a good example.

2-19. A 30-kg (66-lb) child is being mechanically ventilated in the SIMV mode. The following data are available:

Ventilator Settings	Blood Gases
F_{IO_2} 0.45	pH 7.38
Mandatory rate 18	$Paco_2$ 42 torr
Total rate 23	Pao_2 110 torr
V_T 350 mL	HCO_3 23 mEq/L
PEEP 12 cm H_2O	BE 0 mEq/L

Based on these data, which of the following should you do?

    A. Decrease tidal volume
    <u>**B.** Reduce the PEEP</u>
    C. Decrease the rate
    D. Lower the F_{IO_2}

In this scenario, the child's acid-base status and Pco_2 are normal, so no change in ventilation is warranted. The Pao_2 is above normal (hyperoxia) and can be safely lowered if the patient's hemoglobin is acceptable. You can lower the Pao_2 by either lowering the PEEP level *or* lowering the F_{IO_2}. Both answers are right! Which do you choose?

Actually, there is only one correct answer. In this case an F_{IO_2} of 0.45 presents little or no danger to the patient, but a PEEP of 12 cm H_2O is definitely hazardous. Decrease the PEEP first!

The lesson is that when confronted with two or more possible changes in therapy, both of which would have the same good effect, first change the therapy that poses the greatest potential harm to the patient—*back off bad!*

Data Just Don't Jive

Given the number and variety of instruments used to measure and monitor a patient's physiologic status, it is no wonder that the NBRC will test your ability to recognize and/or deal with conflicting data— i.e., numbers that "just don't jive" with each other. Question 2-20 is a good example.

2-20. The following data are obtained for a patient:

Blood Gas Analyzer	CO-Oximeter
pH 7.35	Oxyhemoglobin 97%
$Paco_2$ 28 torr	Carboxyhemoglobin 1%
HCO_3 14 mEq/L	Methemoglobin 1%
BE –10 mEq/L	Hemoglobin 13.8 g/dL
Pao_2 40 torr	
Sao_2 73%	

You should do which of the following?

    A. Report the Sao_2 value as 73%
    B. Report the Sao_2 value as 97%
    C. Recommend administration of bicarbonate
    <u>**D.** Recalibrate the instruments and repeat the analysis</u>

In this example, careful inspection of the data indicates a large discrepancy between the ABG analyzer's Pao_2 and Sao_2 (40 torr and 73%) and the actual oxyhemoglobin reported by the oximeter (97%). *One of these readings must be wrong.* Unfortunately, since no additional information is provided (patient or equipment status), the only good option is to recalibrate the instruments and repeat the analysis.

At the same time, you should probably give the patient supplemental oxygen (just to be sure) while repeating the lab analysis.

Errors, Errors Everywhere!

A little-known NBRC exam specification requires candidates be able to "verify computations and note erroneous data" (Section III-A). Usually the NBRC will offer up 1 to 2 questions that confirm your ability to "check your math" or to recognize plainly incorrect data. Common math error questions focus on equations you use frequently in clinical practice, such as the alveolar air equation and the calculation of compliance or airway resistance on ventilator patients. Also common are errors in reported lab values, as evident in question 2-21.

2-21. The results of an arterial blood gas analysis for a patient who is breathing 100% oxygen are below:

Blood Gases

pH 7.27

$Paco_2$ 44 torr

HCO_3 23 mEq/L

BE +1

Pao_2 598 torr

Sao_2 100%

Which of the following is the likely problem?

 A. Respiratory acidosis
 B. Large physiologic shunt
 C. Metabolic acidosis
 D. <u>Laboratory error</u>

Whenever one option (here D) includes the possibility of an error, check out the numbers! First, the Pao_2 of 598 torr on 100% O_2 is not only possible, but near normal (based on the alveolar air equation). In contrast, the acid-base values are *not* consistent with the underlying relationship that determines pH (the Henderson-Hasselbach equation). In this case, both the $Paco_2$ and HCO_3 are normal. With both these values being within the normal range, the pH also would have to be close to normal, which it clearly is not (pH = 7.27). The only possibility here is a laboratory error.

Don't Know What You're Missing!

In addition to using conflicting or erroneous data in its questions, the NBRC likes to give candidates questions with missing data. These questions are designed to "trap" those inclined to act on insufficient information, while rewarding those who carefully review the data. Question 2-22 illustrates this type of question.

2-22. A doctor asks you to assess if a 75-kg (165-lb) patient with a neuromuscular disorder being mechanically ventilated in the SIMV mode is ready for weaning. You obtain the following data during a bedside ventilatory assessment:

Spontaneous tidal volume	250 mL
Minute ventilation	10 L/min
Vital capacity	750 mL
Max inspiratory pressure (MIP)	–28 cm H_2O

Based on this information, which of the following would you recommend?

    A. Begin a spontaneous breathing T-piece trial
    B. <u>Postpone weaning and reevaluate the patient</u>
    C. Begin weaning using a pressure support protocol
    D. Begin weaning by decreasing the SIMV rate

In this question, many candidates would observe that the patient's vital capacity and MIP are borderline adequate, and conclude that the patient is ready for weaning. *Wrong!* In this case, the minute ventilation and tidal volume data suggest a major problem, but this becomes clear only after identifying and deriving the missing data—the spontaneous breathing rate (spontaneous rate = 10 L/min ÷ 250 mL/breath = 40 breaths/min). This yields a rapid shallow breathing index of 40/0.25 = 160, far above the threshold value of 100 that indicates a potential weaning problem and likely weaning failure. Based on discovery and analysis of the missing data, you would recommend postponing weaning and reevaluating the patient.

    This type of question should make it clear that when given a problem with numeric information, you should *always* review the numbers to see what, if anything, is missing. Then see if you can derive the missing data from the available numbers. Often this is the key to solving these problems.

Jump Back, Jack!

Often the NBRC presents you with a situation in which things go bad (patient worsens, equipment fails, etc.). Just as often, *your* action immediately preceded things going bad. In these cases, the corrective action is usually to reverse course and *undo* what you have done—*jump back, Jack!* Question 2-23 illustrates this principle.

2-23. A surgeon orders an increase in PEEP from 6 to 10 cm H_2O for a post-op patient receiving mechanical ventilation. After you adjust the PEEP setting, you note a rapid fall in the patient's arterial blood pressure and a rapid rise in her heart rate. Which of the following actions would you recommend to the surgeon?

    A. Increase the F_{IO_2} by 10%
    B. Administer a vasopressor
    C. <u>Return the PEEP to 6 cm H_2O</u>
    D. Obtain a stat blood gas

    One of the adverse effects of PEEP is decreased cardiac output (due to increased pleural pressure and decreased venous return). A rapid drop in a patient's blood pressure and rise in heart rate indicate decreased cardiac output. Whenever an adverse response to therapy occurs, your first consideration should be to stop the therapy and restore the patient to his or her prior state; in this case, return the PEEP to its initial level of 6 cm H_2O.

KISS It!

The KISS principle is straightforward: <u>K</u>eep <u>I</u>t <u>S</u>imple, <u>S</u>tupid! When taking an NBRC test, this means that the simplest solution to a problem is often the best. Question 2-24 is a good example of the KISS principle.

2-24. Manual ventilation of a patient with a self-inflating bag-valve-mask device fails to inflate the patient's chest adequately. You should do which of the following?

    A. Intubate and mechanically ventilate the patient
    B. Switch to gas-powered resuscitator with mask
    C. <u>Reposition the patient's head, neck, and mask</u>
    D. Insert a laryngeal mask airway (LMA)

    In this sample troubleshooting question, most options might help resolve the problem. However, option C is the simplest and should at least be tried before moving on to more aggressive options. The lesson here is that whenever one of the options is relatively simple and could provide the solution to the problem at hand, it is probably the correct answer.

Gas Goes In, Gas Comes Out

Almost every NBRC exam includes two or more questions testing your ability to differentiate between leaks and obstructions in equipment, their sources, and their correction. A basic rule of thumb is that *leaks prevent pressure buildup, and obstructions cause pressure buildup.* The classic example is the simple bubble humidifier. Block the tubing outlet while gas is flowing and the pressure pop-off should sound (an obstruction). If the pressure pop-off does not sound, there is a system leak. A similar example is the leak test you perform on a ventilator circuit.

Identifying sources of leaks is simple—any mechanical connection (tubing, nebulizer/humidifier caps, exhalation valves) is a potential source for leakage, as is the patient's airway (mouthpiece, mask, tracheal tube/cuff). To correct a leak, tighten the connection, fix or replace the component, or provide a better airway seal. Question 2-25 provides a good example of a "leaky" question.

2-25. When checking a ventilator, you discover that the set PEEP level cannot be maintained. Which of the following might be causing this problem?

    I. Leak in the tubing
    II. Faulty exhalation valve
    III. Leak around the airway cuff
    IV. Loose humidifier connection

    A. I and II
    B. I and III
    C. II and IV
    D. I, II, III, and IV

According to our rule of thumb, this is definitely a leak scenario. And since any mechanical connection or the patient's airway can be the source of a leak, *all* of the cited problems could be the cause, making D the correct response.

Obstructions can be harder to identify, in part because an obstruction can be complete or partial and because "obstruction" during mechanical ventilation can involve any factor that raises airway pressure (increased resistance or decreased compliance). Correcting or overcoming an obstruction must address the underlying cause. Question 2-26 illustrates this type of question.

2-26. At the bedside of a patient receiving volume-oriented mechanical ventilation, you suddenly observe the simultaneous sounding of the high-pressure and low-volume alarms. Which of following is the most likely cause of this problem?

    A. A leak in the ET tube cuff
    B. A mucous plug in the ET tube
    C. Ventilator circuit disconnection
    D. Development of pulmonary edema

Since this scenario deals with volume-oriented mechanical ventilation, it's best to rely first on a tried and true alarm rule of thumb to identify this problem as being an obstruction:

If the alarm combination is:	Then the problem is:
High pressure/low volume	An obstruction
Low pressure/low volume	A leak

The problem here is that there are two options that involve "obstruction"—the mucous plug and the decreased compliance associated with the development of pulmonary edema. Which to choose? In this case our prior advice on dissecting the question should help. Note the key word *suddenly* in the stem. Although pulmonary edema can develop relatively quickly, it would not change airway pressures suddenly. In contrast, a mucous plug can cause a sudden rise in airway pressure, making B the best choice and correct answer.

Love Those Multiple Trues!

Students tend to hate multiple-true-type questions (the ones with all those answer combinations!). The fact is that most multiple-true questions are easier to answer than simple "ABCD" questions. Why? Because more than any other type of question, multiple trues improve your odds of being correct when you have only partial knowledge of the answer. Question 2-27 demonstrates this important item response concept.

2-27. Which of the following would facilitate clearance of pulmonary secretions in a patient with cystic fibrosis?

     I. Mucomyst
    II. Flutter valve
   III. Atropine
   IV. DNase

  A. I and III
  B. II and IV
  C. <u>I, II, and IV</u>
  D. II, III, and IV

Most candidates will recognize Mucomyst as a mucolytic agent that might facilitate clearance of pulmonary secretions. Based on this partial knowledge, you can eliminate options B and D since they do not include Mucomyst. Alternatively, if based on your partial knowledge you recognize that atropine can dry airway secretion, you can eliminate options A and D since they both include this drug. Note that either of these partial-knowledge approaches immediately improves your odds of getting this question correct from 1 out of 4 (for pure guessing) to 50-50. Then all you need to know is that either DNase *or* a flutter valve can also help, and you can be sure to get this item right!

Treat the Patient, Not the Monitor!

A favorite NBRC "trick" question is to place you in a scenario where patient and monitor data conflict, but action is required. Common forms of this type question include: (1) pulse oximetry data (good) versus bedside assessment of the patient's oxygenation (bad) or (2) ECG (good) versus bedside assessment of the patient's perfusion (bad). Question 2-28 is a good example.

2-28. During a short pause from resuscitation of a child in the emergency department, you cannot palpate a carotid pulse but observe the following rhythm on the ECG monitor (**Figure 2-3**):

Which of the following actions should you take at this time?

  A. <u>Resume cardiac compressions and ventilation</u>
  B. Discontinue compressions and monitor the patient
  C. Recommend cardioversion at 100 Joules
  D. Recommend epinephrine administration

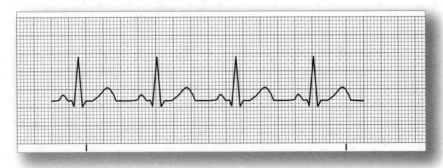

Figure 2-3 ECG Rhythm Observed on Monitor.

Source: Garcia, T. & Miller, G. T. (2004). *Arrhythmia recognition: the art of interpretation.* Sudbury, MA: Jones and Bartlett.

In question 2-28, the likely problem is pulseless electrical activity (PEA). Remembering that the ECG represents only electrical activity and that a patient with no pulse requires resuscitation should make this a "no-brainer." However, over a third of those taking our practice exams decide to go against their better judgment (and their training) and instead treat the monitor. Test smart and don't join that group!

Keeping Order

All NBRC entry-level exams assess your ability to sequence multiple therapies or coordinate your therapy with that of other health professionals. Most of these questions rely on simple common sense— e.g., don't perform postural drainage right after a patient has eaten!

As a special case, you will often be asked in what order to perform combinations of therapy aimed at either getting drugs (e.g., steroids, antibiotics) in or getting secretions out of the airway. In these situations, apply the following rule of thumb:

1. Open 'em up
2. Thin 'em down
3. Clear 'em out

"Open 'em up" means first open the airways, using a bronchodilator. Then administer any other drugs designed for pulmonary deposition (e.g., antibiotics, steroids). "Thin 'em down" means you should next use hydrating or mucolytic agents (bland aerosols, acetylcysteine, DNase) to decrease the viscosity of secretions. "Clear 'em out" means the last step should be to aid in removing the secretions (e.g., directed coughing, postural drainage, suctioning). Question 2-29 illustrates this approach.

2-29. A physician has ordered albuterol (Proventil) and deoxyribonuclease (DNase) by aerosol for a cystic fibrosis patient who also receives postural drainage 3 times a day. You should administer these therapies in which of the following sequences?

    A. Deoxyribonuclease (DNase), postural drainage, albuterol (Proventil)
    B. <u>Albuterol (Proventil), deoxyribonuclease (DNase), postural drainage</u>
    C. Postural drainage, albuterol (Proventil), deoxyribonuclease (DNase)
    D. Deoxyribonuclease (DNase), albuterol (Proventil), postural drainage

Give Me a V; Give Me an O!

Typically the NBRC includes at least half a dozen questions testing your ability to modify ventilator settings properly based on a blood gas report. You simply can't afford to get many of these questions wrong.

First, you need to be able to interpret blood gases properly. Just as important, however, is the need to differentiate between problems of ventilation ("Give Me a V") and problems of oxygenation ("Give Me an O"). This is the secret to slam-dunking these questions.

To help you out in this area, we recommend that you draw a line or mark or circle to separate the blood gas report's ventilation/acid-base data from its oxygenation data. As an example:

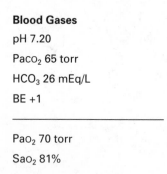

Blood Gases

pH 7.20

$Paco_2$ 65 torr

HCO_3 26 mEq/L

BE +1

———————————

Pao_2 70 torr

Sao_2 81%

Once you have drawn the line, *separately* assess (1) ventilation/acid-base status and then (2) the adequacy of oxygenation. In most cases the NBRC will limit the problem to one or the other—i.e., a problem of ventilation *or* a problem of oxygenation.

If the problem is mainly one of ventilation (as above), either increase or decrease the ventilation, as appropriate. If the problem is mainly oxygenation, you will need to either raise or lower the FIO_2 or adjust PEEP/CPAP. Question 2-30 is an example.

2-30. A 90-kg (198-lb) patient is being ventilated in the postanesthesia care unit (PACU) following upper abdominal surgery. Ventilator settings and arterial blood gas data are below:

Ventilator Settings	Blood Gases
Mode SIMV	pH 7.51
V_T 800 mL	$Paco_2$ 31 torr
Set rate 14/min	HCO_3 24 mEq/L
Total rate 14/min	BE +1
FIO_2 0.40	Pao_2 115 torr
PEEP 5 cm H_2O	Sao_2 99%

You should recommend which of the following?

    A. Increase the FIO_2
    B. <u>Decrease the rate</u>
    C. Decrease the tidal volume
    D. Discontinue the PEEP

Here the problem is clearly one of ventilation, *not* oxygenation. In this case, the patient is being hyperventilated (respiratory alkalosis) and the minute ventilation should be decreased. Since the tidal volume is okay (about 9 mL/kg), you should recommend decreasing the rate.

Alternatively, you may identify the primary problem as one of oxygenation, as evident in question 2-31.

2-31. A 45-year-old 70-kg (154-lb) male with a diagnosis of bilateral pneumonia is receiving volume-controlled ventilation in the SIMV. Ventilator settings and arterial blood gas data are below.

Ventilator Settings	Blood Gases
Mode SIMV	pH 7.35
V_T 700 mL	$Paco_2$ 45 torr
Set rate 6/min	HCO_3 23 mEq/L
Total rate 10/min	BE −1
FIO_2 0.65	Pao_2 55 torr
PEEP 5 cm H_2O	Sao_2 83%

Which of the following should be recommended?

    A. <u>Increase PEEP</u>
    B. Increase the rate
    C. Increase the FIO_2
    D. Add an inspiratory plateau

Since the Pao_2 is less than 60 torr and the Sao_2 is less than 90%, hypoxemia is present. Therefore option A or C could potentially improve oxygenation (a good example of a "double effect" item). Which you choose to raise depends on the underlying cause of the patient's hypoxemia.

To determine the cause and treatment of hypoxemia we recommend you use the "60/60" rule, outlined in **Table 2-7**.

In the scenario in question 2-31, the patient's Pao_2 is less than 60 torr and the Fio_2 is greater than 0.60, so according to the 60/60 rule the cause of the hypoxemia is physiologic shunting. When the cause of the hypoxemia is physiologic shunting, increasing the Fio_2 further will do little good and potential harm (oxygen toxicity). Instead, you need to open up unventilated alveoli (the cause of physiologic shunting). To open up unventilated alveoli, you need to add or increase PEEP/CPAP.

Who's in Charge Here?

These questions typically check to confirm that you know who prescribes respiratory care and who needs to be contacted should a change in care be needed and no protocol exist to manage the patient. Question 2-32 also tests your knowledge of what to do before initiating therapy on a patient.

2-32. A nurse tells you that his patient is scheduled to start chest physiotherapy four times a day this morning and that he would like you to get started before she goes to radiology for a CT scan. Which of the following should you do *first*?

    A. Auscultate and percuss the patient's chest
    B. Initiate therapy after reviewing the X-ray
    C. Interview the patient to obtain a history
    D. <u>Confirm the doctor's order in the chart</u>

Similar questions will ask what to do if you believe a change in therapy is needed, or if the patient asks specific questions regarding his or her diagnosis or prognosis (contact the doctor). Remember, all respiratory care is provided by physician prescription, and (without a protocol) only the physician can change the order.

TAKING THE TEST

Good preparation for any test should also involve consideration of how to take the exam (i.e., strategies to use just before and during actual test administration). Here we provide a few additional pointers specifically applicable to taking the NBRC CRT exam.

Know What to Expect When Reporting to the Testing Center

We recommend that you arrive early for your scheduled test and do something relaxing before actually reporting to the testing center. Note that if you are more than 15 minutes late, you will forfeit your test reservation and will have to reschedule another administration with the NBRC.

In order to sit for the exam, you'll need proper identification. The NBRC currently requires two valid forms of identification that include your name and signature, *one of which must be an official governmental ID with photograph* (e.g., passport, driver's license, military identification card).

If your identification checks out properly, you will be led to a testing room. Note that you are allowed to take only your keys and wallet into the testing room. Test center personnel will provide you with a pencil and scratch paper, which must be returned at the end of the exam.

Table 2-7 60/60 Rule for Oxygenation

Patient's Oxygenation		Cause of Hypoxemia	Best Solution
Pao_2	Fio_2		
> 60 torr	< 0.60	Maldistribution of ventilation	Increase the Fio_2
< 60 torr	> 0.60	Physiologic shunting	Add/increase PEEP/CPAP

To familiarize you with its exam format, the NBRC provides a short practice session before testing begins. This practice session does not affect either the time allotted for the actual exam or your score. Only after you finish or quit the practice session does the actual exam begin.

Once you begin the actual exam, you cannot ask questions. Although you are allowed to take breaks during your exam, break time counts against the total time allotted for your test.

Be Familiar with the Exam Format

Our "know your enemy" guideline applies not just to the content of the CRT exam but to its format. Fortunately, by the time most candidates actually take the NBRC CRT exam, they have taken dozens of similar tests, usually in school. Indeed, most programs require that students pass a computer-based CRT-like exam in order to graduate. You probably already know most of what to expect on the real thing.

As most candidates are aware, all NBRC exams are administered by computer at selected testing centers throughout the United States. The CRT exam is a 3-hour (180-minute) test consisting of 160 multiple-choice questions, of which 140 are scored. The additional 20 test items are what the NBRC terms "pre-test questions" that are being evaluated for use on future exams. You will not know which questions are being scored and which are being pre-tested, so you should try your best on all test items.

The NBRC test software presents one question at a time on the computer screen. As depicted in **Figure 2-4**, each question appears at the top of the screen with the four answer options immediately below. A function bar appears below each question. This bar contains several important buttons and text boxes, and their functions are described in the figure. If you choose to provide comments on specific test questions, the NBRC will apply this information when determining if test score adjustments are needed. For this reason, if you believe that the question you are trying to answer is flawed, be sure to provide a comment that explains why.

To select an option as your answer, you either click your mouse over the corresponding letter (A, B, C, or D) or type in that letter using the keyboard. To change your option choice, simply click on or key in a different letter. Your responses are not registered until you exit the exam for scoring, so you can change your answer to any question at any time during the exam period.

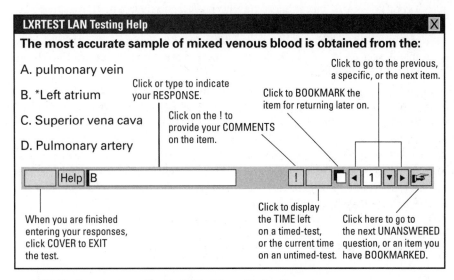

Figure 2-4 NBRC Computer-Based Testing Help Screen.

Source: National Board for Respiratory Care. (2008). *Candidate handbook and application.* Olathe, KS: National Board for Respiratory Care. Reprinted with permission.

Strategies to Employ During the Test

The following strategies should help you perform at your best level when taking the CRT exam:

- Get comfortable
- Answer all questions
- Budget your time
  - Monitor your pace
  - Answer easy questions first
  - Bookmark difficult items and return to them later
  - Use all the available time
- If in doubt, reconsider your answers

Getting comfortable may seem difficult when taking a high-stakes exam, but the preparation this text provides—especially the strategies provided in this chapter—should help allay your test anxiety. Moreover, just like an athlete with pregame "butterflies in the stomach," once you get down to the task at hand, you'll get into the needed rhythm.

Because your score on the CRT exam is based on the number of items you get correct, it is essential that you answer all questions. To do so, you need to develop a good pace and budget your time properly.

Budgeting your time is the single most important strategy when test-taking. You have 180 minutes to answer 160 questions (140 scored and 20 pre-test items), which gives you just over a minute for each question. To keep on pace, you need to be aware of your progress. However, rather than constantly checking the clock, we recommend that you check your progress every 20 to 30 minutes, with the goal of completing, on average, one question per minute. For example, if you check your progress at one hour into the exam, you should have completed about 60 questions.

To further maximize your use of time, you should answer the easy questions first and save the difficult ones for last. However, even if a question appears straightforward, don't rush through it. Spend enough time on each item to read it carefully and apply the strategies we recommend here to select your answer. However, don't linger too long on any one question. In general, if you feel stumped on any given question or know that more than a minute has elapsed, bookmark the item and return to it later.

After completing all the easy questions, use the remaining time to review and answer all your bookmarked items. If you must guess, apply the option selection strategies outlined in this chapter to better your odds of selecting the correct answer.

If time remains after you have answered all the questions, review those items about which you were most unsure. *If an answer was a guess, don't hesitate to reconsider your choice.* Note that this advice is contrary to what most students are taught (i.e., "your first guess is best"). Research consistently indicates that changing answers on multiple-choice exams is more likely to boost your score than lower it.

After you finish the exam, clicking on the COVER button on the function bar will take you to a "cover page," which summarizes how many questions you have answered and how much time you have used. If you have completed all questions and are satisfied with your answers, you can EXIT the exam from this cover page. After exiting the exam, the testing center provides you with your score report. If you have followed the guidance we provide throughout this text, we are confident that you will have passed the exam and achieved your goal of becoming a Certified Respiratory Therapist.

REFERENCES

Aycock, T. (2005). *Test taking strategies.* Meridian Community College, Meridian, MS. Retrieved August 29, 2008, from http://www.mcc.cc.ms.us/nursing/images/test%20taking%20techniques.doc

National Board for Respiratory Care. (2008). *Candidate handbook and application.* Olathe, KS: National Board for Respiratory Care. Retrieved August 29, 2008, from http://www.nbrc.org

Penn State University—Learning Centers. (2001). *Test taking and anxiety.* Retrieved August 29, 2008, from http://www.ulc.psu.edu/studyskills/test_taking.html

Wilkins, R. L., Stoller, J. K., & Kacmarek, R. M. (Eds.) (2009). *Egan's fundamentals of respiratory care* (9th ed.). St. Louis: Mosby.

Patient Data Evaluation and Recommendations

Review Existing Data in Patient Record

CHAPTER

3

Sandra McCleaster and Albert J. Heuer

INTRODUCTION

Patient assessment is the bedrock of quality patient care. Often, the process of patient assessment begins with gathering information from the medical record, also known as the patient's chart. Because the patient's medical record is where most clinical data are documented, efficient and comprehensive assessment requires that you know where to find the relevant information. The medical record contains information relative to past medical history and/or related events. In addition, the results from recently conducted physical exams, lab tests, and imaging studies can also be found there. The medical record also may contain information relating to the future treatment plan (e.g., drug allergies, DNR status). Whether the information relates to the past, present, or future, a proper review of the medical record provides the basis for most clinical decisions or recommendations regarding the patient's care plan. Therefore, before performing therapeutic or diagnostic procedures, you should always review the medical record to verify the doctors' orders, to become familiar with the patient's overall condition, and to review clinical data for potential contraindications. In preparing for the CRT exam, remember that the NBRC expects that you know where to find information in the medical record and how to use this information to optimize patient care.

OBJECTIVES

After completion of this chapter, you should be able to review and determine the relevancy of data in the patient record, including:

1. Past and present medical history
2. Physical exams, including vital signs and physical findings
3. Lab studies such as pulmonary function testing, CBC, electrolytes, coagulation studies, sputum tests, and arterial blood gases
4. Imaging studies, including chest X-rays and MRI, CT, PET, and V/Q scans
5. Monitoring data such as pulmonary mechanics, noninvasive monitoring, and fluid balance
6. Cardiac testing results; most notably ECG and hemodynamic monitoring
7. Maternal, perinatal, neonatal history and data

WHAT TO EXPECT ON THIS CATEGORY OF THE CRT EXAM

Number of questions: about 4 questions, mostly involving the recall of relevant content

WHAT'S NEW FOR 2009

As of July 2009, this section of the NBRC CRT examination includes the following *new content areas*:

- Review patient history:
  - Medication history
  - Patient education (previous)
- Review laboratory data such as:
  - CBC
  - Electrolytes
  - Coagulation studies
  - Culture and sensitivities
  - Sputum Gram stain
- Review monitoring data:
  - Fluid balance
- Review cardiac monitoring:
  - ECG data results (e.g., heart rate, rhythm)
  - Hemodynamic monitoring results
  - Blood pressure
  - CVP
  - Pulmonary artery pressure (PAP)
  - Cardiac output/index
- Review maternal and perinatal/neonatal history and data:
  - Apgar scores
  - Gestational age
  - L/S ratio

PRE-TEST

Carefully respond to each of the following questions. After completing the pre-test, compare your answers to those provided at the end of this chapter. Then thoroughly review each answer's explanation to help understand why it is correct.

3-1. Which of the following specialized imaging tests would be most useful in diagnosing a pulmonary emboli?
A. Chest X-ray
B. Pulmonary function test (PFT)
C. Ventilation-perfusion scan (V/Q scan)
D. Arterial blood gas (ABG)

3-2. While examining a patient in the ICU, you note that he appears somewhat edematous, and the nurse has indicated that the patient's urine output is "minimal." In what section of the medical record would you check to determine the patient's fluid balance (intake vs. output)?
A. Physician orders
B. Consent
C. Lab results
D. Nurses' notes and flow sheet

3-3. Which of the following physical findings would you expect to see in an alert but anxious asthmatic who has just been admitted to the emergency department?
A. Respiratory acidosis
B. Respiratory alkalosis
C. Clubbing
D. Cor pulmonale

3-4. In the lab results section of a patient's medical record, the overall WBC count is shown as 22,000 for a febrile patient who appears acutely ill and in moderate respiratory distress. Which of the following is this patient's most likely diagnosis?
A. Bacterial pneumonia
B. Emphysema
C. Pulmonary embolus
D. Pulmonary fibrosis

3-5. A PET scan would be most useful in the diagnosis of which of the following conditions?
A. Bronchogenic carcinoma
B. Chronic bronchitis
C. Pulmonary fibrosis
D. Smoke inhalation

3-6. Negative inspiratory force (NIF) is useful in the determination of which of the following?
A. Airway resistance
B. Functional residual capacity
C. Respiratory muscle strength
D. Sustained maximal inspiration

3-7. Assessment of a 28-year-old trauma patient reveals diminished breath sounds, asymmetrical chest expansion, severe chest pain, and an SpO_2 of 90%, despite receiving oxygen via cannula at 5 L/min. These findings are most consistent with what diagnosis?
A. Complete airway obstruction
B. Pneumothorax
C. Viral pneumonia
D. Pleural effusion

3-8. A 23-year-old firefighter is admitted with suspected smoke inhalation. You place him on a nonrebreathing mask. What is the most appropriate method of monitoring his oxygenation?
A. Arterial blood gas analysis
B. CO-oximetry
C. Pulse oximetry
D. Calculation of $P(A-a)O_2$

3-9. The ratio of lecithin to sphingomyelin, or L/S ratio, is a test to determine fetal lung maturity. Such a test may be done in the later stages of pregnancy, and the values will initially be noted in the *lab results* section of the mother's medical record. Approximately what ratio is associated with the onset of mature surfactant production?
A. 2:1
B. 20:1
C. 1:2
D. 1:20

3-10. Sputum culture and sensitivity would be indicated in the evaluation of which of the following clinical conditions?
A. Pulmonary edema
B. Bacterial pneumonia
C. Bronchiectasis
D. Empyema

WHAT YOU NEED TO KNOW: ESSENTIAL CONTENT

The Patient Record

The patient record contains a variety of clinical information. Knowing where to find this information quickly will allow you to provide optimal care in an efficient manner. Although the actual organization of information within the sections of a medical record may vary slightly by institution, there is reasonable uniformity in how patient charts are organized. **Table 3-1** lists the major sections of the typical patient record and the information that may be found in each section.

While a complete review of the medical record is important to many aspects of respiratory therapy, the NBRC will expect that you are especially familiar with selected patient data. In particular, the relevant sections include the patient history, physical exam, pulmonary function tests (PFTs), arterial blood gas tests (ABGs), imaging studies, and an array of monitoring data, as described in more detail below.

Table 3-1 Where to Find Clinical Information in the Patient Record[a]

Section of Patient Record	Information Located in That Section
Admitting sheet/face sheet	Patient's next-of-kin, address, religion, and employer; health insurance information.
Patient history	Past and present medical history; family, social, and medical history, including at-home medications as well as demographics.
Progress notes	Discipline-specific notes on a patient's progress and treatment plan, generally entered at frequent (daily) intervals by physicians and allied health professionals such as respiratory therapists, dieticians, and social workers.
Physician's orders	Doctors' diagnostic and therapeutic orders, including those pertaining to respiratory care. All incomplete or unclear orders should be clarified with the prescribing physician.
Informed consent	Consent forms signed by the patient (and witness) for various diagnostic and therapeutic procedures, including those for bronchoscopy and surgery.
DNR/advanced directives	Properly signed and witnessed do-not-resuscitate (DNR), do-not-intubate (DNI), and/or advanced directives.
Lab results	CBC counts (including WBCs), ABGs, electrolytes, coagulation studies (PT and INR), and cultures (sputum, blood, and urine).
Imaging studies (radiology and nuclear medicine)	X-rays (including chest X-rays) and CT, MRI, angiography, PET, and V/Q scans.
Therapy/respiratory therapy	Respiratory therapy charting; results of PFTs and sleep study results; as an alternative to being in lab results section, ABGs may also be in this section. Documentation related to other disciplines, such as physical and occupational therapy, may be included.
ECGs and ultrasound studies	The results of electrocardiograms (ECG/EKGs), echocardiograms, and general ultrasound studies.
Nurses' notes and flow sheet	Nurses' subjective and objective record of the patient's condition, including vital sign trending and fluid intake/ output (I & O) and hemodynamic monitoring such as CVP, PAP, and PCWP.

a. A neonate's medical record may have a section dedicated to *birth history*, or this information will be included in the *patient history* section of the chart.

Patient History

Your review of patient demographics and history can provide important clinical clues relating to the patient's chief complaint(s), which can be essential in helping make a differential diagnosis. Your review of a patient's demographics and history may also uncover important information relevant to the patient's current illness, including past medical conditions or surgeries; occupational exposure to toxins, irritants, or carcinogens; or a history of tobacco or alcohol use. Logically, these data are typically located in the *patient history* section of the medical record, and your review of it should focus on the following items.

Demographic Data

Factors such as a patient's place of residence and age may be relevant in that some respiratory conditions tend to be more common in certain age groups, geographic locations, and ethnic groups.

History of Present Illness

The patient's chief complaint, description of symptoms, frequency, duration, quality, severity, onset, and features that aggravate or alleviate discomfort are often important in diagnosis and treatment.

Past Medical History

Surgeries, treatments for cancer and heart disease, and congenital and childhood conditions also may be relevant.

Medication History

This section provides a complete listing of the medication, dosages, and frequencies of all medications that the patient has been taking.

Family Disease History

This section describes the health status of blood relatives that may be useful in considering diseases with hereditary tendencies.

Occupational History

Work history is noted here with particular emphasis on occupations that may be linked to respiratory dysfunction, such as mining, chemical production, and work involving asbestos.

Social History

Smoking and tobacco usage may contribute to respiratory disorders and should be noted along with alcohol or drug use, social activities, hobbies, recreational activities, and pets.

Patient Education History

This section outlines education that the patient (or caregiver) has previously received from a health care professional regarding his or her medical condition and treatment(s), including medications.

Physical Examination Relative to the Cardiopulmonary System

In addition to reviewing the patient's medical history and other pertinent aspects of the chart, you should pay close attention to the results of the patient's physical examination, laboratory studies, PFT and ABG results, imaging studies, and other relevant monitoring data. This information can provide you with insight as to the patient's current condition and response to therapy. The recorded information related to the physical exam of the patient will include vital signs; the results of inspection, auscultation, and percussion; as well the characteristics of any sputum production.

Vital Signs

The diagnostic value of vital signs can be maximized by comparing the recorded values to age-specific normals and the patient's baseline, as well as by trending them over a period of time. These values may be found in various sections of the chart, including the respiratory therapy or *nurses' notes and flow sheet* section of the chart. You will need to know the age-specific normal values summarized in **Table 3-2**.

Lab Results

Pertinent test results that you need to assess include those from the complete blood count (CBC), electrolytes, and clotting tests. **Table 3-3** lists normal lab values for adult patients and summarizes the significance of test results. In addition to the normal values, some common examples of abnormal findings that you may find in the lab results section of the medical record include:

- Elevated overall white blood cell (WBC) count, or differential WBC values such as neutrophils and bands, often suggests an acute bacterial infection.
- Abnormal red blood cells (RBCs) impact the oxygen-carrying capacity of the blood. Increased RBCs (polycythemia) may be associated with chronic hypoxemia while decreased levels may be associated with bleeding or anemia.
- Low serum potassium (hypokalemia) may lead to certain dysrhythmias, such as premature ventricular contractions (PVCs), and may be associated with respiratory muscle weakness. Certain respiratory medications, such as albuterol, may lower serum potassium.

Table 3-2 Normal Vital Signs

	Adult	Child (Preschool Age)	Infant
Temperature	98.6°F or 37.0°C	37.5°C	37.5°C
Pulse	60–100 beats/min	80–120 beats/min	90–170 beats/min
Respiratory rate	12–20 breaths/min	20–25 breaths/min	35–45 breaths/min
Blood pressure	< 120/80 mm Hg	94/52 mm Hg	84/52 mm Hg
Pulse oximetry	> 92%	> 92%	> 92%

Table 3-3 Normal Lab Values for Adults

Test	Normal Value[a]	Significance
Hematology		
Red blood cells (RBC)	M 4.6–6.2 × 10–6/mm^3 F 4.2–5.4 × 10–6/mm^3	Oxygen transport Response to hypoxemia Degree of cyanosis
Hemoglobin	M 13.5–16.5 g/dL F 12.0–15.0 g/dL	Oxygen transport Response to hypoxemia Degree of cyanosis
Hematocrit	M 40–54% F 38–47%	Hemoconcentration (high) Hemodilution (low)
White blood cells (WBC)	4500–11,500/mm^3	Infection (high)
Platelets	150,000–400,000/mm^3	Slow blood clotting (low) Check before ABG
Prothrombin time (PT)	12–14 seconds	Slow clotting (high) Check before ABG
Partial thromboplastin time (PTT)	25–37 seconds	Slow clotting (high) Check before ABG
Clinical Chemistry		
Sodium	137–147 mEq/L	Acid–base/fluid balance
Potassium	3.5–4.8 mEq/L	Metabolic acidosis (high) Metabolic alkalosis (low) Cardiac arrhythmias (low)
Chloride	98–105 mEq/L	Metabolic alkalosis (low)
Blood urea nitrogen (BUN)	7–20 mg/dL	Renal failure (high)
Creatinine	0.7–1.3 mg/dL	Renal disease (high)
a. Normal lab values may vary slightly depending upon the specific source of such information.		

- Blood work, known as coagulation studies, may reveal prolonged clotting times. Abnormally long prothrombin time (PT) and partial thromboplastin time (PTT) indicate that a patient may be prone to excessive bleeding associated with ABG sampling or tissue samples obtained via bronchoscopy.
- Additional lab studies may detect the presence of cardiac enzymes such as creatine kinase, associated with damaged heart muscle from a recent myocardial infarction.

Physical Examination of the Chest

This aspect of patient assessment includes inspection, palpation, auscultation, and percussion of the chest. This information may be found in the progress notes or respiratory therapy sections of the chart and are summarized below.

- Inspection: Visual exam of the chest for scars, chest contour, and abnormalities including increased AP diameter, pectis excavatum, and kyphoscoliosis.
- Palpation of the chest: Touching of the chest to evaluate lung structures and function, including symmetry, expansion, fremitus (vibrations felt at the chest wall).
- Auscultation: Listening to lung sounds, especially for the presence of abnormal breath sounds, which may signify a clinical abnormality such as:
  - Wheezing (bronchial obstruction, inflammation, asthma)
  - Rhonchi (presence of secretions)
  - Misplaced bronchial sounds (pneumonia)
  - Crackles/rales (pulmonary edema, atelectasis [late inspiratory])
  - Diminished breath sounds with prolonged expiration (COPD or asthma)
- Percussion: Tapping the surface of the skin to evaluate underlying soft tissue, most notably the lung and diaphragm. The following sounds are most clinically significant:
  - Normal resonance (moderately low-pitched sound, commonly heard over normal lung tissue)
  - Dull note (high pitched, short duration, not loud, heard over consolidation or atelectasis)
  - Hyperresonance (low pitched, loud, longer duration heard over hyperinflated lungs from asthma or COPD [bilateral] or pneumothorax [unilateral])

Sputum Analysis

The presence as well as characteristics of a patient's sputum, including the amount, color, consistency, and odor, may provide important clinical clues. For example, thick, green, foul-smelling secretions may indicate the presence of a bacterial lung infection. If you detect abnormal characteristics associated with an acute respiratory condition such as pneumonia or acute bronchitis, consider recommending a sputum Gram stain and culture and sensitivity if one has not recently been obtained. A Gram stain test permits general classification of a microbe (e.g., cocci, rods), and the culture and sensitivity test allows more specific identification of both the specific microbe(s) and medications that may be effective in treating infections caused by them.

Subjective sputum characteristics are often found in the *respiratory therapy* section of the medical record, and the results of formal laboratory sputum analysis are generally found in the *lab results* section of the chart. Sputum assessment is discussed in more detail in Chapters 4 and 13.

Pulmonary Function Testing Results

Pulmonary function testing (PFT) involves measuring a patient's air-flow, volumes/capacities, and gas diffusion by having the patient perform a variety of inspiratory and expiratory maneuvers with a variety of specialized equipment. If such a test has been done, a copy of the results is generally kept in the *respiratory therapy* section of the patient's medical record. These results will often reveal information relevant to the presence or absence of an obstructive disorder such as asthma or chronic obstructive pulmonary disease (COPD), a restrictive disorder including any one of several neuromuscular diseases, or a condition affecting gas diffusion.

Table 3-4 Restrictive Versus Obstructive Disease

Category of Disorder	Examples	Impact on Flows and Volumes	Typical Measurements
Restrictive	Neuromuscular, pulmonary fibrosis	↓ volumes	FVC, IRV, ERV, RV, TLC
Obstructive	Asthma, COPD	↓ flows	FEV_1, PEFR, FEF_{25-75}, $FEF_{200-1200}$, ↓ FEV_1/FVC
Combined: restrictive and obstructive	Cystic fibrosis	↓ volumes and ↓ flows	As noted above

Categorizing PFT Results

Most pulmonary diseases may be categorized as restrictive, obstructive, or combined disorders. **Table 3-4** summarizes the primary features of these categories of disorders. Predicted PFT values are primarily a function of a patient's height, sex, and age. The degree of impairment can be determined by comparing actual PFT results with predicted values, resulting in a percentage predicted. From there, the results can be categorized as being normal or mildly, moderately, or severely impaired, as follows:

Normal	80–120%
Mild	60–79%
Moderate	40–59%
Severe	< 40%

It also should be noted that, in general, an increase in flows of 15% or more after bronchodilator therapy suggests significant reversibility to obstructive disorder.

Diffusion Capacity

Diffusion capacity is generally measured via the inhalation of a trace amount of carbon dioxide (CO_2) and expressed as DLCO. Normal levels are approximately 25 mL/min/mm Hg. A lower than normal diffusion capacity may be found in such disorders as pulmonary fibrosis and emphysema, but it may be increased with a higher than normal concentration of red blood cells, known as polycythemia.

Arterial Blood Gas (ABG) Results

Analysis of an arterial sample provides precise measurement of acid–base balance and of the patient's ability to oxygenate and remove carbon dioxide from the blood. You should review the patient's medical records for ABG results, which can complement other medical data and help you form a complete picture of the patient's respiratory status. ABG results are typically found with other lab results or in the *respiratory therapy* section of the medical record. The following are some considerations you should keep in mind while reviewing ABG results in the medical record.

Normal Ranges

Before reviewing these results in the patient record, you should know the normal ranges for the commonly reported parameters for adults breathing room air as listed in **Table 3-5**.

Interpreting Primary Acid–base Disturbances

We recommend that you first interpret the acid–base status, then evaluate oxygenation separately. To determine the basic acid–base status, you need consider only two parameters, the pH and $Paco_2$.

As indicated in **Figure 3-1**, you first determine whether the pH is normal (7.35–7.45), low (< 7.35; academia), or high (> 7.45; alkalemia). After judging the pH, you then assess the $Paco_2$. A normal $Paco_2$ in the presence of a normal pH indicates normal acid–base balance. If, in contrast, the pH is low, the primary disturbance must be either respiratory acidosis (high $Paco_2$) or metabolic acidosis ($Paco_2 \le 45$

Table 3-5 Normal ABG Ranges

Parameter	Normal Range
pH	7.35–7.45
Paco$_2$	35–45 torr
Pao$_2$	80–100 torr
HCO$_3$ (bicarbonate)	22–26 mEq/L
BE (base excess)	–2 ± 2
SO$_2$ (calculated via PO$_2$ noted above)	95–100%

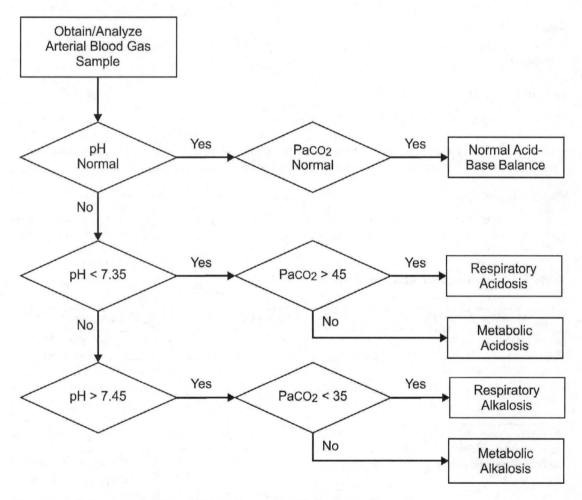

Figure 3-1 Interpretation of Simple Acid–Base Disturbances.

torr). With a high pH, the primary disturbance must be either respiratory alkalosis ($Paco_2 < 35$ torr) or metabolic alkalosis ($Paco_2 \geq 35$ torr).

Interpreting Severity of Hypoxemia

Basic ABG interpretation also requires that you recognize the different categories of hypoxemia. You can categorize the severity of hypoxemia as follows:

Mild	60–79 torr
Moderate	40–59 torr
Severe	< 40 torr

Of course this interpretation depends in part on whether the patient is breathing supplemental O_2. For example, if a patient's Pao_2 is less than 60 torr when breathing a high concentration of oxygen ($\geq 60\%$), most clinicians would categorize this level of hypoxemia as severe. You also should note that as an alternative to the Pao_2 or Sao_2 from an ABG, it is common to monitor oxygenation noninvasively via pulse oximetry, as subsequently described in this text.

Common Abnormalities

For the CRT exam, you should be able to recognize common abnormalities in ABG results, as noted in **Table 3-6**.

Imaging Studies

A variety of imaging studies permit clinicians to see inside the human body without the risk of an invasive procedure. The most common imaging study for most pulmonary patients is the chest X-ray. There is usually a separate section in the medical record for X-ray results or imaging studies. In examining a patient record, it is important for you to review the results of all imaging studies summarized here.

Chest X-Ray (Radiograph)

Chest X-rays are performed to evaluate the lungs and thoracic bones for presence of abnormalities and disease. Chest X-rays are useful in screening for a routine hospital admission or identifying pul-

Table 3-6 Common ABG Abnormalities

Underlying Disorder	Typical ABG Result	Interpretation
Moderate to severe COPD with CO_2 retention	pH 7.36 $Paco_2$ 58 torr Pao_2 62 torr HCO_3 mEq/L BE ±7	Fully compensated respiratory acidosis with mild hypoxemia.
Pneumonia, pulmonary emboli, or any other condition associated with moderate or severe hypoxemia	pH 7.52 $Paco_2$ 27 torr Pao_2 48 torr HCO_3 22 mEq/L BE –1	Uncompensated respiratory alkalosis with moderate hypoxemia. The alkalosis may be a result of tachypnea associated with hypoxemia.
Uncontrolled diabetes with ketoacidosis	pH 7.30 $Paco_2$ 28 torr Pao_2 96 torr HCO_3 14 mEq/L BE –10	Partially compensated metabolic acidosis with normal oxygenation.

monary conditions including lung cancer, pneumonia, tuberculosis, respiratory distress syndrome, degenerative and reactive processes, trauma, and surgical changes. The chest film is also used to evaluate the heart size and great vessels. Details on chest X-ray interpretation are included in Chapters 4 and 13 of this text.

Specialized Imaging Tests

In addition to the chest X-ray, there are several other imaging tests, the results of which may be found in the patient's record. **Table 3-7** summarizes the major specialized imaging tests.

Monitoring Data

The following is a host of data that relates to, and may impact, the pulmonary status of the patient. With the exception of fluid balance, which is generally located in the *nurses' notes and flow sheet*, you may find this information in the *respiratory therapy* or *progress notes* sections of the medical record.

Fluid Balance

A patient's fluid balance is the relationship between fluid intake, mainly from drinking and intravenous infusion, and outputs, primarily from urination. It is normally noted in the *nurses' notes and flow sheet* section of the medical record. The normal fluid intake and output for adults is 1–2 L/day, or 25–50 ml/hr. A positive fluid balance results from excessive intake (intravenous fluid resuscitation) and/or decreased output (renal insufficiency/failure) and may contribute to pulmonary or peripheral edema and hypertension. A negative fluid balance is generally due to insufficient hydration and/or excessive urine output from medications such as diuretics or xanthines (theophylline) and may lead to hypotension and low cardiac output. Other factors, such fluid loss from severe vomiting or diarrhea, as well as the absolute humidity of inspired gases, may also have an impact on fluid balance.

Pulmonary Mechanics

Maximal inspiratory pressure (MIP) or negative inspiratory force (NIF) is used to measure a patient's ventilatory muscle strength. The patient is required to generate negative pressure against an occluded airway. Most commonly, you may use this test in two specific situations. First, it may be used to monitor the presence of progressive respiratory muscular weakness seen in many neuromuscular patients. Second, it is used to assess the readiness of patients for weaning from mechanical ventilation. Nega-

Table 3-7 Specialized Imaging Studies

Imaging Test	Description
CT scan (computer-enhanced radiography)	Facilitates evaluation of abnormalities of the lungs, mediastinum, pleura, and chest wall as well as in diagnosing pulmonary emboli.
MRI (magnetic resonance imaging)	Highly detailed evaluation of the chest for pathology, including the heart, major vessels, mediastinum, lungs, and chest wall. There are several contraindications to MRI, including morbidly obese patients and those with a device such as cardiac pacemaker or intracranial aneurysm clips, depending on metallurgical composition.
PET (positron emission tomography)	Creates "metabolic images" of body tissues via uptake of small amounts of a radioactive tracer injected into the patient. Detects metabolic cellular changes and can help identify rapidly growing cells such as those found in lung cancer.
Angiography	By injection of contrast medium, permits evaluation of arterial abnormalities such as arterial aneurysm, pulmonary embolism, or tumors.
Ventilation-perfusion (V/Q) scan	Angiography (noted above) to examine lung perfusion and an image of the distribution of ventilation via inhalation of radiolabeled gas (xenon 133). Useful in diagnosing pulmonary emboli.

tive 20 to –25 (–20 to –25 cm H₂O) is the threshold for instituting either mechanical ventilation for a spontaneously breathing patient who is worsening or weaning for one already on mechanical ventilation who may be improving.

Vital capacity (VC) is also used for the monitoring of neuromuscular strength and weaning attempts. Unlike the MIP/NIF maneuver, an accurate VC is highly dependent on patient cooperation. For most patients, VC should be at least 15 ml/kg normal body weight.

Respiratory Monitoring

Patients who are at risk for ventilatory failure should have frequent monitoring of bedside parameters to determine if their condition is deteriorating. **Table 3-8** summarizes key thresholds for respiratory monitoring.

Pulmonary Compliance

Loss of lung compliance (C$_L$) is associated with diseases that cause the lung to become "stiff." These disorders include pulmonary fibrosis and acute respiratory distress syndrome (ARDS). Loss of compliance is indicated by rising plateau pressures on mechanically ventilated patients. Normal lung compliance in an adult is 100–200 mL/cm H₂O but may be decreased in patients with ARDS or significant atelectasis.

Airway Resistance

Airway resistance (R$_A$) is associated with obstructive airway problems such as asthma and bronchitis. An increase in R$_A$ can be seen in ventilator patients by a widening in the difference between peak and plateau airway pressures. An abrupt increase in R$_A$ may suggest a sudden change such as a mucous plug or obstructed artificial airway whereby a more gradual increase in R$_A$ may indicate a bronchospasm or accumulation of airway secretions over time.

Work of Breathing

Work of breathing (WOB) is a measurement of the energy utilized in the process of breathing. The precise measurement is quite complex and involves the use of an esophageal pressure-volume curve. The normal range for healthy adults is 0.030–0.050 kg/m/L. More common than this sophisticated measurement, a cluster of bedside clinical findings such as accessory muscle use, tachypnea, and an overall distressed appearance may strongly suggest an increase in WOB. In general, WOB may be elevated in a variety of conditions such as asthma, COPD, and ARDS.

V$_D$/V$_T$

V$_D$/V$_T$ describes the ratio of deadspace to tidal volume. Normally about 30%, a V$_D$/V$_T$ ratio greater than 60% indicates wasted ventilation and a need for mechanical ventilation. Conditions such as pulmonary emboli and emphysema increase the V$_D$/V$_T$.

Table 3-8 Respiratory Monitoring Thresholds

Parameter	Threshold
V$_T$	3–4 mL/lb *ideal* body weight
VC	< 15 mL/kg of normal body weight[a]
MIP/NIF	–20 to –25 cm H₂O[a]
RR	12–20 breaths/min
V̇$_E$	5–7 L/min (amount of air exhaled in one minute)
V$_{alv}$	V̇$_E$ – V$_{D\ anat}$ (anatomical deadspace: 1 mL/lb ideal weight)
a. Represents the common threshold for mechanical ventilation.	

Capnography

Capnography measures exhaled carbon dioxide. The most common measure provided is the end-tidal CO_2, or $ETCO_2$. The $ETCO_2$ is usually 5–10 mm Hg less than $paCO_2$. A normal capnogram will appear as a square wave pattern. An increase in $ETCO_2$ suggests hypoventilation or increased metabolism and may warrant additional tests such as an ABG.

Pulse Oximetry

Pulse oximetry (SpO_2) uses the principle of infrared light absorption to monitor arterial blood oxygenation noninvasively. The measured SpO_2 values may appear in several locations in the medical record, including the progress notes, lab values, as well as respiratory or nursing notes. The normal range for an adult patient breathing room air is 95–100%. However, patients with certain pulmonary abnormalities such as moderate to severe COPD may have baseline SpO_2 readings in the 88–92% range. Standard pulse oximetry is *not* accurate for measuring oxygenation in victims of carbon monoxide (CO) poisoning, and readings may be affected by movement, skin pigmentation, and peripheral circulation.

CO-oximetry

CO-oximetry uses the principle of spectrophotometry (multiple light waves) to measure relative blood concentrations of oxyhemoglobin, caroxyhemoglobin, methhemoglobin, and reduced hemoglobin. Look for these measurements in place of pulse oximetry in cases of suspected carbon monoxide poisoning.

Transcutaneous Monitoring

Transcutaneous monitoring continuously measures diffusion of gases through the skin and is used primarily for neonates. Transcutaneous diffusion occurs through the use of a heated electrode usually applied to the leg, abdomen, or trunk that must be calibrated and maintained at 43–44°C. Readings should be compared with arterial blood gas values.

Cardiac Monitoring

Within the medical record you will also find clinical data related to the patient's cardiac status. In general, this information includes electrocardiograms (ECGs), echocardiograms, and hemodynamic monitoring results. ECG "strips" reflecting the patient's heart rate and rhythm, as well as the physician's interpretation of them, is often located in the *ECGs and ultrasound studies* section of the patient record. This section generally also contains the results of ultrasound studies, including echocardiograms of the patient's heart. If the patient's hemodynamic status is being monitored invasively through a central venous or pulmonary artery pressure catheter, these values, including central venous pressures (CVP) and pulmonary artery pressure (PAP), are generally reflected in the *nurses' notes and flow sheet* portion of the medical record. While the interpretation of cardiac monitoring values is reviewed in Chapter 4 of this text, **Table 3-9** lists the normal hemodynamic values for adults.

Maternal History and Perinatal and Neonatal History and Data

Maternal History and Data

The medical record or chart of a pregnant mother is similar to that of most other patients in that much of the information is located in the sections of the chart described in Table 3-1. For example, blood tests such as CBC results will be found in the *lab results* section of the chart, and the mother's history will be located in the *patient history* section. However, some of the data in these sections will differ in that they may be unique to pregnancy. A prime example of this is the lecithin to sphingomyelin ratio, or *L/S ratio*, which is used to determine fetal lung maturity. Generally, this ratio reaches 2:1 (twice as much lethicin than sphingomyelin) near week 35 of gestation, which corresponds to the onset of mature surfactant production. The L/S ratio is generally noted in the *lab results* section of the mother's medical record. Another example of how the maternal medical record is somewhat unique from records for other patients is the type of information recorded in the *patient history* section. Proper prenatal care is heavily reliant on documenting a thorough maternal history, including factors that may place the

Table 3-9 Normal Hemodynamic Values (Adults)

Parameter	Normal Value/Range[a]
Systolic blood pressure	< 120 mm Hg
Diastolic blood pressure	< 80 mm Hg
Mean arterial blood pressure	80–100 mm Hg
Central venous pressure (CVP)	< 6 mm Hg
Right atrial pressure	2–6 mm Hg
Right ventricular pressure, systolic	20–30 mm Hg
Right ventricular pressure, diastolic	2–6 mm Hg
Pulmonary artery pressure, systolic	20–30 mm Hg
Pulmonary artery pressure, diastolic	6–15 mm Hg
Pulmonary artery pressure, mean	10–20 mm Hg
Pulmonary artery wedge pressure, mean	4–12 mm Hg
Cardiac output (CO)	4.0–8.0 L/min
Cardiac index (CI)	2.5–5.0 L/min/m^2
Stroke volume (SV)	60–130 mL/beat
Stroke index (SI)	30–50 mL/beat/m^2
Ejection fraction (EF)	65–75%
Systemic vascular resistance (SVR)[b]	900–1400 dyne·sec·cm^{-5}
Pulmonary vascular resistance (PVR)[b]	110–250 dyne·sec·cm^{-5}

a. Normal values and ranges vary by laboratory, norms used, and/or reference source.
b. To convert resistance measures from dyne·sec·cm^{-5} to mm Hg/L/min, divide by 80.

mother and/or neonate at risk. These factors relate to maternal demographic and socioeconomic factors, the general medical and obstetric history, and the current obstetric status. **Table 3-10** summarizes the major factors associated with high-risk pregnancies.

Perinatal and Neonatal Data

Once the neonate is born, a separate medical record is established for the newborn. Some of the information from the mother's medical record, such as the maternal history, is copied and transferred into the neonate's chart. Other data are reflective of the delivery and the clinical status of the neonate at birth and will be included in the *birth history* or *patient history* section of the neonate's chart. Birth and delivery information that will be recorded in this section of the chart includes the delivery position of the neonate, the presence of meconium, as well as the baby's initial color, muscle tone, and heart rate. Based on these and other factors, the neonate will often be classified in a general sense as "vigorous," with a favorable initial assessment, or "nonvigorous" if they are in distress. Any unusual interventions or treatment immediately following the birth, such as the administration of positive pressure ventilation or other resuscitative efforts, will also be noted.

At 1 and 5 minutes after birth, the Apgar score is determined in order to assess and document the status of the newborn. The score is based on five variables, each rated from 0 to 2, with scores ranging from 10 for a stable, responsive neonate to a minimum of 0 if stillborn. Though this score is generally not used to determine medical intervention, it is useful in documenting a newborn's clinical status and somewhat predictive of clinical outcomes.

Table 3-10 High-Risk Pregnancy Factors

Category	Factors
Socioeconomic factors	Low income and poor housing
	Unwed status, especially adolescent (under 16 years old)
	Minority status
	Obese or underweight prior to pregnancy
	Height less than 5 feet
	Familial history of inherited disorders
Obstetric history	History of infertility
	History of infant malformation or birth injury
	History of miscarriage, stillbirth, or ectopic pregnancy
	High parity (many children)
	History of premature or prolonged labor
Maternal medical history	History of low birth weight infant
	Cardiac, pulmonary, or renal disease
	Diabetes or thyroid disease
	Gastrointestinal or endocrine disorder
	History of hypertension or seizures
	History of venereal and other infectious diseases
	Weight loss greater than 5 pounds
Current obstetric status	Surgery during pregnancy
	Absence of prenatal care
	Rh sensitization or maternal anemia
	Excessively large or small fetus
	Preeclampsia or premature labor
	Premature membrane rupture or vaginal bleeding
Habits	Postmaturity
	Smoking
	Regular alcohol intake
	Drug use or abuse

During the first few hours or days of life, the neonate's gestational age will be estimated using either the Dubowitz or Ballard assessment tools. While these two methods are about equally accurate, Dubowitz exam uses 11 physical and 10 neurologic signs, and the more streamlined Ballard exam relies on only 6 physical and 6 neurological signs.

The clinical uses of the gestational age assessment tools and the Apgar scoring system are discussed in more detail in Chapter 4 of this text.

COMMON ERRORS TO AVOID

You can improve your score by avoiding these mistakes:

- Don't forget to review the patient's medical record, including physician's orders, *before* you administer any respiratory care.
- Do *not* follow MD's order in the patient's record if there is an apparent error. Instead, contact the physician and clarify and correct the order.
- Avoid making recommendations based on information in one section of the patient's record. Instead, review and interpret an array of patient data to formulate a complete clinical assessment to assist with the differential diagnosis and treatment plan.
- Avoid reviewing only the most recent clinical data in the medical record. Instead, review data over time for trends and clues regarding the patient's progress.
- Avoid utilizing clinical data that are seemingly erroneous (SpO_2 of 80% for a patient resting comfortably) or grossly inconsistent with other results. If necessary, recommend that a test or procedure be repeated.
- For a patient with a central venous or pulmonary artery pressure catheter, don't forget to check central venous pressures (CVP) and pulmonary artery pressure (PAP), which will generally be noted in the *nurses' notes and flow sheet*. The normal values for CVP and PAP are less than 6 mm Hg and 20–30 mm Hg (systolic) / 6–15 mm Hg (diastolic), respectively.
- Never initiate or continue CPR and resuscitative efforts for a patient with a properly executed and current DNR order or advanced directive indicating the patient's desire not to be resuscitated.
- Never review a patient's medical record solely for the purpose of confirming orders. Instead, be mindful that potentially valuable patient data exists in all sections of the patient's chart.

SURE BETS

In some situations you can always be sure of the right approach to a clinical problem or scenario:

- Always review the medical record before performing respiratory procedures to ensure the physician order has been written and to become familiar with the patient's overall condition and potential contraindications.
- Always clarify incomplete or unclear orders with the prescribing physician.
- Always review trends in vital signs and other clinical data to gain insight regarding the patient's response to therapy and to monitor overall progress, or lack thereof.
- In reviewing clinical data in the patient record, always remember that the normal ranges often vary by age. For example, the normal heart rate for an adult is 60–100 beats/min, while that for a newborn is 90–170 beats/min.
- When reviewing pulmonary function results, always keep in mind that a *restrictive disorder* is characterized by a reduction in volumes and capacities and relatively normal (or somewhat higher) flows, and a significant *obstructive disorder* will result in reduced flows and higher residual capacity and total lung capacity.
- Always remember that if the medical record indicates an increase in both PIP and plateau pressure, this suggests a loss of compliance (stiffening lung). However, an increase in PIP generally means an increase in airway resistance, often due to airway obstruction.
- Always remember that the patient's fluid intake and output is generally noted on the *nurses' notes and flow sheet* and that the normal fluid intake and output for adults is 1–2 L/day, or 25–50 ml/hr.
- If the medical record indicates that a patient has excessive secretions, always note the amount, consistency, color, and odor of such secretions and consider recommending that a Gram stain and culture and sensitivity be obtained.
- If the patient record indicates that the vital capacity (VC) is at or below 15 ml/kg normal body weight and/or the negative inspiratory force (NIF) is less than –20 to –25 cm H_2O, or a review of trending reveals a rapid deterioration in these values, then you should always consider recommending intubation and mechanical ventilation.

- When reviewing a patient's medical record, always try to recognize the cluster of clinical signs and symptoms associated with certain conditions. For example, a patient with moderate emphysema will often present as barrel-chested, with dyspnea on exertion and an ABG that reflects a compensated respiratory acidosis.
- Always remember that when reviewing the radiologist's interpretation of a chest X-ray, radiolucency is seen as darkness on the image and associated with the presence of air. Opacities are seen as whiteness and generally mean the absence of air (solid tissue or fluid) and may be associated with atelectasis, consolidation, ARDS, or a tumor.
- Always remember that certain conditions, such as acute asthma or pneumonia, may cause hyperventilation due to hypoxemia, resulting in an uncompensated respiratory alkalosis (increased pH and decreased Pco_2). With appropriate oxygen therapy, hyperventilation will often subside and $Paco_2$ normalize.
- Always remember that the Apgar score is used to assess and document the status of the newborn at 1 and 5 minutes after birth, with scores ranging from 10 for a stable, responsive neonate to a minimum of 0 if stillborn. In contrast, during the first few hours or days of life, the neonate's gestational age is estimated using either the Dubowitz or Ballard tools.

PRE-TEST ANSWERS AND EXPLANATIONS

Below are this chapter's pre-test answers and explanations. Be sure to review each answer's explanation thoroughly to help you understand why it is correct. If the explanation is still unclear to you, review the chapter contents or the references and/or refer to this chapter's supplemental resources on the CD.

3-1. **Correct Answer: C.** Ventilation-perfusion scan (V/Q scan). A chest X-ray and an ABG might be useful in detecting an abnormality, but not specifically a pulmonary emboli. Pulmonary function tests (PFTs) may reveal abnormal flows and volumes/capacities but no perfusion problems inherent in a pulmonary emboli. A ventilation-perfusion scan would show a lack of blood flow due to emboli (a clot) in the blood pulmonary circulation. Ventilation to lung regions would be shown as well.

3-2. **Correct Answer: D.** Nurses' notes and flow sheet. A patient's fluid balance is the relationship between fluid intake and outputs primarily from urination. It is normally noted in the *nurses' notes and flow sheet* section of the medical record. The normal fluid intake and output for adults is 1–2 L/day, or 25–50 ml/hour. A positive fluid balance results from excessive intake and/or decreased output and may contribute to pulmonary or peripheral edema and hypertension. A negative fluid balance is generally due to insufficient hydration and/or excessive urination from medications such as diuretics or theophylline and may lead to hypotension and low cardiac output.

3-3. **Correct Answer: B.** Respiratory alkalosis. Asthmatics typically present with respiratory alkalosis. Shortness of breath and accompanying hypoxemia cause the patient to increase his rate of breathing and alkalosis occurs. It is important to note here that once hypoxemia is relieved by the administration of supplemental oxygen, patient's $Paco_2$ and pH will normalize.

3-4. **Correct Answer: A.** Bacterial pneumonia. The elevated WBCs suggest a bacterial infection. The respiratory distress further points to a respiratory infection such as bacterial pneumonia. In addition, the other choices are not infectious processes, and therefore you would not likely see elevated WBCs.

3-5. **Correct Answer: A.** Bronchogenic carcinoma. A PET scan is a nuclear imaging technique used in the diagnosis/staging/management of tumors and cancer. The answer choice *bronchogenic carcinoma* describes lung cancer.

3-6. **Correct Answer: C.** Respiratory muscle strength. Negative inspiratory force (NIF) or maximal inspiratory pressure (MIP) is used for the bedside assessment of respiratory muscle strength. You probably know that it is a measurement of pressure only. Since airway resistance is a measurement of pressure divided by flow, and since functional residual capacity and sustained maximal inspiration are measurements of volume, the process of elimination leaves *muscle strength* as the only correct answer.

3-7. **Correct Answer: B.** Pneumothorax. Both viral pneumonia and pleural effusion can be ruled out as correct answers as they are not related to trauma. Breath sounds, though diminished, can be heard, and chest expansion, though asymmetrical, is present; both of these are not consistent with a complete airway obstruction. The physical assessment is consistent with the correct answer, pneumothorax.

3-8. **Correct Answer: B.** CO-oximetry. In the case of smoke inhalation, carbon monoxide (CO) binds to the hemoglobin molecule in place of oxygen. Neither ABGs, pulse oximetry, or calculation of A-a gradient will indicate how much oxygen is bound to hemoglobin. Any victim of suspected smoke inhalation *must* be monitored with CO-oximetry.

3-9. **Correct Answer: A.** 2:1. The lecithin to sphingomyelin ratio, or *L/S ratio*, is used to determine fetal lung maturity. Generally, this ratio reaches 2:1 (twice as much lethicin as sphingomyelin) near week 35 of gestation, which corresponds to the onset of mature surfactant production. The L/S ratio will generally be noted in the *lab results* section of the mother's medical record.

3-10. **Correct Answer: B.** Bacterial pneumonia. Sputum culture and sensitivity are used to identify microorganisms and their most appropriate drug therapy. Bacterial pneumonia is the obvious infectious process in the choice of answers.

REFERENCES

Butler, T. J., Close, J. R., & Close, R. J. (1998). *Laboratory exercises for competency in respiratory care*. Philadelphia: FA Davis.

Kasmarek, R. M., Dimas, S., & Mack, C. W. (2005). *The essentials of respiratory care* (4th ed.). St. Louis: Mosby.

Wilkins, R. L., Dexter, J. R., & Heuer, A. J. (2009). *Clinical assessment in respiratory care* (6th ed.). St. Louis: Mosby.

Wilkins, R. L., Stoller, J. K., & Kacmarek, R. M. (Eds.) (2009). *Egan's fundamentals of respiratory care* (9th ed.). St. Louis: Mosby.

Wyka, K. A., Mathews, P. J., & Clark, W. F. (2002). *Foundations of respiratory care*. Albany: Delmar.

Collect and Evaluate Pertinent Clinical Information

Craig L. Scanlan and Robert L. Wilkins

INTRODUCTION

Patient assessment is one of the most important skills needed to perform as a competent respiratory care provider. Obtaining pertinent clinical information at the bedside helps you determine the patient's medical condition, develop the proper treatment plan, and evaluate the patient's response to the therapy. Since respiratory therapists are the ones at the bedside providing treatment and monitoring the patient, their assessment skills and knowledge must be excellent if the patient is to receive the best possible care. The CRT exam has numerous questions about collecting and interpreting clinical information for patients with cardiopulmonary disease. Your success on the exam depends heavily on your knowledge in this area.

OBJECTIVES

After completion of this chapter, you should demonstrate the knowledge needed to:

1. Assess the patient's overall cardiopulmonary status by:
   a. Inspection
   b. Palpation
   c. Percussion
   d. Auscultation
2. Integrate common physical examination findings
3. Interview the patient to obtain essential information regarding the patient's:
   e. Level of consciousness, ability to cooperate, and emotional state
   f. Level of pain
   g. Breathing difficulties and exercise tolerance
   h. Cough and sputum production
   i. Nutritional status
   j. Social history
   k. Advance directives
4. Assess the patient's learning needs
5. Review and interpret chest and lateral neck radiographs
6. Perform and interpret the results of selected diagnostics procedures

WHAT TO EXPECT ON THIS CATEGORY OF THE CRT EXAM

Number of questions: 18
Level of questions: about 35% recall, 60% application, and 5% analysis

WHAT'S NEW FOR 2009

As of July 2009, this section of the NBRC CRT examination includes the following *new content areas*:

- Assessing a patient's overall cardiopulmonary status by inspection to determine:
  - Airway assessment (e.g., macroglossia, neck range of motion)
  - Apgar score, gestational age, transillumination of chest
- Assessing a patient's overall cardiopulmonary status by percussion
- Interviewing a patient to determine nutritional status
- Reviewing a chest radiograph to determine the position of indwelling tubes and catheters
- Reviewing lateral neck radiographs (e.g., to diagnose epiglottitis, foreign body)
- Performing and/or interpreting the results of:
  - Arterialized capillary blood sampling (covered in Chapter 13)
  - Timed walk test (e.g., 6-minute walk test [6MWT])
  - Oxygen titration with exercise
  - Cardiopulmonary calculations (e.g., $P(A-a)O_2$, V_D/V_T [covered in Chapter 20])
  - Hemodynamic monitoring (e.g., blood pressure, CVP)
  - Arterial line insertion (covered in Chapter 13)
  - Stress testing (e.g., ECG, pulse oximetry)
  - CPAP/BiPAP™ titration during sleep

PRE-TEST

Carefully respond to each of the following questions. After completing the pre-test, compare your answers to those provided at the end of this chapter. Then thoroughly review each answer's explanation to help understand why it is correct.

4-1. Which of these conditions is associated with jugular venous distension?
- **A.** Cor pulmonale
- **B.** Pneumonia
- **C.** Simple pneumothorax
- **D.** Septic shock

4-2. You palpate the patient's neck and notice that the trachea is shifted to the patient's left. Which of the following conditions could explain this finding?
- **A.** Left ventricular enlargement
- **B.** Left upper lobe collapse
- **C.** Right lower lobe collapse
- **D.** Pleural effusion on the left

4-3. On reviewing the results of the attending physician's physical examination of a patient's chest, you note "a dull percussion note and bronchial breath sounds—LLL." All of the following are potential problems *except*:
- **A.** Infiltrates
- **B.** Atelectasis
- **C.** Consolidation
- **D.** Pneumothorax

4-4. You hear bronchial breath sounds over the patient's right middle lobe. What condition is probably present?
- **A.** Emphysema
- **B.** Asthma
- **C.** Pneumonia
- **D.** Pleural effusion

4-5. Upon exam of an acutely dyspneic and hypotensive patient, you note the following (all limited to the left hemithorax): reduced chest expansion, hyperresonance to percussion, absence of breath sounds and tactile fremitus, and a tracheal shift to the right. These findings suggest:
A. Left-sided pneumothorax
B. Left-sided consolidation
C. Left lobar obstruction/atelectasis
D. Left-sided pleural effusion

4-6. During an interview with your patient you determine that she is disoriented to time, place, and person. What may explain this finding?
A. Respiratory alkalosis
B. Severe hypoxemia
C. Metabolic acidosis
D. Hyperthermia

4-7. To assess the level of pain that a 2-year-old child is experiencing during a procedure, you would do all of the following *except*:
A. Look for facial grimacing
B. Ask for the mother's judgment
C. Use a numeric pain scale
D. Observe for crying

4-8. During an interview with your patient you discover that he gets short of breath at night when he lays down so he often sleeps with several pillows propping his head up. What symptom is present?
A. Apnea
B. Orthopnea
C. Platypnea
D. Orthodeoxia

4-9. A patient complains that she has a chronic cough usually accompanied by sputum production. This information indicates that the patient probably has which of the following conditions?
A. Acute asthma
B. Chronic bronchitis
C. Pulmonary emphysema
D. Bacterial pneumonia

4-10. All of the following are associated with a patient being at risk for malnutrition *except*:
A. Recent weight gain
B. Being significantly underweight
C. Having poor dietary habits
D. Inability to prepare own food

4-11. Which of the following aspects of a patient's social history is most important in the diagnosis of lung disease?
A. Marital status
B. Cultural background
C. Education
D. Occupational history

4-12. You come upon an elderly patient who is unresponsive and is not breathing. You had heard from her nurse that she had discussed with her physician whether or not to a have a do-not-resuscitate (DNR) order in her chart. You should:
A. Check the patient's chart for a DNR order/advanced directive
B. Immediately call a code and begin resuscitation efforts
C. Contact the nurses' station and ask how best to proceed
D. Call a "slow code" (i.e., apply basic CPR, but not ACLS)

4-13. The best way to determine whether or not a patient has learned the information needed to understand how her disease impacts on lung function would be to:
A. Have her take a multiple-choice quiz
B. Discuss the information with her family
C. Have her "teach" the information back to you
D. Have her perform a return demonstration

4-14. You note on inspection of an anterior-posterior (AP) chest radiograph that the left hemidiaphragm is elevated above normal. Which of the following is the most likely cause of this abnormality?
A. Right pleural effusion
B. Right tension pneumothorax
C. Right phrenic nerve paralysis
D. Right lower lobe pneumonia

4-15. An AP X-ray of a 3-year-old child with wheezing and stridor shows an area of prominent subglottic edema, but the lateral neck X-ray appears normal. What is the most likely problem?
A. Croup
B. Foreign body
C. Epiglottitis
D. Cystic fibrosis

4-16. On reviewing an ECG printout you note widened QRS complexes. Which of the following is the most likely cause of this problem?
A. atrial fibrillation
B. first-degree heart block
C. sinus arrhythmia
D. bundle branch block

4-17. A 150-lb patient is breathing at a frequency of 20 breaths/min, with a tidal volume of 550 mL. What is his estimated *alveolar* ventilation per minute?
A. 11.00 L/min
B. 8.00 L/min
C. 3.00 L/min
D. 14.00 L/min

4-18. You obtain a bedside vital capacity (VC) of 400 mL on a cooperative 50-kg female patient receiving ventilatory support in the CMV mode. Which of the following conclusions can you draw from this finding?
A. The patient's VC is normal for her size and weight.
B. The patient cannot sustain prolonged spontaneous ventilation.
C. The patient is in acute hypoxemic respiratory failure.
D. The patient has a generalized obstructive disease process.

4-19. When performing bedside spirometry on a 46-year-old man who is six feet tall, you obtain a peak flow measurement of 3.3 L/sec. Which of the following are possible explanations for this finding?
I. The patient's peak flow is within normal limits.
II. The patient is not exerting full effort.
III. The patient has expiratory flow obstruction.
IV. The patient has poor pulmonary gas distribution.
A. I only
B. II and III
C. II, III, and IV
D. III only

4-20. A patient's bedside spirometry results (as compared to normal) are as follows: FVC decreased, FEV_1 normal, and $FEV_1\%$ increased. What is the most likely problem?
A. An obstructive disorder
B. Poor patient effort
C. A restrictive disorder
D. Within normal limits

4-21. A patient has a vital capacity of 3200 mL, a functional residual capacity of 4500 mL, and expiratory reserve volume of 1200 mL. What is her residual volume (RV)?
A. 8900 mL
B. 2000 mL
C. 3300 mL
D. 5700 mL

4-22. After performing comprehensive pulmonary function testing on a patient, you note the following results:

Test	% Predicted
$FEV_1\%$	50
RV	150
TLC	135
D_{LCO}	60

Which of the following interpretations is most consistent with these findings?
A. The patient has pulmonary fibrosis.
B. The patient has pulmonary emphysema.
C. The patient has chronic bronchitis.
D. The patient is not exerting maximum effort.

4-23. An apnea monitor on a premature infant indicates an abnormal *decrease* in respiratory rate and an abnormal *increase* in heart rate. What is the most likely cause of this problem?
A. Hypoxemia
B. Apnea of prematurity
C. Periodic breathing
D. Motion/activity artifact

4-24. In analyzing overnight oximetry data, a desaturation event represents a decrease in SpO_2 of what amount?
A. 2% or more
B. 3% or more
C. 4% or more
D. 5% or more

4-25. You conduct a 6-minute walk test (6MWT) on four patients before and after participation in a pulmonary rehabilitation program. Based on the 6-minute walking distance (6MWD) data provided below, for which of these patients has the program been effective in improving their functional capacity?

Patient	Pre-Program 6MWD	Post-Program 6MWD
A.	200 m	210 m
B.	150 m	200 m
C.	250 m	270 m
D.	400 m	430 m

4-26. As measured on the Borg scale, which of the following exertion levels is appropriate for titrating a COPD patient's O_2 flows to support exercise?
A. Weak/light exertion (rating of 2)
B. Somewhat strong exertion (rating of 4)
C. Very strong exertion (rating of 7)
D. Maximal exertion (rating of 10)

4-27. To assess gas exchange at the tissues you would sample blood from which of the following?
A. Systemic artery
B. Central vein
C. Pulmonary artery
D. Peripheral vein

4-28. A patient has a pulmonary capillary wedge pressure (PCWP) of 18 mm Hg. All of the following are potential causes for this finding *except*:
A. Hypovolemia
B. Mitral valve stenosis
C. Positive end-expiratory pressure
D. Left ventricular failure

4-29. Based on the results of cardiopulmonary exercise testing, which of the following patients most likely has a ventilatory limitation to exercise?

Patient	VO_{2max}	Anaerobic Threshold	Breathing Reserve
A.	Decreased	Decreased	Normal
B.	Decreased	Normal	Normal
C.	Normal	Increased	Increased
D.	Decreased	Normal	Decreased

4-30. A patient undergoing CPAP titration during sleep exhibits three obstructive apnea events during a 5-minute observation interval at a pressure of 8 cm H_2O. What would be the appropriate action at this time?
A. Switch the patient to BiPAP™ with EPAP = 8 cm H_2O and IPAP = 12 cm H_2O
B. Increase the CPAP to 10 cm H_2O for 5 minutes and continue observation
C. Discontinue the titration trial and place the patient on nasal O_2 at 2 L/min
D. Decrease the CPAP to 6 cm H_2O for 5 minutes and continue observation

WHAT YOU NEED TO KNOW: ESSENTIAL CONTENT

Assess the Patient's Overall Cardiopulmonary Status by Inspection

Inspection involves assessing the patient's appearance, with emphasis on identifying signs associated with abnormal respiratory structure or function. In regard to inspection, the NBRC expects you to be proficient in evaluating a patient's general appearance, examining the airway, and evaluating cough and sputum production. In addition, you should be able to apply gestational age assessment, Apgar scoring, and transillumination to assess an infant's overall cardiopulmonary status.

General Appearance

Table 4-1 summarizes the major observations and their implications arising from bedside inspection of the patient. Table 4-1 makes the important distinction between central and peripheral cyanosis (often tested on the CRT exam). Central cyanosis represents a condition of low arterial hemoglobin (Hb) saturation associated with poor oxygenation of the blood by the lungs, usually evident as a bluish discoloration of the mucous membranes of the *lips and mouth*. Assuming a normal Hb concentration, central cyanosis generally appears when SaO_2 drops below 80%, corresponding to a PaO_2 of about 45 torr.

Table 4-1 Signs Observed During Patient Inspection and Their Implications

Sign	Observation	Potential Implications
General		
Body habitus	Weak/emaciated (cachexia)	General ill health/malnutrition
Position	Sitting/leaning forward	Respiratory distress
	Always elevated with pillows	Orthopnea, congestive heart failure
Respiratory rate	Tachypnea	Respiratory distress, restrictive disease
Breathing pattern	Prolonged exhalation	Expiratory obstruction (asthma, COPD)
	Prolonged inspiration	Upper airway obstruction (croup, epiglottitis)
	Rapid and shallow	Loss of lung volume (atelectasis, pulmonary fibrosis, ARDS, acute pulmonary edema)
	Kussmaul's breathing (deep and fast)	Diabetic ketoacidosis
	Biot's breathing (irregular breathing with periods of apnea)	Increased intracranial pressure
	Cheyne Stokes breathing (waxing and waning)	Central nervous system (CNS) diseases or severe congestive heart failure (CHF)
Speech pattern	Interrupted	Respiratory distress
Skin	Diaphoretic (sweating)	Fever, increased metabolism, acute anxiety
Facial expression	Anxious	Fear, pain
Personal hygiene	Poor	Illness affecting patient's daily activities
Sensorium	Depressed	Poor cerebral oxygenation, degenerative brain disorders, drugs/drug overdose
Head/Neck		
Nose	Nasal flaring (especially in infants)	Increased work of breathing
Lips/oral mucosa	Central cyanosis	Arterial hypoxemia
Lips	Pursed-lip breathing	Expiratory airway obstruction
Jugular veins	Distended	Right heart failure (cor pulmonale)

(continues)

Table 4-1 Signs Observed During Patient Inspection and Their Implications (continued)

Sign	Observation	Potential Implications
Thorax		
Configuration	Barrel chest	COPD
	Kyphoscoliosis	Severe restrictive lung defect
Muscle activity	Accessory muscle use	Increased work of breathing, loss of normal diaphragm function
	Abdominal paradox	Diaphragmatic fatigue, increased work of breathing
	Retractions	Reduced lung volume, low lung compliance, increased work of breathing
Extremities		
Digits	Clubbing	Bronchogenic carcinoma, COPD, chronic cardiovascular disease
Capillary beds	Peripheral cyanosis	Poor perfusion

Peripheral cyanosis or *acrocyanosis* is due to poor blood flow, can occur in the presence of normal Hb saturation, and tends to appear *only* in the extremities. *When observed together with coolness of the extremities, peripheral cyanosis is a sign of circulatory failure.*

Regardless of type, the intensity of cyanosis increases with the amount of Hb in the blood. For this reason, patients with high Hb content (polycythemia) can be cyanotic yet still have adequate arterial oxygen content. Conversely, patients with low Hb content (anemia) can be severely hypoxic before cyanosis ever appears.

Airway Assessment

As a component of respiratory system inspection, you should also assess the patient's airway. Knowledge of the physical characteristics of a patient's airway can help determine the cause of other physical or history findings, such as snoring and sleep apnea. Airway assessment can also help you determine whether special procedures or equipment will be needed should the patient require insertion of an artificial airway. To assess the airway, you should:

1. Inspect the patient's external nose and note any asymmetry or deformities
2. Test for nasal patency by occluding each nostril in turn and asking the patient to breathe in
3. Inspect the nasal cavities (use a nasal speculum and penlight if needed) for a deviated septum, edema, erythema, bleeding, or lesions
4. Have the patient open his or her mouth as widely as possible and extend the tongue; look for the presence of dentures or other dental appliances such as bridges and inspect the oral and pharyngeal anatomy (tongue, hard palate, soft palate, uvula, tonsillar pillars, etc.)
5. Inspect the neck for length and circumference; have the patient flex and extend the neck as far as possible while you view the motion from the side

Table 4-2 outlines the potential significance of the most common observations associated with the assessment of a patient's airway.

Cough and Sputum Production

Cough and sputum production are two important and related respiratory symptoms. **Table 4-3** (see page 69) describes some of the common types of cough and their likely causes. As indicated in Table 4-3, several conditions are associated with production of sputum, such as COPD, infections,

Table 4-2 Inspection of the Airway

Area	Observation	Significance
Nostrils/nasal cavity	Broken, misshapen, swollen nose Occluded nasal passages Deviated septum	Compromised nasal route for O_2 or airway insertion
Oral cavity and pharynx	Dentures or dental appliances present	Potential aspiration risk; may need to be removed for airway access
	Macroglossia (large tongue)	Associated with difficult intubation and may impair aerosol delivery via the mouth
	Mallampati classification of pharyngeal anatomy: *Class 1:* Full visibility of tonsils, uvula, and soft palate *Class 2:* Visibility of hard and soft palate, upper portion of tonsils, and uvula *Class 3:* Soft and hard palate and base of the uvula are visible *Class 4:* Only hard palate visible	Class 4 is associated with difficult intubation as well as a higher incidence of sleep apnea
Neck	Short/thick	Difficult endotracheal intubation; difficult trachostomy tube fit
	Poor range of motion (patient cannot touch tip of chin to chest and/or cannot extend neck)	Difficult BVM ventilation; difficult endotracheal intubation

bronchiectasis, lung abscess, and asthma. Because sputum represents respiratory tract secretions that are *abnormal* in volume or consistency, sputum assessment should be included in the evaluation of the patient's overall history and also be conducted whenever secretion clearance takes place. Typically you evaluate the volume, color, consistency, and odor of expectorated sputum.

When interviewing patients about the volume of sputum production, you can help them estimate how much they produce by using familiar measures such as a teaspoon (about 5 mL), tablespoon (about 15 mL), or shotglass full (about 1 oz. or 30 mL). More precise quantification of volume can be obtained using a sputum cup calibrated with mL markings. *As a rule of thumb, sputum production in excess of 30 mL/day indicates the need for airway clearance.*

In terms of color, sputum is typically described as being either clear/white, pinkish, red, yellow, or green. Sputum consistency is typically described as being thin/watery, frothy, or thick/viscous. Regarding odor, foul-smelling or *fetid* sputum indicates tissue necrosis. In combination, color, consistency, and odor help describe the sputum "type" as being mucoid, mucopurulent, purulent, or bloody. As indicated in **Table 4-4**, this assessment can help you identify the likely underlying disorder.

Neonatal Inspection

The NBRC expects that you comprehend the basic procedures involved in neonatal inspection, including the Apgar score, gestational age assessment, and the use of transillumination to help detect pneumothoraces in neonates.

Apgar Score

The Apgar score (**Table 4-5**; see page 70) is used to assess the status of the newborn infant, usually at 1 and 5 minutes after birth. The score has five dimensions (**A**ppearance, **P**ulse, **G**rimace, **A**ctivity,

Table 4-3 Common Types of Coughs with Likely Causes

Description	Likely Causes
Acute (< 3 wks)	Postnasal drip, allergies, and infections (especially common cold, bronchitis, laryngitis)
Chronic (> 3 wks) or recurrent (adults)	Postnasal drip, asthma, gastroesophageal reflux, chronic bronchitis, bronchiectasis, COPD, TB, lung tumor, Angiotensin-Converting Enzyme (ACE) inhibitors, left heart failure
Recurrent (children)	Viral bronchitis, asthma, allergies
Barking	Epiglottitis, croup, influenza, laryngotracheal bronchitis
Brassy or hoarse	Laryngitis, laryngeal paralysis, laryngotracheal bronchitis, pressure on laryngeal nerve, mediastinal tumor, aortic aneurysm
Wheezy	Bronchospasm, asthma, cystic fibrosis, bronchitis
Dry	Viral infections, inhalation of irritant gases, interstitial lung diseases, tumor, pleural effusion, cardiac conditions, nervous habit, radiation or chemotherapy
Dry progressing to productive	Atypical pneumonias, Legionnaires' disease, pulmonary embolus, pulmonary edema, lung abscess, asthma, silicosis, emphysema (late phase), smoking, AIDS
Chronic productive	Bronchiectasis, chronic bronchitis, lung abscess, asthma, fungal infections, bacterial pneumonias, TB
Paroxysmal (especially at night)	Aspiration, asthma, left heart failure
Positional, especially when lying down	Bronchiectasis, left heart failure, chronic postnasal drip or sinusitis, gastroesophageal reflux with aspiration
Associated with eating or drinking	Neuromuscular disease of the upper airway, esophageal problems, aspiration

Adapted from: Wilkins, R. L., Sheldon, R. L., & Krider, S. J. (2005). *Clinical assessment in respiratory care* (5th ed.). St. Louis, MO: Mosby.

Table 4-4 Sputum Assessment

Type of Sputum	Color and Consistency	Likely Conditions
Mucoid	Clear/white, thin to thick	Asthma
Mucopurulent	Clear to yellowish, thick	Chronic bronchitis, cystic fibrosis, pneumonia (blood streaked)
Purulent	Yellow to green, thick	Aspiration pneumonia, bronchiectasis (fetid/foul smelling, may separate into layers if left standing), lung abscess (fetid/foul smelling, may separate into layers if left standing)
Bloody	Pink to red/dark red, thin (unless coagulated)	Tuberculosis (red), lung cancer (red), pulmonary infarction (red), pulmonary edema (pink, watery, frothy)

Adapted from: MacIntyre, N. R. (1990). Respiratory monitoring without machinery. *Respiratory Care, 35,* 546–553.

Table 4-5 Apgar Score

Parameter	Acronym	0	1	2
Color	Appearance	Blue or pale	Pink body with peripheral cyanosis (acrocyanosis)	Completely pink
Heart rate	Pulse	Absent	< 100 beats/min	> 100 beats/min
Reflex irritability[a]	Grimace	Unresponsive	Grimace when stimulated	Active movement, crying, coughing
Muscle tone	Activity	Flaccid, limp	Some flexion of extremities	Active movement
Respiratory effort	Respirations	Absent	Slow, irregular, weak, gasping	Crying, vigorous breathing

a. Catheter in nares or tactile stimulation.

Respirations), each rated from 0 to 2, with a maximum score of 10 (stable, responsive infant) to a minimum of 0 (stillborn infant).

In general, an Apgar score of 7 to 10 is considered normal, and an increase in the score between 1 and 5 minutes indicates clinical improvement and a good response to therapy. Scores of 4, 5, and 6 are intermediate and usually indicate the need for more intensive support. Although infants with Apgar scores of 0 to 3 usually undergo aggressive resuscitation efforts, these scores should not be used to dictate resuscitation procedures. Also, needed interventions at birth should never be delayed in order to obtain the Apgar score.

Gestational Age

Normal gestation lasts 38–42 weeks. Besides being helpful in predicting delivery date, knowledge of the gestational age of the fetus provides information essential in anticipating perinatal problems and establishing sound care plans.

Gestational age can be estimated either before or after birth. **Table 4-6** summarizes the three methods that can be used to estimate the gestation age of a fetus before birth. After birth, determination of gestational age involves careful assessment of selected neuromuscular and physical characteristics using methods developed by Dubowitz and Ballard over the past 30 years. This assessment is normally conducted by a neonatologist or nurse practitioner within 30–40 hours after birth. Although respiratory therapists do not normally conduct this assessment, you should be familiar with its components.

Figure 4-1 depicts the Ballard Gestational Age Assessment and scoring system. The neuromuscular component addresses the following six areas:

- Posture: How does the infant hold his or her arms and legs?
- Square window: How much can the infant's hands be flexed toward the wrist?
- Arm recoil: How much do the infant's arms "spring back" to a flexed position?
- Popliteal angle: How far do the infant's knees extend?
- Scarf sign: How far can the elbows be moved across the infant's chest?
- Heel to ear: How close can the infant's feet be moved to the ear?

The physical component also addresses six areas:

- Skin: ranges from sticky and red to cracking or peeling to leathery
- Lanugo (soft body hair): absent in immature babies, then appears with maturity, and then disappears again with postmaturity
- Plantar (foot soles) surface: heel-to-toe length and presence of creases, ranging from absent to covering the entire foot, depending on the maturity

Table 4-6 Methods Used to Estimate Gestation Age Before Birth

Method	Measurement	Comments
Time since last menses	Weeks since end of last normal menstrual period + 2	Traditional but unreliable
Ultrasonography	1. Crown to rump length up to 14th week (table lookup) 2. Fetal head diameter (biparietal diameter) between 14th and 20th week of gestation (table lookup)	Accurate and reliable
Biochemical analysis (measurement of amniotic fluid phospholipid levels)[a]	1. Lecithin/sphingomylein (L/S) ratio > 2.0 2. Presence of phosphatidylglycerol (PG) 3. Lecithin/albumin (L/A) ratio ≥ 40.0 mg/g	Fetal maturity indicated by L/S ratio > 2; presence of PG; or L/A ratio > 40.0 mg/g
a. Used primarily to indicate fetal lung maturity and/or predict Infant Respiratory Distress Syndrome.		

NEUROMUSCULAR MATURITY

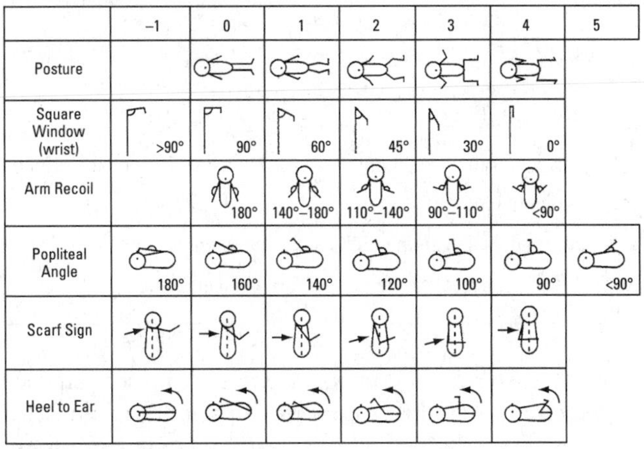

	−1	0	1	2	3	4	5
Posture							
Square Window (wrist)	>90°	90°	60°	45°	30°	0°	
Arm Recoil		180°	140°−180°	110°−140°	90°−110°	<90°	
Popliteal Angle	180°	160°	140°	120°	100°	90°	<90°
Scarf Sign							
Heel to Ear							

MATURITY RATING

score	weeks
−10	20
−5	22
0	24
5	26
10	28
15	30
20	32
25	34
30	36
35	38
40	40
45	42
50	44

PHYSICAL MATURITY

Skin	sticky; friable; transparent	gelatinous; red; translucent	smooth; pink; visible veins	superficial peeling and/or rash; few veins	cracking; pale aeas; rare veins	parchment; deep cracking; no vessels	leathery; cracked; wrinkled
Lanugo	none	sparse	abundant	thinning	bald areas	mostly bald	
Plantar surface	heel-toe 40−50 mm: −1 <40 mm: −2	>50 mm; no crease	faint red marks	anterior transverse crease only	creases ant. 2/3	creases over entire sole	
Breast	imperceptible	barely perceptible	flat areola; no bud	stippled areola; 1−2 mm bud	raised areola; 3−4 mm bud	full areola; 5−10 mm bud	
Eye/ear	lids fused loosely: −1 tightly: −2	lids open; pinna flat; stays folded	sl. curved pinna; soft; slow recoil	well-curved pinna; soft but ready recoil	formed and firm; instant recoil	thick cartilage; ear stiff	
Genital male	scrotum flat; smooth	scrotum empty; faint rugae	testes in upper canal; rare rugae	testes descending; few rugae	testes down; good rugae	testes pendulous; deep rugae	
Genitals female	clitoris prominent; labia flat	prominent clitoris; small labia minora	prominent clitoris; enlarging minora	majora and minora equally prominent	majora large; minora small	majora cover clitoris and minora	

Figure 4-1 Ballard Gestational Age Assessment.

Modified from: Ballard, J. L., Novak, K. K., & Denver, M. (1979). A simplified score for assessment of fetal maturation in newborn infants. *Journal of Pediatrics, 95,* 769–774.

- Breast: the thickness and size of breast tissue and areola (the darkened ring around each nipple)
- Eyes and ears: eyes fused or open and curvature and stiffness of the outer ear tissue (pinna)
- Genitals, male: presence of testes and appearance of scrotum, from smooth to wrinkled
- Genitals, female: appearance and size of the clitoris and the labia

Scores are summed across both components to yield a composite score. A composite score of 10 or less indicates significant prematurity (≤ 28 weeks' gestation). An infant born at full term (38–42 weeks) typically scores in the 35–45 range, with higher values indicating a post-term baby.

Transillumination of Chest

Transillumination is a quick and sensitive procedure used in infants to help detect pneumothorax. You should recommend transillumination for any high-risk infant (especially those receiving positive pressure ventilation) with clinical signs of pneumothorax, including retractions, tachypnea, cyanosis, hypotension, and asymmetrical chest motion.

Transillumination involves placing a specialized high-intensity fiberoptic cold light source on the external chest wall. Normally only the skin about 1 cm around the light will illuminate, forming a halo. If instead the chest "lights up," a pneumothorax is likely. The basic transillumination procedure is outlined in the accompanying box.

Transillumination Procedure

1. Make the room as dark as possible

2. Place the infant in the supine position

3. Switch on the light to the brightest setting

4. Hold the light against the infant's skin along the midaxillary line about halfway down the chest on the affected side

5. Observe whether or not the chest illuminates (lights up)

6. Repeat the assessment on the same side at the midclavicular line halfway down the chest

7. Repeat the assessment on the opposite side of the chest to compare the degree of illumination

---

If only one side of the chest lights up, then a pneumothorax is probably present on that side. If both sides of the chest illuminate poorly, then a pneumothorax is probably not present. However, negative results do not rule out a pneumothorax. This is because transillumination can miss small pneumothoraces and may be of limited value in large babies. For this reason, if the results of transillumination are negative but the infant still exhibits symptoms of pneumothorax, you should recommend an immediate chest X-ray.

Assess the Patient's Overall Cardiopulmonary Status by Palpation

Palpation applies the sensation of touch to evaluate underlying structure and function. Palpation is performed to: (1) evaluate heart rate, rhythm, and force, (2) assess tracheal position, (3) evaluate vocal/tactile fremitus, (4) estimate thoracic expansion, and (5) assess the skin and tissues of the chest and extremities.

Heart Rate, Rhythm, and Force

Palpation can provide valuable information about the heart's rate, rhythm, and force. You obtain this information by palpating both a peripheral pulse (usually the radial) and an apical pulse, over the precordium (area of anterior thorax over the heart).

You palpate the peripheral pulse to measure a patient's heart rate while obtaining the vital signs. Commonly, the radial pulse is selected. Other locations for palpating the peripheral pulse include the carotid, brachial, femoral, and popliteal (behind the knee) arteries.

Heart Rate

Normal ranges for heart rates by age group are specified in Chapter 3. Based on this knowledge, you determine whether the rate is normal or if the patient has tachycardia or bradycardia. **Table 4-7** outlines the most common causes of tachycardia and bradycardia.

Heart Rhythm

To detect if the pulse is regular or irregular, you may need to palpate it for a full minute. Minor irregularities are common, particularly in young people (sinus arrhythmia). If, however, you believe that a significant irregularity exists, repeat your assessment with a second clinician simultaneously measuring the apical rate via palpation or auscultation over the heart. If the apical rate is higher than that obtained peripherally, a *pulse deficit* exists. A pulse deficit usually indicates a cardiac arrhythmia, such as atrial fibrillation or flutter, PVCs, or heart block.

Strength of Pulse

Careful assessment of the peripheral pulse can reveal variation in its strength. **Table 4-8** summarizes the most common findings and their likely causes.

Palpating the Precordium

You palpate the precordium to assess the location and strength of the heart's point of maximum impulse (PMI). The normal PMI is located at or near the fifth intercostal space, midclavicular line. Variations in the strength or position of the PMI indicate abnormalities. A weak impulse may indicate hyperinflation (as with COPD) or decreased cardiac contractility. Abnormally strong pulsations and/or a shift in the PMI downward and to left suggest left ventricular hypertrophy. Also, the PMI tends to move when the mediastinum is displaced. For example, the PMI tends to shift *toward* areas of atelectasis, and *away from* space-occupying lesions such as pneumothoraces or pleural effusions.

Table 4-7 Common Causes of Abnormal Heart Rates

Abnormality	Common Causes
Tachycardia	Fever
	Hypoxemia
	Pain
	Shock
	Anemia
	Cardiac arrhythmias
	Hyperthyroidism
	Thyrotoxicosis
	Drug effects: B-adrenergic agents; cholinergic blocking agents (e.g., atropine); stimulants (e.g.,nicotine, caffeine); illicit drugs (e.g., amphetamines, cocaine)
Bradycardia	Vasovagal reflex
	Cardiac arrhythmias
	Increased intracranial pressure
	Hypothyroidism
	Hypothermia
	Electrolyte imbalances
	Drug effects: B-adrenergic blockers; calcium-channel blockers; digoxin; antiarrhythmic agents

Table 4-8 Summary of Pulse Findings

Type	Description	Causes
Strong	Easy to palpate	Increased stroke volume (e.g., exercise)
Weak or thready	Hard to palpate	Decreased cardiac contractility; decreased circulating blood volume; loss of vascular tone (e.g., septic shock); aortic stenosis
Bounding	Rapid/strong initial pressure rise followed by a quick fall-off	Aortic insufficiency; patent ductus arteriosus; atherosclerosis
Pulsus alternans	Pulse alternates in strength from beat to beat	Left-sided heart failure/CHF
Pulsus paradoxus	Pulsations vary with the breathing cycle, such that weaker pulses are felt during inspiration	Severe airway obstruction (status asthmaticus); constrictive pericardial disease (e.g., cardiac tamponade)

Tracheal Position

Normally, the trachea lies in the midline of the neck. Because it connects to the structures enclosed in the mediastinum, tracheal deviations away from the midline are due to the same problems that cause the PMI to shift position. In general, the trachea shifts *toward areas of collapse/atelectasis* and *away from space-occupying lesions* such as pneumothoraces, large effusions, and tumors.

Fremitus

Fremitus refers to vibrations that you can feel by palpating the chest. There are two types of fremitus that you need to be familiar with: rhonchial fremitus and vocal fremitus.

Rhonchial fremitus is caused by vibrations created as air moves through large airways containing excess secretions. You detect rhonchial fremitus by placing the flat of your hand on the chest to either side of the sternum. Typically, rhonchial fremitus diminishes or clears with coughing or after effective suctioning.

Vocal fremitus represents the transmission of voice sounds from the larynx, through the airways and to the chest wall. You assess vocal fremitus by having the patient repeat the word "ninety-nine" while you palpate the chest wall. In general, vocal fremitus increases in those conditions in which lung tissue density increases, such as pneumonia (consolidation) and atelectasis. In contrast, overall sound transmission and vocal fremitus tend to decrease in obese patients and those with COPD. More locally, vocal fremitus decreases whenever and wherever the lungs are separated from the chest wall, as occurs with pneumothorax and pleural effusion. Last, vocal fremitus also tends to decrease over areas where the underlying lung lobe or segment is obstructed by a mucous plug or foreign body.

Thoracic Expansion

Palpation can help determine whether the chest expands equally on both sides during deep inhalation. To do so anteriorly, place your hands over the lower lateral chest wall, with the thumbs extended along the lower rib margins. On the back, you position your hands over the posterolateral chest with the thumbs meeting at about the eighth thoracic vertebra. When the patient takes a full, deep breath, each thumb should move an equal distance of about 1–2 inches from the midline. Lesser or unequal movement is abnormal. You will often see a bilateral reduction in chest expansion in COPD patients and those with neuromuscular disorders. Unilateral reduction in chest movement (on the affected side) tends to occur with lobar pneumonia, atelectasis, pleural effusion, and pneumothorax.

Skin and Soft Tissues

You can palpate the skin and soft tissues to determine temperature and assess for crepitus, edema, capillary refill, and tenderness.

Peripheral Skin Temperature

When the heart fails to circulate enough blood, the blood vessels in the arms and legs constrict in order to help direct flow to the vital organs. With less blood flow, the extremities tend to cool. For this reason, hands and feet that are cool when palpated usually indicate poor perfusion.

Crepitus

Especially in patients receiving positive pressure ventilation, gas can leak from the lungs or airways into the tissues around the head, neck, and chest, forming fine subcutaneous bubbles. This condition is termed *subcutaneous emphysema*. When palpated, these gas bubbles produce a crackling sensation called *crepitus*. Although subcutaneous emphysema by itself normally is harmless, it often occurs in conjunction with a pneumothorax. For this reason, *if you detect crepitus, be sure to assess the patient for a pneumothorax and immediately communicate your findings to the patient's physician*. Many would recommend getting a chest X-ray whenever crepitus occurs in a patient receiving positive pressure ventilation.

Dependent Edema

Many patients with chronic respiratory or cardiac disease exhibit gravity-dependent tissue edema, typically in the feet and ankles (pedal edema). This type of edema is most associated with right ventricular failure (cor pulmonale), although it also occurs in congestive heart failure. In these patients, when you firmly press on their edematous tissue with a finger, it "pits" or indents. The degree of pitting is usually rated on a 3-point scale, with +3 being the most serious. In general, the farther up the legs the edema can be detected, the more severe the heart failure.

Capillary Refill

You assess capillary refill by pressing firmly on a patient's fingernails, then releasing the pressure and noting how quickly blood flow returns. When cardiac output is reduced and digital perfusion is poor, capillary refill is slow, taking 3 or more seconds.

Abdominal Palpation

You can palpate the abdomen for evidence of distension and tenderness. Abdominal distension and pain can restrict movement of the diaphragm, impair coughing and deep breathing, and contribute to respiratory insufficiency. Typically, the right upper quadrant of the abdomen is palpated for tenderness and to estimate the size of the liver. Abdominal tenderness and an enlarged liver may be seen in patients with chronic cor pulmonale. This condition is called *hepatomegaly*.

Assess the Patient's Overall Cardiopulmonary Status by Percussion

In a complete thoracic exam, you should systematically percuss the lung fields on both sides of the chest, being sure to avoid bony structures and female breasts. To move the scapulae out of the way for posterior percussion, have the patient raise his or her arms.

Percussion over normal air-filled lung tissue produces a relatively low-pitched and easily heard hollow sound, called *normal resonance*. A percussion sound that is louder and lower pitched than normal is referred to as *increased resonance* and typically occurs in patients with hyperinflation (acute asthma, COPD) or a pneumothorax. A percussion note that is short, muted, and higher pitched than normal is termed *dull* or *flat*. The decreased resonance associated with a dull percussion note occurs due to increased lung tissue density, as observed in patients with pneumonia, atelectasis, or lung tumors. Decreased resonance to percussion also occurs when fluid accumulates in the pleural space, as with a pleural effusion or hemothorax.

Percussion over the lower posterior thorax also can help you assess the position of the diaphragm and its range of motion. As you percuss downward over the lower lung fields, the sound will change from a normal to a dull note, indicating the level of the diaphragm. The difference between the maximum inspiratory and expiratory levels represents the full range of diaphragm motion, which in adults should be about 5–7 cm. Patients with neuromuscular disorders affecting this muscle and those with severe pulmonary hyperinflation typically have a decreased range of diaphragm motion.

Assess the Patient's Overall Cardiopulmonary Status by Auscultation

You auscultate the thorax with a stethoscope to identify normal or abnormal lung and heart sounds. In general, you should use the stethoscope's diaphragm for auscultation of higher-pitched breath sounds, whereas the bell is recommended to listen to lower-pitched heart sounds.

Breath Sounds

Characteristics of the normal breath sounds are described in **Table 4-9**. These sounds are normal only if noted at the specified location. Normal sounds identified at abnormal locations are abnormal! For example, bronchial breath sounds are considered abnormal when heard over peripheral lung regions. They tend to replace normal vesicular sounds when lung tissue increases in density, as in atelectasis and pneumonia/consolidation.

Breath sounds are decreased or diminished when the patient's breathing is shallow or slow. A decrease in breath sound intensity also occurs when airways are obstructed or the lung tissue is hyperinflated, as in asthma or COPD. Air or fluid in the pleural space and obesity can also reduce breath sounds.

Abnormal or *adventitious* breath sounds include crackles (rales), rhonchi, wheezes, and stridor. Chapter 13 provides details on the characteristics and causes of these adventitious sounds.

Heart Sounds

Normal heart sounds are generated when the heart valves close. The first heart sound, or *S1*, signals closure of the mitral and tricuspid valves following ventricular contraction. The second heart sound, or *S2*, occurs with closure of the pulmonic and aortic valves. You listen to heart sounds to assess the apical heart rate and to identify gross abnormalities in structure or function.

When the peripheral pulses are difficult to palpate, you should assess the *apical rate* by direct auscultation of heart sounds at the PMI. As with palpation, you also can use auscultation to compare the apical rate to that palpated at a peripheral artery in order to determine if a pulse deficit is present.

The intensity or loudness of heart sounds diminishes in conditions that impair sound transmission between the heart and the exterior chest wall, such as pulmonary hyperinflation, pleural effusion, pneumothorax, and obesity. Heart sounds also are diminished in cases of heart failure, hypotension, and shock. In contrast, heart sound intensity can increase when there is partial obstruction to outflow from the ventricles, as in mitral stenosis (affecting S1) and pulmonary hypertension (affecting S2). Heart sounds may also be louder than normal in children and thin-chested patients. Variation in the intensity of heart sounds, especially S1, occurs with cardiac arrhythmias that alter ventricular filling, such as atrial fibrillation and complete heart block.

You will sometimes hear a third heart sound (S3), occurring just after S2. The presence of this extra sound creates a galloping pattern, often equated with the saying the word "Kentucky" (S1 = ken; S2 = tuc; S3 = ky). S3 is commonly present in many normal children and also can be heard in well-conditioned athletes. Its presence in older patients usually indicates congestive heart failure.

Table 4-9 Normal Breath Sounds

Breath Sound	Description	Normally Heard at (Location)
Vesicular	Low-pitched soft sounds; heard primarily during inhalation, with only a minimal exhalation component	Periphery of lungs
Bronchial	High-pitched loud, tubular sounds with an expiratory phase equal to or longer than the inspiratory phase	Over trachea
Bronchovesicular	Moderate pitch and intensity; equal inspiratory and expiratory phases	Around upper sternum (anterior); between scapulae (posterior)

Cardiac murmurs indicate turbulent flow through a heart valve, which occurs when either a valve fails to properly close (causing backflow or regurgitation) or outflow from the valve is obstructed (stenosis). Systolic murmurs are heard when either an atrioventricular (AV) valve allows backflow or a semilunar valve restricts outflow. Diastolic murmurs occur with semilunar valve regurgitation or AV valve stenosis.

Auscultatory Assessment of Blood Pressure

You also apply auscultation skills when measuring blood pressure (known as the noninvasive occlusion method). As you deflate the blood pressure cuff, you listen for the *Korotkoff sounds* that occur as the blood flows turbulently through the partial obstruction created by the cuff. The pressure at which the Korotkoff sounds first appear is the systolic pressure, while the point at which these sounds suddenly become muffled and disappear is the diastolic pressure.

In patients with normal blood pressure, auscultation of these sounds is relatively easy and provides accurate data. However, there are several common situations deserving special consideration when using auscultation for noninvasive blood pressure measurement. These are summarized in **Table 4-10**.

Integrating Physical Examination Findings

When assessing or reviewing a patient's physical exam findings, proper interpretation demands that you integrate the results of inspection, palpation, percussion, and auscultation. **Table 4-11** summarizes the major physical findings associated with various common clinical disorders.

Table 4-10 Special Considerations in Noninvasive Measurement of Blood Pressure

Problem	Caused By	Solution(s)
Inaudible blood pressure	Poor technique	Use proper technique.
	Severe hypotension or shock	Consider arterial line monitoring.
	Venous engorgement (due to repeated measurements)	For venous engorgement, remove the cuff and have the patient raise his or her arm over the head for 1–2 minutes before repeating the measurement.
Irregular cardiac rhythms	Atrial fibrillation, frequent PVCs, heart block	Make several measurements and use the average.
Auscultatory gap	A silent interval between the systolic and diastolic pressure sounds that if not recognized can result in underestimation of the systolic pressure or overestimation of the diastolic pressure; usually caused by hypertension	Measure and record *three* pressures: (1) the opening systolic or "snap" pressure, (2) the pressure at which continuous pulses again are heard, and (3) the diastolic pressure.
Paradoxical pulse (*pulsus paradoxus*)	A larger than normal drop (> 6–8 mm Hg) in systolic pressure during inspiration seen in patients with severe airway obstruction (such as acute asthma) or in conditions that impair ventricular filling (such as cardiac tamponade)	To measure paradoxical pulse, slowly deflate the cuff until you hear sounds *only on exhalation* (point 1). Then reduce the cuff pressure again until you can hear sounds throughout the breathing cycle (point 2). The difference in pressures between points 1 and 2 is the paradoxical pulse measurement.

Table 4-11 Physical Findings Associated with Various Common Clinical Disorders

Abnormality	Inspection	Palpation	Percussion	Auscultation
Asthma	Use of accessory muscles	Reduced expansion	Increased resonance	Expiratory wheezing
COPD	Increased AP diameter; use of accessory muscles	Reduced expansion	Increased resonance	Diffuse decrease in breath sounds; early inspiratory crackles
Consolidation (pneumonia or tumor)	Inspiratory lag	Increased fremitus	Dull note	Bronchial breath sounds; crackles
Pneumothorax	Unilateral expansion	Decreased vocal fremitus	Increased resonance	Absent breath sounds
Pleural effusion	Unilateral expansion	Absent vocal fremitus	Dull note	Absent breath sounds
Atelectasis	Unilateral expansion	Absent vocal fremitus	Dull note	Absent breath sounds
Diffuse interstitial fibrosis	Rapid shallow breathing	Often normal; increased fremitus	Slight decrease in resonance	Late inspiratory crackles
Upper airway obstruction (croup, foreign body, etc.)	Labored breathing	Often normal	Often normal	Inspiratory and/or expiratory stridor

Interview the Patient

Interviewing provides essential information about a patient's (1) level of consciousness, ability to co-operate, and emotional state, (2) experience of pain, (3) breathing difficulties, (4) activities of daily living (including exercise tolerance), (5) social history, and (6) advance directives.

Level of Consciousness, Ability to Cooperate, and Emotional State

You can quickly assess patients for their level of consciousness, or "sensorium," by asking them the time of day, where they are, and who they are. Alert patients are well oriented as to time, place, and person, or "oriented × 3." The most common reasons for a patient not being well oriented to time, place, and person are neurologic injury, pharmacologic sedation, and severe hypoxemia or hypercapnia. *In general, only alert patients can be expected to cooperate and fully participate in their own care.*

If a patient is alert, you also should try to assess his or her emotional state during the interview. Patients in a normal emotional state will usually respond with alternating facial expressions appropriate to the conversation; describe themselves as well adjusted, generally happy, or appropriately concerned about their present condition; and appear either relaxed or moderately anxious. Patients in an abnormal emotional state typically appear depressed or overly anxious, as evident by irritability, difficulty focusing, breathlessness, dizziness, trembling, palpitations, and/or chest pain. In general, patients in an abnormal emotional state will be difficult to manage until their anxiety can be resolved.

Whenever encountering patients who are not alert, you should objectively assess their level of consciousness using the Glasgow Coma Scale (**Table 4-12**). To apply this scale, you assess the patient's eye, verbal, and motor responses and assign a numeric value to each component. The three values are summed to yield a composite score, with the lowest possible value being 3 (deep coma) and the highest being 15. Relative impairment is interpreted as follows:

- Mild impairment: 13–15
- Moderate impairment: 9–12
- Severe impairment (coma): < 8

Table 4-12 Glasgow Coma Scale

	1	2	3	4	5	6
Eyes	Does not open eyes	Opens eyes in response to painful stimuli	Opens eyes in response to verbal stimuli	Opens eyes spontaneously	n/a	n/a
Verbal	Makes no sounds	Incomprehensible speech	Utters inappropriate words	Confused, disoriented	Oriented, converses normally	n/a
Motor	Makes no movements (flaccid)	Extension to painful stimuli	Abnormal flexion to painful stimuli	Flexion/withdrawal to painful stimuli	Localizes painful stimuli	Obeys commands

Experience of Pain

To determine if an alert patient is experiencing pain, ask the question, "Are you having any pain or discomfort now?" If the patient answers yes, then she is in pain.

When soliciting a patient's description of pain, you should try to quantify its intensity using an objective measure. For alert adults, a numeric rating scale is a good objective measure of pain severity. Patients are asked to rate the severity of their current pain on a scale ranging from 0 to 10, where 0 signifies "no pain" and 10 represents "the worst possible pain." Patients can use the same scale to pinpoint their maximum tolerable level of pain.

A numeric pain scale may not be useful for young children or patients who are unable to express themselves. As an alternative, you can interview family members to get information about pain history, typical behaviors when the patient has pain, and activities that may cause or worsen the patient's pain. Without such information, you may have to rely on observing related patient behaviors, such as moaning, and looking for facial expressions that indicate severe pain, such as grimacing or tearing.

After you determine the severity of pain, you should try to assess how much it interferes with the patient's daily activities. A similar 10-point scale can be used to make this assessment, with 0 signifying "no interference" and 10 signifying "unable to carry out usual activities." Whenever a patient complains of an interference level above 4, you should report this finding to the patient's attending physician.

Breathing Difficulties

The evaluation of patients' dyspnea, orthopnea, work of breathing, and exercise tolerance is a critical skill for all respiratory therapists. Dyspnea and orthopnea are clinical *symptoms* that must be evaluated by interviewing or questioning the patient. The work of breathing and exercise tolerance are clinical *signs* that must be detected and quantified by the health professional.

Dyspnea and Orthopnea

Dyspnea is defined as the patient's sensation of uncomfortable breathing or breathlessness. *Orthopnea* is the patient's sensation of uncomfortable breathing when lying down, which typically is relieved by elevating the thorax—with multiple pillows if in bed—or by sitting or standing up. Both dyspnea and orthopnea are associated with cardiac or pulmonary disorders.

The most common method used to quantify a patient's dyspnea is the modified Borg Scale (**Table 4-13**). Like the pain scale, the Borg Scale is a simple 0–10 point numeric scale, with 0 representing no sensation and 10 representing maximal. As indicated in Table 4-13, the Borg Scale can be used to assess both a patient's perceived level of dyspnea *or* degree of exertion and is always applied in association with a predefined level of activity (e.g., exercise test level, end of 6-minute walk).

Table 4-13 Modified Borg Scale

Rating	For Rating Dyspnea	For Rating Exertion
0	Nothing at all	Nothing at all
0.5	Very, very slight (just noticeable)	Very, very weak (just noticeable)
1	Very slight	Very weak
2	Slight	Weak (light)
3	Moderate	Moderate
4	Somewhat severe	Somewhat strong
5	Severe	Strong (heavy)
6		
7	Very severe	Very strong
8		
9	Very, very severe (almost maximal)	Very, very strong (almost maximal)
10	Maximal	Maximal

To administer the Borg Scale to assess a patient's dyspnea, have the patient stop the activity, review the scale ratings, and select the number corresponding to his or her degree of breathing difficulty being experienced at that moment.

Work of Breathing

Abnormal work of breathing is a clinical *sign*. In combination, the following observations should indicate to you that a patient is experiencing an abnormally high work of breathing:

- Tachypnea
- Thoracic-abdominal dysynchrony ("seesaw" motion)
- Use of accessory muscles

Exercise Tolerance

The gold standard for assessing a patient's exercise tolerance is a graded cardiopulmonary exercise test. A less rigorous but very useful alternative method for objectively evaluating exercise tolerance is the 6-minute walk test. Both of these tools are discussed later in this chapter.

A simpler measure that you can employ to assess a patient's exercise tolerance via interview is the American Thoracic Society (ATS) Breathlessness Scale (**Table 4-14**). The ATS Breathlessness Scale is designed to help you quantify the point at which a patient develops dyspnea during common daily activities. By inquiring as to when breathlessness is first noticed by the patient, you can assign a rating of 0–4 to the symptom, with a descriptive term for each level. For example, a patient who reports sensing breathlessness only when hurrying on level ground or walking up a slight hill would receive an ATS rating of 1 (indicating slight dyspnea).

Nutritional Status

A comprehensive nutritional assessment—which involves the collection of history and physical data, physical and physiologic measurements, and the evaluation of assorted lab tests—is usually conducted by a clinical nutritionist or the patient's doctor. However, since nutritional status can have a major impact on the outcome of respiratory care, you need to gather enough information to assess a patient's risk for malnutrition. Obvious physical signs associated with severe malnutrition include a weak or emaciated appearance (cachexia); generalized edema (anasarca); cracked lips (cheilosis); dry, scaly skin; and listlessness. For patients lacking obvious signs of malnutrition, a series of basic interview

Table 4-14 American Thoracic Society Breathlessness Scale

Grade	Degree	Description of Breathlessness
0	None	Not troubled with breathlessness except with strenuous exercise
1	Slight	Troubled by shortness of breath when hurrying on level ground or walking up a slight hill
2	Moderate	Walks slower than people of the same age on level ground because of breathlessness or has to stop for breath when walking at own pace on level ground
3	Severe	Stops for breath after walking about 100 yards or after a few minutes on level ground
4	Very severe	Too breathless to leave the house or breathless when dressing and undressing

questions that focus on recent weight changes and dietary habits can suffice. Typical questions include the following:

- What is the patient's average weight and weight range during the past month, year, five years? Is there a history of major weight gain or loss? If so, did this involve any special dieting?
- What specific foods does the patient eat and in what amounts? Has there been any recent change in appetite?
- What is the patient's eating pattern (e.g., three meals/day, smaller meals more often)?
- How much fluid does the patient take in daily (estimated)?
- Is the patient able to afford and obtain the desired/needed foods?
- Does the patient prepare his or her own food? If so, are there any preparation problems (e.g., fatigue, poor vision, lack of appliances or clean water)? If not, is the food to his or her liking?
- Does the patient have any problem with chewing or swallowing?
- What is the patient's perception of his or her own nutritional status?

Based on answers to these questions, you should be able to identify patients at risk for malnutrition. This would include any patient who:

- Is significantly underweight (< 90% predicted body weight)
- Has had recent weight loss of 10% or more of usual body weight
- Has poor dietary habits or inadequate food intake (due to any cause)
- Is impoverished, isolated, or unable to prepare own food

If you identify a patient at risk for malnutrition, you should share this information with the patient's doctor and/or refer the patient to a dietitian or clinical nutritionist.

Social and Occupational History

A complete interview includes questions about a patient's social and occupational history. These questions should focus on obtaining relevant information addressing the following key elements:

- Marital status and family relationships
- Cultural and religious influences
- Living situation and social support
- Education, employment, finances
- Occupational history
- Diet, exercise, and other habits
- Social activities, hobbies, and recreation
- Tobacco, alcohol, or drug use (substance abuse)
- Satisfaction/stress with life situation

Note that due to its importance in diagnosis of certain lung diseases, the occupational history is often considered a separate category of interview.

Tobacco Use/Smoking History

To determine smoking history, you first ask patients if they are current smokers, are former smokers, or have never smoked. You also need to determine if the habit involves primarily cigarettes, cigars, or pipe smoking. For former smokers, determine how long ago they quit. For current or former cigarette smokers, quantify their smoking history in *pack-years* as follows:

pack-years = daily packs of cigarettes smoked × number of years smoking
Example: A 38-year-old patient has been smoking 1-1/2 packs per day for 20 years.
pack-years = 1.5 × 20 = 30 pack-years

Cigarettes smoked per day (1 pack = 20 cigarettes) also is a good indicator of nicotine dependence, along with how soon after waking the patient smokes the first cigarette. Patients who smoke more than a pack a day and must immediately have their first cigarette upon waking are heavily nicotine dependent.

Substance Abuse

Substance abuse refers to any continued harmful use of a drug or chemical (including alcohol) that results in repeated adverse social consequences (e.g., failure to meet work, family, or school obligations; interpersonal conflicts; legal problems). People can abuse illegal drugs, legal over-the-counter drugs, prescription medications, and common chemicals such as alcohol or glue.

According to the *Diagnostic and Statistical Manual for Mental Disorders* (DSM-IV-TR), symptoms of substance abuse include one or more of the following occurring during a given 12-month period:

- Substance use resulting in a recurrent failure to fulfill work, school, or home obligations (e.g., work absences, substance-related school suspensions, neglect of children)
- Substance use in physically hazardous situations such as driving or operating machinery
- Substance use resulting in legal problems such as drug-related arrests
- Continued substance use despite negative social and relationship consequences

Other physical signs and symptoms of substance abuse depend on the specific drug class. For example, amphetamine abuse is associated with a rapid heartbeat, elevated or depressed blood pressure, dilated pupils, weight loss, inability to sleep, confusion, and occasional paranoid psychotic behavior.

To help identify substance abuse during a patient interview, you should ask the following two questions (from Brown et al., 2001):

1. Have you felt you wanted or needed to cut down on your drinking or drug use in the past year?
2. In the past year, have you ever drunk or used drugs more than you meant to?

A positive response to either of these two questions indicates current substance abuse.

Advance Directives and DNR Orders

Unless otherwise informed, you can legally presume that your patients want life-saving treatment. Indeed, *whenever in doubt or when written orders are not present, you should always initiate emergency life support or resuscitation when needed.* However, in order to ensure that your actions are consistent with your patients' desires, you should include in your initial interview questions focusing on any advance directives they have specified.

An advance directive allows patients to specify the health care choices they want made should they become unable to make informed decisions. Because you have a legal obligation to follow advanced directives, you need to be aware if your patient has formally made these arrangements, usually via either a living will or durable power of attorney. A living will limits the level of care that patients desire should they become incapacitated and terminally ill. A durable power of attorney (also called a proxy directive) gives a spouse, relative, or friend the legal authority to make health care decisions for the patient. Normally, both types of advance directives are obtained when a patient is admitted to the hospital and can be found in the patient's chart (see Chapter 3).

Do-not-resuscitate (DNR) orders represent a special type of advance directive in which patients specify that no resuscitation should be attempted should they suffer cardiorespiratory arrest. This request can come directly from the patient or from his or her legal proxy or surrogate. After obtaining informed consent from the patient or proxy, the attending physician places the DNR order in the chart.

Patients can change or revoke an advance directive or DNR order at any time, as long as they are able to think rationally and communicate their wishes clearly. Although such changes normally must be made in writing, patients can communicate their desires orally to medical personnel or to family members or friends. Should a patient or their surrogate ask you to change or revoke an advance directive or DNR order, you must *immediately* notify the attending physician, who must either cancel the DNR order or have the new request replace any prior written documentation.

Assess the Patient's Learning Needs

The provision of effective patient education is a standard of the Joint Commission, the accrediting body for hospitals. According to the Joint Commission, patient education should be designed to foster healthy behaviors and increase patients' involvement in their health care decisions.

Assessment of a patient's learning needs, abilities, preferences, and readiness to learn is the first step in patient education. Normally, this is performed via a comprehensive educational assessment conducted at the time of admission to a care unit and is documented in the patient's chart. **Figure 4-2** provides an example of a patient/family educational documentation form.

Patient/Family Education Record

Teaching/Learning Assessment	Assessment of Patient Ability to Learn		Assessment of Patient Readiness to Learn	
Speaks English? ☐ Y ☐ N If no, primary language _____ Preferred Learning Method: ☐ Listening ☐ Television ☐ Doing ☐ Demonstration ☐ Reading ☐ Other (specify) _____	☐ No barriers noted ☐ Cannot assess Specific barriers noted: ☐ Physical ☐ Emotional ☐ Cognitive ☐ Motivational ☐ Cultural ☐ Language ☐ Religious ☐ Developmental ☐ Other: _____		Receptive to learning? Patient: ☐Y ☐N ☐NA Other ☐Y ☐N ☐NA (specify) _____ Capable of learning? Patient: ☐Y ☐N ☐NA Other ☐Y ☐N ☐NA	
Date	**What Was Taught**	**To Whom**	**How (Method)**	**Response**	**Signature**

Acceptable Abbreviations	
What	D/C = discharge instruction; EQ = equipment; REHAB = rehabilitation techniques; MED = drugs
To Whom	PT = patient; SP = spouse; PR = parent; SO = significant other (e.g., other family member, partner, etc)
How	D = demonstration; T = television/video; V = verbal instructions; W = written materials;
Response	AV = attentive verbal response; RD = return demonstration; DI = seems disinterested; NR = needs reinforcement

Figure 4-2 Example of a Patient/Family Educational Documentation Form.
Typically, such forms include an assessment of the patient's learning ability and needs as well as documentation of the education provided to meet those needs.

As indicated on this form, you first need to determine if there is any potential language barrier that might impact on teaching and learning. If so, you may need to enlist an English-speaking family member for assistance or secure a translator.

You then should determine the patient's preferred learning method. This can be accomplished by having patients tell you about something they recently learned and how they learned it, or how they would have preferred learning it. Hints as to preferred ways of learning can also be gleaned from questions about the patient's field of work and hobbies.

The next step is to identify any barriers that might affect patient learning, as revealed by chart review and/or patient interview. **Table 4-15** outlines the most common barriers to patient learning and suggests ways to address them when they occur. Note the importance of gaining family assistance in overcoming many of these limiting factors.

After identifying potential barriers to learning, you should assess the patient's readiness to learn. Especially useful in this regard are the explicit desires of patients to learn more about their condition or its management. In addition, careful listening can help determine a patient's readiness to learn. When patients are ready to learn, they tend to express discomfort with their current abilities or situation.

Table 4-15 Accommodating Common Barriers to Patient Learning

Barrier to Learning	Accommodations
Age (young child)	Keep teaching/learning episodes short Use "fun and games" approach Enlist family assistance
Reduced level of consciousness	Postpone until patient becomes alert Apply methods that don't require cooperation
Presence of pain	Recommend analgesia Postpone until pain management is effective
Presence of anxiety	Postpone until anxiety management is effective Enlist family assistance Recommend anxiolytic therapy
Physical limitations	Ascertain specific limitations Apply methods that circumvent limitation Enlist family assistance
Educational level (low)	Emphasize oral (vs. written) instruction Adjust language level as appropriate Provide written materials at 5th- to 8th-grade reading level
Potential language barrier	Enlist family assistance Secure translator
Cultural or religious factors	Ascertain key factors affecting care Modify to accommodate Enlist family assistance
Vision difficulty	Have patient wear glasses Emphasize sound and touch Enlist family assistance
Hearing difficulty	Have patient use hearing aid Emphasize visualization and touch Enlist family assistance

Table 4-16 Evaluating Patient Learning

What Change You Are Evaluating	How to Evaluate the Change
Patient knowledge	Teach-back
Patient skill level	Return demonstration
Patient attitudes	Discussion with patient and/or family

The last step is to determine the patient's specific learning needs as related to the care you will provide. To do so you need to interview the patient, using terms and language appropriate to the patient's ability to understand. This interview should address the following baseline questions:

- Does the patient understand his or her current condition?
- Is the patient knowledgeable about his or her medications?
- Is the patient familiar with the procedures you will implement?
- Is the patient familiar with the equipment you plan to use?

If answers to any of these questions indicate a shortcoming or "knowledge gap," you have identified a learning need. In addition to identifying needs, you also should try to discover the patient's "wants" (i.e., any specific things the patient desires to learn more about). In combination, these needs and wants should provide the basis for setting mutually agreed-to education goals with patients and their families.

After implementing any patient learning activity, you need to evaluate the results and document the intervention in the patient's chart. As outlined in **Table 4-16**, how you evaluate a patient learning episode depends on whether your focus was on improving knowledge, developing skills, or changing attitudes.

With the teach-back method, you simply ask patients to repeat in their own words the information you are trying to get them to understand. A return demonstration is similar to the teach-back method, except the focus is on patients actually "going through the motions" of a procedural skill after you have demonstrated it to them. Attitudinal change is more difficult to assess, usually requiring probing questions and open discussion with the patient and/or key family members. Alternatively, changes in a patient's behavior related to critical attitudes may be used as indicators of success.

As with all patient interventions, patient education episodes should be documented in the medical record. Such documentation must include who was taught (patient and/or family), what was taught, how it was taught, and the relevant outcomes of learning (Figure 4-2).

Review and Interpret the Chest Radiograph

Chapter 3 outlines the various imaging studies commonly used in the diagnosis and management of respiratory disorders. Chapter 13 specifies the characteristics of the common abnormalities seen on chest radiographs. Here we outline the process of reviewing a chest X-ray, including some key features to look for during assessment. The basic steps in review of a chest X-ray are outlined in the accompanying box.

Reviewing the Chest Radiograph

If reviewing an actual negative, the side marker (left or right) should identify proper orientation of the film. Key features will reveal the projection (PA or AP) and whether the patient was at full inspiration when the film was taken. A proper axis (lack of rotation) can be judged by confirming structural symmetry about the spine.

- A right-side marker should appear on the left side of the film when viewing it, and vice versa; if in doubt, confirm the position of the heart's apex and gastric air bubble—both normally appear on the patient's left side.

Basic Steps in Review of a Chest X-Ray

1. Obtain the chest X-ray film; verify identification (patient, date) and orientation (using side marker)

2. Identify the view of the film (AP or PA)

3. Review the entire film for symmetry and identify:

   a. Clavicles, scapulae, and ribs

   b. Spinal column (note whether it is midline)

   c. Lungs, right and left

   d. Level of hemidiaphragms and costophrenic angles (sharp or blunted)

   e. Gastric air bubble

   f. Breast shadows

4. Trace the outline of each rib, noting the angle and any fractures or other abnormalities

5. Observe the tracheal position

6. Identify the carina and the mainstem bronchi

7. Examine the hila for size and position

8. Identify the lung markings

9. Identify the aortic knob and the heart shadow

10. Estimate the cardiothoracic ratio

11. Note the presence and position of any artificial airways or catheters

12. State an overall impression of the film

- In an AP view the scapulae can be visualized behind the lungs; in a PA view the scapulae are clear of the lung fields.
- At normal full inspiration, the diaphragm should be at the level of the sixth rib anteriorly and tenth rib posteriorly.
- Rotation is minimal if the spine is in the midline (confirmed when the medial ends of the clavicles are equidistant to spinous processes of the vertebral column).

Position of or Change in Hemidiaphragms

Table 4-17 summarizes key findings related to the position or appearance of the hemidiaphragms.

Tracheal Position

Consistent with normal findings during palpation, the trachea as visualized on X-ray should lie in the midline of the neck, overlying the spinal column on the AP view. Tracheal deviations away from the midline on X-ray are due to the same problems that cause a shift of the PMI. In general, the trachea can be seen on X-ray shifting *toward* areas of collapse/atelectasis and *away from* space-occupying lesions such as pneumothoraces, large effusions, and tumors.

Table 4-17 Abnormalities Associated with Changes in the Position or Appearance of the Hemidiaphragms

Appearance or Position	Likely Problem
Blunted costophrenic angles (affected side)	Lower-lobe pneumonia, pleural effusion
Flattened (affected side)	Hyperinflation, tension pneumothorax
Elevated (affected side)	Phrenic nerve paralysis, hepatomegaly
Air under diaphragms (differentiate from normal gastric air bubble)	Perforated gastrointestinal tract

Position of Endotracheal or Tracheostomy Tubes

Taking an AP chest X-ray is the most common method used to confirm proper placement of an endotracheal or tracheostomy tube. Ideally, the tube tip should be positioned about 4–6 cm above the carina. This normally corresponds to a location between thoracic vertebrae T2 and T4, or about the same level as the superior border of the aortic knob.

Lung Fields

Key to understanding markings on a chest film is the fact that a radiograph is a negative. This means that areas of increased whiteness or *radiopacity* indicate poor penetration of X-rays through high-density objects, such as bone or consolidated tissue. In contrast, areas of darkness or *radiolucency* indicate good penetration of X-rays through low-density matter such as air. **Table 4-18** lists the most common causes of radiopacity and radiolucency seen on a chest radiograph. Details on the specific radiograph findings associated with these abnormalities are provided in Chapter 13.

Position of Indwelling Tubes, Catheters, and Foreign Objects

Objects visible on a chest radiograph that do not originate from the patient are called *foreign bodies*. Foreign bodies include those appearing by accident or trauma—such as an aspirated tooth or bullet—and purposefully placed medical devices. Aspiration of small objects into the airway is the most common source of accidental foreign bodies, especially in children. This possibility should always be considered in the differential diagnosis of airway obstruction in children and is justification for recommending both a chest and lateral neck X-ray (covered in the next section of this chapter).

Other than some plastics, most foreign bodies are more dense than human tissues. For this reason, these objects appear radiopaque on an X-ray, with their shape often helping to identify their origin. For example, an aspirated small coin will appear as a solid white, round object on a radiograph. Likewise, medical devices such as surgical staples are easily identifiable by their shape and position.

In contrast, the lower density of plastic medical devices, such as ET tubes and intravascular catheters, would make them hard to visualize on an X-ray. This problem is overcome by embedding radiopaque markers in these devices. **Table 4-19** outlines common medical devices that may be visualized on a chest X-ray, including relevant comments about each item.

Review Lateral Neck Radiographs

When used in combination with a chest radiograph, lateral neck X-rays are useful in assessing for upper-airway obstruction, especially in children. The most common causes of upper-airway obstruction in children are aspirated foreign bodies and infection. As indicated previously, high-density aspirated foreign bodies are readily visualized on X-ray. Some plastic foreign bodies may be harder to identify and often require laryngoscopy or bronchoscopy to confirm and resolve.

In terms of serious upper-airway infections in pediatric patients, croup and epiglottis are the most common. **Table 4-20** (see page 89) compares the typical radiographic findings in these two conditions.

Table 4-18 Common Pulmonary Abnormalities Altering the Density of the Lung Fields on a Chest Radiograph

Increased Radiodensity	Increased Radiolucency
Atelectasis	Pulmonary emphysema
Consolidation	Pneumothorax
Interstitial lung disease	Pneumomediastinum
Pulmonary infiltrates/edema	Pneumopericardium
Pleural effusion	Subcutaneous emphysema
Lung/mediastinal tumors	Pulmonary interstitial emphysema
Calcification	

Table 4-19 Medical Devices Visualized on the Chest Radiograph

Devices	Comments
Extrathoracic	
ECG leads	Three electrodes (below the right and left clavicles and to the left of the patient's lower sternum) and lead wires typically are visible.
Clamps, syringes, and other instruments	May be on top of or under patient but can appear to be "inside" thorax and thus confuse interpretation.
Ventilator circuits, heating wires, temperature sensors	Adult circuits normally exhibit typical corrugated appearance; wires/sensors may be confused with intrathoracic devices such as pacemakers.
Breast implants	May be either unilateral or bilateral; shadows can be confused with lung pathology.
Intrathoracic	
Thoracostomy (chest) tubes	Used to evacuate fluid or air from the pleural space. To evacuate air (pneumothorax) tube normally is positioned anterosuperiorly, and to evacuate fluid, posteroinferiorly.
Endotracheal tubes	Tube tip should be 4–6 cm above the carina, or between thoracic vertebrae T2 and T4.
Nasogastric tubes	Used for feeding or gastric drainage; should be seen passing through the mediastinum and diaphragm into the stomach. *Misplacement of a feeding tube high in the esophagus or in the trachea can result in massive aspiration.*
Central venous catheter	Used for hemodynamic monitoring, administering fluids and medications, and parenteral nutrition; should be seen in the superior vena cava or right atrium.
Pulmonary artery catheter	Used for hemodynamic monitoring and administering fluids and medications; accurate wedge pressure measurement requires the catheter tip be visualized in the lower lobe, ideally posteriorly. Improper placement can result in false readings (e.g., pressure in the alveoli pressure instead of the pulmonary veins/left atrium).
Implanted cardiac pacemakers and cardioverter/defibrillators	Pulse generator most often implanted and visualized below the clavicle; one (ventricular) or two (ventricular + atrial) pacing wires should be seen coursing through the superior vena cava into the respective heat chamber(s).
Sternal wires	Sternal wires are the most common way of reattaching the two halves of the sternum after median sternotomy for coronary artery bypass surgery; appear on the chest radiograph as several opaque "tied" loops running up and down the sternum.
Cardiac valve replacements (prostheses)	Made from natural pig or human tissue or materials such as metal, plastic, or Dacron. On X-ray, prosthetic valves appear in the same location as what they replace (mitral and aortic being the most common). Metal "ball and cage" (Starr-Edwards) valves are most easily visualized on a radiograph.
Intra-aortic counterpulsation balloon device (IACB or IABP)	Consists of an inflatable balloon about 25 cm long, the tip of which normally can be visualized just distal to the left subclavian artery in the descending thoracic aorta.

Table 4-20 Radiographic Findings: Croup Versus Epiglottitis

	Condition	
	Croup	*Epiglottitis*
Chest film (AP)	"Steeple sign" (i.e., narrowed and tapering airway below larynx due to subglottic edema); tracheal dilation may be present if the film was taken during expiration	Usually appears normal (little or no evidence of subglottic involvement)
Lateral neck film	May appear normal (little or no evidence of supraglottic involvement)	"Thumb sign" due to prominent shadow caused by swollen epiglottis

Perform and Interpret Results of Selected Diagnostic Procedures

Twelve-lead ECG

Health care providers use the data obtained from a 12-lead ECG to assess rhythm disturbances, determine the heart's electrical axis, and identify the site and extent of myocardial damage.

Performing

Chapter 6 provides details on the use and troubleshooting of ECG machines. The basic procedure for obtaining a 12-lead ECG is outlined in the accompanying box. As detailed in Chapter 6, a good ECG tracing should have a stable isoelectric baseline and no extraneous noise or AC interference.

Basic 12-Lead ECG Procedure

1. Turn on machine (plug into outlet if AC powered) and confirm its operation

2. Place patient appropriately in supine or semi-Fowler's position

3. Have patient remove all jewelry or metal

4. Instruct patient to relax completely

5. Apply clean limb electrodes to muscular areas of arms and legs

6. Place chest leads in proper locations:

    a. V1: Fourth intercostal space, right sternal margin

    b. V2: Fourth intercostal space, left sternal margin

    c. V3: Midway between V2 and V4

    d. V4: Fifth intercostal space, left midclavicular line

    e. V5: Fifth intercostal space, left anterior axillary line

    f. V6: Sixth intercostal space, left midaxillary line

7. Ensure patient comfort and respect patient privacy and modesty

8. Calibrate machine

9. Run test strip

10. Inspect rhythm strip for:

    a. Wandering baseline

    b. 60-cycle (AC) artifact

    c. Noise due to muscle tremor artifact or poor electrode contact

    d. Disconnected lead or intermittent loss of signal

11. Run complete 12-lead ECG to obtain a good tracing

Interpreting

Although you may have received training in interpreting a full 12-lead ECG, *this skill is not tested on the CRT exam*. However, you may be expected to identify common abnormalities from a rhythm strip. To do so, you systematically assess the rate, rhythm, P waves, the PR interval, QRS complex, QT interval, ST segment, and T-waves.

The easiest way to estimate heart rate is to use the "Rule of 300." **Figure 4-3** demonstrates this rule. As long as the rhythm is regular, you can estimate the heart rate by (1) counting the number of *large* boxes between two consecutive R waves (the R-R interval) and then (2) dividing this number into 300. For example, if the R-R interval spans four large boxes, the rate is 300 ÷ 4 = 75 beats/min. **Table 4-21** summarizes key findings defining major abnormalities in rhythm, P waves, the PR interval, QRS complex, QT interval, ST segment, and T-waves and their most common causes.

Bedside Assessment of Ventilation

Bedside assessment of ventilation involves measurement of a patient's tidal volume, rate of breathing, minute volume, vital capacity, and maximum inspiratory and expiratory pressures (**Table 4-22**; see page 92). You should recommend measuring these parameters when the need exists to:

- Assess the progress of diseases affecting respiratory muscle strength (e.g., neuromuscular disorders)
- Evaluate a patient's potential need for mechanical ventilation
- Assess a patient's readiness for weaning from mechanical ventilation

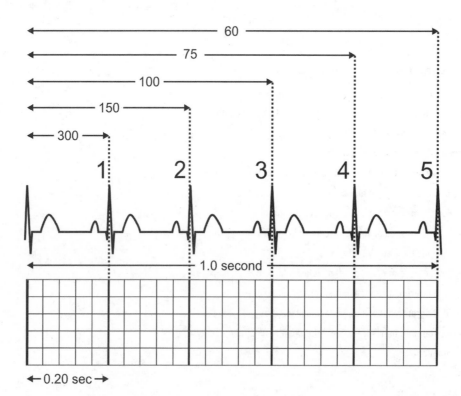

Figure 4-3 Using the Rule of 300. With the ECG machine set at the standard recording speed of 25 mm/second, each little 1 mm box represents 0.04 sec and each large box represents 5 × 0.04, or 0.20 sec. Therefore, if a QRS complex were to occur with each large box, then the R-R interval would be 0.20 sec, and the rate would be 5 beats/sec × 60 sec/min, or 300 beats/min. As long as the rhythm is regular, dividing 300 by the number of big boxes spanned by the R-R interval provides a good estimate for any cardiac rate. For example, if the R-R interval spans three large boxes, the rate would be approximately 300 ÷ 3 = 100/min.

Table 4-21 Major ECG Abnormalities and Their Common Causes

Abnormal ECG Findings	Common Causes
P waves—abnormal	Left or right atrial hypertrophy, PACs
P waves—absent	Atrial fibrillation
P-P interval—variable	Sinus arrhythmia
PR interval—prolonged (> 0.20 sec)	First-degree or Mobitz-type I A-V block
R-R interval—shortened (< 0.60 sec)	Tachycardia (R-R sec or rate > 100/min)
R-R interval—prolonged (> 1.00 sec)	Bradycardia (R-R > 1.00 sec or rate < 60/min)
R-R interval—variable (> 0.12 sec or > 10% variation)	Sinus arrhythmia; atrial fibrillation; 2nd-degree heart block (Type I)
QRS complex—widened (> 0.12 sec)	PVC, right or left bundle branch block, ventricular fibrillation, hyperkalemia
QT interval—prolonged (> 0.45 sec)	MI, electrolyte imbalance, antiarrhythmics, tricyclic antidepressants
QT interval—shortened (< 0.30 sec)	Electrolyte imbalance, digoxin
ST segment—depressed (≥ 0.2 mV in chest leads)	Myocardial ischemia, acute MI, ventricular hypertrophy, conduction disturbances, hyperventilation, hypokalemia digoxin
ST segment—elevated (≥ 0.2 mV in chest leads)	Myocardial ischemia, acute MI, conduction disturbances, ventricular hypertrophy, hyperkalemia, digoxin
T wave—tall	Hyperkalemia, acute MI, conduction disturbances, ventricular hypertrophy
T wave—small, flattened, or inverted	Myocardial ischemia, hyperventilation, anxiety, left ventricular hypertrophy, digoxin, pericarditis, pulmonary embolism, conduction disturbances, electrolyte imbalances
U wave—prominent	Hypokalemia, hypomagnesemia, ischemia

In combination, tidal volume, rate, and minute volume affect the efficiency of ventilation and work of breathing. You typically obtain a patient's tidal volume and minute volume using a mechanical respirometer attached to a one-way valve, as described in Chapter 6.

A patient's vital capacity indicates how well the entire ventilatory apparatus works together, including lung and chest wall interaction *and* respiratory muscle function. You measure the slow vital capacity using either a mechanical respirometer or a bedside electronic spirometer. To obtain the slow vital capacity, you instruct the patient to inhale as deeply as possible (*deeper, deeper, deeper...*) and then exhale slowly and completely for as long as possible (*more, more, more...*) or until no volume increment is observed for at least 2 seconds. This procedure should be repeated at least two additional times to ensure maximum effort.

A patient's maximum inspiratory and expiratory pressures represent the strength of the inspiratory and expiratory muscles. You measure maximum inspiratory pressure (MIP) using an aneroid manometer, with the one-way valve configured to allow exhalation but not inspiration. With this setup, the patient will "buck down" toward RV on each successive breath, at which point a maximum inspiratory effort is ensured. Since this technique can cause extreme anxiety in alert patients, you should provide a careful and reassuring explanation. Measurement of maximum expiratory pressure (MEP) is also measured with an aneroid manometer but does not require the one-way valve setup.

Table 4-22 Bedside Ventilation Parameters

Measure (Abbreviation)	Definition	Approximate Adult Normal	Weaning Threshold
Tidal volume (VT)	Volume of gas inhaled or exhaled on each breath	5–7 mL/kg predicted body weight (PBW)	> 5 mL/kg
Rate (f)	Number of breaths inhaled or exhaled in one minute	12–20/min	< 30–35/min
Minute volume ($\dot{V}_E$)	Total volume of air exhaled per minute; equals breathing rate times tidal volume (f × VT)	5–10 L/min (depends on body size/metabolic rate)	> 4 L/min < 10 L/min
Vital capacity (VC)	Maximum volume of gas exhaled after a maximum inhalation (may be measured during either a slow or a forced exhalation)	70 mL/kg PBW	> 10–15 mL/kg
Maximum inspiratory pressure (MIP, NIF, P$_{I}$max)	Maximum pressure generated against airway occlusion at or near residual volume (RV) after successive inspiratory efforts for 15–25 sec	–80 to –120 cm H_2O	< –25 cm H_2O
Maximum expiratory pressure (MEP, PEmax)	Maximum pressure generated by forced exhalation against airway occlusion at or near total lung capacity (TLC)	> +150 cm H_2O	> +60 cm H_2O

In obtaining these measures, a few key points bear emphasis:

- To compute the tidal volume, count the rate of breathing over a one-minute collection interval and divide the minute volume by the breath frequency (i.e., VT = $\dot{V}_E$ ÷ f).
- Because mechanical respirometers can be damaged by high flows (> 60 L/min), they should not be used to measure *forced* vital capacity.
- The slow vital capacity and maximum expiratory pressure measurements require cooperation and thus *cannot be measured on unconscious patients.*

A typical example of the bedside measurement of these parameters is outlined in the accompanying box.

Measurements, Computations, and Interpretations

Measurements. You obtain the following measures on a 100-kg male patient during a spontaneous breathing trial for weaning from mechanical ventilation:

$\dot{V}_E$ = 11.4 liters

f (rate) = 38

(slow) VC = 800 mL

MIP = –18 cm H_2O

MEP = +35 cm H_2O

Computations. Your computations would be as follows:

VT = 11.4 ÷ 38 = 0.3 L, or 300 mL

VT (ml/kg) = 300/100 = 3 mL/kg

VC (mL/kg) = 800 ÷ 100 = 8 mL/kg

(continues)

Interpretation. Based on these data, the patient likely needs continued ventilatory support and cannot be weaned at this time. This conclusion is based on the following:

- The tidal volume is below the weaning threshold of 5 mL/kg
- The minute ventilation exceeds the high weaning threshold of 10 L/min
- The rate of breathing exceeds the threshold of 30–35 breaths/min
- The vital capacity is below the threshold of 10 mL/kg
- The MIP and MEP are below their threshold values

In combination, the low vital capacity and poor MIP indicate inadequate ventilatory reserves. The low MEP indicates inadequate expiratory muscle strength, needed for spontaneous coughing. Last, the high rate and low tidal volume together indicate a rapid, shallow breathing pattern that is likely causing both an increase in deadspace (wasted) ventilation as well as an increased work of breathing (see text for details).

A useful quantitative measure of rapid, shallow breathing is the *rapid shallow breathing index* (RSBI). You compute the RSBI by dividing the patient's rate of breathing by the average tidal volume in liters, i.e., RSBI = f ÷ V_T (L). For example, using the same data collected in the boxed example of a patient's spontaneous breathing trial, you would compute the RSBI as follows:

$$\text{RSBI} = f \div V_T \text{ (L)}$$
$$\text{RSBI} = 38 \div 0.3$$
$$\text{RSBI} \approx 127$$

In general, *an RSBI of less than 100 is a good predictor of a patient's ability to be weaned from mechanical ventilation.* In our example, the patient's RSBI is well above 100, indicating that the likelihood of successful weaning is poor at this time.

The reason a fast and shallow breathing tends to increase deadspace ventilation is evident in the formula for alveolar minute ventilation, *which is often tested on the CRT exam.* The alveolar minute ventilation is the volume of "fresh" gas (gas *not* mixed with expired carbon dioxide) reaching the alveoli per minute. To compute the alveolar minute ventilation, you simply multiply a patient's rate of breathing (f) times the difference between the tidal volume and the physiologic deadspace per breath:

$$\dot{V}_A = f(V_T - V_D)$$

Unless otherwise indicated, *you should assume a deadspace of about 1 mL per pound of predicted body weight.* Using the above formula and assuming a 125-lb. patient breathing at a rate of 15 breaths/min with a tidal volume of 400 mL, you would compute this patient's alveolar minute ventilation as follows:

$$\dot{V}_A = f(V_T - V_D)$$
$$\dot{V}_A = 15 \times (400 - 125) = 4125 \text{ mL}$$

In this case, about 69% of the patient's ventilation per minute is fresh gas (4125/6000), with the remaining 31% consisting of wasted or deadspace ventilation (6000 − 4125 = 1875 mL). Thirty percent deadspace ventilation (per breath or per minute) is considered about normal.

To demonstrate the effect that rapid shallow breathing would have on the amount of deadspace ventilation in this patient, let's double her rate of breathing but halve her tidal volume, keeping her minute ventilation constant at 6000 mL/min:

$$\dot{V}_E = 30 \times 200 \text{ mL} = 6000 \text{ mL/min}$$
$$\dot{V}_A = 30 \times (200 - 125) = 2250 \text{ mL}$$

Even though the patient's minute ventilation remains unchanged, the rapid shallow breathing pattern has doubled her deadspace ventilation per minute (6000 − 2250 = 3750 mL). Now only about 38% (2250/6000) of the patient's minute ventilation consists of fresh gas. Since the alveolar P_{CO_2} is directly proportional to the amount of deadspace ventilation, this patient's arterial P_{CO_2} will rise.

As a rule of thumb, *high rates and low tidal volumes result in the highest deadspace ventilation per minute, while low rates and high tidal volumes waste the least amount of ventilation per minute.*

Lung Mechanics and Ventilator Graphics

More sophisticated measures of ventilatory mechanics can be provided on patients being supported by critical care ventilators equipped with graphic displays. These measures include estimates of total compliance and airway resistance and plotting of pressure-volume and flow-volume loops during breathing. Details on these advanced monitoring tools are provided in Chapter 13.

Peak Expiratory Flow Rate (PEFR)

The peak expiratory flow rate (PEFR) is the maximum flow generated when a patient executes a forced expiration, and it is used as a basic test of airway obstruction. However, because the PEFR is a highly effort-dependent measure, it is not used for definitive diagnosis of pulmonary impairment but instead considered a supplemental monitoring tool. For this reason, you should measure a patient's PEFR only when necessary to:

- Monitor the effect of bronchodilator therapy (using pre- and post-test measures)
- Assess the severity of asthma symptoms
- Detect early changes in asthma control that require adjustments in treatment

Often the patient makes these measurements at home and records them in a log. Inspection of this log can help health professionals assess the pattern of a patient's symptoms and his or her response to therapy.

Performing

Typically, you measure a patient's PEFR with a peak flow meter and report the value in L/sec or L/min (BTPS). *To convert L/sec to L/min, multiply by 60; to convert L/min to L/sec, divide by 60.*

In order to make this measurement, the patient must be able to follow simple instructions and coordinate breathing with use of the metering device. Critical data needed for interpretation include the patient's height and weight. In addition, you should obtain the patient's smoking history and information on current medications, including bronchodilators and steroids. Key points in performing the procedure and ensuring valid data include the following:

- The meter should be set to zero before the test.
- The meter should be properly positioned (some devices are accurate only when held level).
- The patient ideally should stand up straight.
- The patient must inhale fully to total lung capacity (TLC).
- The mouthpiece should be inserted between the teeth, above the tongue.
- The patient should form a tight seal around the mouthpiece with the lips.
- The patient should exhale in a strong, sharp burst with maximum force (active coaching may be needed).
- Full exhalation is not needed unless the FVC is being measured at the same time.
- The measurement should be repeated until three values are obtained that vary by less than 10%
- Record the highest of the three values.

Interpreting

Normal values for PEFR are based on sex, age, and height. **Table 4-23** lists the common ranges of normals cited in the literature by patient age and sex. In general, low values for PEFR indicate an expiratory flow obstruction. However, because test results are so dependent on patient effort and starting lung volume, you should always consider the possibility of either poor effort ("malingering") or poor technique whenever the patient's value is significantly below the predicted normal.

Table 4-23 Normal Ranges for PEFR

Patient Category	Range of Normals	
	L/min	L/sec
Adult males	450–750 L/min	8–12 L/sec
Adult females	350–530 L/min	6–9 L/sec
Children (depends on height)	150–450 L/min	3–8 L/sec

When measuring peak flow before and after bronchodilator therapy, be sure to give the drug time to reach its full effect before taking the post-test measure, typically 20–30 minutes. Upon completing the post-test measure, you then compute the percent change from the baseline pre-test as follows:

$$\% \text{ change} = \frac{\text{Post} - \text{pre}}{\text{pre}} \times 100$$

where "post" is the patient's post-test/after bronchodilator peak flow and "pre" is the pre-test/before bronchodilator value for this measure.

For example, if a patient has a peak flow before use of a bronchodilator of 6.1 L/sec and a value of 7.5 L/sec after treatment, his % change would be:

$$\% \text{ change} = \frac{7.5 - 6.1}{6.1} \times 100$$

$$\% \text{ change} = 23\%$$

A change of 15–20% indicates a significant improvement in airway caliber. If you record lesser changes, you should recommend an increase in the dose or frequency of the prescribed bronchodilator.

When measuring peak flow to assess the severity of asthma symptoms, you need to compute the % predicted value for the patient. The formula for computing a patient's % predicted value for any pulmonary function parameter is as follows:

$$\% \text{ predicted} = \frac{\text{actual}}{\text{predicted}} \times 100$$

where "actual" is the patient's measured value and "predicted" is the normal value of that parameter for that specific patient (as determined by nomogram or equation).

Note that in asthma management we often substitute the patient's *personal best* value for the predicted value in computing the % predicted measure. A patient's personal best PEFR is the highest value achieved over a 2-week asymptomatic period.

For example, if a patient's personal best PEFR is 6.5 L/sec and her actual measured value is 4.0 L/sec, then her % predicted would be:

$$\% \text{ predicted} = \frac{4.0}{6.5} \times 100$$

$$\% \text{ predicted} = 62\%$$

As indicated in **Table 4-24**, when a patient presents to the emergency department with a history of asthma and corresponding symptoms, the % predicted PEFR can help determine the severity of the exacerbation and proper course of therapy.

Table 4-24 Severity and Recommended Therapy Associated with Declines in PEFR

% Predicted or % Personal Best	Relative Severity (Including Symptoms)	Recommended Therapy
> 80%	Mild	Short-acting beta-agonist (SABA) bronchodilator Vital sign monitoring
50–80%	Moderate	O_2 to keep saturation > 90% SABA Consider anticholinergic + oral steroids
< 50%	Severe	Admit to hospital O_2 to keep saturation > 90% SABA + anticholinergic + oral steroids Consider epinephrine Frequent vital sign monitoring

Bedside Spirometry

Bedside spirometry involves the measurement of the forced vital capacity and related measures (e.g., PEFR, FEV_t, FEF_{25-75}) at the bedside using a portable electronic spirometer. Chapter 6 provides details on the selection, use, and troubleshooting of bedside spirometers. Here we focus on performing and interpreting the results of bedside spirometry.

Performing

Like the measurement of peak flow, forced expiratory volume measurements depend on proper patient performance, as instructed and coached by the clinician. The accompanying box outlines a basic procedure designed to help ensure accurate and reproducible results.

Bedside Spirometry Procedure

1. Make sure your spirometer is turned on and insert new mouthpiece or sensor; some disposable sensors include individual calibration information that must be inputted or scanned into the computer module before testing

2. Be sure to input all requested patient data accurately, typically including age, sex, height, ethnicity, and smoking history

3. Remove candy, gum, and/or dentures from the patient's mouth and loosen any tight clothing

4. Patient may sit or stand, but be consistent and record the patient's position

5. Demonstrate the procedure using your own mouthpiece/sensor, being sure to show:

    a. How to hold the sensor steady/avoid jerky motions (can cause flow errors)

    b. How deeply to inhale

    c. How to correctly place the mouthpiece on top of the tongue

    d. How fast and long to exhale (at least 6 seconds)

6. Use nose clips to prevent patient leaks

7. Have the patient perform the maneuver while you carefully observe test performance:

    a. Ensure that the patient breathes in as deeply as possible (to full inspiratory capacity)

    b. Have the patient forcibly **blast** the breath out, as fast and as long as possible

    c. Loudly prompt **more, more, more** until the subject has exhaled **for at least 6 seconds** (patients with severe COPD may take up to 15 seconds to fully exhale)

    d. Carefully observe the patient for poor technique and correct as needed

8. Repeat the procedure until you have three acceptable maneuvers (may require 4–8 efforts)

9. Print and review the results

Interpreting and Applying the Results

Figure 4-4 outlines the basic process for interpreting the results of bedside spirometry. Because the results depend on proper patient performance, the first step is always to assess test validity, as described in Chapter 7. Assuming valid test results, you first compare the patient's FVC, FEV_1, and FEV_1% to the normal values for the patient being tested. The FVC and FEV_1 are considered normal (N) if the patient's values are at least 80% of the predicted values. A normal FEV_1% is 70% or more for all patients. As indicated in **Table 4-25**, by comparing these three values, you can immediately categorize the type of impairment present.

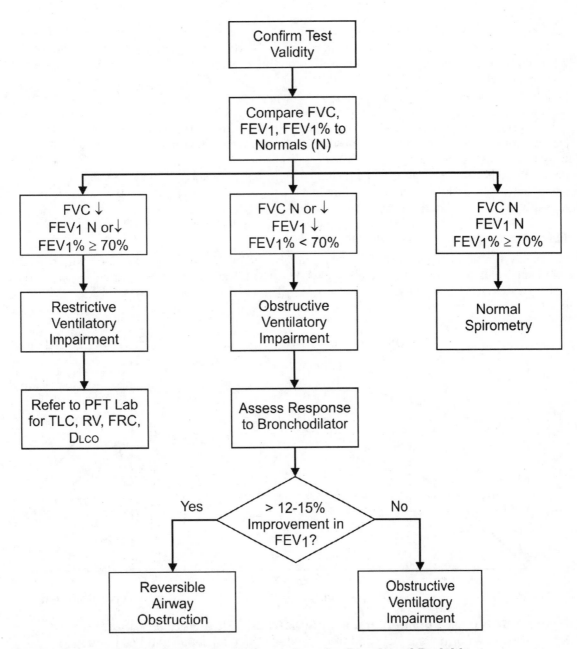

Figure 4-4 Basic Procedure for Interpreting the Results of Bedside or Ambulatory Spirometry.

Adapted from: Barreiro, T. J. & Perillo, I. (2004). An approach to interpreting spirometry. *American Family Physician, 69,* 1107–1114.

Table 4-25 Bedside Spirometry Categorization of Pulmonary Function Impairment

Parameter	Normal	Obstructive	Restrictive	Mixed
FVC (% predicted)	N	↓ or N	↓	↓
FEV$_1$ (% predicted)	N	↓	↓ or N	↓
FEV$_1$% (N ≥ 70%)	N	↓	↑ or N	↓

Notes: N = normal; ↓ = decreased; ↑ = increased. For obstructive impairments, judge severity by either % predicted FVC or FEV$_1$ as follows: 70–79% mild; 60–69% moderate; 50–59% moderately severe; 35–49% severe; and < 35% very severe.

Graphic analysis should always supplement numeric assessment. Depending on the spirometer used, the FVC graph may be volume vs. time or flow vs. volume. **Figure 4-5** compares the typical normal, obstructive, and restrictive patterns seen on these two types of spirograms.

If analysis indicates an obstructive ventilatory impairment, you should recommend assessing the patient's response to bronchodilator therapy, with repeat spirometry timed to correspond to the peak response time of the drug being used, usually after 20–30 minutes. If the patient's FEV$_1$ improves by at least 12–15% (and ≥ 200 mL in adults), then the obstruction is classified as reversible, as in asthma. Lesser improvement indicates that the obstruction is not reversible, as in most forms of COPD.

If analysis indicates a restrictive or mixed ventilatory impairment, you should recommend the patient undergo a full evaluation in the pulmonary function laboratory, to include static lung volumes and a diffusing capacity assessment. In combination, these tests will help differentiate among the various causes of restriction detected at the bedside.

Pulmonary Function Laboratory Studies

Pulmonary function laboratory studies include the same FVC measurements assessed with bedside spirometry, plus static lung volumes (TLC, FRC, VC, IC, ERV, and RV) and sometimes the lung's diffusing capacity.

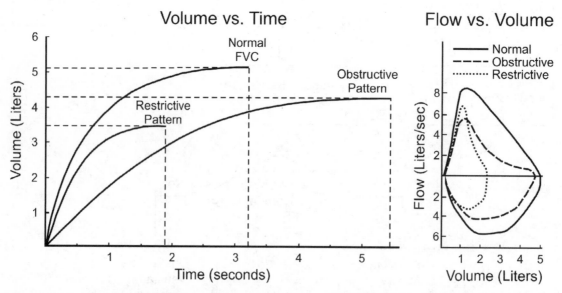

Figure 4-5 Typical Volume Versus Time (left) and Flow Versus Volume (right) Spirograms. A normal subject can forcibly exhale the vital capacity (FVC) in about 3 seconds while patients with obstructive conditions may require 6 or more seconds for complete exhalation. Patients with restrictive conditions typically have reduced expiratory volumes but may exhibit near normal expiratory flows. Their absolute FEV$_1$ values usually are below normal, but their FEV$_1$% may be normal or even high.

Performing

Static lung volumes and the DLCO are measured separately. The key static lung volume from which the others are derived is the functional residual capacity (FRC). If the FRC is known, both the RV and TLC are computed as follows:

$$RV = FRC - ERV$$
$$TLC = FRC + IC$$

Table 4-26 describes the three common methods used to measure FRC in pulmonary function laboratories. Note that whereas the helium dilution and nitrogen washout methods both measure the actual FRC (lung volume communicating with the airways), body plethysmography measures the total thorax gas volume (TGV). Normally the FRC and TGV are equal. A TGV that exceeds the FRC indicates the presence of "trapped" gas that is not in communication with the airways, as in seen in bullous emphysema.

The diffusing capacity of the lung (DLCO) is assessed by measuring the transfer of carbon monoxide from the lungs into the pulmonary capillaries. The *single breath* test is the most common procedure, key elements of which include the following:

- The patient performs an expiratory reserve volume maneuver, exhaling completely to RV.
- The patient inspires from RV to TLC a gas mixture of 21% O_2, 10% He, and 0.3% CO.
- The patient holds his or her breath for 10 seconds.
- The first portion of the patient's exhalation is discarded (to avoid the anatomical deadspace).
- Thereafter a sample of 0.5–1.0 L of expired gas is collected and analyzed for % He and % CO.
- The test is repeated after at least a 4-minute wait until results are within 5% or 3 mL/minute/mm Hg.
- Reported measures include the DLCO in mL/min/mm Hg (Hb and HbCO corrected), the alveolar volume (VA, an estimate of TLC), the ratio of DLCO to VA, and the inspiratory VC.

Prediction equations based on age, gender, height, and weight are used to compute normal values, with the "typical" normal single-breath DLCO ranging between 25 and 30 mL/minute/mm Hg. The DLCO is low in conditions that actually impair alveolar-capillary membrane diffusion (as in pulmonary fibrosis) or decrease surface area (as in emphysema). The DLCO can also be less than normal when Hb levels, pulmonary capillary blood flow, or alveolar volumes are reduced. Increases in DLCO occur with increased Hb (as in secondary polycythemia), pulmonary blood flow, and alveolar volume, and during exercise.

The severity of impairment in pulmonary diffusion capacity is judged against the patient's predicted normal, with values in the 60–80% range representing mild impairment, between 40% and 60% being a moderate abnormality, and less than 40% of normal indicating a severe problem.

Interpreting and Applying the Results

Once the results of the FVC, static lung volume, and diffusing capacity tests are known, the nature of the impairment can be determined systematically. **Figure 4-6** (see page 102) provides a basic algorithm for interpreting pulmonary lab test results based on just four measures: the FEV_1%, the (slow) vital capacity (VC), the total lung capacity (TLC), and the diffusing capacity (DLCO). You assess the FEV_1% first, followed by the VC, TLC, and then (if needed) the DLCO.

A less than normal FEV_1% indicates either an obstructive disorder or a mixed obstructive and restrictive disorder. For obstructive disorders, the DLCO differentiates between emphysema (low DLCO) and other forms of airway obstruction—such as asthma or chronic bronchitis—in which the DLCO is normal. To differentiate asthma from chronic bronchitis you should recommend a pre-/post-bronchodilator assessment or (in advanced labs) a methacholine challenge.

When you determine that the FEV_1% is at or above normal, the patient has either normal pulmonary function or a restrictive disorder. In these cases, look for a low TLC to identify a restrictive disorder. Again, the DLCO helps you differentiate between the two most common types of restrictive disorders, with a normal or high value suggesting a chest wall or neuromuscular problem and a low value consistent with interstitial lung diseases that limit diffusing capacity, such as pulmonary fibrosis.

Table 4-26 Comparison of Methods Used to Measure Functional Residual Capacity (FRC)

Method	Description	Key Points
Helium dilution (closed circuit method)	• At the end of a normal resting expiration (FRC), patient is connected to spirometer containing 5–10% He and then breathes normally • CO_2 is chemically absorbed by soda lime crystals • O_2 is added to keep the end-expiratory level constant (about 3.5 mL/kg/min or 0.25 L/min for the average patient) • Test continues until equilibration is achieved (i.e., % He constant [< 0.02% change] over a 2-minute period or after 10 minutes) • FRC calculated based on initial and final % He, the volume of He and O_2 added to the system, and the system deadspace	• Spirometer must be leak free and He analyzer properly calibrated • Some patients cannot maintain a good mouth seal or cooperate adequately for the time needed to complete the test • Perforated eardrums, tracheostomies, and transtracheal O_2 catheters will cause He leakage and invalidate test results • Test validity depends on proper starting point (i.e., end of a normal resting expiration) • After the FRC is obtained, the VC, IC, ERV, and IRV should be measured • Variation on repeat studies of 500 mL or more or obvious leaks during the test invalidate test results • FRC may be underestimated in individuals with air trapping • Hypercapnia and/or hypoxemia may occur if CO_2 is not adequately removed or if O_2 is not added to the system
Nitrogen washout (open circuit method)	• At the end of a normal resting expiration (FRC), patient is connected to a 100% O_2 reservoir • Expired N_2 and expired volume are measured continuously • Test continues for 7 minutes or until % N_2 falls below 1.0% (in patients with air trapping, the time period needs to be extended) • FRC computed based on total expired volume and final % N_2	• System must be leak free and N_2 analyzer properly calibrated • Some patients cannot maintain a good mouth seal or cooperate adequately for the time needed to complete the test • Ventilatory drive may be depressed in some patients who breathe 100% O_2 • Initial alveolar N_2 concentration of 80% can be assumed if patient has been breathing room air for at least 15 minutes • Test validity depends on proper starting point, i.e., end of a normal resting expiration • After the FRC is obtained, the VC, IC, ERV, and IRV should be measured • A minimum of 15 minutes should elapse before test is repeated • Variation on repeat studies of 500 mL or more, any obvious leaks during the procedure (as evidenced by an increase in expired % N_2) invalidate test results

(continues)

Table 4-26 Comparison of Methods Used to Measure Functional Residual Capacity (FRC) (continued)

Method	Description	Key Points
Body box (body plethysmography)	• Patient sits in closed chamber • Transducers measure chamber pressure, mouth pressure, and flow • A mouthpiece shutter occludes the airway at end-expiration • The patient "pants" against the closed shutter, alternately compressing and expanding the gas in the thorax *and* the chamber • Changes in chamber pressure due to thoracic volume changes are proportional to changes in alveolar gas pressure • Volume of gas in thorax is computed according to Boyle's law $(P_1V_1 = P_2V_2)$	• Careful calibration of multiple transducers is required • Measure total thoracic gas volume (TGV), which may differ from FRC • Usually measured together with airway resistance/conductance • Claustrophobic patients may not tolerate procedure • Test validity requires proper panting (as evidenced by "closed" P-V loops); patients should pant at a constant rate of about 1 cycle/sec and press their hands against their cheeks to avoid "bowing" • TGV should be averaged from a minimum of 3–5 separate, acceptable panting maneuvers • After the FRC is obtained, the VC, IC, ERV, and IRV should be measured • Overestimation of TGV can occur in patients who pant with their accessory muscles (compresses abdominal gas) or those with severe airway obstruction • Difference between TGV and FRC measured by He dilution or N_2 washout is due to gas volume that is not in communication with the airways (e.g., cysts or bullae, as in emphysema)

Blood Gases and Related Measures

Obtaining and interpreting arterial blood gas and arterialized capillary blood samples, as well as related noninvasive measures such as pulse oximetry, transcutaneous monitoring, and capnography, can be tested on this section of the CRT exam. However, most questions in these areas focus on the application of this information to patient care. For this reason, we cover these topics primarily in Chapter 13 (Evaluate and Monitor Patient's Objective and Subjective Responses to Respiratory Care).

Apnea Monitoring

Apnea monitoring is designed to warn caregivers of life-threatening respiratory and cardiac events, most often in neonates. Apnea monitors use two electrodes placed on the chest wall to detect respiratory movements via changes in electrical impedance, with most units also able to detect heart rate via the ECG signal. On bedside monitors, impedance changes are displayed as a continuous waveform that is equivalent to the cycle of chest wall motion, with the respiratory rate also provided. Although you can use the displays and alarms on these systems to warn of adverse events, you should always confirm a patient's status by visual inspection at the bedside.

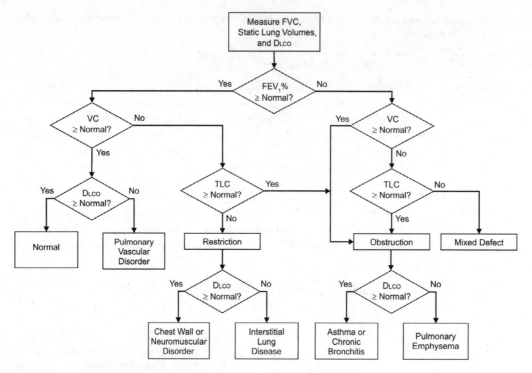

Figure 4-6 Interpretation of Pulmonary Lab Test Results.

Less than normal is < 70% for the FEV₁%, and < 80% predicted for the VC, TLC, and DLCO.

Adapted from: Pellegrino, R., Viegi, G., Brusasco, V. et al. (2005). Interpretative strategies for lung function tests. *European Respiratory Journal, 26,* 948–968.

Apnea monitoring is indicated in neonates at risk for recurrent apnea, bradycardia, and hypoxemia. This procedure may also be considered for infants:

- Receiving drug therapy (e.g., caffeine) for a history of apnea and bradycardia
- With bronchopulmonary dysplasia, especially those requiring supplemental oxygen
- With symptomatic gastroesophageal reflux (GER)
- Born to a substance-abusing mother if clinically symptomatic
- With a trach or an airway abnormality that increases the risk of obstruction
- With neurologic or metabolic disorders affecting respiratory control

Older children and adults may also require apnea monitoring, especially those with conditions affecting the control of breathing. Because impedance changes measure only chest wall movement and not air flow, simple apnea monitoring cannot detect airway obstruction and thus should *not* be used to assess patients for obstructive sleep apnea–hypopnea syndrome (SAHS). Patients suspected of obstructive sleep apnea should undergo overnight oximetry and/or laboratory polysomnography.

Performing

Key points in performing apnea monitoring include the following:

- Set the low/high heart rate alarm limits (typically 80–220 for infants).
- Set the apnea time alarm limit (typically 20 seconds).
- For event recording:
  - Clear memory and set the desired option for waveform recording
  - Set the event log limits for low/high heart rate and apnea time
- Secure the electrodes on the right and left side of the chest, midway between the nipple line and the midaxillary line where the greatest chest motion is occurring.
- Connect the patient cable, turn the monitor on, and confirm a successful system check.
- Confirm that the monitor signals match the patient's heart and respiratory rate.

Interpreting

You can use an apnea monitor's event recording (chest motion, heart rate trend, ECG) to identify the following conditions:

Apnea	The cessation of respiratory air flow. The respiratory pause may be central (no respiratory effort), obstructive, or mixed. Short (< 10 sec) periods of central apnea can be normal for all ages.
Pathologic apnea	Apnea occurring for longer than 20 seconds or associated with cyanosis, abrupt marked pallor, hypotonia, or bradycardia (< 80–100 beats/min in neonates).
Periodic breathing	A breathing pattern characterized by three or more respiratory pauses > 3 seconds duration with < 20 seconds of respiration between pauses. Periodic breathing is not associated with cyanosis or changes in heart rate and can be a normal event.

To differentiate among the various causes for altered respiratory rate, you compare the apnea monitor's impedance signal to the heat rate, as summarized in **Table 4-27**. Note that apnea monitoring cannot identify the cause of apnea (central vs. obstructive) nor by itself identify related symptoms (e.g., cyanosis, abrupt marked pallor, hypotonia, choking, or gagging).

Overnight Pulse Oximetry

Overnight or *nocturnal* oximetry uses a recording pulse oximeter to record changes in SpO_2 and heart rate while the patient is sleeping. Overnight oximetry can help identify patients with obstructive SAHS and assess their response to therapy. In addition, overnight oximetry can determine whether serious desaturation occurs in certain COPD patients during sleep.

Performing

Key points in performing overnight oximetry include the following:

- Set up and verify equipment operation:
  - Set the device to TREND monitoring and select the planned period (e.g., 8 hrs).
  - If settable, adjust the capture rate to the shortest allowable (usually 2–6 sec).
  - Confirm that there is sufficient memory to capture the data for the planned period.
  - If needed, turn LOW alarm off and begin trend monitoring.
- Instruct and prepare the patient (remove artificial fingernails and nail polish).
- Attach sensor and begin recording.
- Return in the morning to gather the data.
- If conducted in the home:
  - Provide simple step-by-step written instructions for the patient and family.
  - Demonstrate proper setup and operation of the equipment on the patient.
  - Require a return demonstration to verify its proper use.
  - Provide a phone number where the patient can get help.

Table 4-27 Interpretation of Apnea Monitoring Signals

Respirations	Heart Rate	Likely Significance
Absent	Decreased	Pathologic apnea
Decreased	Increased	Hypoxemia[a]
Decreased/irregular	Unchanged	Periodic breathing
Increased	Increased	Motion/activity artifact
a. Confirmed via simultaneous pulse oximetry.		

Once the data have been gathered, you must transfer them to a computer for permanent storage and analysis. This is normally done by connecting the oximeter to the computer's serial communication data port (RS 232 or USB) and running the applicable data acquisition software.

Interpreting

Figure 4-7 provides a 5-hour segment of a typical overnight oximetry trend graph for a patient being assessed for SAHS. The graph includes both the SpO_2 and the pulse rate, as well as marks indicating potential periods of motion artifact (to help eliminate false-positive desaturations). This graph shows several major periods of desaturation, visible as "valleys" in the SpO_2 trend, associated with increases in the heart rate. *A desaturation event occurs when the SpO_2 drops by 4% or more.* The average number of desaturation events per hour of sleep is defined as the *oxygen desaturation index* (ODI). Oximetry software typically reports the total number of desaturation events and the ODI, along with the percentage of time that the SpO_2 was below a given percentage, most commonly 90%.

In general, an ODI of 15 or more desaturation events/hour indicates the presence of SAHS. In these cases, a follow-up polysomnography exam is not needed to confirm the diagnosis or begin therapy, except as may be required to titrate CPAP treatment (described subsequently). Patients suspected of sleep-disordered breathing who exhibit fewer than 15 desaturation events per hour should undergo full laboratory polysomnography to diagnose SAHS and help determine its cause.

In COPD patients, falls in arterial O_2 saturation may occur in the absence of apnea, hypopnea, or heavy snoring. For this reason, the ODI is not as useful in assessing COPD patients' nocturnal desaturation. Instead, Medicare allows nocturnal oxygen therapy if:

1. Nocturnal oximetry demonstrates a drop in SpO_2 below 88% or greater than 5%
2. The patient has signs or symptoms of hypoxemia (e.g., impaired cognitive process, insomnia)

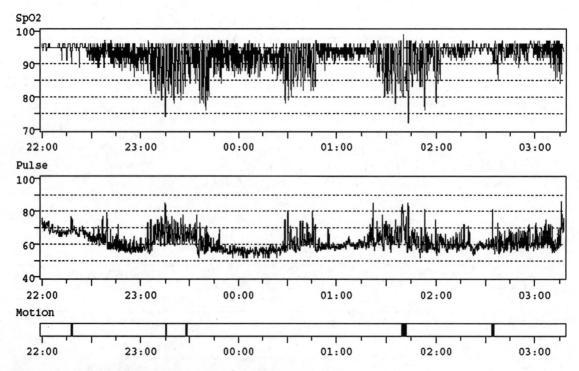

Figure 4-7 Overnight Oximetry Trend Graph.

Source: Courtesy of Sleep Solutions, Inc. Glen Burnie, MD.

These criteria are essentially the same as for continuous long-term oxygen therapy (LTOT) in COPD ($SaO_2 \leq 88\%$ or $PaO_2 \leq 55$ torr on room air). When documented nocturnal desaturation is associated with complications such as pulmonary hypertension, daytime somnolence, and cardiac arrhythmias, it is best to consider continuous O_2 therapy, as opposed to just supplemental O_2 at night. For those already certified for continuous LTOT who also exhibit nocturnal desaturation, the liter flow can be titrated upward in 1-L/min increments until the nighttime SpO_2 consistently exceeds 88% and no further desaturation events occur.

Titration of CPAP or BiPAP During Sleep

Once a patient is diagnosed with SAHS, most physicians will order a continuous positive airway pressure (CPAP)/bilevel positive airway pressure (BiPAP™) titration study to assess the effectiveness of this therapy and tailor its level to the patient's needs. Titration studies can be manually conducted via laboratory polysomnography or using an unattended auto-CPAP system.

Manual Titration of CPAP or BiPAP

Typically, a manual CPAP/BiPAP™ titration is indicated after either a full night or a 3-hour polysomnography study confirms the diagnosis of SAHS, normally based on documenting an apnea-hypopnea index (AHI) of fewer than 15 events/hr (see **Table 4-28** for pertinent sleep study event definitions). If the 3-hour polysomnography exam is used for diagnosis, the remainder of the night is used to conduct the CPAP/BiPAP™ titration, a procedure called a *split-night study*.

Regardless of the approach taken, you should ensure that all patients undergoing CPAP/BiPAP™ titration should first receive appropriate instructions (with demonstration), be carefully fitted with a comfortable mask, and be given the time needed to get use to the device. Once this is accomplished, the basic titration procedure commences as follows:

- Start CPAP at 4 cm H_2O (a higher pressure can be used if the patient complains of "not getting enough air" or cannot fall asleep).
- Maintain each CPAP pressure level for an observation interval of at least 5 minutes.
- If *any* of the following events occur during the observation interval, increase the CPAP level by at least 1 cm H_2O:
  - ≥ 2 obstructive apneas
  - ≥ 3 hypopneas
  - ≥ 5 respiratory effort–related arousals (RERAs)
  - ≥ 3 min of loud snoring
- Continue increasing the CPAP level until the obstructive events are abolished or controlled, or until you reach the maximum CPAP level of 20 cm H_2O.

Table 4-28 Definitions Related to Sleep Studies

Term	Definition
Obstructive apnea	A cessation of airflow for at least 10 seconds during which there is continued effort to breathe
Central apnea	A cessation of airflow for at least 10 seconds during which there is *no* effort to breathe
Hypopnea	A reduction in air flow of at least 30% from baseline lasting at least 10 seconds and associated with significant oxygen desaturation (> 3–4%)
Respiratory-effort related arousal (RERA)	A sequence of breaths with increasing respiratory effort leading to an arousal from sleep
Apnea-hypopnea index (AHI)	The average number of apneas and hypopneas occurring per hour of sleep
Respiratory disturbance index (RDI)	The average number of apneas, hypopneas, and RERAs occurring per hour of sleep

- Quantify the level of control obtained with CPAP using the respiratory disturbance index (RDI), which equals the total number of apneas, hypopneas, and RERAs occurring per hour of sleep.
- Base your determination of the degree of control at the selected pressure on an observation interval of at least 15 minutes, which should include a period of rapid eye movement (REM) sleep in the supine position. Consider control:
  ○ *Optimal* when the titrated CPAP level reduces the RDI to less than 5 and REM sleep is not continually interrupted by spontaneous arousals
  ○ *Good* when the titrated CPAP level reduces the RDI to 10 or less (or by 50% if the baseline RDI was less than 15) and REM sleep is not continually interrupted by arousals
  ○ *Adequate* when at the titrated CPAP level the RDI remains above 10 but is reduced 75% from baseline and REM sleep is not continually interrupted by spontaneous arousals
- If (1) the patient cannot tolerate high CPAP pressures, (2) there are continued obstructive respiratory events at higher levels of CPAP (> 15 cm H_2O), or (3) the patient exhibits periods of central sleep apnea during titration, consider a trial of BiPAP™:
  ○ Start at EPAP = 4 cm H_2O and IPAP = 8 cm H_2O
  ○ Recommended minimum IPAP-EPAP differential = 4 cm H_2O
  ○ Recommended maximum IPAP-EPAP differential = 10 cm H_2O
  ○ Recommended maximum IPAP = 30 cm H_2O
  ○ Raise EPAP to abolish obstructive events
  ○ Raise IPAP to abolish hypopnea and snoring
  ○ If events persist at maximum tolerated IPAP, increase EPAP in 1-cm H_2O increments

Auto-CPAP

Some modern CPAP units incorporate a mode in which the CPAP pressure is automatically optimized to abolish or control obstructive events. Typically these units monitor pressure, flow, and system leaks using a pneumotachograph and pressure transducer (see Chapter 6). Using this input data, a computer algorithm identifies the nature of the event and adjusts the pressure accordingly. For example, the algorithm may identify apnea as an 80% reduction in flow lasting at least 10 seconds. Based on a defined number of repeat occurrences of this event, the device will begin a programmed step-up in CPAP pressure until the problem resolves or the preset maximum pressure is reached. **Figure 4-8** provides a trend graph of CPAP pressure and obstructive events over a 7-hour period that demonstrates how auto-CPAP functions.

Although current evidence suggests that auto-CPAP titration is as good as that done with polysomnography, the American Academy of Sleep Medicine (AASM) specifies several limitations and cautions regarding the use of these devices. Current AASM recommendations are as follows:

- Auto-CPAP devices should not be used to diagnose obstructive sleep apnea.
- Auto-CPAP devices may be used during polysomnography to identify the optimum pressure.
- Auto-CPAP devices should not be used therapeutically on patients having significant comorbidities, such as:
  ○ Congestive heart failure
  ○ COPD
  ○ Central sleep apnea
  ○ Hypoventilation syndromes
- Patients being treated with auto-CPAP must be followed up closely to assess treatment effectiveness and safety.
- Reevaluation and a standard attended CPAP titration should be performed if the symptoms of a patient receiving auto-CPAP do not resolve or the treatment otherwise appears ineffective.

6-Minute Walk Test

The 6-minute walk test (6MWT) measures the distance in meters that a patient can quickly walk on a flat surface in 6 minutes. It evaluates how well the body as a whole responds to exertion and is used to determine overall functional capacity or changes in capacity due to therapy in patients with moderate to severe heart or lung disease. **Table 4-29** summarizes the indications for the 6MWT.

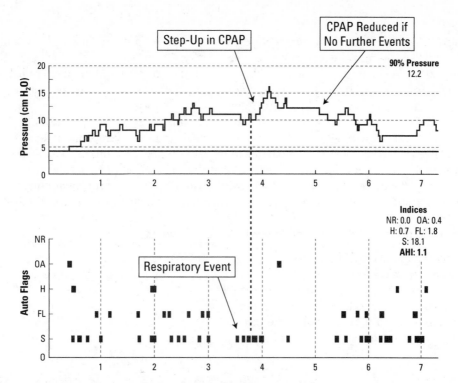

Figure 4-8 Trend Graph of Auto-CPAP (REMstar Auto). The occurrence of a respiratory event (snoring) 4 hours into sleep triggers a programmed step-up in CPAP pressure until the problem resolves, at which point the pressure is incrementally reduced if no additional events occur.

Abbreviations: NR: Nonresponsive Apnea/Hypopnea; OA: Obstructive Apnea; H: Hypopnea; FL: Flow Limitation; S: Snore; AHI: Apnea/Hypopnea Index (which is the sum of OA + H).
Source: Graph courtesy of Philips Respironics, Murrysville, PA.

The 6MWT should *not* be performed on patients who have either had a myocardial infarction or experienced unstable angina during the month prior to the test. Relative contraindications include (1) a resting heart rate greater than 120 beats/min, (2) a systolic blood pressure greater than 180 mm Hg, or a diastolic blood pressure greater than 100 mm Hg.

In terms of limitations, the 6MWT does not measure maximum oxygen uptake nor help identify either the cause of dyspnea or the factors limiting a patient's exercise tolerance. If such information is needed, you should recommend a comprehensive cardiopulmonary exercise test.

Table 4-29 Indications for the 6-Minute Walk Test (6MWT)

Functional Status (Single Measurement)	Pre- and Post-Treatment Comparisons
COPD	Lung transplantation
Cystic fibrosis	Lung resection
Heart failure	Lung volume reduction surgery
Peripheral vascular disease	Pulmonary rehabilitation
Fibromyalgia	COPD
Effects of aging	Pulmonary hypertension
	Heart failure

Performing

To maximize reliability of the 6MWT results, the ATS has developed a standardized protocol that health professionals should follow. The first consideration is the walking course itself, which must be 30 meters (about 100 ft.) in length. If conducted in the hospital, the course should have minimal traffic, no stairwell/elevator exits, and both a clearly set starting line and a turnaround point, with the distance between them marked carefully in 3-meter increments.

In terms of equipment, you will need a countdown timer or stopwatch, a movable chair, and a recording worksheet. **Figure 4-9** provides a 6MWT worksheet like that recommended by the ATS.

You will also need a sphygmomanometer to measure blood pressure, as well as a visual Borg Scale to assess the patient's dyspnea and level of exertion. If used, a pulse oximeter must be lightweight and not have to be held by the patient while walking. Last, for potential emergencies, you must also have immediate access to a source of oxygen, an automated electronic defibrillator (AED), and a telephone.

To prepare for the 6MWT, patients should do the following:

- Wear comfortable clothing
- Wear appropriate shoes for walking
- Use their usual walking aids (e.g., cane, walker)
- Follow their usual medical regimen
- Eat a light meal (if desired) before the test
- Avoid vigorous exercise for 2 hours prior to the test

6-Minute Walk Test			Walk #:		Date:										
Patient Name:			**Patient ID:**					**Gender:** M F							
Race/ Ethnicity:			**Height (cm):**		**Weight (kg):**			**Blood Pressure:**							
Medications taken before the test (dose and time):															
Supplemental O$_2$ during the test?				No	Yes	Flow L/min:			Device:						
Lap counter	1	2	3	4	5	6	7	8	9	10	11	12	13	14	15
					Start/Baseline					**End of Test**					
Time															
Heart Rate															
SpO$_2$															
Dyspnea (Borg Scale)															
Fatigue (Borg Scale)															
Stopped or paused before 6 minutes?				Yes	No	Reason:									
Other symptoms at end of exercise:		☐ Angina ☐ Dizziness		☐ Hip or leg pain ☐ Diaphoresis		☐ Ashen appearance ☐ Other:									
Number of laps:		x 60 m/lap	+ partial lap of		m	=		Total distance (6MWD)							
Predicted 6MWD:			m	% Predicted (actual/predicted)				%							
Comments:															
Interpretation:															
Test Administrator (Name):				**Signature:**											

Figure 4-9 Recording and Documentation Form for the 6-Minute Walk Test as Recommended by the American Thoracic Society.

Adapted from: American Thoracic Society. (2002). ATS statement. Guidelines for the six-minute walk test. *American Journal of Respiratory and Critical Care Medicine, 166,* 111–117.

If the patient has had a recent resting ECG, the results should be reviewed by a physician before the 6MWT. For patients with a history of stable angina on exercise, make sure they take their angina medication before the test and have rescue nitrates available. For patients on supplemental O_2, it should be provided at the prescribed rate using the same portable system normally used.

According to the American Thoracic Society, a "warmup" period or practice walk before the actual test is not necessary. Instead, the ATS recommends you carefully implement a standard test protocol, as outlined in the accompanying box.

American Thoracic Society 6-Minute Walk Protocol

1. Have the patient sit at rest for at least 10 minutes before the test starts

2. Assemble all equipment (lap counter, timer/stopwatch, Borg Scale, recording worksheet)

3. With the patient at rest, gather the needed demographic data and measure/record the vital signs

4. If Spo_2 is to be monitored, record the baseline value

5. Have the patient stand and rate his or her baseline dyspnea and exertion levels using the Borg Scale

6. Move to the starting point and set the timer/stopwatch to zero

7. Position the patient at the starting line and provide the ATS-recommended demonstration and instructions (see the source document for details)

8. Start the timer as soon as the patient starts to walk

9. Do not walk with the patient and remain at the starting line while you watch the patient and carefully tally and record the completed laps (1 lap = down and back to the starting line)

10. At the completion of each lap, make sure the patient sees you tallying the lap by exaggerating your body action (like using a stopwatch at a race)

11. At the end of each minute, provide encouragement to the patient and specify the remaining available time

12. After exactly 6 minutes, firmly say "Stop!" and then walk to the patient and use a bean bag or piece of tape to mark the stop point on the floor—if the patient appears exhausted, provide a chair for sitting

13. Repeat the Borg Scale assessment of dyspnea and exertion levels, being sure to remind the patient of their prior ratings; in addition, ask: "What, if anything, kept you from walking farther?"

14. If using a pulse oximeter, record the end-of-walk Spo_2 and pulse rate from the oximeter and then remove the sensor

15. Record the number of laps and additional distance covered in the final partial lap, if any

16. Calculate and record the total distance walked, rounding to the nearest meter

17. Congratulate the patient on good effort

Source: American Thoracic Society. (2002). ATS statement. Guidelines for the six-minute walk test. *American Journal of Respiratory and Critical Care Medicine, 166*, 111–117.

You should immediately stop a 6MWT if the patient develops chest pain, intolerable dyspnea, leg cramps, staggering, diaphoresis, or a pale or ashen appearance. In these cases, sit the patient in the chair, retake the vital signs, administer O_2 as appropriate, and arrange for a physician assessment. Once you are sure the patient is stable, record the time stopped, distance walked, and the reason the patient could not continue.

Interpreting

The outcome measure for the 6MWT is the 6-minute walking distance, or 6MWD. Prediction equations for the 6MWD have been developed but are not very useful in assessing those with moderate to severe heart or lung disease. In general, a 6MWD that is less than 500–600 meters provides a useful preliminary screening threshold for identifying an abnormal functional capacity. However, a low 6MWD is not diagnostic of any specific condition. In patients who exhibit a low 6MWD, further pulmonary and cardiac function tests are needed to identify the cause of the impairment. If you are using the 6MWT to assess medical or surgical interventions, you should expect at least a 10–20% *improvement* in the 6MWD to consider the treatment effective.

Cardiopulmonary Exercise Testing

Cardiopulmonary exercise testing involves analysis of gas exchange and cardiac function at rest and during incremental levels of exercise on a treadmill or bicycle ergometer. Parameters directly measured typically include tidal volume, respiratory rate, SpO_2, O_2 consumption, CO_2 production, blood pressure, heart rate, 12-lead ECG, and patient workload. If precise assessment of arterial oxygen saturation and/or blood lactic levels is required, blood samples may be obtained and analyzed during the procedure.

Cardiopulmonary exercise testing is specifically indicated to:

- Detect or assess the prognosis of coronary artery disease (CAD)
- Differentiate cardiac versus pulmonary limitations to increased work capacity
- Evaluate exercise capacity in patients being considered for heart transplantation
- Evaluate a patient's response to therapy intended to increase exercise tolerance
- Determine the intensity of exercise training in rehabilitation programs
- Detect the presence of exercise-induced bronchospasm or its response to therapy
- Determine the degree of hypoxemia or desaturation that can occur with exercise
- Assess cardiopulmonary fitness in disability evaluations

According to the American College of Cardiology, absolute contraindications against cardiopulmonary exercise testing include the following:

- Acute myocardial infarction (within 2 days)
- Uncontrolled heart failure
- Unstable angina
- Uncontrolled cardiac arrhythmias
- Severe aortic stenosis
- Acute pulmonary embolus or infarction
- Acute myocarditis or pericarditis
- Acute aortic dissection

Relative contraindications against cardiopulmonary exercise testing include electrolyte abnormalities, severe hypertension, and any mental or physical impairment that prevents adequate test performance, including uncooperativeness.

Performing

Cardiopulmonary exercise testing normally is performed under physician supervision in a cardiac or exercise physiology lab. Ideally, patients should previously have had a pulmonary function workup.

Your role may involve equipment setup; patient preparation, assessment, and monitoring; and sampling and analysis of arterial blood. In terms of equipment, in addition to the treadmill or bicycle ergometer, you need to obtain, assemble, and confirm proper operation of the following devices:

- Pneumotachometer
- Patient interface (nonrebreathing valve with mouthpiece or mask)
- Metabolic cart (O_2 + CO_2 analyzer)
- 12-lead ECG machine
- Pulse oximeter
- ABG sampling and analysis equipment
- Sphygmomanometer

Also, a fully stocked crash cart with a defibrillator, cardiac drugs, O_2, and suction and airway equipment must be in the testing area, with all staff involved trained in advanced life support.

In most cases, patients scheduled for an exercise test should be told to take their regular medications and avoid strenuous activity the day of the test. In addition, you should instruct patients to avoid caffeine, smoking, or eating for at least 2 hours prior to the test and to wear loose, comfortable clothing and non-slip footwear suitable for walking, such as sneakers.

In terms of assessment and monitoring during cardiopulmonary exercise testing, you may be involved in measuring common ventilatory parameters; inspired and expired O_2 and CO_2 concentrations; heart rate, blood pressure, blood gas, and lactate levels; and patient symptoms.

If blood analysis is indicated, you normally obtain a sample at rest and then at peak exercise, but you may sometimes need to draw specimens at each step in the protocol. Samples can be obtained via arterial puncture or an indwelling cannula. If you have difficulty drawing blood at the peak exercise level, a sample obtained within 10–15 seconds after the end of the test is satisfactory. Pulse oximetry should be used primarily to warn of gross desaturation during testing ($SpO_2 < 88\%$) or to help titrate supplemental O_2 during the procedure.

If you are asked to assess the patient's perceived level of exertion, you should use the Borg Scale (Table 4-13). Typically this assessment is conducted at the end of each step in the test procedure.

The most common type of cardiopulmonary exercise evaluation is the incremental work rate test. Although the basic steps can vary, they usually include those outlined in the accompanying box.

Basic Incremental Cardiopulmonary Exercise Test Procedure

1. Obtain appropriate medical and medication history and PFT results

2. Measure the patient's height and weight

3. Place and secure the ECG leads (a net vest may be needed to minimize motion artifact)

4. Obtain a baseline resting 12-lead ECG

5. Select a good site for and place and secure the pulse oximetry probe

6. Tape a sphygmomanometer cuff in place and obtain a baseline blood pressure

7. If ordered, obtain a baseline arterial blood sample (ABG/lactate level)

8. Instruct the patient in the operation of the treadmill or cycle ergometer

9. Familiarize the patient with the breathing interface and confirm proper, leak-free fit

10. Have the patient breathe through the system at rest for 2–3 minutes, until stable

11. Provide 2–3 minutes of unloaded warmup activity, e.g., 1–2 mph, 0% grade on treadmill

12. Apply the prescribed protocol to increment patient workload

13. Measure blood pressure, heart rate, SpO_2, Borg exertion rating, and symptoms (if any) toward the end of each graded interval

14. End test when:

    a. Vo_{2max} or maximum steady-state heart rate achieved (stop at end of that stage)

    b. The patient cannot continue due to exhaustion

    c. An abnormal or hazardous response occurs

15. If ordered, obtain an arterial blood sample at or immediately following test cessation

16. Provide 2–3 minutes of unloaded cool-down activity, e.g., 1–2 mph, 0% grade

17. Continue to monitor blood pressure and heart rate until they return to baseline

18. Have the patient stop activity

19. If assessing for exercise-induced bronchospasm, immediately obtain spirometry measures

---

In terms of incrementing patient workload, there are several different bicycle and treadmill protocols used, with the most common increasing exercise intensity by 1–2 *metabolic equivalents* (METs) at each stage. A MET is an objective measure of workload representing one's resting oxygen consumption per minute (Vo_2), equal to 3.5 mL/kg of body weight.

The normal end of the procedure occurs when the patient cannot continue due to exhaustion and asks to stop. According to the American Heart Association, abnormal or hazardous patient responses that justify terminating an exercise test include the following:

- A drop in systolic blood pressure greater than 10 mm Hg from baseline when accompanied by other evidence of ischemia such as ECG changes
- A hypertensive response (systolic blood pressure > 250 mm Hg and/or diastolic > 115 mm Hg)
- Moderate to severe angina
- Increasing nervous system symptoms such as ataxia, dizziness, or near-syncope
- Signs of poor perfusion, such as cyanosis or pallor
- Sustained ventricular tachycardia or other serious arrhythmias
- Major ST segment changes
- Severe wheezing or dyspnea

Interpreting

CRT exam questions on exercise test interpretation likely will focus on identifying the primary factors limiting a patient's exercise tolerance.

The gold standard for assessing overall exercise capacity is the maximum uptake of oxygen per minute (VO_{2max}). In general, if patients can attain their predicted VO_{2max} and a heat rate at or near their normal maximum (HRmax) at peak exercise capacity, the study results are considered normal. Typically, these patients will also be able to increase their ventilation in proportion to metabolic demands and maintain normal arterial oxygen saturations at their peak exercise levels.

The primary indicator of an abnormal cardiopulmonary exercise test is a low VO_{2max}. As a rule of thumb, a VO_{2max} less than 15 mL/kg or the patient's inability to achieve at least 5 METs during maximum exercise represents poor exercise capacity.

Poor exercise capacity can be due to poor physical conditioning or an abnormal disease state, typically either a cardiovascular or a pulmonary disorder. To determine which of these is the primary factor limiting exercise capacity requires more information. The key measures needed to identify the cause of poor exercise capacity are summarized in **Table 4-30**.

Low exercise capacity due to *poor conditioning* is associated with a low VO_{2max} but a normal anaerobic threshold (> 40% of the VO_{2max}). These patients generally also exhibit a greater than normal heat rate at their peak exercise capacity.

Patients in whom a *cardiovascular disorder is the primary limiting factor for exercise* have a reduced *anaerobic threshold* and a higher than predicted heart rate at peak exercise capacity. In addition, these patients are distinguished by a *low O_2 pulse*. The O_2 pulse is the product of the heart's stroke volume and the arterial-venous O_2 content difference, or $C(a-v)O_2$. The reduced O_2 pulse in those with cardiovascular disease is due primarily to their inability to augment stoke volume in proportion to increased exercise demands.

Patients in whom a *pulmonary disorder is the primary limiting factor for exercise* may be able to increase cardiac stoke volume during exertion. However, these patients usually cannot increase their ventilatory capacity sufficiently to meet their exercise demands. This ventilatory limitation to exercise often makes it impossible for the patient even to reach his or her anaerobic threshold.

This limitation is most evident in the measure called *breathing reserve*. Breathing reserve represents the difference between one's maximum voluntary ventilation (MVV) and the maximum ventilation achieved at peak exercise capacity ($\dot{V}E_{max}$). For comparison between patients, the breathing reserve is computed as a proportion or percentage using the following formula:

$$\textbf{Breathing reserve} = [1 - (\dot{V}E_{max}/MVV)]$$

If the patient's MVV was not measured, you can estimate it from the FEV_1 as follows:

$$MVV \approx FEV_1 \times 40$$

Normal individuals have a breathing reserve of at least 30%, meaning that at peak exercise they are using only about two-thirds or less of their MVV to meet their metabolic demands. Patients with

Table 4-30 Key Parameters Associated with Exercise Limitation

Measurement	Definition	Normal Values at Peak Exercise Capacity	Poor Conditioning	Cardiovascular Disorders	Pulmonary Disorders
VO_{2max}	Maximum uptake of oxygen at peak exercise capacity	Men: 35–90 mL/kg/min Women: 25–75 mL/kg/min	↓	↓	↓
Anaerobic threshold	Exercise intensity beyond which progressive increases in blood lactate occur	> 40% VO_{2max}	N	↓	N
HRmax	Maximum heart rate at peak exercise capacity	220 – age	↑	↑	↓
Breathing reserve	Proportion of MVV that is unused after reaching maximum minute ventilation at peak exercise	> 30%	N	N	↓
Spo_2	O_2 saturation (pulse oximetry)	> 88%	N	N	May ↓
O_2 pulse	Oxygen consumption per heart beat at peak exercise capacity	Men: > 12 mL/beat Women: > 8 mL/beat	N	↓	N

Abbreviations: VO_2, oxygen consumption; HR, heart rate; MVV, maximum voluntary ventilation

Symbols: N, Normal; ↑, increased; ↓, decreased

pulmonary disorders that limit exercise typically exhibit breathing reserves less than 30%. In addition, these patients also may exhibit a reduced Sao_2 during exercise. This occurs most often in those with advanced COPD and interstitial lung diseases who have marginal blood oxygenation at rest. **Figure 4-10** summarizes the uses of these measures to differentiate among the conditions limiting exercise capacity.

If the test is being done to detect exercise-induced asthma, look for a 20% drop in FEV_1 post-exercise. If the test is being conducted to justify participation in a pulmonary rehabilitation program, the patient's VO_{2max} should be less than 75% of predicted, with a breathing reserve less than 30%. When the test is performed to evaluate a patient's response to therapy, there is no need to repeat the full incremental test each time. Instead, subsequent tests can be conducted at a fixed submaximal level, typically 50–70% of the rate achieved when performing the maximum workload procedure.

Oxygen Titration with Exercise

According to the American Association for Respiratory Care (AARC), O_2 titration with exercise is indicated to:

- Assess the adequacy of arterial oxygenation during exercise in patients who are clinically suspected of desaturation, especially those with pulmonary disease who complain of dyspnea on exertion or have a decreased D_{LCO} and/or low Pao_2 at rest
- Determine the optimal amount of supplemental O_2 to treat desaturation previously documented to have occurred during exertion such as by the 6MWT

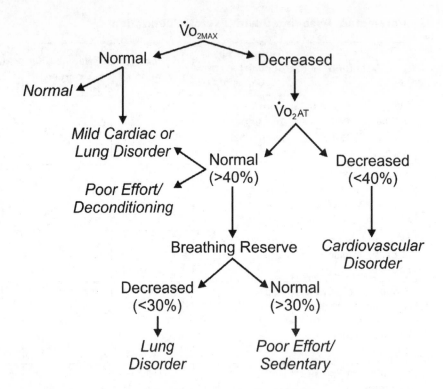

Figure 4-10 Differentiating Among the Conditions Limiting Exercise Capacity.

Contraindications and patient preparation are also basically the same as for cardiopulmonary stress testing, with the additional cautions against performing this test on patients with a resting SpO_2 less than 85% on room air. Technically, the inability to obtain either accurate pulse oximetry data or an arterial sample (via puncture or cannulation) will rule out this procedure.

Performing

O_2 titration with exercise can be performed in PFT or exercise labs, pulmonary rehabilitation centers, clinics, and physicians' offices. Often this test is performed during cardiopulmonary stress testing and requires the same basic equipment, except for the metabolic cart. Ideally, the patient's exercise levels should be quantified using a treadmill. If a treadmill is not available, a step test or the 6MWT can be substituted. A cycle ergometer is not recommended for O_2 titration. This is because *patients' O_2 needs during exercise must be established while carrying the portable system they use or that is planned for use.* Heart rate monitoring via pulse oximeter is mandatory; ECG monitoring should be used if at all possible. Because pulse oximetry provides indirect assessment of arterial O_2 saturation, the AARC recommends that the SpO_2 be validated by arterial sampling and co-oximetry. If a co-oximeter is not available, measurement of the PaO_2 via standard blood gas analysis can suffice.

The basic procedure is depicted in **Figure 4-11**. After gathering relevant patient data, you obtain a baseline SaO_2 on room air (or the patient's prescribed resting O_2 liter flow). If the SaO_2 is less than 85% you terminate the protocol and record the reason. For patients continuing on, you have them begin walking and slowly increase their activity until it replicates the highest intensity they will likely perform in the home environment, usually equivalent to a 3 or 4 on the Borg rating of perceived exertion (Table 4-13). After having the patient maintain this activity level for at least 3 minutes, you re-measure the SaO_2 (or SpO_2 if calibrated against the SaO_2). If the patient's O_2 saturation at the peak activity level is less than or equal to 88%, the patient does not need any additional oxygen and the test can be terminated. If, in contrast, the patient's SaO_2 drops by 2% or more or if the SaO_2 is less than 88% ($PaO_2 \leq$ 55 torr), increment the O_2 flow by 1 L/min (up to 6 L/min). After stabilization on the new O_2 flow for 3 minutes, reassess the SaO_2 while the patient continues to exercise. Repeat this procedure until the

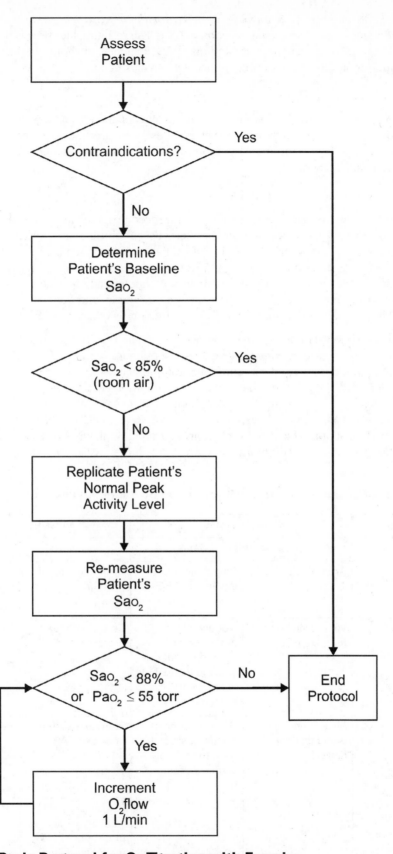

Figure 4-11 Basic Protocol for O$_2$ Titration with Exercise.

Sao_2 is *at least* 88% or the Pao_2 is above 55 torr. *To provide an extra margin of safety, the AARC recommends setting the target Sao_2 during titration to 93%.* The resulting liter flow is that needed to prevent arterial desaturation during regular exertion by the patient and should be the value prescribed by the ordering physician for use during applicable activities.

Hemodynamic Monitoring

Hemodynamic monitoring involves bedside measurements obtained from indwelling systemic arterial, central venous, or pulmonary artery (PA) catheters. These measures include both blood samples and vascular pressures and flows. **Table 4-31** outlines the key information that hemodynamic monitoring provides by sampling location.

Performing

In regard to performing to hemodynamic monitoring procedures, the NBRC is likely to focus on arterial line insertion; general aspects of indwelling catheter use, troubleshooting, and infection control; and the interpretation of the data obtained. Insertion of arterial lines is covered in Chapter 13. Chapter 6 provides details on the use and troubleshooting of pressure-measuring devices. Here we focus on the specific aspects of indwelling catheter use, including troubleshooting and infection control. The following sections address interpretation of vascular pressure, blood sample, and flow data.

General considerations that apply to the proper use of indwelling catheters include the following:

- For accurate pressure measurements, you need to ensure that the transducer is at the same level as the pressure it measures; for central venous and pulmonary artery pressures this level is the patient's *plebostatic axis* (i.e., intersection of the fourth intercostal space with the midaxillary line).
- Both CVP and PCWP are affected by changes in intrathoracic pressure during spontaneous and positive pressure breathing; to minimize this effect, make your measurements at end-expiration.
- Do not remove patients from PEEP/CPAP to measure CVP or PCWP; if PEEP is less than or equal to 10 cm H_2O, simply obtain the end-expiratory reading; if PEEP is greater than 10 cm H_2O, apply the following correction formula: corrected value = measured value – [.5 × (PEEP/1.36)].

Table 4-31 Hemodynamic Monitoring Information by Sampling Location

Location	Blood Collection		Pressure Monitoring	
	Sample	*Reflects*	*Pressure(s)*	*Reflects*
Systemic artery	Arterial blood	Pulmonary gas exchange (ABGs)	Systemic arterial pressure	LV afterload Vascular tone Blood volume
Central vein	Venous blood (unmixed)	Not useful for assessing gas exchange, but can be used instead of venipuncture for most lab tests	Central venous pressure (CVP)	Fluid volume Vascular tone RV preload
Pulmonary artery (PA)	Mixed venous blood (balloon deflated)	Gas exchange at the *tissues;* can be used to compute cardiac output (Fick method)	Pulmonary artery pressure (PAP)	RV afterload Vascular tone Blood volume
			Pulmonary capillary wedge pressure or PCWP (balloon inflated)	LV preload
Notes: LV = left ventricle; RV = right ventricle.				

- To obtain a valid blood sample from an indwelling catheter, you first need to remove fluid from the "deadspace" of the system (i.e., by using a separate syringe to aspirate the flush solution until whole blood appears); only then do you obtain the blood sample.
- When sampling mixed venous blood from a PA catheter, you must be sure the balloon is deflated and the sample is withdrawn slowly (otherwise you may get arterialized blood).
- In order to avoid clot formation in the transducer, stopcock, and connecting tubing, you need to briefly flush all indwelling catheter systems after obtaining a blood sample.

Unfortunately, indwelling catheters are a common cause of bloodstream infections. To help avoid this problem, the Centers for Disease Control have established guidelines for preventing catheter-related infections. Key recommendations provided in those guidelines include the following:

- Equipment
  - Use a catheter with the minimum number of ports needed to manage the patient
  - Use an antimicrobial-impregnated catheter for expected long-term use (> 5 days)
  - Use a sterile disposable transducer whenever possible
- Insertion
  - Use aseptic technique, including maximal sterile barrier precautions (cap, mask, sterile gown, sterile gloves, and a large sterile sheet)
  - Use a 2% chlorhexidine preparation for skin antisepsis during insertion (an iodophor, or 70% alcohol, is an acceptable alternative)
- Care of the insertion site
  - Use sterile gauze or a sterile, transparent, semipermeable dressing to cover the site
  - Replace the catheter site dressing when it becomes damp, loosened, or visibly soiled or when inspection of the site is necessary
  - Replace gauze dressings every 2 days and transparent dressings at least every 7 days
  - Do *not* apply topical antibiotics on insertion sites (except when using dialysis catheters) because of their potential to promote fungal infections and antimicrobial resistance
- Use
  - Keep all components of the pressure monitoring system sterile
  - Observe proper hand-hygiene procedures and use aseptic technique whenever obtaining blood samples or manipulating system components
  - Replace transducers and other external system components every 96 hours
- Surveillance
  - Record the operator, date, and time of catheter insertion/removal and dressing changes
  - Regularly monitor catheter sites visually or by palpation through the intact dressing
  - If a patient has tenderness at the insertion site, fever without obvious source, or other signs indicating sepsis, remove the dressing to examine the site
- Catheter removal/replacement
  - Promptly remove any intravascular catheter that is no longer essential
  - To prevent catheter-related infections, do not routinely replace catheters
  - Replace catheters only if the patient is hemodynamically unstable or infection is suspected

If you are responsible for monitoring vascular pressures obtained via indwelling catheters, you will likely encounter several common problems, including unexpectedly high or low pressure readings, damped or absent pressure waveforms, and signal artifact. **Table 4-32** outlines these problems and their solutions.

Interpreting Pressures

To interpret vascular pressures, you must first know the normal values in both the systemic and pulmonary circulations and their significance. **Table 4-33** (see page 119) summarizes the normal ranges and causes of abnormally high and low systemic arterial, central venous, right heart, and pulmonary artery pressures.

In general, pressures rise above normal due to increased cardiac activity (increased contractility and/or rate), hypervolemia, distal vasoconstriction, or flow obstruction. Pressures fall below normal due to decreased cardiac activity, hypovolemia, or distal vasodilation.

Table 4-32 Troubleshooting Vascular Lines

Problem/Causes	Solution
Unexpectedly High or Low Venous/PA Pressure Readings	
Change in transducer reference level	Position transducer at plebostatic axis (midchest)
Damped Pressure Waveform	
Catheter tip against vessel wall	Pull back, rotate, or reposition catheter while observing pressure waveform
Partial occlusion of catheter tip by clot	Aspirate clot with syringe and flush with heparinized saline (< 2–4 mL)
Clot in stopcock or transducer	Disconnect and flush stopcock and transducer; if no improvement, change stopcock and transducer
Air bubbles in transducer or connector tubing	Disconnect transducer and flush out air bubbles
Absent Waveform/No Pressure Reading	
Catheter occluded	Aspirate blood from line
Catheter out of vessel	Notify doctor and prepare to replace line
Stopcock off patient	Position stopcock correctly
Loose connection	Tighten loose connection
Transducer not connected to monitor	Check and tighten cable connection
Monitor set to zero, cal, or off	Make sure monitor set to proper function/display
Incorrect scale selection	Select appropriate scale (arterial = high; venous = low)
Signal Artifact	
Patient movement	Wait until patient is quiet before taking a reading
Electrical interference	Make sure electrical equipment is connected and grounded correctly
Catheter fling	Notify doctor to reposition catheter

In critical care settings, vascular pressures are often measured and displayed continuously on a monitor at the bedside. **Figure 4-12** (see page 120) provides an example of a display of systemic arterial pressure, CVP, and the accompanying ECG, as well as an annotated single cycle depicting the key events.

Although most hemodynamic monitors compute mean vascular pressures, the NBRC often tests your ability to estimate these measures. You estimate both the systemic and pulmonary arterial mean pressures using the following formula:

Estimated mean pressure = diastolic + 1/3 (systolic – diastolic)

For example, the mean arterial pressure of a patient with a systolic value of 110 mm Hg and a diastolic value of 70 mm Hg would be:

Estimated mean pressure = 70 + 40/3 = 17 + 13.2 ≈ 83 mm Hg

The NBRC also may test your knowledge of vascular pressures as related to PA catheter ("Swan-Ganz") insertion. As indicated in **Figure 4-13** (see page 121), as the catheter is advanced from the right atrium (equivalent to CVP pressure), through the right ventricle, into the pulmonary artery, and then "wedged" into a small artery, distinct pressure changes occur. It is these distinct pressure changes that inform the doctor where the catheter is and whether it is properly positioned.

Table 4-33 Vascular Pressures: Normal Ranges and Causes of Abnormalities

Measurement	Normal Range	Increased	Decreased
Systemic arterial pressure	Systolic: < 120 mm Hg (120–139 mm Hg = prehypertension) Diastolic: < 80 mm Hg (80–89 mm Hg = prehypertension)	Increased LV contractility (e.g., inoptropes) Vasoconstriction (e.g., alpha adrenergics) Increased blood volume Increased cardiac rate Arteriosclerosis Essential hypertension	LV failure (e.g., MI, CHF) Vasodilation (e.g., alpha blockers) Hypovolemia Decreased cardiac rate Arrhythmias Shock
Mean systemic arterial pressure	80–100 mm Hg	Any factor increasing arterial pressure	Any factor decreasing arterial pressure
Central venous/right atrial pressure	< 6 mm Hg	Increased venous return/hypervolemia RV failure (e.g., cor pulmonale) Tricuspid or pulmonary valve stenosis Pulmonary hypertension Hypoxemia (e.g., COPD) Pulmonary embolism Cardiac tamponade/ constrictive pericarditis Positive pressure ventilation Pneumothorax	Vasodilation Hypovolemia Shock Spontaneous inspiration
Pulmonary artery (PA) pressure	Systolic: 20–30 mm Hg Diastolic: 6–15 mm Hg	Increased RV contractility Hypervolemia Pulmonary hypertension Hypoxemia (e.g., ARDS, COPD) Pulmonary embolism Left ventricular failure Cardiac tamponade Mitral stenosis Vasoconstriction (e.g., vasopressors)	RV failure Vasodilation (e.g., nitric oxide, sildenafil) Hypovolemia
Mean PA pressure	10–20 mm Hg	Any factor increasing PA pressures	Any factor decreasing PA pressures
Pulmonary capillary wedge pressure (PCWP)	4–12 mm Hg	LV failure/cardiogenic shock Hypervolemia Cardiac tamponade/ constrictive pericarditis Mitral stenosis Positive pressure ventilation/PEEP Pneumothorax	Hypovolemia Shock other than cardiogenic Spontaneous inspiration

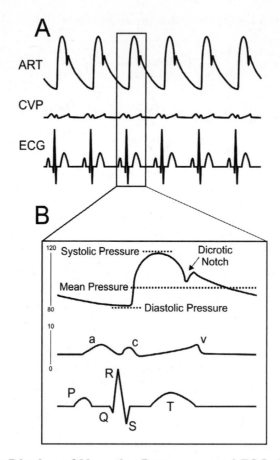

Figure 4-12 Monitor Display of Vascular Pressures and ECG. From top to bottom, view A displays the systemic arterial pressure (ART), CVP, and ECG at a normal sweep speed. View B extracts a single cycle run at a higher sweep speed. Note first that the rapid rise in arterial pressure is due to ventricular contraction, which immediately follows the ECG QRS complex. The peak and low points of the arterial waveform correspond respectively to the systolic and diastolic pressures, with the dicrotic notch indicating aortic valve closure. The difference between the systolic and diastolic pressures equals the pulse pressure, normally about 40 mm Hg in the systemic circulation. Critical care monitors also often display the computed average or mean arterial pressure (MAP). Due to its lower pressure, the CVP waveform is displayed on a different pressure scale. At high scan speed (view B), three distinct waves can be visualized. The "a" wave corresponds to the rise in pressure due to atrial contraction, which closely follows the P wave of the ECG. The "c" wave reflects ventricular contraction and bulging of the closed tricuspid valve back into the atrium. The "v" wave corresponds to the increase in pressure occurring as the right atrium refills.

Initially the CVP/RA (right atrial) pressure is displayed. As the catheter passes through the tricuspid valve into the right ventricle (RV), systolic pressures rise sharply, due to right ventricular contraction. As the catheter passes through the pulmonary valve into the pulmonary artery (PA), the diastolic pressures rise and a dicrotic notch appears, caused by pulmonary valve closure. As the catheter advances further and "wedges" into a small pulmonary artery, pulse pressure variations disappear. This pressure is the pulmonary capillary wedge pressure (PCWP). PCWP reflects left atrial pressure, which in turn normally equals left ventricular end-diastolic pressure or LV preload.

Note that after confirming the wedge position, the catheter must be withdrawn slightly to restore PA pressures. Thereafter, measurement of PCWP is obtained by inflating the balloon at the catheter's tip, which has the same effect as actual wedging.

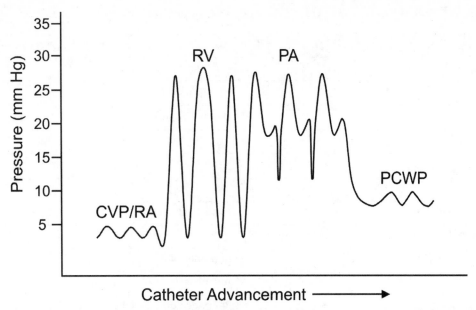

Figure 4-13 Monitor Display of Typical Vascular Pressures During Insertion of a Pulmonary Artery Catheter ("Swan-Ganz").

Interpreting Blood Sample Data

Blood obtained from an arterial line provides standard ABG data. The blood obtained from the distal port of a PA catheter is mixed venous blood, useful in assessing tissue oxygenation. When obtained concurrently, arterial and mixed venous samples can be used to compute cardiac output and the amount of physiologic shunting occurring in the pulmonary circulation.

To assess how well the tissues are getting oxygenated, we need to know *how much oxygen is left over after the blood leaves the capillaries.* We call this measure the *mixed venous oxygen content*, or Cvo_2. With a normal Hb, Pao_2, and cardiac output, the Cvo_2 ranges between 14 and 16 mL/dL, equivalent to an Svo_2 between 68% and 77% at a Pvo_2 of 38–42 torr.

The NBRC will often assess your understanding of mixed venous oxygen content as it relates to both tissue oxygen delivery *and* demand. Oxygen delivery is simply the product of the arterial oxygen content time cardiac output ($Cao_2 \times CO$). For the body as a whole, oxygen demands equal oxygen consumption, or Vo_2. The relationship between oxygen delivery and demand is best understood as based on the Fick equation for cardiac output:

$$CO = \frac{\dot{V}o_2}{C(a\text{-}v)o_2 \times 10}$$

where CO equals the cardiac output in L/min, Vo_2 equals the whole-body O_2 consumption in mL/min, and $C(a\text{-}v)o_2$ equals the difference between the arterial and mixed venous blood oxygen content, in ml/dL. Rearranging the formula to solve for Cvo_2 helps explain what causes this blood value to increase or decrease:

$$Cvo_2 = Cao_2 - \frac{\dot{V}o_2}{CO \times 10}$$

According to this formula, Cvo_2 will rise if either of the factors responsible for O_2 delivery increases—i.e., if there is an increase in arterial O_2 content or cardiac output. Cvo_2 also will rise if O_2 consumption decreases (all else being equal). In contrast, Cvo_2 will fall if either arterial O_2 content or cardiac output decreases or if O_2 consumption increases. **Table 4-34** demonstrates these relationships

Table 4-34 Clinical Conditions Associated with Changes in CvO$_2$

Low CvO$_2$	
↑ Oxygen delivery[a]	Anemia, hemorrhage
↑ Hb	Hypoxia, suctioning
↑ SaO$_2$	Hypovolemia, shock
↑ CO	Arrhythmias
↓ Oxygen demand[a]	Hyperthermia, pain, shivering, seizures
High CvO$_2$	
↑ Oxygen delivery	Hyperoxia (↓ FiO$_2$)
↓ Oxygen demand	↓ Hb
	Hypothermia
	Anesthesia
	Pharmacologic paralysis
	Cyanide poisoning[b]
	Sepsis[b]

a. Oxygen delivery = CO × CaO$_2$; oxygen demand = whole-body VO$_2$.

b. In both cyanide poisoning and sepsis, CvO$_2$ can be higher than normal, even though tissue hypoxia may be present. For this reason, in patients with pathologic conditions that decrease oxygen demand, mixed venous lactate or pyruvate levels may be a better indicator of the state of tissue oxygenation.

and summarizes the common clinical conditions associated with changes in mixed venous oxygen content.

In general, with a normal Hb level, *if the SvO$_2$ is less than 50% or the PvO$_2$ is less than 27 torr, the patient has impaired tissue oxygenation.* An SvO$_2$ below 30% (corresponding to a PvO$_2$ of about 27 torr) can lead to unconsciousness and permanent organ damage.

Instead of using the CvO$_2$ alone, many clinicians prefer to use the difference between the arterial and mixed venous oxygen content to assess tissue oxygenation. Normally, the C(a-v)O$_2$ is less than 7.0 mL/dL. Again, according to the Fick equation, C(a-v)O$_2$ will increase if oxygen consumption increases or cardiac output decreases. In contrast, *C(a-v)O$_2$ decreases when oxygen consumption falls or cardiac output increases.*

Concurrently obtained arterial and mixed venous samples also can be used to compute the percentage of physiologic shunting occurring in the pulmonary circulation. Shunting occurs in the lungs when venous blood bypasses ventilated alveoli and returns unchanged into the left (arterial) side of the circulation. Shunting *always* lowers arterial oxygen content, in direct proportion to the percentage of cardiac output bypassing ventilated alveoli. Due to design "flaws" in the pulmonary and cardiac circulations, small anatomic shunts (3–5%) are normal. Shunting above this level is abnormal.

The true physiologic shunt in the lungs is computed using the following equation:

$$\% \text{ shunt} = \frac{Cc'O_2 - CaO_2}{Cc'O_2 - CvO_2}$$

where Cc'O$_2$ equals the "ideal" pulmonary end-capillary oxygen content, CaO$_2$ equals the arterial oxygen content, and CvO$_2$ equals the mixed venous oxygen content. You calculate arterial and mixed venous blood contents in the usual manner (as described in Chapter 20). To determine the Cc'O$_2$, you must substitute the alveolar PO$_2$ (PAO$_2$) into the formula for calculating total O$_2$ content.

Fortunately, the NBRC will not test your ability to compute the % shunt using the true shunt equation. Instead, you will be expected to *estimate* the % shunt based on the alveolar-arterial oxygen tension gradient, or $P(A-a)O_2$. Assuming a normal $C(a-v)O_2$, one can estimate the percent shunt of a patient breathing 100% oxygen as follows:

$$\% \text{ shunt} = \frac{P(A\text{-}a)O_2 \times 0.003}{[P(A\text{-}a)O_2 \times 0.003 + 5]}$$

where the $P(A-a)O_2$ is the alveolar-arterial oxygen tension gradient and 5 is the normal $C(a-v)O_2$ in mL/dL. Rather than perform this computation, you instead can apply the rule of thumb provided in the accompanying box.

Estimating the Percent Shunt [assumes PaO_2 > 100 torr and $C(a-v)O_2$ = 5]

Rule of Thumb: Breathing 100% oxygen, every 100 torr $P(A-a)O_2$ equals about a 5% shunt.

Example: A patient breathing 100% O_2 has a $P(A-a)O_2$ of 300 torr. What is her approximate % shunt?

Solution: 300/100 = 3

Approximate % shunt = $3 \times 5 = 15\%$

Interpreting Flows and Resistances

Cardiac output (CO) is the total volume flow of blood per minute through the circulation. It is the simple product of the average stroke volume (SV) times the heart rate (HR) in beats per minute, i.e.,

$$\text{CO (mL/min)} = \text{SV (mL/beat)} \times \text{HR (beats/min)}$$

Direct monitoring of stroke volume at the bedside is difficult. Instead, to measure CO at the bedside we use flow data obtained via a pulmonary artery catheter. Although the Fick method (previously described) can be used, it has largely been replaced by the thermal dilution technique. The thermal dilution technique determines cardiac output by measuring blood temperature changes that occur between two points on the PA catheter. The traditional method involves rapidly injecting a cool saline solution (at least 10°C cooler than body temperature) into the right atrial port of the catheter. A newer method is to use a catheter that heats the blood using a thermal filament on its surface that can provide continuously updated measurements without injections. In either case, a computer measures the rate of temperature change, from which it calculates the cardiac output.

Using one of these methods, we observe that adult cardiac output typically varies between 4 and 8 L/min. This large range is due to the fact that cardiac output depends on body size—in particular, body surface area. For this reason, interpretation of cardiac output must be adjusted for body surface area. We call this measure the cardiac index (CI) and compute it as follows:

$$\text{CI} = \frac{\text{CO}}{\text{BSA}}$$

where CI is the cardiac index in L/min/m², CO is the cardiac output in L/min, and BSA is the body surface area as estimated using the Dubois nomogram or its prediction equation.

Knowledge of the cardiac output, heart rate, CVP, mean arterial and pulmonary arterial pressures, and PCWP allows computation of several other hemodynamic parameters, as defined in **Table 4-35**.

Table 4-35 Common Hemodynamic Parameters

Parameter	Formula	Normal Range
Cardiac output (CO)	n/a – Fick or thermal dilution value	4–8 L/min
Cardiac index (CI)	CI = CO (L/min) ÷ BSA	2.5–5 L/min/m^2
Stroke volume (SV)	SV = CO (mL/min) ÷ HR	60–130 mL/beat
Stroke (SI)	SI = CI ÷ HR or SV/BSA	30–50 mL/m^2
Systemic vascular resistance (SVR)	SVR = [(MAP – CVP) ÷ CO] × 80	900–1400 dyne·sec·cm^{-5} 15–20 Wood units[a]
Pulmonary vascular resistance (PVR)	PVR = [(MPAP – PCWP) ÷ CO] × 80	110–250 dyne·sec·cm^{-5} 1–3 Wood units

Abbreviations: BSA, body surface area (m^2); HR, heart rate (beats/min); MAP, mean arterial pressure (systemic, mm Hg); CVP, central venous pressure (mm Hg); MPAP, mean pulmonary artery pressure (mm Hg); PCWP, pulmonary capillary wedge pressure (mm Hg).

a. The units used to measure vascular resistance (dyne·sec·cm^{-5}) are cgs units. The factor of 80 converts the traditional "Wood" units (mm Hg/L/min) to the corresponding cgs units.

The NBRC will expect you to know the normal ranges for adult cardiac output, cardiac index, and stroke volume and to be able to compute a patient's cardiac index (given the CO and BSA) and stroke volume (given the CO and heart rate). In addition, you should be able to interpret all the values in Table 4-35. See the accompanying box for a simple example.

Simple Hemodynamic Computations and Interpretation

Problem: Given a patient with a cardiac output of 4 L/min, heart rate of 100/min, and a body surface area of 2.0 m^2, compute his stroke volume and cardiac index.

Solution:

Stroke volume

$$SV \text{ (mL)} = CO \text{ (mL/min)} \div HR$$
$$SV = 4000 \div 100 = 40 \text{ mL}$$

Cardiac index

$$CI \text{ (L/min/m}^2) = CO \div BSA$$
$$CI = 4 \div 2 = 2 \text{ L/min/m}^2$$

Interpretation: The patient's stroke volume and cardiac index are both below normal. Decreased stroke volume is associated with decreased cardiac contractility (e.g., an MI) or increased afterload (e.g., vasoconstriction).

To interpret vascular resistance measures, you need to understand the concept involved. As with resistance to gas flow through a tube, vascular resistance represents a change in pressure per unit flow:

$$R = \frac{\Delta P}{\dot{V}}$$

where R is resistance, ΔP is the pressure difference across the tube, and $\dot{V}$ is the flow. In terms of vascular resistance, the "tubes" are the systemic and pulmonary circulations. In both circulations, the flow equals the cardiac output. For the systemic circulation, the pressure difference is that between the start (mean arterial pressure) and end (CVP) of the system. Likewise, ΔP across the pulmonary circulation equals the starting mean PA pressure minus the ending left ventricular end-diastolic pressure (LVEDP), which is equivalent to the PCWP.

The causes of increased vascular resistance are complex. With the exception of those conditions causing hypervolemia or affecting cardiac contractility, essentially all the factors specified in Table 4-33 as increasing pressures in the systemic and pulmonary circulations are caused by increased vascular resistance—e.g., hypertension (systemic or pulmonary), arteriosclerosis, hypoxemia (pulmonary circulation only), and vasopressor drugs. You should also note that one of the body's responses to cardiogenic and hypovolemic shock (which both *decrease* systemic and pulmonary vascular pressures) is to increase vascular resistance by vasoconstriction.

Putting It All Together

In terms of basic hemodynamics, the NBRC often will ask a question or two that require you to integrate your knowledge of pressure, flow, and resistance parameters as related to common clinical conditions. **Table 4-36** outlines the typical hemodynamic changes you will see in selected critically ill patients. The accompanying box provides an example interpretation.

Simple Hemodynamic Computations

Problem: Measurements taken via a pulmonary artery catheter on a patient with a decreased cardiac output and low arterial blood pressure indicate the following:

- Increased CVP
- Increased pulmonary artery pressure (PAP)
- Increased pulmonary capillary wedge pressure (PCWP)

Interpretation: The increased CVP and PAP could be due to LV failure/cardiogenic shock, pulmonary hypertension, or pulmonary embolism. However, the elevated PCWP is most consistent with LV failure/cardiogenic shock.

Table 4-36 Hemodynamic Changes in Common Clinical Conditions

Condition	SAP	CVP	CO	PAP	PCWP	PVR	SVR
Dehydration/hypovolemic shock	↓	↓	↓	↓	↓	↑	↑
LV failure/cardiogenic shock	↓	↑	↓	↑	↑	↑	↑
Septic shock	↓	↓	↑ (early)	↓	↓	↓	↓
Neurogenic shock	↓	↓	↓	↓	↓	↓	↓
Pulmonary hypertension	N	↑	N or ↓	↑	N	↑	N
Pulmonary embolism	↓	↑	↓	↑	N or ↓	↑	↑

Abbreviations: N, normal; ↑, increased; ↓, decreased; SAP, systemic arterial pressure; CVP, central venous pressure; CO, cardiac output; PAP, pulmonary artery pressure; PCWP, pulmonary artery wedge pressure; PVR, pulmonary vascular resistance; SVR, systemic vascular resistance.

COMMON ERRORS TO AVOID

You can improve your score by avoiding these mistakes:

- Don't assume that all that wheezes are asthma; patients with congestive heart failure may also exhibit wheezing due to peribronchial edema.
- Don't assume that a lack of central cyanosis means satisfactory oxygenation; a patient with anemia can be severely hypoxemic without cyanosis.

- Never delay needed interventions for a newborn in order to assess Apgar scores.
- Do not use a numeric pain scale with young children or patients who are unable to express themselves.
- Do not attempt patient education until all major barriers to learning have been resolved.
- Do not use mechanical (vane-type) respirometers to measure forced vital capacities.
- Do not try to determine the nature of a patient's pulmonary impairment based on the peak expiratory flow measure.
- Never accept bedside spirometry results until you have three acceptable maneuvers.
- Do not use apnea monitoring or auto-CPAP to assess patients for obstructive apnea.
- Do not use the 6MWT to identify the cause of a patient's dyspnea or exercise intolerance.
- Avoid cardiopulmonary exercise testing in patients with uncontrolled heart failure or unstable angina.
- Do not use a cycle ergometer when titrating a patient's supplemental O_2 needs.
- Do not remove patients from PEEP/CPAP to measure CVP or PCWP.
- Never forget to deflate the balloon of a pulmonary artery catheter.
- To prevent infection, do not routinely replace indwelling catheters.

SURE BETS

In some situations you can always be sure of the right approach to a clinical problem or scenario:

- Always consider peripheral cyanosis, coolness of the extremities, and slow capillary refills as signs of circulatory failure.
- Always consider recommending airway clearance for patients whose sputum production exceeds 30 mL/day.
- Always think pulmonary edema when a patient has pink, frothy secretions.
- Always remember that the trachea and PMI shift toward areas of atelectasis and away from space-occupying lesions such as pneumothoraces or pleural effusions.
- If you detect crepitus, always consider the possibility of pneumothorax (and immediately communicate your findings to the doctor).
- When you detect a pulse deficit, you can be sure there is a cardiac arrhythmia, such as atrial fibrillation.
- Recognize that only alert patients can cooperate and fully participate in their own care.
- Always consider a patient to be comatose if the Glasgow score is less than 8.
- Tachypnea, thoracic-abdominal dysynchrony, and the use of accessory muscles always indicate increased work of breathing.
- Whenever in doubt regarding DNR status, always initiate emergency life support or resuscitation when needed.
- When reading an X-ray, always verify patient identification and film orientation.
- Always consider foreign body aspiration as a possibility in the differential diagnosis of airway obstruction in children (and as justification for recommending both chest and lateral neck X-rays).
- High breathing rates and low tidal volumes always increase deadspace ventilation per minute.
- To consider a change in a pulmonary flow parameter to be clinically significant, expect at least a 15% improvement from baseline.
- The primary indicator of an abnormal cardiopulmonary exercise test is a low VO_{2max}.
- For accurate vascular pressure measurements, ensure that the transducer is at the same level as the pressure it measures, typically the patient's plebostatic axis.

PRE-TEST ANSWERS AND EXPLANATIONS

Below are this chapter's pre-test answers and explanations. Be sure to review each answer's explanation thoroughly to help you understand why it is correct. If the explanation is still unclear to you, review the chapter contents or the references and/or refer to this chapter's supplemental resources on the CD.

4-1. **Correct answer: A.** Cor pulmonale. Cor pulmonale is right heart failure due to chronic lung disease. Right heart failure occurs when chronic hypoxemia elevates the pulmonary vascular resistance and puts a strain on the right ventricle to pump blood through the constricted pulmonary capillaries. Right heart failure causes venous blood to back up into the neck veins.

4-2. **Correct answer: B.** Left upper lobe collapse. Volume loss in the upper lobe will pull the trachea toward the collapsed lung. In this case the trachea has shifted to the left indicating that either volume loss has occurred on the left or a tumor on the right is pushing the trachea to the left.

4-3. **Correct answer D.** Pneumothorax. A patient with a dull percussion note and bronchial breath sounds on chest examination most likely has either pulmonary infiltrates, atelectasis, or consolidation of the affected area. A pneumothorax normally results in a hyperresonant percussion note.

4-4. **Correct answer: C.** Pneumonia. Bronchial breath sounds normally are heard only over the trachea. When heard over the lung periphery, consolidation (due to pneumonia) is present. Consolidation of the lung allows the turbulent flow sounds of the larger airways to pass directly through the lung as attenuation is reduced.

4-5. **Correct answer: A.** Left-sided pneumothorax. An acutely ill patient with dyspnea, hypotension, unilateral findings of reduced chest expansion, a hyperresonant percussion note, absence of breath sounds and tactile fremitus, and a tracheal shift to the right has most likely suffered a large pneumothorax on the affected side. If the pneumothorax is severe enough to disrupt cardiac function, blood pressure will also fall.

4-6. **Correct answer: B.** Severe hypoxemia. An abnormal sensorium is often caused by a lack of adequate oxygenation to the brain. Severe hypoxemia reduces the oxygen available to the brain and leads to confusion. An abnormal sensorium in any patient should be assumed to be caused by hypoxia until proven otherwise.

4-7. **Correct answer: C.** Use a numeric pain scale. A numeric pain scale is *not* useful for young children or patients who cannot express themselves. The best way to assess the pain level of a young child is to get the input of a family member. Without such information, you may have to rely on observing patient behaviors that indicate severe pain, such as moaning, crying, or grimacing.

4-8. **Correct answer: B.** Orthopnea. Orthopnea is present when the patient has difficult breathing upon lying down. In most cases this is due to pulmonary edema filling the lungs when the patient assumes a horizontal position. Keeping the patient's head up during sleep with the use of pillows reduces the collection of fluid in the lungs.

4-9. **Correct answer: B.** Chronic bronchitis. Chronic bronchitis is defined primarily by its symptoms: chronic cough and sputum production.

4-10. **Correct answer: A.** Recent weight gain. Any patient who (1) is significantly underweight; (2) has recently lost a significant amount of weight; (3) has poor dietary habits or inadequate food intake; or (4) is impoverished, isolated, or unable to prepare his or her own food is at high risk for malnutrition. Weight gain is not normally associated with malnutrition.

4-11. **Correct answer: D.** Occupational history. Of the items listed, occupational history is most important in the diagnosis of lung disease. Many lung diseases are associated with inhalation of dust or toxic chemicals in the work setting.

4-12. **Correct answer: B.** Immediately call a code and begin resuscitation efforts. If there is any doubt regarding a DNR order or if written orders are not present, start resuscitation efforts. Formal or informal directives such as "slow code" or "code gray" bypass the patient's rights and are generally inappropriate.

4-13. Correct answer: C. Have her "teach" the information back to you. Teach-back is the best way to determine whether a patient has learned critical information related to his or her care. A return demonstration is appropriate for procedural skills, whereas discussion is the best method for assessing attitudinal change.

4-14. Correct answer: C. Right phrenic nerve paralysis. An elevated hemidiaphragm indicates phrenic nerve paralysis on the affected side or hepatomegaly (generally right side only). Pleural effusions blunt the costophrenic angles, whereas hyperinflation tends to flatten the hemidiaphragms, as does tension pneumothorax (on the affected side).

4-15. Correct answer: A. Croup. Croup is the most likely problem. On an AP X-ray, croup is characterized by the "steeple sign"—i.e., a narrowed and tapering airway below larynx due to subglottic edema. Typically, the lateral neck X-ray in these patients is normal (showing little or no evidence of supraglottic involvement).

4-16. Correct answer: D. Bundle branch block. QRS complexes appear wider than normal (> 0.12 sec) in PVCs, bundle branch block, ventricular fibrillation, and hyperkalemia.

4-17. Correct answer: B. 8.00 L/min. The formula for alveolar minute ventilation is $\dot{V}_E = f \times (V_T - V_D)$. In this case the physiologic deadspace is estimated at 1 mL/lb ideal body weight, or 150 mL. Substituting the patient's values for f, V_T, and estimated V_D, we compute an alveolar minute ventilation of $20 \times (550 - 150) = 8000$ mL/min, or 8.00 L/min.

4-18. Correct answer: B. The patient cannot sustain prolonged spontaneous ventilation. This patient has a VC of about 8 mL/kg (400 mL/50 kg). A normal VC is about 65–75 mL/kg. Values below 65–75 mL/kg indicate a restrictive disorder, which may be due to neuromuscular weakness, acutely decreased lung volumes, or interstitial lung disease. When the VC drops below 10–15 mL/kg it is unlikely that a patient can support prolonged spontaneous ventilation.

4-19. Correct answer: B. II and III. Normal adult male peak flows range between 8 and 12 L/sec, while adult female normal peak flows range between 6 and 9 L/sec. This patient's peak flow is considerably below normal, which generally indicates an expiratory flow obstruction. However, the peak flow test is highly effort dependent. For this reason, poor effort should always be considered when peak flow results are below predicted norms.

4-20. Correct answer: C. A restrictive disorder. A patient with a decreased FVC, normal FEV_1, and increased $FEV_1\%$ is exhibiting the classic pattern of a restrictive pulmonary disorder—i.e., decreased volumes and normal (or increased) flows.

4-21. Correct answer: C. 3300 mL. The functional residual capacity (FRC) equals the sum of the residual volume and the expiratory reserve volume (FRC = RV + ERV). Rearranging this equation (to solve for RV) yields RV = FRC − ERV. In this case, RV = 4500 − 1200, or 3300 mL.

4-22. Correct answer: B. The patient has pulmonary emphysema. The low $FEV_1\%$ and higher than normal TLC and RV confirm an obstructive disorder with hyperinflation (emphysema, chronic bronchitis, acute asthma, etc.). Among these obstructive disorders, only patients with emphysema exhibit a low D_{LCO}, due to the destruction of the alveolar capillary membrane.

4-23. Correct answer: A. Hypoxemia. A decreased respiratory rate in combination with an increased heart rate in a neonate most likely indicates hypoxemia, which should be confirmed by pulse oximetry or an ABG.

4-24. Correct answer: C. 4% or more. Most sleep disorder specialists agree that a desaturation event represents a decrease in saturation of 4% or more. The total number of these desaturation events per hour is the oxygen desaturation index (ODI).

4-25. **Correct answer: B.** Patient B. When using the 6MWT to assess medical or surgical interventions, you should expect at least a 10–20% improvement in the 6MWD to consider the treatment effective. Only patient B has more than a 10% improvement in this measure of functional capacity [(200 − 150)/150 = 33% improvement].

4-26. **Correct answer: B.** Somewhat strong exertion (rating of 4). For patients continuing on, you have them initiate walking and slowly increase their activity until it replicates the highest intensity they will likely perform in the home environment, usually equivalent to a 3 to 4 on the Borg rating of perceived exertion.

4-27. **Correct answer: C.** Pulmonary artery. To assess gas exchange at the tissues, you need to assess blood after it leaves the capillaries. For the body as a whole, you need to wait until after all the blood from all the capillary beds mixes together, which is complete only in the pulmonary artery.

4-28. **Correct answer: A.** Hypovolemia. A pulmonary capillary wedge pressure (PCWP) of 18 mm Hg is higher than the normal pressure of 4–12 mm Hg. All of the causes listed except hypovolemia can increase PCWP. Hypovolemia tends to lower *all* vascular pressures.

4-29. **Correct answer: D.** Patient D. All patients with poor exercise capacity have a reduced Vo_{2max}. In addition, patients with a pulmonary limitation to exercise tend to have a normal anaerobic threshold (if it can be reached) but a decreased breathing reserve. Patients with a cardiovascular limitation to exercise typically have a reduced anaerobic threshold but a normal breathing reserve. In the presence of a low Vo_{2max}, poor effort is revealed by a normal anaerobic threshold and breathing reserve.

4-30. **Correct answer: B.** Increase the CPAP to 10 cm H_2O for 5 minutes and continue observation. If any of the following events occur during a CPAP titration observation interval (up to the maximum protocol pressure, typically 20 cm H_2O), you should increase the CPAP level by at least 1 cm H_2O: ≥ 2 obstructive apneas, ≥ 3 hypopneas, ≥ 5 RERAs, ≥ 3 min of loud snoring.

REFERENCES

American Association for Respiratory Care. (1996). Spirometry, 1996 update. *Respiratory Care, 41,* 629–636.

American Association for Respiratory Care. (2001). Clinical practice guideline. Exercise testing for evaluation of hypoxemia and/or desaturation. 2001 revision and update. *Respiratory Care, 46,* 514–522.

American College of Cardiology/American Heart Association Task Force on Practice Guidelines, Committee on Exercise Testing. (2002). *2002 guideline update for exercise testing.* Bethesda, MD: American College of Cardiology.

American Society of Anesthesiologists. (2003). Practice guidelines for pulmonary artery catheterization: An updated report by the American Society of Anesthesiologists Task Force on Pulmonary Artery Catheterization. *Anesthesiology, 99,* 988–1014.

American Thoracic Society. (2002). ATS statement: Guidelines for the six-minute walk test. *American Journal of Respiratory Critical Care Medicine, 166,* 111–117.

American Thoracic Society. (2005). *Pulmonary function laboratory management and procedure manual* (2nd ed.). New York: American Thoracic Society.

Bickley, L. S. & Szilagyi, P. G. (2004). *Bates' guide to physical examination and history taking* (8th ed.). Philadelphia: Lippincott, Williams & Wilkins.

Brown, R. L., Leonard, T., Saunders, L. A., & Papasouliotis. (2001). A two-item conjoint screen for alcohol and other drug problems. *Journal of the American Board of Family Practice, 14,* 95–106.

Centers for Disease Control and Prevention. (2002). Guidelines for the prevention of intravascular catheter-related infections. *Morbidity and Mortality Weekly Report, 51,* RR-10 (August 9).

Expert Panel on Thoracic Imaging. (2006). *Routine chest radiograph.* Reston, VA: American College of Radiology.

Fuhrman, T. M. (2004). Be aware of advanced directives. *NBRC Horizons, 30*(4), 2.

The Joint Commission. (2007). *The Joint Commission guide to patient and family education* (2nd ed.). Chicago: The Joint Commission.

Kushida, C. A., Chediak, A., Berry, R. B., et al. (2008). Clinical guidelines for the manual titration of positive airway pressure in patients with obstructive sleep apnea. *Journal of Clinical Sleep Medicine, 4*, 157–171.

Kwiatkowski, C. A., Touger-Decker, D., & O'Sullivan-Maillet, J. Nutritional aspects of health and disease. In Scanlan, C. L., Wilkins, R. L., & Stoller, J. K. (Eds.). *Egan's fundamentals of respiratory care* (7th ed.). St. Louis, MO: Mosby, 1999.

MacIntyre, N. R. (1990). Respiratory monitoring without machinery. *Respiratory Care 35*, 546–553.

Morgenthaler, T. I. (2008). Practice parameters for the use of autotitrating continuous positive airway pressure devices for titrating pressures and treating adult patients with obstructive sleep apnea syndrome: An update for 2007. *Sleep, 31*, 141–147.

Pellegrino, R., Viegi, G., Brusasco, V., et al. (2005). Interpretative strategies for lung function tests. *European Respiratory Journal, 26*, 948–968.

Wilkins, R. L., Dexter, J. R., & Heuer, A. J. (2009). *Clinical assessment in respiratory care* (6th ed.). St. Louis, MO: Mosby.

Wilkins, R. L., Stoller, J. K., & Kacmarek, R. M. (Eds.) (2009). *Egan's fundamentals of respiratory care* (9th ed.). St. Louis: Mosby.

Recommend Procedures to Obtain Additional Data

Craig L. Scanlan

INTRODUCTION

Other than providing therapy to your patients, your role as a respiratory therapist often will involve making recommendations to others in order to improve the outcomes of care. Making recommendations related to enhancing *therapeutic* outcomes is covered in Chapter 15. However, the NBRC also expects that you have the knowledge to recommend needed *diagnostic procedures* for your patients. In previous versions of the CRT exam, assessment of this knowledge was integrated into other sections of the test. The NBRC now considers this area important enough to deserve its own separate section on the CRT exam, beginning in July 2009.

OBJECTIVES

After completion of this chapter, you should demonstrate the knowledge needed to recommend the following diagnostic procedures:

1. Radiographic and other imaging studies
2. Diagnostic bronchoscopy
3. Sputum Gram stain, culture, and sensitivities
4. Bronchoalveolar lavage
5. Pulmonary function testing
6. Lung mechanics
7. Blood gas analysis, pulse oximetry, and transcutaneous monitoring
8. Capnography
9. Electrocardiogram
10. Hemodynamic monitoring
11. Sleep studies

WHAT TO EXPECT ON THIS CATEGORY OF THE CRT EXAM

Number of questions: 4
Level of questions: about 25% recall, 75% application

WHAT'S NEW FOR 2009

This is an entirely new section of the NBRC CRT exam, first included in the July 2009 test administration. With the exception of recommending blood gas analysis, pulse oximetry, and transcutaneous O_2/CO_2 monitoring, all content in this section also is new.

PRE-TEST

Carefully respond to each of the following questions. After completing the pre-test, compare your answers to those provided at the end of this chapter. Then thoroughly review each answer's explanation to help understand why it is correct.

5-1. A patient admitted to the emergency department is suspected of having suffered pulmonary injury due to inhalation of toxic fumes. To determine the location and extent of potential injury you would recommend which of the following procedures?
   A. V/Q scan
   B. Chest X-ray
   C. Blood gas analysis
   D. Fiberoptic bronchoscopy

5-2. Your patient in the ICU is suspected of having developed a bacterial ventilator-associated pneumonia. Which of the following procedures would you recommend as best able to diagnose the cause of this problem?
   A. Sputum culture and sensitivity
   B. Chest X-ray
   C. Bronchoalveolar lavage
   D. CT scan

5-3. To estimate the metabolic rate of a patient receiving mechanical ventilation, you would recommend:
   A. Hemoximetry
   B. ABG analysis
   C. Capnography
   D. Maximum voluntary ventilation

5-4. To evaluate and follow the course of a patient with interstitial lung disease, which of the following pulmonary function testing procedures would you recommend?
   A. Diffusing capacity (DLCO)
   B. He dilution FRC and TLC
   C. Forced expiratory volumes/flows
   D. Methacholine challenge test

5-5. Which of the following tests of lung mechanics would you recommend to detect the presence of auto-PEEP on a patient receiving ventilatory support?
   A. Pressure-volume loop
   B. Flow-volume loop
   C. Static compliance (inspiratory hold)
   D. Airway resistance (inspiratory hold)

5-6. The wife of a patient receiving postoperative incentive spirometry asks if this therapy will help get rid of his snoring, daytime sleepiness, and morning headaches. In communicating this information to the patient's surgeon, you would recommend which of the following diagnostic procedures?
   A. Lateral neck X-ray
   B. Arterial blood gas
   C. Polysomnography
   D. Diffusing capacity

5-7. To continuously monitor the adequacy of ventilation of a patient in the ICU being supported by mask BiPAP™, you would recommend which of the following?
   A. Transcutaneous P_{CO_2}
   B. Pulse oximetry
   C. ABG analysis
   D. Capnography

5-8. As you are fitting him with a nonrebreathing mask, a 62-year-old patient in the emergency department complains of severe chest pain. Which of the following tests would you first recommend for this patient?
   A. Arterial blood gas (ABG)
   B. Electrocardiogram (ECG)
   C. V/Q scan
   D. Bedside spirometry

5-9. To assess tissue oxygenation in a patient with ARDS, you would recommend which of the following?
  A. A CVP line
  B. A pulmonary artery catheter
  C. An arterial line
  D. Pulse oximetry

5-10. You would recommend consideration of all of the following imaging modalities for diagnosing a patient suspected of having a pulmonary embolism *except*:
  A. V/Q scan
  B. AP chest X-ray
  C. Computed tomography (CT scan)
  D. Pulmonary angiography

WHAT YOU NEED TO KNOW: ESSENTIAL CONTENT

Radiographic and Other Imaging Studies

Imaging studies that you may be expected to recommend include chest and lateral neck X-rays; computed tomography (CT), magnetic resonance imaging (MRI), and positron emission tomography (PET) scans; pulmonary angiography; ultrasound imaging; and V/Q scans. **Table 5-1** outlines the primary reasons for recommending these imaging studies for your patients.

Diagnostic Bronchoscopy

According to the AARC, you should recommend diagnostic bronchoscopy whenever the need exists to:

- Assess lesions of unknown etiology that appear on the chest X-ray film
- Evaluate recurrent atelectasis or pulmonary infiltrates
- Assess the patency of the upper airway
- Investigate the source of hemoptysis
- Evaluate unexplained cough, localized wheeze, or stridor
- Follow up on suspicious or positive sputum cytology results
- Obtain lower respiratory tract secretions, cell washings, or biopsies for cytologic or microbiologic assessment
- Determine the location and extent of injury from toxic inhalation or aspiration
- Evaluate problems associated with artificial airways—e.g., tube placement or tracheal damage
- Facilitate endotracheal tube insertion during difficult intubations
- Locate/clear mucus plugs causing lobar or segmental atelectasis
- Remove abnormal endobronchial tissue by forceps, basket, or laser
- Remove foreign bodies from the airway (although rigid bronchoscopy is preferred)

Just as important as knowing the indications for diagnostic bronchoscopy is awareness of the contraindications. According to the AARC, you should recommend *against* performing diagnostic bronchoscopy in patients who:

- Cannot be adequately oxygenated during the procedure due to severe refractory hypoxemia
- Have a bleeding disorder that cannot be corrected
- Have severe obstructive airway disease
- Are hemodynamically unstable

Bronchoalveolar Lavage

Bronchoalveolar lavage (BAL) is a diagnostic procedure that involves the instillation and immediate removal of sterile normal saline solution into a lung segment via the suction channel of a fiberoptic bronchoscope. The withdrawn fluid then undergoes chemical, cytologic, and/or microbiologic assessment.

According to the American Thoracic Society, BAL is indicated in patients with the following problems:

- Nonresolving pneumonia
- Unexplained lung infiltrates (interstitial and/or alveolar)
- Suspected alveolar hemorrhage

Table 5-1 Recommending Imaging Studies

Modality	Recommend To	Comments
Chest X-ray	• Evaluate signs and symptoms of respiratory and cardiovascular disorders • Follow known chest disease processes to assess progression or improvement • Monitor patients receiving ventilatory support • Monitor patients after thoracic surgery • Assess surgical risk in patients with cardiac or respiratory symptoms • Comply with government requirements for chest radiography, as in occupational lung disease • Confirm proper placement of endotracheal tubes, CVP and PA catheters, and NG and chest tubes	Although getting a chest X-ray after thoracentesis is common, the American College of Radiology recommends this procedure only if a pneumothorax is suspected (e.g., if air rather then fluid is aspirated during the procedure).
Neck X-ray	• Help diagnose causes of stridor and respiratory distress in children (e.g., croup vs. epiglottitis) • Detect the presence of aspirated foreign bodies • Detect retropharyngeal abscesses and hematomas • Confirm adenoid hypertrophy	AP vs. lateral neck films are taken to differentiate croup from epiglottitis; however, the classic AP-view "steeple sign" described for croup is not specific to that disorder and can be absent.
Thoracic CT	• Evaluate abnormalities identified by chest X-ray (e.g., interstitial lung disease and pulmonary nodules) • Stage lung cancer • Detect tumor metastases to the lung • Detect mediastinal masses/nodes • Detect pulmonary embolism (CT angiography) • Detect and evaluate aortic aneurysm • Assess trauma to thoracic organs and structures	Patient cooperation is essential because the patient must remain motionless during the procedure. Helical CT angiography may replace V/Q scans as screening test for pulmonary embolism.
Thoracic MRI	• Evaluate the heart, major vessels, and lungs for pathology • Assess the chest wall and surrounding soft tissues for abnormalities • Evaluate posterior mediastinal masses • Detect and evaluate aortic aneurysm • Detect/assess mediastinal, vascular, and chest-wall metastasis of lung cancer • Stage lung cancer in patients who are allergic to radiographic contrast media	Patient lies motionless during the procedure. Contraindicated for patients with pacemakers, metallic surgical clips or heart valves, or infusion or chemotherapy pumps. Ventilatory support must be provided manually (BVM) or via a ventilator certified for use in strong magnetic fields. MRI is less accurate than CT for assessing lung parenchyma disease.

(continues)

Table 5-1 Recommending Imaging Studies (continued)

Modality	Recommend To	Comments
PET scan	• Differentiate malignant vs. benign masses • Assess tumor metastases • Assess tumor response to therapy • Determine tumor biopsy site(s) • Detect and localize impaired blood flow to the myocardium	Often combined with CT scanning to enhance diagnostic accuracy. Most common use in pulmonary medicine is to diagnose, stage, and evaluate treatment of non–small cell lung cancer.
Pulmonary angiography	• Evaluate the pulmonary arteries for pulmonary embolism, stenosis, AV malformation, or aneurysm	Contraindicated in patients with bleeding abnormalities (high PT or PTT), extremely high blood pressure, or shock. Being replaced by CT angiography.
V/Q scan	• Detect and quantify effect of pulmonary embolism • Assess regional pulmonary blood flow in patients undergoing lung resection surgery	Patient must be able to cooperate during the test (e.g., breathe through a mouthpiece, hold the breath for 10 seconds or more, and remain still for about 15 minutes).
Transthoracic ultrasound	• Detect free fluid in the thorax (pleural or pericardial effusion, hemithorax, etc.) • Detect pneumothorax • Detect mediastinal masses • Detect pulmonary atelectasis or consolidation • Assess the pleural surfaces for pleuritis or granulomatous processes • Assess thoracic wall lesions and rib masses • Assess trauma to the diaphragm, heart, and large thoracic blood vessels, as well as fractures of the ribs and sternum • Guide thoracentesis and percutaneous needle biopsies	Generally ineffective in imaging tissues or organs *through* aerated lung tissue or pneumothorax.

BAL also is one of the best tools available to diagnose bacterial ventilator-associated pneumonia (VAP) and can be helpful in confirming a diagnosis of various lung cancers (squamous cell, small cell carcinoma, and adenocarcinoma). The only major contraindication to BAL is a predisposition for bleeding.

Sputum Gram Stain, Culture, and Sensitivity

You should recommend a sputum Gram stain and culture and sensitivity (C&S) on any patient suspected of having a respiratory tract infection such as pneumonia and for whom focused antibiotic therapy might be needed. By identifying whether the organisms are primarily Gram+ or Gram−, the Gram stain can be used to as a general guide to initial antibiotic therapy. By determining which *specific* antibiotics the organisms are susceptible to, the subsequent C&S study can help the doctor decide on the most appropriate drug or drugs to prescribe for the patient. Because organism identification by culturing can require 2 or more days, this method is being replaced by more rapid techniques such as antibody and DNA testing.

Pulmonary Function Testing

Pulmonary function testing ranges from simple bedside assessment of peak flows to computerized plethysmographic measurement of airway resistance and thoracic gas volume. **Table 5-2** outlines the primary reasons why you would recommend each of these tests for your patients.

Lung Mechanics

The term "lung mechanics" broadly refers to the physical properties of the lungs and thorax. More specifically, lung mechanics reflect the relationships among pressure, volume, and flow as related to the elastic and frictional forces opposing ventilation. Elastic resistance to ventilation is measured as *compliance* of the lungs, thorax, and lungs/thorax combined. Frictional opposition to ventilation is measured

Table 5-2 Recommending Common Pulmonary Function Tests

Specific Test	Recommend To
Peak expiratory flow rate (PEFR)	• Monitor asthma patients' airway tone over time (via diary) • Assess changes in airway tone in response to bronchodilator therapy (usually performed by the patient)
Bedside spirometry	• Screen for lung dysfunction suggested by history and physical indicators or abnormal diagnostic tests (e.g., ABGs or X-rays) • Assess changes in lung function in response to treatment • Assess the risk for surgical procedures known to affect lung function
Pre-/post-bronchodilator spirometry (bedside or lab)	• Confirm need for therapy • Individualize the patient's medication dose • Determine patient status during acute and long-term drug therapy • Determine if a change in dose, frequency, or medication is needed
Laboratory spirometry (FVC volumes and flows)	• Quantify the severity and prognosis associated with lung or chest wall disease • Follow-up on bedside spirometry results that are not definitive (e.g., restrictive conditions) • Assess the potential pulmonary effects of environmental or occupational exposures • Monitor for adverse reactions to drugs with known pulmonary toxicity • Assess the degree of pulmonary impairment for rehabilitation placement or disability claims
Maximum voluntary ventilation (MVV)	• Assess the integrated function of the airways, lungs, thoracic cage, and respiratory muscles • Evaluate preoperative pulmonary function • Predict breathing reserve for exercise testing • Evaluate respiratory disability
Functional residual capacity (FRC) and total lung capacity (TLC)	• Evaluate the degree of hyperinflation in obstructive abnormalities • Determine volume of gas-trapped gas cysts or bullae (requires comparison of He dilution or N_2 washout to body plethysmography determination of thoracic gas volume)

(continues)

Table 5-2 Recommending Common Pulmonary Function Tests (continued)

Specific Test	Recommend To
Carbon monoxide diffusing capacity (DLco)	• Evaluate and follow the course of parenchymal and interstitial lung diseases such as pulmonary fibrosis, pneumoconiosis, and sarcoidosis • Evaluate and follow the course of emphysema and cystic fibrosis • Differentiate among chronic bronchitis, emphysema, and asthma in patients with obstructive patterns • Quantify the degree of pulmonary impairment for disability claims • Evaluate cardiovascular disorders affecting diffusion or pulmonary blood flow • Evaluate the pulmonary effects of systemic diseases such as rheumatoid arthritis and lupus • Evaluate the effects of drugs known to cause pulmonary damage, such as amiodarone and bleomycin • Help predict arterial desaturation during exercise in patients with lung disease
Bronchial provocation (methacholine challenge test)	• Exclude a diagnosis of airway hyperreactivity • Evaluate occupational asthma • Assess the severity of airway hyperresponsiveness • Determine the relative risk of developing asthma • Assess response to therapeutic interventions
Airway resistance (body plethysmography)	• Evaluate airway responsiveness to provocation • Identify the specific type and severity of obstructive lung disease • Localize the primary site of flow limitation

as *airway resistance*. How you measure these mechanical properties on mechanically ventilated patients is discussed in Chapter 13. Here we focus on *why* you would recommend measuring lung mechanics.

The four most common measures of lung mechanics obtained on mechanically ventilated patients are static compliance, airway resistance, the pressure-volume curve, and the flow-volume curve. Most often, static compliance and airway resistance are computed using the end-inspiratory occlusion method (inspiratory hold). Pressure-volume and flow-volume curves are generated by the ventilator's sensors and can be continuously displayed on a graphics screen. **Table 5-3** summarizes when you should recommend each of these measures of lung mechanics on patients receiving ventilatory support.

Blood Gas Analysis, Pulse Oximetry, and Transcutaneous Monitoring

No aspect of bedside assessment is more important in respiratory care than the monitoring and evaluation of oxygenation, ventilation, and acid–base status. These processes are best assessed by measuring relevant blood parameters, either invasively (by arterial sampling) or noninvasively through the skin or in the expired air.

Oxygenation of arterial blood can be assessed by blood gas analysis (ABGs), hemoximetry, pulse oximetry, and transcutaneous Po_2 monitoring (mainly in infants and children). Ventilation can be assessed by ABGs or transcutaneous monitoring of Pco_2 (capnography also can be used to assess ventilation and is discussed here in a separate section). Full assessment of acid-base status requires an ABG. However, the ventilatory component of acid-base balance can be determined noninvasively by measuring either the transcutaneous or end-tidal Pco_2. **Table 5-4** outlines the key indications for these various measurements, as recommended by the AARC.

Regarding these measurement methods, ABG analysis is always the gold standard against which all other measures are compared. *If the goal is the most accurate evaluation of oxygenation, ventilation, and acid-base status, always recommend ABG analysis.*

Table 5-3 Recommending Measures of Lung Mechanics

Measure	Recommend To
Static compliance	• Regularly monitor patients during patient-ventilator system check • Detect trends in patients subject to rapid changes in lung "stiffness" (e.g., ARDS, pulmonary edema)
Airway resistance	• Regularly monitor patients during patient-ventilator system check • Detect trends in patients subject to rapid changes in airway caliber (e.g., asthma)
Pressure-volume curve	• Detect trends in patients subject to rapid changes in lung "stiffness" (e.g., ARDS, pulmonary edema [*slope* of curve]) • Detect trends in patients subject to rapid changes in airway caliber (e.g., asthma [*width* of curve]) • Detect suspected overinflation ("beaking" appearance) • Determine optimum PEEP level (just above lower inflection point)
Flow-volume curve	• Assess response to bronchodilator therapy (changes in peak expiratory flow and slope of expiratory flow curve) • Detect auto-PEEP (expiratory flow does not return to baseline before start of next breath)

Table 5-4 Indications for Various Invasive and Noninvasive Blood Measurement

Method	Indications
Blood gas analysis	• Evaluate ventilation ($Paco_2$), acid-base (pH, $Paco_2$, and HCO_3), and oxygenation ($Paco_2$) status • Assess the patient's response to therapy and/or perform diagnostic tests (e.g., O_2 therapy, exercise testing) • Monitor severity and progression of a documented disease process
Hemoximetry (CO-oximetry)	• Determine *actual* blood O_2 saturation (as opposed to that computed with a simple blood gas analyzer) • Measure abnormal Hb levels (HbCO, metHb, and sulfhemoglobin)
Pulse oximetry	• Monitor the adequacy of arterial oxyhemoglobin saturation • Quantify the response of arterial oxyhemoglobin saturation to therapeutic intervention or to diagnostic procedure (e.g., bronchoscopy) • Comply with mandated regulations or recommendations by authoritative groups (e.g., anesthesia monitoring)
Transcutaneous monitoring ($Ptco_2$, $Ptcco_2$)	• Continuously monitor the adequacy of arterial oxygenation and/or ventilation • Continuously monitor for excessive arterial oxygenation (hyperoxia) • Quantify real-time changes in ventilation and oxygenation due to diagnostic or therapeutic interventions • Assess functional shunts or determine the response to an O_2 challenge in patients with congenital heart disease

The only real limitations of ABG analysis are that (1) it does not measure actual hemoglobin content or saturation and (2) it does not reveal the presence of abnormal hemoglobins, such as carboxyhemoglobin (HbCO). If you need accurate measures of any of these parameters, you *must* use or recommend hemoximetry (CO-oximetry). The most common patient scenario in which you should recommend hemoximetry is smoke inhalation/CO poisoning. In addition, you should recommend hemoximetry when you need to calibrate pulse oximetry reading (SpO_2) against the actual arterial saturation.

Often called the "fifth vital sign," pulse oximetry is the most widely used measure of blood oxygenation. However, *it should never be substituted for ABG analysis or hemoximetry when the clinical situation demands accurate assessment of blood oxygenation.* You should also recommend *against* reliance on pulse oximetry data for patients with poor peripheral perfusion and when there is a need to monitor for or warn of hyperoxemia, as when protecting a premature infant against retrolental fibroplasia.

Traditionally, transcutaneous PO_2 and PcO_2 monitoring has been limited to infants and small children in need of continuous monitoring of oxygenation and ventilation. However, recent research indicates that the $PtcCO_2$ can be reliably measured in hemodynamically stable adults, making it a good choice for continuous monitoring of ventilation when capnography is unavailable or impractical—e.g., during noninvasive ventilation. However, the calibration time and long warm-up period needed when applying a new transcutaneous sensor to any patient means that this method should never be recommended to assess oxygenation in emergencies.

Capnography

As indicated above, capnography (expired CO_2 analysis) is an alternative method for noninvasively assessing a patient's ventilation. You should recommend capnography when the need exists to:

- Noninvasively monitor the effectiveness ($PETCO_2$) and efficiency ($PaCO_2$-$PETCO_2$) of ventilation, usually during mechanical ventilation
- Monitor the severity of pulmonary disease and assess the response to therapies intended to lower physiologic deadspace and/or better match ventilation to perfusion (V/Q)
- Determine endotracheal tube placement (tracheal vs. esophageal intubation)
- Monitor levels of therapeutically administered CO_2 gas
- Measure CO_2 production (to assess metabolic rate)
- Provide graphic data useful in evaluating the ventilator-patient interface

Note first that the AARC recommends *against* using capnography on all patients receiving mechanical ventilation. Second, in terms of endotracheal intubation, simple colorimetric CO_2 detectors are sufficient to help determine tube placement, which precludes the need for a capnograph just for this purpose.

Regarding graphic evaluation of the ventilator-patient interface, end-tidal CO_2 trend analysis can indicate potential hyper/hypoventilation, which should be confirmed by ABG analysis. Analysis of the shape of the capnogram at high sweep speed also can be helpful in identifying conditions such as circuit rebreathing, esophageal intubation, and maldistribution of ventilation. More detail on the analysis of the capnogram is provided in Chapter 13.

Electrocardiography

You should recommend obtaining a 12-lead electrocardiogram to:

- Screen for heart disease (e.g., CAD, left ventricular hypertrophy)
- Rule out heart disease in surgical patients
- Evaluate patients with chest pain
- Follow the progression of patients with CAD
- Evaluate heart rhythm disorders (using rhythm strips)

A 12-lead ECG also can be used to help assess the effect of metabolic disorders associated with electrolyte disturbances—in particular, calcium and potassium imbalances.

Hemodynamic Monitoring

Hemodynamic monitoring ranges from simple and safe noninvasive methods, such as auscultatory assessment of arterial blood pressure, to complex and hazardous invasive techniques, such as pulmonary artery catheterization. In general, the more critically ill the patient, the greater the need for invasive hemodynamic monitoring.

Noninvasive Blood Pressure Measurement

As a component of the vital signs, blood pressure should be measured noninvasively on a regular basis on all patients. The frequency of measurement varies according to the patient's cardiovascular stability. Automated noninvasive bedside systems allow setting of measurement intervals as short as every 5 minutes.

Invasive Hemodynamic Monitoring

Although the decision to insert an indwelling catheter is a medical one, you need to be aware of the circumstances in which your patients could benefit from hemodynamic monitoring. Likewise, given the many hazards and complications associated with invasive hemodynamic monitoring, you must be knowledgeable of the contraindications against the use of indwelling catheters. This knowledge is particularly important for arterial lines ("A-lines"), which are often recommended, inserted, and removed by respiratory therapists. **Table 5-5** summarizes the key indications and contraindications for indwelling catheters by location.

Sleep Studies

Sleep studies that respiratory therapists might recommend include overnight pulse oximetry and polysomnography.

Overnight Oximetry

You should recommend overnight oximetry to:

- Help identify patients with obstructive sleep apnea–hypopnea syndrome (SAHS)
- Help assess SAHS patients' response to therapy, such as CPAP
- Identify whether serious desaturation occurs in COPD patients during sleep

In terms of diagnosing SAHS, the gold standard is laboratory polysomnography, which includes oximetry. However, polysomnography is expensive and not readily available to all patients with suspected sleep-disordered breathing. In comparison, overnight oximetry is readily available, inexpensive, and can be performed in the patient's home.

In regard to screening those with COPD, it is well known that some of these patients experience large drops in arterial O_2 saturation during sleep. In general, the occurrence of nocturnal desaturation in these individuals can be predicted from their daytime saturation or PO_2 levels and is probably due to hypoventilation occurring during periods of REM sleep. When considering screening COPD patients for possible nocturnal desaturation, the focus should be on those with hypercapnia, erythrocytosis, and/or evidence of pulmonary hypertension.

Polysomnography

In general, you should recommend polysomnography for patients who complain of or exhibit signs or symptoms associated with sleep-disordered breathing (e.g., daytime somnolence and fatigue, morning headaches, pulmonary hypertension, and polycythemia). According to the AARC, polysomnography is specifically indicated in patients with:

- COPD whose daytime Pao_2 exceeds 55 torr and whose condition includes one or more of the following complications: pulmonary hypertension, right heart failure, polycythemia, or excessive daytime sleepiness
- Chest wall or neuromuscular restrictive disorders and whose condition includes one or more of the following complications: chronic hypoventilation, polycythemia, pulmonary hypertension, disturbed sleep, morning headaches, daytime somnolence, and fatigue

Table 5-5 Indications and Contraindications for Indwelling Catheters

Indications	Contraindications
Systemic Arterial Monitoring	
• To continuously monitor arterial pressure in unstable/hypotensive patients • To continuously monitor patients receiving vasoactive drugs • To obtain frequent ABGs to assess patients in respiratory failure or receiving mechanical ventilation	• Inadequate collateral arterial circulation (negative Allen test) • Evidence of infection or peripheral vascular disease in the selected limb • Severe coagulopathy (e.g., platelet count < 50,000 or PTT > 37 sec) • Presence of a surgical/dialysis shunt in the selected arm (consider contralateral limb)
Central Venous Monitoring	
• To monitor central venous pressure/right ventricular function in unstable or hypotensive patients • To provide volume resuscitation (*note:* a 14- or 16-gauge peripheral IV is equivalent) • To infuse drugs that can cause peripheral phlebitis (e.g., certain vasopressors and chemotherapeutic agents) • To provide a route for total parenteral nutrition (TPN) • To perform plasmapheresis or hemodialysis • To introduce transvenous pacing wires • To provide venous access in patients with poor peripheral veins	• Evidence of infection at the insertion site • Distorted anatomy at the insertion site (e.g., vascular injury, prior surgery, radiation therapy, rib/clavicle fractures, chest wall deformity) • Suspected injury to the superior vena cava • Severe coagulopathy (e.g., platelet count < 50,000 or PTT > 37 sec [*note:* the subclavian vein cannot be compressed to stop bleeding]) • Presence of intravascular pacemaker or vena cava filter • Severe obesity (causing technical difficulties) • Bullous lung disease (high risk of pneumothorax)
Pulmonary Artery Monitoring	
• To identify the cause of various shock states • To identify the cause of pulmonary edema • To diagnose pulmonary hypertension • To diagnose valvular disease, intracardiac shunts, cardiac tamponade, and pulmonary embolus • To monitor and manage complicated myocardial infarction • To assess the hemodynamic response to therapies • To manage multiple organ failure and/or severe burns • To manage hemodynamic instability after cardiac surgery • To optimize fluid and inotropic therapy • To measure tissue oxygenation and selected hemodynamic indices, including cardiac output • To perform atrial and ventricular pacing (specialized PA catheters)	• Wolff-Parkinson-White syndrome (PA catheters can induce arrhythmias) • Left bundle branch block (due to the risk of complete heart block) • Tricuspid or pulmonary valve endocarditis, stenosis, or mechanical prosthesis • Right heart mass (thrombus and/or tumor) • Infection at the insertion site • The presence of an RV assist device, transvenous pacemaker, or defibrillator • Severe coagulopathy (e.g., platelet count < 50,000 or PTT > 37 sec)

- Disorders of respiratory control with chronic hypoventilation (daytime $Paco_2$ > 45 torr) or whose illness is complicated by pulmonary hypertension, polycythemia, disturbed sleep, morning headaches, daytime somnolence, and fatigue
- Nocturnal cyclic brady or tachyarrhythmias, nocturnal AV conduction abnormalities, or ventricular ectopic beats that increase during sleep
- Excessive daytime sleepiness or sleep maintenance insomnia
- Snoring associated with observed apneas and/or excessive daytime sleepiness

Polysomnography is also indicated to help diagnose certain neurologic and movement disorders such as restless leg syndrome and nocturnal seizures, as well as parasomnias like sleepwalking. Last, polysomnography is used to assess the adequacy of sleep-related interventions, including titrating CPAP in patients with obstructive sleep apnea and determining the BiPAP™ levels for patients with central sleep apneas or respiratory insufficiency due to chronic neuromuscular disorders, such as amyotrophic lateral sclerosis.

COMMON ERRORS TO AVOID

You can improve your score by avoiding these mistakes:

- Never recommend diagnostic bronchoscopy in patients who are hemodynamically unstable or cannot be adequately oxygenated during the procedure due to severe refractory hypoxemia.
- Never let pulse oximetry data substitute for ABG analysis or hemoximetry when the clinical situation demands accurate assessment blood oxygenation.
- Never use a capnograph to verify endotracheal tube placement when simpler methods (such as colorimetric CO_2 detectors) are available.
- Never recommend or insert a radial arterial line when the Allen test indicates inadequate collateral circulation on that side.

SURE BETS

In some situations you can always be sure of the right approach to a clinical problem or scenario:

- You should always recommend a sputum Gram stain and culture and sensitivity on any patient suspected of having a respiratory tract infection.
- To determine if a change in the dose or frequency of administration of an aerosolized bronchodilator is needed, always recommend pre-/post-bronchodilator spirometry.
- To assess the presence and severity of restrictive abnormalities, always recommend both TLC/FRC measurement and the diffusing capacity test (DLCO).
- Always recommend ABG analysis whenever the need exists to evaluate ventilation, acid–base balance, and/or oxygenation status.
- Always recommend CO-oximetry for patients suspected of suffering smoke inhalation.
- Always recommend polysomnography for patients who complain of or exhibit signs or symptoms associated with sleep-disordered breathing, such as daytime somnolence and fatigue.

PRE-TEST ANSWERS AND EXPLANATIONS

Below are this chapter's pre-test answers and explanations. Be sure to review each answer's explanation thoroughly to help you understand why it is correct. If the explanation is still unclear to you, review the chapter contents or the references and/or refer to this chapter's supplemental resources on the CD.

5-1. **Correct answer: D.** Fiberoptic bronchoscopy. Injury from toxic inhalation or aspiration most immediately affects the airways. In these patients the location and extent of injury is best determined initially using fiberoptic bronchoscopy.

5-2. Correct answer: C. Bronchoalveolar lavage. A sputum culture and sensitivity could help diagnose this problem. However, bronchoalveolar lavage (BAL) is one of the best tools available to diagnose bacterial ventilator-associated pneumonia (VAP) and is thus the better choice for this patient. According to the American Thoracic Society, bronchoalveolar lavage (BAL) is indicated in patients with nonresolving pneumonia, unexplained lung infiltrates (interstitial and/or alveolar), and suspected alveolar hemorrhage.

5-3. Correct answer: C. Capnography. Capnography (expired CO_2 analysis) is used primarily to noninvasively monitor the effectiveness (P_{ETCO_2}) and efficiency (P_{aCO_2}-P_{ETCO_2}) of ventilation, usually during mechanical ventilation. Most capnographs can also compute the accumulated volume of CO_2 over time if the expired minute ventilation is known or measured. CO_2 production per minute is one measure of metabolic activity, the other being O_2 consumption.

5-4. Correct answer: A. Diffusing capacity (D_{LCO}). The primary indication for the carbon monoxide diffusing capacity (D_{LCO}) test is to evaluate and follow the course of parenchymal and interstitial lung diseases such as pulmonary fibrosis, pneumoconiosis, and sarcoidosis. In addition, the D_{LCO} test can be used to differentiate among the various patterns of airway obstruction (emphysema patients typically have a low D_{LCO}) and is helpful in following the course of emphysema and cystic fibrosis. The D_{LCO} test also can help predict arterial desaturation during exercise in patients with lung disease.

5-5. Correct answer: B. Flow-volume loop. Of the tests listed, only the flow-volume loop would help detect the presence of auto-PEEP on a patient receiving ventilatory support. When viewing the flow-volume loop of a patient with auto-PEEP, you will note that the expiratory flow does not return to baseline before the start of the next breath.

5-6. Correct answer: C. Polysomnography. You should recommend polysomnography for patients who complain of or exhibit signs or symptoms associated with sleep-disordered breathing (e.g., daytime somnolence and fatigue, morning headaches, pulmonary hypertension, and polycythemia).

5-7. Correct answer: A. Transcutaneous P_{CO_2} analysis. Although traditionally used only with infants and children, recent research indicates that the transcutaneous P_{CO_2} is an accurate measure of ventilation in hemodynamically stable adults, making it a good choice for continuous monitoring of ventilation when capnography is unavailable or impractical (e.g., during noninvasive ventilation).

5-8. Correct answer: B. Electrocardiogram (ECG). You should recommend obtaining an electrocardiogram to screen for heart disease, rule out heart disease in surgical patients, evaluate patients with chest pain, follow the progression of patients with CAD, and evaluate heart rhythm disorders.

5-9. Correct answer: B. A pulmonary artery catheter. To assess how well the tissues are getting oxygenated, we need to know how much oxygen is *left over* after the blood leaves the capillaries. This measure, called the mixed venous oxygen content (C_{vO_2}), can be obtained only from the distal port of a pulmonary artery catheter.

5-10. Correct answer: B. AP chest X-ray. A standard chest X-ray is not useful in detecting a pulmonary embolism. Pulmonary angiography has been the gold standard, along with V/Q scanning. However, more recently, CT angiography and transthoracic ultrasound have become accepted noninvasive tools for diagnosing pulmonary embolism.

REFERENCES

American Association for Respiratory Care. (1995). Clinical practice guideline. Assessing response to bronchodilator therapy at point of care. *Respiratory Care, 40*, 1300–1307.

American Association for Respiratory Care. (1999). Clinical practice guideline. Single-breath carbon monoxide diffusing capacity. 1999 update. *Respiratory Care, 44*, 539–546.

American Association for Respiratory Care. (2001). Clinical practice guideline. Blood gas analysis and hemoximetry. 2001 revision and update. *Respiratory Care, 46,* 498–505.

American Association for Respiratory Care. (2001). Clinical practice guideline. Methacholine challenge testing. 2001 revision and update. *Respiratory Care, 46,* 523–530.

American Association for Respiratory Care. (2003). Clinical practice guideline. Capnography/capnometry during mechanical ventilation. 2003 revision and update. *Respiratory Care, 48,* 534–539.

American Association for Respiratory Care. (2004). Clinical practice guideline. Transcutaneous blood gas monitoring for neonatal and pediatric patients. 2004 revision and update. *Respiratory Care, 49,* 1070–1072.

American Association for Respiratory Care. (2007). Clinical practice guideline. Bronchoscopy Assisting. 2007 revision and update. *Respiratory Care, 52,* 74–80.

American Association of Sleep Medicine. (2005). Practice parameters for the indications for polysomnography and related procedures: An update for 2005. *Sleep, 28,* 499–519.

Aquino, S. L., Kahn, A., Batra, P. V., et al. (2006). *Expert panel on thoracic imaging. Routine chest radiograph.* Reston, VA: American College of Radiology.

Equipment Application and Cleanliness

Manipulate Equipment by Order or Protocol

Craig L. Scanlan

INTRODUCTION

Manipulate Equipment by Order or Protocol represents the single biggest section of the NBRC CRT exam, with the largest number of analysis-level questions. Historically, it is also one of the areas with which candidates have had the most difficulty. There are two primary reasons for this difficulty. First, this section covers a very broad scope of equipment, some of which you may not use on a daily basis. Second, whereas principles of equipment operation are emphasized in school, the focus in this section is on selecting, adjusting, and troubleshooting equipment (e.g., application and analysis).

Consistent with the importance and difficulty of this section of the exam, this chapter is the largest and most comprehensive in the text. For each category of equipment, we present clear guidelines on selecting, using, and troubleshooting the applicable devices. This information will not only help you score high on questions in this category but also help you do well on other sections of the exam that might have equipment-related questions. For this reason, we recommend returning here whenever you need to clarify how to use equipment properly.

OBJECTIVES

After completion of this chapter, you should demonstrate the knowledge needed to select, use, and troubleshoot the following equipment by order or protocol:

1. Oxygen administration devices
2. Humidifiers, nebulizers, and mist tents
3. Resuscitation devices
4. Ventilators, CPAP devices, and breathing circuits
5. Artificial airways
6. Vacuum systems, suction, and pleural drainage devices
7. Gas cylinders, reducing valves, flowmeters, and O_2 blenders
8. Point-of-care blood gas analyzers
9. Incentive breathing devices
10. Percussors and vibrators
11. Positive expiratory pressure (PEP) and vibratory PEP devices
12. Manometers
13. Bedside pulmonary function devices
14. CO, He, O_2, and specialty gas analyzers
15. ECG monitors and 12-lead ECG machines
16. Noninvasive oximetry monitoring devices
17. Aerosol drug-delivery systems
18. Bronchoscopes

WHAT TO EXPECT ON THIS CATEGORY OF THE CRT EXAM

Number of questions: 22
Level of questions: about 20% recall, 50% application, and 30% analysis

WHAT'S NEW FOR 2009

As of July 2009, this section of the NBRC CRT examination includes the following *new equipment topics*:

- High-flow nasal cannula
- Speaking tubes and valves
- Laryngeal mask airway (LMA)
- Esophageal-tracheal Combitube®
- Oxygen-conserving devices, e.g., reservoir cannula, pulse-dose
- Oxygen concentrators and air compressors
- Oxygen hoods
- ECG monitors
- CO, He, O_2, and specialty gas analyzers
- Bronchoscopes

PRE-TEST

Carefully respond to each of the following questions. After completing the pre-test, compare your answers to those provided at the end of this chapter. Then thoroughly review each answer's explanation to help understand why it is correct.

6-1. You measure an oxygen concentration of 55% being delivered by an air-entrainment mask set to deliver 31% oxygen. Which of the following actions is most appropriate?
  A. Add an aerosol collar to the mask
  B. Decrease the oxygen input flow
  C. Check the entrainment ports
  D. Increase the oxygen input flow

6-2. Which of the following is the approximate total output flow delivered from a 35% air-entrainment mask operating at 8 L/min?
  A. 12 L/min
  B. 48 L/min
  C. 52 L/min
  D. 72 L/min

6-3. You observe that the reservoir bag on a patient receiving O_2 at 10 L/min does not deflate at all when the patient inspires. What should you do *first*?
  A. Tell the patient to breathe deeper
  B. Decrease the O_2 flow to 6 L/min
  C. Check the mask for a snug fit
  D. Remove mask valve flaps

6-4. Which of the following is the most probable cause of insufficient mist in a croup tent?
  A. Decreased temperature within the canopy
  B. Insufficient ice in the cooling chamber
  C. Inadequate size of the tent
  D. A clogged capillary tube in the nebulizer

6-5. A physician specifies in her respiratory orders the following objective for a patient with an artificial airway: "to overcome the patient's humidity deficit." Which of the following aerosol generators should you select for this patient?
  A. Small-volume sidestream jet nebulizer
  B. Large-reservoir heated jet nebulizer
  C. Small-particle aerosol generator (SPAG)
  D. Metered-dose inhaler (MDI)

6-6. During CPR, the oxygen reservoir bag of a bag-valve manual resuscitator collapses during the refill phase. You can correct this problem by:
  A. Shortening the bag refill time
  B. Increasing O_2 flow to the bag
  C. Increasing the rate of compression
  D. Increasing the volume delivery

6-7. While a patient is being ventilated with a bag-valve resuscitator, the bag fills rapidly and collapses on minimal pressure, although little chest movement by the patient is noted. The cause of the problem may be which of the following?
A. Absence of the inlet valve
B. Excessive oxygen flow
C. Plugged endotracheal (ET) tube
D. Plugged inlet valve

6-8. An intubated adult patient with severe expiratory airway obstruction requires ventilatory support. Which of the following factors is most important in selecting a ventilator for this patient?
A. Ability to compensate for airway interface leaks
B. Variable flow control and adjustable I:E ratios
C. Ability to run on 12-volt DC (battery) power
D. Certification for use during MRI procedures

6-9. Which of the following types of breathing circuits should you select when assembling a home-care ventilator?
A. Dual-limb "Y" circuit
B. Single-limb circuit with expiratory balloon valve
C. Single-limb circuit with leakage-type exhaust port
D. Single-limb circuit without any valve

6-10. To provide a low to moderate concentration of oxygen to a patient receiving nasal BiPAP™ via a device that uses a turbine or blower to generate pressure, you should:
A. Connect the BiPAP™ device to a 50-psi O_2 outlet
B. Apply a nasal cannula to the patient under the mask
C. Bleed supplemental O_2 from a flowmeter into the circuit
D. Add a reservoir bag to the BiPAP™ breathing circuit

6-11. Which of the following alarm conditions indicates a potential system leak when delivering volume-oriented ventilatory support?
A. High volume + low pressure
B. Low volume + high pressure
C. High volume + high pressure
D. Low volume + low pressure

6-12. A patient with a chronic neuromuscular condition requires nocturnal positive pressure ventilation over the long term. Which of the following airways should you recommend for this patient?
A. Oral ET tube
B. Fenestrated tracheostomy tube
C. Laryngeal mask airway
D. Standard tracheostomy tube

6-13. Which of the following would indicate an obstruction in the ET tube of a patient who is being mechanically ventilated by a volume-cycled ventilator?
I. High pressure is required to deliver the volume
II. The low-pressure alarm is sounding
III. A suction catheter cannot be passed
A. I and III only
B. I and II only
C. I, II, and III
D. II and III only

6-14. Prior to intubation in an emergency, injection of air into the pilot line fails to inflate the cuff. You should:
A. Check the cuff for leaks
B. Check the valve on the pilot line
C. Replace the ET tube
D. Inspect the pilot line for patency

6-15. Resistance is encountered while suctioning through a size 6-mm ID ET tube with a 14-Fr catheter. Which of the following is the most appropriate action for you to take?
A. Lubricate the catheter
B. Use a 10-Fr catheter
C. Turn the patient's head
D. Instill normal saline solution

6-16. All of the following could cause suctioning to stop suddenly during tracheobronchial aspiration *except*:
A. Disconnected tubing
B. Clearance of secretions
C. A full suction reservoir
D. A mucous plug in the catheter

6-17. About how many hours will an H-cylinder of oxygen last if it has 1100 psig and is emptying at a flow of 8 L/min?
A. 0.6 hours
B. 8.2 hours
C. 7.2 hours
D. 0.7 hours

6-18. After attaching a yoke connector to an E-size cylinder and opening the cylinder valve, you notice a leak at the gas outlet. Which of the following are possible causes for this leak?
   I. The gas outlet bushing is missing or damaged
   II. Missing pin-indexed safety system (PISS) pins
   III. The yoke hand screw is not tight enough
A. I and II only
B. II and III only
C. I and III only
D. I, II, and III

6-19. While obtaining an arterial sample for analysis using a point-of-care analyzer, you should do all of the following *except*:
A. Analyze the sample within 3 minutes
B. Place the sample in an ice slush
C. Thoroughly mix the sample
D. Prevent sample exposure to air

6-20. An alert 55-year-old patient who two days earlier had abdominal surgery has moderate basilar crackles on the left side, a respiratory rate of 13 breaths/min, and an SpO_2 of 96% on nasal cannula at 2 L/min. The surgeon is concerned that the patient may be developing atelectasis. Which of the following approaches should you select to manage this patient?
A. Intermittent positive pressure breathing
B. Incentive breathing therapy
C. Postural drainage and percussion
D. Aerosolized bronchodilator therapy

6-21. To apply vibrations to a patient when using an electrically powered percussor during postural drainage, you should use the _____ available frequency and apply during _____ only.
A. Highest; exhalation
B. Lowest; exhalation
C. Highest; inhalation
D. Lowest; inhalation

6-22. After setting up a flow-resistor expiratory airway pressure (PEP) device for a patient with postoperative atelectasis, you note that the system does not generate *any* pressure during active patient expiration. Your first action in this case should be to:
A. Dispose of the device and get a new one
B. Recheck and tighten all connections
C. Select and connect a larger orifice
D. Have the patient exert less expiratory effort

6-23. You can use a fluid column pressure manometer for all of the following *except*:
A. To measure atmospheric pressure
B. To measure static pressures
C. To calibrate other manometers
D. To measure rapid pressure changes

6-24. You need to measure the forced vital capacity (FVC) of an adult patient at the bedside. Which of the following devices should you select to make this measurement?
A. A computerized electronic spirometer with flow sensor
B. Strain-gauge pressure transducer and amplifier
C. Mechanical turbine-type volumeter/Wright respirometer
D. Water-sealed bell spirometer with high-speed kymograph

6-25. Upon inspection of a portable spirometer's FVC curve obtained on an adult outpatient, you determine that the back extrapolated volume is excessive. Prior to repeating the maneuver, which of the following instructions should you provide to the patient?
A. "Don't hesitate"
B. "Blast out faster"
C. "Blow out longer"
D. "Breathe deeper"

6-26. After setting up a 12-lead ECG on a patient, you note a noisy and unstable signal. All of the following would help to resolve this problem *except*:
   A. Verifying that the leads are connected properly
   B. Checking the ECG main lead cable for damage
   C. Turning off filtering of extraneous electrical activity
   D. Confirming that the patient is staying motionless

6-27. To spot check a patient's oxygen saturation at the bedside, you should select which of the following?
   A. Oxygen analyzer
   B. Hemoximeter
   C. Transcutaneous monitor
   D. Pulse oximeter

6-28. A neonatal intensive care unit (NICU) nurse calls you to check an infant on a transcutaneous P_{O_2}/P_{CO_2} monitor due to a rapid rise in Ptc_{O_2} and concurrent fall in Ptc_{CO_2} to below 10 torr. The most likely cause of this problem is:
   A. The presence of peripheral vasoconstriction
   B. A defective sensor or sensor membrane

   C. Interference due to bright ambient lighting
   D. Air leakage around the sensor's adhesive ring

6-29. A 2-year-old child is admitted to the emergency department with severe asthmatic symptoms. The attending physician orders a bronchodilator that is available in both solution and MDI preparations. Which of the following is the best delivery system for this drug to this patient?
   A. Breath-actuated MDI with mask
   B. Small-volume nebulizer (SVN) with mouthpiece
   C. MDI with holding chamber and a mask
   D. SVN using the "blow by" technique

6-30. Which of the following is the preferred delivery method for cromolyn sodium to young children?
   A. MDI with mask
   B. Small-volume nebulizer
   C. MDI with holding chamber
   D. Dry powder inhaler

WHAT YOU NEED TO KNOW: ESSENTIAL CONTENT

Oxygen Administration Devices

According to the American Association for Respiratory Therapy (AARC), you should select or recommend oxygen therapy in the following situations:

- Documented hypoxemia (Pa_{O_2} < 60 torr or Sa_{O_2} < 90% on room air)
- Signs of hypoxemia (e.g., dyspnea, tachypnea, tachycardia, cyanosis, confusion)
- Severe trauma
- Acute myocardial infarction
- Short-term therapy or surgical intervention (e.g., post-anesthesia recovery)

Available Devices

Most O_2 devices are categorized as being either low- or high-flow systems. **Table 6-1** summarizes these devices, their flow settings, F_{IO_2} ranges, advantages, disadvantages, and best use.

Low-Flow Devices

Low-flow devices include standard nasal cannulas and masks. These devices deliver O_2 at *flows that are less than the patient's inspiratory flow*, so that the O_2 is always diluted with some room air. **Table 6-2** (see page 153) summarizes factors affecting the amount of air dilution and the F_{IO_2} in low-flow systems.

Table 6-1 Common Oxygen Administration Devices

Device	Flow	FIO$_2$ Range	Advantages	Disadvantages	Best Use
Low Flow					
Standard nasal cannula	¼–8 L/min (adults) ≤ 2 L/min (infants)	22–45%	Can be used on adults, children, and infants Easy to apply Disposable Low cost Well-tolerated	Unstable, easily dislodged High flows uncomfortable Can cause dryness/ bleeding Polyps, deviated septum may block flow	Stable patient needing low FIO$_2$ Home care patient requiring long-term therapy
Simple mask	5–10 L/min	35–50%	Can be used on adults, children, and infants Quick, easy to apply Disposable; inexpensive	Uncomfortable Must be removed for eating Prevents radiant heat loss Blocks vomitus in unconscious patients	Emergencies Short-term therapy requiring moderate FIO$_2$
Partial rebreathing mask	6–10 L/min (prevent bag collapse)	40–70%	Same as for simple mask Moderate to high FIO$_2$s	Same as for simple mask Potential suffocation hazard	Emergencies Short-term therapy requiring moderate to high FIO$_2$s
Nonrebreathing mask	Minimum 10 L/min (prevent bag collapse)	60–80%	Same as for simple mask High FIO$_2$s	Same as for simple mask Potential suffocation hazard	Emergencies Short-term therapy requiring high FIO$_2$s
High Flow					
Air-entrainment mask	Varies; output should be > 60 L/min to ensure FIO$_2$	24–50%	Easy to apply Disposable Inexpensive Stable, precise FIO$_2$s	Limited to adult use Uncomfortable Noisy Must be removed for eating FIO$_2$ ≥ 0.35 not ensured FIO$_2$ varies with back pressure	Unstable patient requiring precise, low FIO$_2$

(continues)

Table 6-1 Common Oxygen Administration Devices (continued)

Device	Flow	F_{IO_2} Range	Advantages	Disadvantages	Best Use
Air-entrainment nebulizer	10–15 L/min input; output should be > 60 L/min to ensure F_{IO_2}	28–100%	Provides temperature control and extra humidity	F_{IO_2} < 28% or ≥ 0.35 not ensured F_{IO_2} varies with back pressure High infection risk	Patients with artificial airways requiring low to moderate F_{IO_2}s via T-tube or trach mask; post extubation (aerosol mask)
High-flow nasal cannula	1–40 L/min adults; 1–20 L/min children; 1–8 L/min infants	24–95%	Easy to apply Stable, precise F_{IO_2}s Provides gas at BTPS without condensation Meets/exceeds nonrebreather performance Decreases anatomic deadspace (CO_2 washout)	Requires special (proprietary) cannulas and heating/humidification system Can create occult CPAP Potential electrical risks Some units associated with contamination/infection	As an alternative to a nonrebreathing mask in patients requiring precise moderate to high F_{IO_2}; including those with claustrophobia or facial burns Patients with traumatic or postop hypothermia patients requiring heliox or NO therapy

Adapted from: Wilkins, R. L., Stoller, J. K., & Scanlan, C. L. (2003). *Egan's fundamentals of respiratory care,* (8th ed.). St. Louis: Mosby.

Table 6-2 Factors Affecting the F_{IO_2} of Low-Flow Oxygen Systems

Less Air Dilution Higher F_{IO_2}	More Air Dilution Lower F_{IO_2}
Device related	
Higher O_2 input	Lower O_2 input
Reservoir present (mask)	Reservoir absent (cannula)
Leak present (masks)	Leak absent (masks)
Valves present (masks)	Valves absent (masks)
Patient related	
Lower inspiratory flow	Higher inspiratory flow
Lower tidal volume	Higher tidal volume
Slower rate of breathing	Faster rate of breathing
Smaller minute volume	Larger minute volume

Note that the F_{IO_2} ranges described in Table 6-1 for low-flow systems are estimates only. *For normal adults receiving nasal O_2, we estimate that each L/min of O_2 raises the F_{IO_2} by about 4%.* For example, a patient on a nasal cannula at 2 L/min would have an estimated F_{IO_2} of about 29% (21 + 8). However, given the large number of factors affecting the F_{IO_2}s, you never can be sure exactly how much O_2 a patient is receiving from a low-flow system. For this reason, you should always rely on evaluating the patient's actual response to therapy, as described in Chapter 13.

Special consideration is required when continuous low-flow oxygen therapy is prescribed for patients in the home and ambulatory care settings (refer to Chapter 19). In these settings, we try to make the most efficient use of the available oxygen and/or extend the time available to patients when using portable O_2. Both goals are accomplished using *oxygen-conserving devices.*

Oxygen-conserving devices are designed to overcome the inefficiency of standard nasal cannulas, which typically waste about 1/2 to 2/3 of the delivered O_2. This waste can be minimized either by (1) providing a reservoir to accumulate the O_2 normally lost during exhalation (continuous-flow systems), or (2) providing the flow *only when needed*, i.e., during inspiration (intermittent-flow systems). **Table 6-3** identifies the currently available O_2-conserving devices according to these categories.

Compared with standard nasal cannulas, these devices can reduce O_2 usage by 50–75%. For an ambulatory patient carrying a full D cylinder, that difference would extend the available time of usage from about 1½ hours up to 5 hours.

Reservoir cannulas employ a small reservoir (either below the nose or at chest level) that stores O_2 during exhalation and releases it during inhalation. Unfortunately, many patients object to the appearance of these devices and fail to comply with their prescribed use, especially outside the home.

A transtracheal O_2 catheter delivers oxygen directly into the trachea through a small neck stoma. In this case, the reservoir is the trachea and lower airway itself. Given that catheter placement involves a surgical procedure and that comprehensive education and ongoing support are required to ensure proper and safe patient usage, transtracheal O_2 therapy has fallen into disfavor.

Due to the many limitations of continuous-flow O_2-conserving devices, intermittent-flow systems have become the equipment of choice for improving the efficiency of O_2 delivery in the ambulatory care setting. As indicated in Table 6-3, intermittent-flow O_2-conserving devices include pulse-dose and demand-flow systems. These devices are electronically or pneumatically controlled systems that use a sensor to detect the onset of inspiration and trigger a valve to deliver O_2 only during that phase of breathing. Whereas pulse-dose systems deliver a rapid flow or "bolus" of O_2 at the start of inspiration, demand-flow systems deliver O_2 continuously throughout the inspiratory cycle, but at a lower flow.

Unfortunately, manufacturers of O_2-conserving devices each have their own protocol to set and adjust these systems. As a rule of thumb, *when switching patients from a standard nasal cannula to an O_2-conserving device, you should start them out at 1/2 the original flow and then adjust the flow to achieve the desired saturation, as determined by pulse oximetry.* This should be done both at rest and under the work or exertion levels that the patient will commonly encounter day to day.

In terms of troubleshooting these systems, responsibility for action generally will be with the patient. For this reason the cardinal troubleshooting rule is that *whenever patients suspect a problem, they must switch to a backup supply of continuous O_2 via nasal cannula at the equivalent liter flow* (2–3 times that of the O_2-conserving device). More in-depth troubleshooting guidelines for electrically controlled pulse-dose O_2-delivery systems are provided in **Table 6-4**.

High-Flow Devices

High-flow devices deliver an O_2 mixture at *flows* greater *than the patient's inspiratory flow*, thereby generally ensuring a fixed and stable F_{IO_2}. Most high-flow systems function on the principle of air entrainment. Air entrainment occurs when source O_2 is driven through a high-velocity gas jet, which draws

Table 6-3 Oxygen-Conserving Devices

Continuous-Flow Systems	Intermittent-Flow Systems
Reservoir cannulas	Pulse-dose systems
Transtracheal catheter	Demand-flow systems

Table 6-4 Troubleshooting Common Problems with Electrically Controlled Pulse-Dose O$_2$-Delivery Systems

Problem	Possible Causes	Remedies
Low battery light flashes	Batteries are low	Replace old batteries with new batteries
Alarm stays on	Batteries are low	Replace old batteries with new batteries
	No inspiration is sensed	Turn unit off then back on to reset alarm Check all cannula and tube connections to ensure they are tight and not kinked or otherwise obstructed Adjust cannula to ensure a comfortable fit, then initiate inspiration
Hissing sound coming from inside device	Pressure from oxygen regulator is too high	Reduce pressure to recommended level
No oxygen is delivered	Nasal cannula is not adjusted properly	Check all cannula and tubing connections to ensure they are tight Adjust the cannula to fit comfortably in the nares
	Kinks in delivery tubing	Check all tubing to ensure there are no kinks, bends, obstructions, or objects putting pressure on the tube
	Oxygen source is turned off	Check all tubing connections and ensure oxygen source is turned on
Oxygen is delivered continuously	Selector knob is set to continuous flow	Check selector to ensure it is set to pulse mode
	Unit is in bypass mode due to failure to sense inspiration	Turn unit off then back on to reset alarm Check all cannula and tube connections to ensure they are tight and not kinked or otherwise obstructed Adjust cannula to ensure a comfortable fit, then initiate inspiration

in air through surrounding ports and mixes it with pure oxygen. Bigger ports and/or smaller jets cause more air dilution, lower O$_2$ concentrations, and higher total flows, while smaller ports and/or bigger jets cause less air dilution and higher O$_2$ concentrations, but lower total flows.

Based on different port and jet size combinations, air-entrainment devices are designed to mix air and O$_2$ at specific ratios in order to achieve a given O$_2$ concentration, ranging from 24% to 80%. **Table 6-5** provides the approximate air-to-oxygen mixing ratios for common O$_2$ concentrations delivered by air-entrainment systems, as well as their total output flows based on a sample O$_2$ input of 10 L/min (for illustration). Note that *changing the O$_2$ input flow does not alter the air/O$_2$ ratio or delivered O$_2$% by air-entrainment systems.*

Table 6-5 Air-to-O$_2$ Ratios and Total Flow Output of Air-Entrainment Devices at Common O$_2$ Concentrations

Air-to-Oxygen Ratio	O$_2$%	Total Ratio Parts	Total Flow[a] at 10 L/min O$_2$ Input
0.3:1	80	1.3	13
0.6:1	70	1.6	16
1:1	60	2	20
1.7:1	50	2.7	27
3:1	40	4	40
5:1	35	6	60
7:1	31	8	80
10:1	28	11	110
25:1	24	26	260

a. Total flow (air + oxygen) in L/min computed by multiplying the O$_2$ input flow (L/min) by the total ratio parts. Changing input flow does not alter the air/O$_2$ ratio or delivered O$_2$%.

As evident in Table 6-5, because entrainment devices dilute source oxygen with air, they *always* provide less than 100% oxygen. More important is the fact that *the higher the delivered O$_2$% from an air-entrainment device, the lower its total flow*. For example, Table 6-5 shows that the same air-entrainment nebulizer with an O$_2$ input of 10 L/min delivers a total flow of 60 L/min when set to 35%, but only 16 L/min when set to 70%.

It is the total flow of air-entrainment devices that determines their performance. Specifically, *if the total flow output of the device drops below a patient's inspiratory flow, additional air dilution will occur and the F$_{IO_2}$ becomes variable*. You can observe this problem directly in some patients receiving O$_2$ therapy via an air-entrainment nebulizer and T-tube or aerosol mask. In these cases, you will observe the mist completely disappearing from the device's open port(s) during inspiration. The mist is disappearing because the patient's inspiratory flow exceeds that delivered by the device, resulting in additional air dilution and an F$_{IO_2}$ lower than that set on the device. In these situations, what is labeled as a high-flow system becomes a low-flow system, delivering a variable F$_{IO_2}$.

How much total flow is enough to ensure a stable F$_{IO_2}$? Because patients' inspiratory flows vary greatly, *the best way to ensure a stable F$_{IO_2}$ is to provide a total flow of at least 40 L/min*. As indicated in Table 6-5, for an input flow of 10 L/min, this occurs only at or below the 40% O$_2$ settings. Total output flow can be boosted somewhat by increasing the O$_2$ input flow (*this does NOT affect the air/O$_2$ ratio or O$_2$%*). However, especially with air-entrainment nebulizers, the input flow is limited by the back pressure created at the jet, typically to 12–15 L/min. According to Table 6-5, then, the maximum flow one could expect from an air-entrainment nebulizer set to 70% with an input flow of 16 L/min is about 24 L/min (1.6 × 16), which may not meet the inspiratory flow needs of many patients, especially those who are critically ill and/or have high minute volumes.

An alternative high-flow approach that does not depend on air entrainment is the *high-flow nasal cannula* system. These systems typically include a blender to provide variable F$_{IO_2}$s, a high-flow flowmeter, a heating/humidification system to maintain BTPS conditions at the airway, an O$_2$ sensor, and specialized cannula delivery tubing that uses heated wires or coaxial warming to prevent condensation. In concept, by providing warm, humidified gas to the airway, a high-flow nasal cannula system helps overcome the problems associated with delivering high flows via a standard cannula. The higher available flows (up to 40 L/min in adults) minimize air entrainment, which allows for moderate to high F$_{IO_2}$s. As an added benefit, high-flow nasal cannulas "wash out" CO$_2$ from the anatomic deadspace of the upper airway, thus increasing the efficiency of ventilation. **Table 6-6** provides the approximate F$_{IO_2}$s that high-flow nasal cannulas can provide to adults at various flows.

Table 6-6 Approximate Adult FIO₂s Provided by High-Flow Nasal Cannulas

Flow (100% O₂)	Approximate FIO₂
10 L/min	60%
15 L/min	80%
20 L/min	90%
30 L/min	95%

Because the heating/humidification systems used with high-flow cannulas employ sensors and computerized alarm indicators like those used with ventilator humidifiers, troubleshooting these devices is also similar. Note that a low-temperature alarm often occurs temporarily when the water reservoir is changed. A persistent high-temperature warning is more serious and generally requires that the device be discontinued or replaced. *If no replacement system is available, you should substitute an O₂ modality that matches the high-flow system's FIO₂ as closely as possible—e.g., a nonrebreathing mask if delivering high FIO₂s.* Additional serious alarms requiring your immediate attention are those signaling an out-of-range O₂%, failure of the gas supply, or empty water reservoir.

O₂ Therapy Enclosures

O₂ enclosures (isolettes, hoods, and tents) represent a separate category of O₂-delivery systems. Generally you use O₂ enclosures only with infants and children. **Table 6-7** provides a summary of these devices, including their flow settings, advantages, disadvantages, and best use.

Table 6-7 Oxygen Therapy Enclosure Systems

Device	Flow	FIO₂ Range	Advantages	Disadvantages	Best Use
Oxyhood	≥ 7 L/min	21–100%	Full range of FIO₂s	Difficult to clean, disinfect	For infants requiring supplemental oxygen
Isolette	8–15 L/min	40–50%	Provides temperature control	Expensive, cumbersome Unstable FIO₂ (leaks) Difficult to clean, disinfect Limits patient mobility Fire hazard	For infants requiring supplemental oxygen and precise thermal regulation
Tent/ croupette	12–15 L/min	40–50%	Provides concurrent aerosol therapy	Expensive, cumbersome Unstable FIO₂ (leaks) Requires cooling Difficult to clean, disinfect Limits patient mobility Fire hazard	For toddlers or small children requiring low to moderate FIO₂s and bland aerosol

Adapted from: Wilkins, R. L., Stoller, J. K., & Scanlan, C. L. (2003). *Egan's fundamentals of respiratory care.* (8th ed.). St. Louis: Mosby.

O₂ Device Selection

As a general rule, sicker patients require higher and more stable F_{IO_2}s, whereas less acutely ill patients usually can be managed with lower, less exact F_{IO_2}s. **Table 6-8** provides guidance in selecting an O₂-delivery system based on these factors.

In terms of patient age, you should provide oxygen to newborns and infants via either an oxyhood or an isolette at the lowest F_{IO_2} required to maintain adequate oxygenation, with proper *warming and humidification* of the delivered gas (to ensure a neutral thermal environment). High-flow cannulas (at 1–8 L/min) are also a viable option for these small patients.

Most toddlers or small children needing a low to moderate F_{IO_2} can accept a standard nasal cannula, to be used in conjunction with a *calibrated low-flow flowmeter*. If the child cannot tolerate a nasal cannula, you may need to recommend using an O₂ tent/croupette. Providing high F_{IO_2}s to toddlers or small children can be a major problem, since they often do not tolerate masks. If they can tolerate a cannula, consider using a high-flow cannula system at 5–20 L/min to provide the high F_{IO_2}. Alternatively, you may need to recommend sedation or intubation for the child so that O₂ can be provided via a T-tube.

Table 6-9 summarizes and applies these concepts to the selection of specific O₂-delivery systems in a variety of common clinical scenarios you will likely see on the NBRC CRT exam.

O₂ Device Assembly and Use

Most O₂-therapy appliances are disposable single-use devices that require minimal assembly. The following guidelines apply to their assembly and use:

- Should any assembly be required, carefully follow the manufacturer's recommended procedure.
- Use a simple bubble humidifier for low-flow systems set to deliver more than 4 L/min.
- Make sure all threaded components are properly seated and tightened.
- When using a standard heated humidifier or any aerosol system to deliver oxygen, be sure to use large-bore (22 mm/7/8" ID) corrugated tubing (to help prevent condensate from obstructing the delivery system).
- Make sure that all tubing connections are snug.

O₂ Device Troubleshooting

According to the AARC, all O₂-delivery systems should be checked at least once per day. More frequent checks with an oxygen analyzer should be performed in systems that are susceptible to variation in F_{IO_2}

Table 6-8 Selecting an Oxygen Administration Device Based on Desired F_{IO_2} and Stability

Desired O₂%	Needed Stability in Delivered O₂%	
	Stable/Fixed	*Variable*
Low (< 35%)	Air-entrainment mask Air-entrainment nebulizer High-flow cannula with blender	Standard nasal cannula Isolette (infant) Tent/croupettes (child)
Moderate (35–60%)	Air-entrainment nebulizer High-flow cannula with blender	Simple mask Isolette (infant) Tent/croupettes (child)
High (> 60%)	Multiple air-entrainment nebulizers in parallel Oxyhood (infant) High-flow cannula with blender	Partial rebreather Nonrebreather

Adapted from: Wilkins, R. L., Stoller, J. K., & Scanlan, C. L. (2003). *Egan's fundamentals of respiratory care* (8th ed.) St. Louis: Mosby.

Table 6-9 O₂ Device Selection Scenarios

Patient Scenario	Recommended O₂-Delivery System
A stable adult medical patient needing a moderate F_{IO_2}	Nasal cannula, 4–6 L/min
A patient admitted to emergency department with chest pain and a suspected MI	Nonrebreathing mask, > 10 L/min OR high-flow nasal cannula (≥ 20 L/min)
A patient just extubated from ventilatory support on 30% O₂	Air-entrainment nebulizer, 30–50% and T-tube
An unstable COPD patient requiring a precise low F_{IO_2}	Air-entrainment mask, 24% or 28%
A postop patient with an ET requiring a moderate F_{IO_2}	Air-entrainment nebulizer, 30–50%, and T-tube with open reservoir OR high-flow nasal cannula (≤ 20 L/min)
A stable post-op patient with a trach needing low F_{IO_2}	Air-entrainment nebulizer, 30–35%, and trach collar
An ICU patient with a high minute volume needing high F_{IO_2}	Two air-entrainment nebulizers in parallel, 50–70%, and T-tube with open reservoir OR high-flow nasal cannula (≥ 30 L/min)
A stable 2-year-old child needing a low F_{IO_2}	Nasal cannula ¼–2 L/min with calibrated low-flow flow meter
An infant requiring short-term supplemental O₂	Simple O₂ mask
An infant requiring high F_{IO_2}s and temperature control	Oxyhood with servo-controlled heated humidification system. High-flow nasal cannula (1–8 L/min)
A small child requiring moderate F_{IO_2}s and bland aerosol	Croup tent with supplemental O₂

(such as blending systems) or when applied to unstable patients, those with ET or tracheal tubes, or those requiring high F_{IO_2}s.

Table 6-10 summarizes the most common problems that you may encounter when checking low-flow O₂-therapy devices, along with the causes and potential solutions.

Table 6-11 (see page 161) summarizes the most common problems that you may encounter with high-flow O₂ therapy devices, along with the causes and potential solutions. Note in particular that an obstruction to flow downstream from any air-entrainment device *decreases* air entrainment, resulting in a higher delivered O₂ concentration but a lower overall flow, with an unpredictable effect on the patient.

As indicated in Table 6-7, the primary problems you will encounter with O₂ therapy enclosures are (1) inability to maintain the desired F_{IO_2} and (2) proper temperature regulation.

The most common problem with O₂ enclosures is a lower than desired oxygen concentration. If the O₂ level in an enclosure is lower than desired, check for and correct any major leaks and ensure that the flow is sufficient to maintain the desired O₂%. A related problem occurs when an infant or child must be removed from an O₂-therapy enclosure for a procedure. In these cases, you should be prepared to provide an equivalent O₂ concentration via an alternative device, such as a simple mask. Although rare, you may also encounter an O₂% that is higher than desired, especially in isolettes. The most common cause of this problem is a clogged air inlet filter, which should be replaced.

Careful regulation of O₂-delivery temperatures is critical for newborn infants in order to maintain a neutral thermal environment. For infants in oxyhoods, overheating can cause dehydration, while underheating can cause apnea and increase O₂ consumption. For this reason, the best way to ensure a neutral thermal environment in an oxyhood is to use a servo-controlled heated humidifier system with

Table 6-10 Troubleshooting Common Problems with Low-Flow O₂ Therapy Devices

Problem/Clue	Cause(s)	Solution
Nasal Cannulas		
No gas flow can be felt coming from the cannula	Flow meter not on System leak Humidifier down tube obstructed	Adjust flow meter as needed Check connections Repair or replace device
Humidifier pop-off sounding	Obstruction distal to humidifier Flow set too high Obstructed naris	Find and correct obstruction Lower flow Use alternative O₂ appliance
Patient complains of soreness over lip or ears	Irritation/inflammation due to appliance straps/loops	Loosen straps Place cotton balls at pressure points Use alternate device
Masks		
Patient constantly removes mask	Claustrophobia Confusion	Use alternative device Restrain or sedate patient
No gas flow detected	Flow meter not on System leak	Adjust flow meter as needed Check connections
Humidifier pop-off sounding	Obstruction distal to humidifier High input flow Jammed inspiratory valve	Find and correct obstruction Omit humidifier (short term) Repair or replace mask
Reservoir bag collapses when the patient inhales	Inadequate flow	Increase flow
Reservoir bag remains inflated during inhalation	Large mask leak Inspiratory valve jammed/reversed	Correct leak Repair or replace mask
Patient develops erythema over face/ears	Irritation/inflammation due to appliance or straps	Reposition mask/straps Place cotton balls over ear pressure points Provide skin care

appropriate high- and low-temperature alarms. See this chapter's section on *Ventilators, CPAP Devices, and Breathing Circuits* for a discussion of the special problems encountered when using heated-wire circuits to deliver gas to infants under radiant warmers or in incubators.

Because tents and croupettes impair radiant heat loss, the problem in using these devices is providing sufficient cooling, not heating. The temperature in most modern enclosures is electronically maintained by a thermostatically controlled refrigeration system. Some old-style oxygen tents and croupettes lack this feature and depend solely on high flows to prevent heat buildup

Of course, all O₂-therapy devices present a potential fire hazard, with O₂ enclosures being the most dangerous in this regard. To minimize the risk of fire with these devices, you must keep all electrical equipment out of the enclosure.

Humidifiers, Nebulizers, and Mist Tents

A *humidifier* is a device that adds molecular water to gas. Most often, this occurs via simple evaporation from a water surface. Alternatively, a *nebulizer* can be used to generate and disperse small particles of water into the air (a bland water aerosol) to provide additional water content.

Table 6-11 Troubleshooting Common Problems with High-Flow O_2 Therapy Devices

Problem/Clue	Cause(s)	Solution
Air-Entrainment Masks		
Patient's SaO_2 lower than expected	Inadequate total flow	Increase input flow Check for/correct any flow obstructions
	Inadequate O_2 concentration	Switch to higher % device
Patient complains of dryness	Inadequate water vapor content	Use aerosol collar + air-driven nebulizer to increase humidification
Air-Entrainment Nebulizers		
Patient's SaO_2 lower than expected	Inadequate total flow (only for high O_2% settings, i.e., > 35–40%)	Maximize input flow Add open reservoir to expiratory side of T-tube Connect multiple nebulizers together in parallel Provide inspiratory reservoir with one-way expiratory valve Set nebulizer to low O_2% and bleed-in extra O_2 Use a specialized high-flow/high O_2% generator
Delivered O_2% higher than set or expected	Obstruction to flow in circuit	Drain tubing condensate Check/correct kinking or other outlet obstructions

Humidifiers and Humidification

There are three primary types of humidifiers, defined mainly by the method of exposing gas to water gas: bubble humidifiers, passover humidifiers, and heat and moisture exchangers (HMEs). A bubble humidifier disperses small bubbles of the gas being humidified through a water reservoir. A passover humidifier directs gas over the surface of a water reservoir for evaporation. There are two common types of passover humidifiers: the wick type and the membrane type.

Both bubble and passover humidifiers can be used either to humidify inspired oxygen delivered via O_2-therapy appliances or to humidify gases delivered by mechanical ventilators. Both types of devices are considered *active humidifiers* and may incorporate heating elements and reservoir feed systems.

Many CRT candidates have difficulty with questions related to humidifier water vapor output and delivery system condensation. The following are the key facts and concepts that you need to know to address exam questions about humidification systems.

- All modern humidifiers saturate the gas passing through them (achieve 100% relative humidity).
- The actual water vapor content (absolute humidity) delivered to the patient depends on:
  - The humidifier's operating temperature (the higher the temperature, the greater the absolute humidity)
  - Whether the gas leaving the humidifier warms, cools, or remains at the same temperature
- Condensation in the delivery system occurs only if the gas leaving the humidifier cools on the way to the patient.

Figure 6-1 demonstrates these concepts in three delivery systems using (A) an unheated humidifier, (B) a heated humidifier, and (C) a heated humidifier with heated wires in the delivery circuit. Due to evaporative cooling, the unheated humidifier operates at temperatures below those in the room (10°C). Although the gas leaving is 100% saturated with water vapor, it has low water vapor content (about 10 mg/L). As it passes through the delivery tubing, the surrounding room temperature *warms* it up to 20°C. This increases the capacity of the gas to hold water vapor, but not its content. As a result, *no condensation occurs in the circuit, and the relative humidity provided to the patient decreases* (to about 54%). Although this is adequate for patients receiving medical gases via the nose/upper airway, it is not sufficient for patients with artificial tracheal airways.

For these patients, the simple solution is to heat the humidifier, which raises the water vapor content delivered to the patient (example B). However, now the gas leaving the humidifier will be *cooled* by the lower room temperature. To offset this cooling and achieve BTPS conditions (100% relative humidity at 37°C) at the patient's airway, we must set the humidifier's operating temperature substantially higher than 37°C, in this example 45°C. *As this hot, saturated gas transverses the cooler delivery circuit, significant condensation occurs in the tubing.* If not removed, this condensate can block the tubing or be aspirated by the patient.

The solution to the problem of condensate when using heated humidifiers is simple: prevent cooling in the circuit. As demonstrated in example C, this is accomplished using heated wires. Since the heated wires prevent cooling, the operating temperature of the humidifier can be set at the same level desired at the airway (generally 32–35°C). *As long as the heated wires maintain this gas temperature constant throughout the circuit, condensation will not occur, and the patient will receive the gas at or near BTPS conditions.*

A simpler and less expensive solution to the problem of rain-out in ventilator circuits is to use a heat and moisture exchanger (HME). HMEs function much like the nose in that they capture a portion of the patient's expired water vapor via condensation and humidify the inspired gas via evaporation of this condensate. HMEs require no heating or water reservoir system and are thus referred to as *passive humidifiers*. However, because they depend on bidirectional flow for proper function, HMEs are used only to condition inspired gas in ventilator circuits. Details on humidification during mechanical ventilation are provided in Chapter 10.

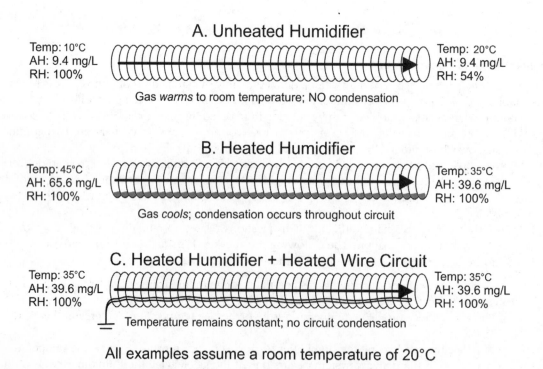

A. Unheated Humidifier

Temp: 10°C
AH: 9.4 mg/L
RH: 100%

Temp: 20°C
AH: 9.4 mg/L
RH: 54%

Gas *warms* to room temperature; NO condensation

B. Heated Humidifier

Temp: 45°C
AH: 65.6 mg/L
RH: 100%

Temp: 35°C
AH: 39.6 mg/L
RH: 100%

Gas *cools*; condensation occurs throughout circuit

C. Heated Humidifier + Heated Wire Circuit

Temp: 35°C
AH: 39.6 mg/L
RH: 100%

Temp: 35°C
AH: 39.6 mg/L
RH: 100%

Temperature remains constant; no circuit condensation

All examples assume a room temperature of 20°C

Figure 6-1 Comparison of Active Humidification Systems.

Nebulizers

Devices used to generate bland aerosols include large-volume jet nebulizers and ultrasonic nebulizers. **Table 6-12** compares and contrasts these devices in terms of key operating principles and best use.

Specialized high-output jet nebulizers are available to deliver bland aerosols into mist tents. Typically these enclosure systems generate higher flows and water outputs than those designed for application to the airway. Because heat buildup in enclosures is a problem, these systems always run cool (never heated).

Assembly and Use of Humidifiers and Nebulizers

Humidifiers and nebulizers either come preassembled or require minimal assembly. The following guidelines should help avoid most problems:

- Should any assembly be required, carefully follow the manufacturer's recommended procedure.
- During any assembly, avoid contamination by not touching any internal parts.
- If the device does not come pre-filled, fill its reservoir with sterile H_2O.
- To ensure accurate input flows when using a jet nebulizer as an O_2-delivery system, you must use a compensated Thorpe-tube flowmeter.
- Make sure all threaded components are properly seated and tightened.
- When using a heated humidifier or any aerosol system with adults, be sure to use large-bore (22 mm/7/8" ID) corrugated tubing (to help prevent tubing obstruction from condensate).
- Make sure that all tubing connections are snug.

Troubleshooting Humidifiers and Nebulizers

Common problems with active humidification systems include leaks or obstructions to flow—with heated devices—water vapor condensation, and temperature fluctuations. **Table 6-13** summarizes the

Table 6-12 Operating Principles and Best Uses for Jet and Ultrasonic Nebulizers

Jet Nebulizers	Ultrasonic Nebulizers
Key Operating Principles	
• Produce aerosols via shearing of water into particles at the interface of a high-velocity gas jet and liquid siphon tube • Typically incorporate one or more baffles to remove larger, nonrespirable particles from the suspension • The low pressure created at the gas jet can also be used to entrain air, providing for increased flow and variable F_IO_2 • As with humidifiers, heating the water reservoir will increase total water output	• Produce small (1–3 μ), uniform high-density aerosols using high-frequency sound waves • Need a separate source of gas flow to carry the aerosol suspension to the patient • Do not need or use baffles • Amplitude of the sound waves determines aerosol output (mg/min) • Aerosol density (mg/L) depends on the ratio of amplitude to carrier gas flow (i.e., the greater the amplitude and the lower the gas flow, the higher the aerosol density)
Best Use	
• Patients with ET or trach tubes requiring long-term supplemental humidification • Short-term application to patients with upper-airway edema—e.g., croup or post extubation and to help thin secretions • Short-term application to patients with thick or inspissated secretions • Single-treatment application (heated) to help provoke cough and obtain sputum specimens—may use hypertonic saline	• Short-term application to patients with thick or inspissated secretions • Single-treatment application to help provoke cough and obtain sputum specimens—may use hypertonic saline

Table 6-13 Troubleshooting Common Problems with Active Humidifiers

Problem/Clue	Cause(s)	Solution
Bubble Humidifier		
No gas flow can be felt coming from the cannula	Flow meter not on System leak[a]	Adjust flow meter Check connections
Humidifier pop-off is sounding	Obstruction distal to humidifier Flow is set too high Obstructed naris	Find/correct obstruction Use alternative device Use alternative device
Heated Humidifier		
Intermittent flow or "bubbling" in tubing circuit	Condensation of water vapor	Regularly drain condensate (away from patient) Place water traps at low points in the circuit Employ a heated-wire circuit
Airway temperature too high	Temperature set too high Abrupt decrease in flow Temperature probe not inserted in the circuit Unit was warmed up without flow through the circuit Unit failure	Reset to 32–35°C Ensure proper flow Insert temperature probe in the circuit Let temperature equilibrate with flow before application Replace unit
Airway temperature too low	Unit not plugged in Circuit breaker activated Temperature set too low Cool water added to reservoir Abrupt increase in flow Reservoir low or empty Unit failure	Plug unit into wall outlet Reset circuit breaker Reset to 32–35°C System will readjust Ensure proper flow Refill/replenish reservoir Replace unit
Loss of pressure (during positive pressure ventilation)	Leak in unit or connections	Check/tighten connections Replace unit

a. You can also use the humidifier pop-off to test an oxygen-delivery system for leaks. If you obstruct the system at or near the patient interface and the pop-off sounds, the system is leak-free; failure of the pop-off to sound indicates a leak.

most common problems that you may encounter with humidification devices, along with the causes and potential solutions. **Table 6-14** summarizes the most common problems that you may encounter with nebulizers used to deliver bland aerosols, along with the causes and potential solutions.

Resuscitation Devices

Resuscitation devices are used to provide ventilation and oxygenation in emergency situations and during short patient transports and certain special procedures, such as hyperinflation before and after suctioning. There are three resuscitation devices in common use: (1) self-inflating manual resuscitators (bag-valve-mask systems, or BVMs), (2) gas-powered resuscitators, and (3) mouth-to-valve mask resuscitators.

Table 6-14 Troubleshooting Common Problems with Bland Aerosol Delivery Systems

Problem/Clue	Cause(s)	Solution
Large-Volume Jet Nebulizer		
Inadequate mist output	Inadequate input flow	Increase input flow
	Siphon tube obstruction	Repair or replace unit
	Jet orifice misalignment	Repair or replace unit
Aerosol mist disappears during inspiration (T-tube or mask)	Inadequate flow	Maximize input flow Add open reservoir to expiratory side of T-tube Connect multiple nebulizers together in parallel
Airway temperature too high or too low	Heat setting incorrect	Adjust to ensure 32–35°C at airway
	Malfunctioning heater	Repair or replace unit
Ultrasonic Nebulizer		
No "geyser" produced in nebulizer chamber	Unit not on or connected to line power Circuit breaker tripped Amplitude set too low Inadequate fluid level	Connect unit to line power and turn on Reset circuit breaker Increase amplitude/output Ensure adequate fluid volume
Misting in chamber but no aerosol delivered	Inadequate flow through chamber	Increase flow through chamber
Aerosol density too high/low	Incorrect amplitude or flow setting	Increase density by lowering flow and/or increasing amplitude Decrease density by increasing flow and/or lowering amplitude
Patient's O_2 sat lower than desired	Lack of supplemental O_2	Provide supplemental O_2 flow, adjust to provide desired SpO_2

Resuscitation Device Selection

The following guidelines apply to the selection of resuscitation devices:

- BVMs are the standard and should be your first choice; select the correct size for the patient.
- Use a mouth-to-valve mask resuscitator to ventilate adults when a BVM is not available or fails.
- Do *not* use a gas-powered resuscitator on an infant or child; be careful in applying to adults.

To ensure effective ventilation and avoid overinflation, always select the appropriate BVM with the correct stroke volume and mask size. Typically, manufacturers provide four size/stroke volume combinations: adult (≤ 800 mL), pediatric (≤ 500 mL), infant (≤ 300 mL), and neonatal (≤ 100 mL). Some pediatric, infant, and neonatal models provide a 40-cm H_2O pressure relief valve to help avoid gastric insufflation and barotrauma.

Generally, you would consider a gas-powered resuscitator for an adult only when such factors as small hand size or fatigue would impair provision of adequate ventilation to adults with a BVM. However, malfunction or misuse of these devices has caused severe patient injury, including barotrauma. To avoid complications with these devices, you need to select a device that limits flow to 40 L/min and keeps pressures below 60 cm H_2O.

Resuscitation Device Assembly and Use

Most BVMs are disposable and need minimal assembly. Key considerations in their use include the following:

- Ensure that an O_2 reservoir bag or hose is attached; volume should equal or exceed stroke volume.
- Ensure that the device is connected to a O_2 flowmeter set to the maximum specified by the manufacturer (generally no higher than 15 L/min); in emergency situations never delay ventilation to obtain oxygen.
- If the patient is not intubated, attach an appropriate-size mask to the standard connector.
- If needed and not provided with the unit, attach a PEEP valve to the expiratory port and adjust to the desired level (critical for supporting patients already receiving PEEP).
- As needed for children and infants, connect a pressure manometer to the pressure monitoring port to monitor airway pressures.
- Always test the device for proper function before application (see troubleshooting section).
- To ensure the highest possible O_2 concentration during BVM ventilation, manually slow refilling of the bag (if time permits).

Most mouth-to-valve mask resuscitators come preassembled. If not, assemble as per the manufacturer's instructions. If the mask has an O_2 supply port, attach it to an O_2 source. *Never delay ventilation to obtain oxygen.*

Resuscitation Device Troubleshooting

Before applying a resuscitation device to a patient, check it for proper function. For BVMs, follow these two simple steps:

1. Occlude the patient connector, then squeeze the bag. If the bag has a pressure relief valve, it should pop off. If the bag does not have a pressure relief valve, it should not be possible to compress the bag.
2. Squeeze the bag and then occlude the patient connection. The bag should reinflate via the inlet valve, and any attached O_2 reservoir bag should deflate.

Failure of the first test indicates that either the patient nonrebreathing valve or the bag inlet valve is missing or leaking. Failure of the second test indicates a jammed or malpositioned bag inlet valve. *If the BVM fails either test, replace it immediately.* If no replacement is available, use a mouth-to-valve mask resuscitator or initiate mouth-to-mouth ventilation.

During BVM use, always apply the following troubleshooting guidelines:

- If the valve jams open, check the input flow. If excessive, reduce it to the manufacturer's recommended maximum. If this does not correct the problem, replace the device.
- If secretions or vomitus accumulate and jam the valve, replace the device.
- If a pressure pop-off continually activates, squeeze the bag more slowly. If this fails to lower the airway pressure, consider potential causes (e.g., pneumothorax, endobronchial intubation) before overriding it.

As with BVMs, always be sure to check the function of a mouth-to-valve mask resuscitator's valve before use. If you can inhale through the device's one-way valve, it is either misassembled or malfunctioning. Try quickly reversing the valve. If that does not work, get a replacement device. If no replacement device is available, initiate mouth-to-mouth ventilation.

Ventilators, CPAP Devices, and Breathing Circuits

Ventilators and CPAP Device Selection

Other than cost (*not* assessed on the NBRC CRT exam), four key questions dictate choice of a ventilator or CPAP device:

1. What patient variables apply?
2. Where will the device be used and for how long?

3. How will the device be used?

4. What added capabilities are needed or desired?

Table 6-15 provides common answers to these key questions and guidance on recommending the type of ventilator you should select for each circumstance.

Ventilators and CPAP Device Assembly and Use

Ventilators and CPAP devices require little or no assembly. However, before you apply a ventilator to a patient, you need to select and assemble the appropriate breathing circuit *and* confirm its operation via an operational verification procedure. Ventilator operational verification procedures are described in Chapter 8. Here we focus on the breathing circuit.

All ventilators and CPAP devices use an external tubing circuit to deliver gas from the device to the patient and provide a mechanism to direct exhaled gases out to the atmosphere. Most adult circuits use large-bore (22 mm/7/8″ ID) corrugated tubing. Pediatric and neonatal circuits are typically constructed of smaller-diameter (15 mm ID for children, 10 mm for infants), low-compliance tubing to minimize compressed volume loss. All disposable breathing circuits should come labeled with a compliance factor. This factor is required during computerized ventilator setup to program the device to compensate for compressed volume loss.

In addition, breathing circuits usually include either an active or a passive humidification system and can provide bacterial filtration and monitoring functions. Often the breathing circuit also provides the mechanism to create PEEP/CPAP. Last, specialized oral or nasal patient interfaces may be incorporated into breathing circuits designed for CPAP or noninvasive ventilation (NPPV).

Types of Circuits

There are two general types of breathing circuits: (1) the dual-limb or "Y" circuit, and (2) the single-limb circuit. Single-limb circuits may include a true expiratory valve, a leakage-type exhaust port, or no valve at all. **Table 6-16** (see page 169) summarizes the appropriate use of these different breathing circuits.

Dual-Limb Circuits. **Figure 6-2** (see page 169) shows a typical dual-limb heated-wire breathing circuit, the most common circuit used with general-purpose critical care ventilators. The same basic circuit can be used with continuous-flow CPAP devices. It includes three basic components that together resemble the shape of the letter "Y": (1) an inspiratory limb that delivers fresh gas from the ventilator outlet or humidifier to the patient, (2) a standard 15-mm patient connector/swivel adapter, and (3) an expiratory limb that returns to the inlet/expiratory valve of the ventilator or to the PEEP/CPAP valve in a CPAP circuit. Additional components include one (inspiratory limb only) or two (both limbs) plug connectors for the heated wires, a pressure-sensing line, and 1–2 ports for temperature probes.

The expiratory valve of most critical care ventilators consists of an *internal* electromechanical valve that closes when the machine triggers into inspiration and opens during the expiratory phase. When linked to a pressure transducer and an electronic processing circuit, this valve can also regulate PEEP/CPAP levels by preventing expiration below a specific pressure baseline. Alternatively, when a dual-limb breathing circuit is used to provide continuous-flow CPAP, the expiratory limb is connected to a separate PEEP/CPAP valve, such as an underwater column or spring-loaded disk. With a water-column PEEP/CPAP valve, you simply immerse the expiratory limb of the circuit under water. The PEEP/CPAP level is adjusted by varying how far you immerse the tube under water, with each centimeter equal to 1 cm H_2O PEEP/CPAP. PEEP/CPAP levels with spring-loaded disks are adjusted by altering the tension on the spring.

The mechanical deadspace or rebreathed volume in dual-limb circuits is that between the patient connector/swivel adapter (located at the "tail" of the Y) and the patient's airway. *Any tubing or device (e.g., an HME) added distal to this point will increase mechanical deadspace.*

Single-Limb Circuits. There are two types of single-limb circuits: (1) those with built-in expiratory valves and (2) those with leakage-type exhaust ports. **Figure 6-3** (see page 169) depicts a single-limb breathing circuit with a built-in expiratory valve, as used with most transport ventilators, as well as those used in the home and long-term care settings. As indicated in the figure, single-limb circuits have a separate pneumatic line running from the ventilator to the expiratory valve. This line intermittently

Table 6-15 Selecting a Ventilator or CPAP Device

Question	Answer	Recommended Device
What patient variables apply?	Patient is an infant or small child	Ventilator certified for use on specific age group
	Patient has or needs an artificial tracheal airway	Standard multipurpose ICU ventilator If artificial tracheal airway not needed, select a noninvasive positive-pressure ventilator[a]
	Patient has either a restrictive or obstructive disorder	Ventilator capable of a high driving pressure (> 60 cm H_2O)
	Patient has severe expiratory airway obstruction	Ventilator with variable flow control and adjustable I:E ratios
	Patient has hypoxemic respiratory failure only, adequate ventilation	Consider CPAP-only device with appropriate backup and alarms
Where will the device be used and for how long?	In the acute care setting	Pneumatically powered ventilator For the home- or long-term care setting, select an electrically powered ventilator
	For short-term transport	BVM or simple pneumatically powered transport ventilator (note: for long term consider an electrically powered ventilator capable of running on 12-volt DC)
	During MRI procedures	Pneumatically powered, pneumatically or fluidically controlled ventilator certified for use during MRI procedures
How will the device be used?	On critically ill/unstable patients	Standard multipurpose microprocessor-controlled ICU ventilator For stable home- or long-term care patients, select an electrically powered ventilator with volume-control A/C or IMV, and variable flow
What additional capabilities are needed or desired?	Advanced alarm and monitoring functions	Standard multipurpose microprocessor-controlled ICU ventilator with graphics display For stable home- or long-term care patients, select a ventilator with basic alarms (e.g. vent inoperative, high pressure, disconnect)
	Data analysis/storage and programmability	Standard multipurpose microprocessor-controlled ICU ventilator with graphics display

a. Because the airway interface defines noninvasive positive-pressure ventilation (NPPV), *any* ventilator can be applied noninvasively. However, because NPPV interfaces tend to leak, the ventilator used must be able to compensate for leakage. Moreover, since NPPV normally is applied only to spontaneously breathing patients, the ventilator has to reliably detect and respond to patient inspiratory effort, even with significant leakage. Pressure-support ventilation (PSV) meets both these expectations and thus is the most common mode of NPPV. PSV (with CPAP) can be delivered by most ICU ventilators but more commonly is provided by electrically powered pressure generators, which are less expensive, simpler to use, and more portable than their ICU counterparts.

Table 6-16 Appropriate Use of Common Ventilator/CPAP Circuits

Circuit Type	Appropriate Use
Dual-limb "Y" circuit	Most critical ventilators Continuous-flow CPAP circuit
Single-limb circuit with expiratory valve	Transport and home-care ventilators
Single-limb circuit with leakage-type exhaust port	Noninvasive positive pressure/BiPAP™ ventilators
Single-limb circuit without any valve	Simple home-type CPAP generators

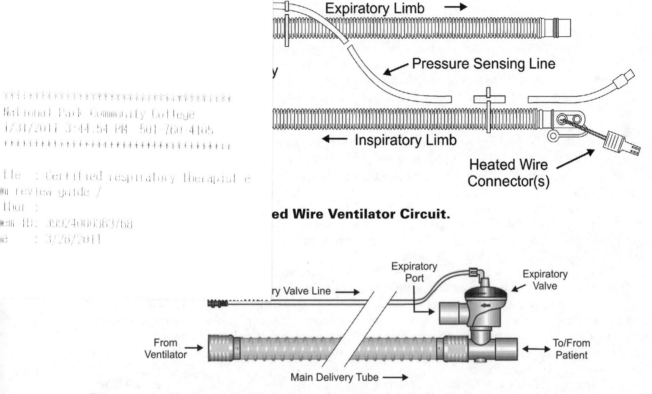

Expiratory Limb →

Pressure Sensing Line

← Inspiratory Limb

Heated Wire Connector(s)

...ed Wire Ventilator Circuit.

Figure 6-3 Single-Limb Breathing Circuit with Built-In Expiratory Valve.

provides the pressure needed to close the expiratory valve during inspiration, which blocks gas outflow during the application of inspiratory positive pressure. At the beginning of expiration, this valve depressurizes and opens to allow expired gases to escape. The expiratory valve also can be used to control or retard expiratory flow or provide CPAP/PEEP. CPAP/PEEP is provided simply by maintaining pressure in the valve's balloon or diaphragm at the desired level throughout expiration. The expiratory valve also provides a standard 22-mm port for the collection or monitoring of expired gases. The mechanical deadspace in these circuits is that between the built-in expiratory valve and patient airway.

Figure 6-4 shows a single-limb circuit with a leakage-type exhaust port, as used with noninvasive positive pressure (NPPV) ventilators/BiPAP™ devices. These circuits are very simple in design, consisting of a single section of large-bore tubing and an open exhaust port, usually either a small orifice or a set of slotted vent holes. The continuous flow that noninvasive positive pressure ventilators provide through the circuit forces expired gas out this exhaust port during exhalation. Combined with the leakage associated with all NPPV interfaces, this simple setup is sufficient to prevent rebreathing of most expired gas, thereby minimizing mechanical deadspace. When provided, PEEP/CPAP is created by the continuous regulation of pressure and system flow/leakage via the ventilator's demand valve.

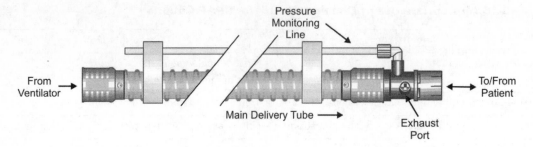

Figure 6-4 Single-Limb Circuit with a Leakage-Type Exhaust Port as Used with Common Noninvasive Positive Pressure Ventilators.

As indicted in Figure 6-4, a single-limb circuit with a leakage-type exhaust port also includes a pressure-monitoring line. This line connects the pressure sensor port of the ventilator to the main tubing at or near the exhaust port. Proper connection of this pressure line is essential in order to ensure adequate ventilator response and pressure maintenance.

Since many NPPV ventilators and BiPAP™ devices use a simple air blower to generate pressure, circuit modification may be needed to provide supplemental oxygen. Typically this is done by placing a small-bore tubing adapter at either the patient interface or the machine outlet. After connecting this adapter to a flowmeter via O_2-delivery tubing, you bleed O_2 into the circuit until the desired level is confirmed by O_2 analysis. Note that high supplemental O_2 flows can interfere with the proper triggering or cycling of some NPPV ventilators. For this reason, you should always follow the manufacturer's recommendations when considering how best to increase the FIO_2 of these devices.

NPPV Interfaces. Connected to this circuit is the NPPV patient interface, the most critical part of the delivery system. **Figure 6-5** depicts the three most common NPPV interfaces: the oronasal mask, nasal mask, and nasal pillows. Oral devices (i.e., combined mouthpieces/lip seals) are also used, primarily in the long-term care and home settings.

There are no set rules for selecting an NPPV patient interface. In the acute care setting, clinical experience suggests that the lower leakage associated with oronasal masks may make them the best choice for short-term treatment of hypoxemic respiratory failure. However, these devices have the most deadspace and thus may be contraindicated for patients with hypercapnic respiratory failure. Oral mouthpieces and lip seals have proved successful in managing patients with chronic hypercapnic respiratory failure in need of intermittent support, such as those with progressive neuromuscular diseases.

Ultimately, the best interface is the one that you and the patient prefer. For this reason, when time allows, you should have several different types and models of devices available for the patient to try. In addition, where available, you should always use sizing tools to help customize the device's fit. Whichever device is selected must be positioned and secured well enough to prevent major leakage, but loose enough to avoid discomfort or pressure sores. To avoid tissue damage during long-term usage, you may need to consider special cushioning materials and/or intermittently using alternative devices.

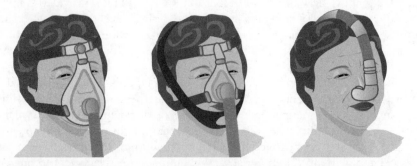

Figure 6-5 Common Noninvasive Positive Pressure Ventilation Patient Interfaces. (A) Oronasal mask. (B) Nasal mask. (C) Nasal pillows.

Circuit Assembly

Proper assembly of the dual- and single-limb breathing circuits involves connecting all components to the proper ventilator outlets and inlets and checking to confirm that all connections are tight and leak-free. Generally, you connect the inspiratory limb to either a HEPA (high-efficiency particulate air) filter at the ventilator's gas outlet or to the outlet side of a heated humidifier. The HEPA filter protects the patient from bacteria that may be present in the inspired gas by trapping particles as small as 0.3 mμ. Because its performance can be affected by condensation, *the HEPA filter must be positioned proximal to any active humidification system*. In order to prevent airborne cross-contamination, some ventilators also place a HEPA filter at or near the expiratory valve, *which must be heated to prevent condensation*.

All patients needing ventilatory support via a tracheal airway require a humidifier system in the ventilator circuit. For these patients, you can provide humidification using either an active heated passover humidifier or a passive HME. To help prevent condensate generated by heated humidifiers from obstructing gas flow, water traps may be placed at low points in the circuit limbs. If a heated-wire circuit is used, the wire connector(s) must be plugged into the low-voltage outlets provided on the humidifier. *If an HME is used for humidification, it must be placed to ensure bidirectional flow (i.e., distal to the patient connector/swivel adaptor in a dual-limb circuit and between the expiratory valve and patient airway in a single-limb circuit)*. Details on humidification during invasive ventilatory support are provided in Chapter 10.

Circuit Testing. After the circuit is connected to the ventilator and all accessories are in place, you should confirm circuit integrity by running a leak test. On a microprocessor-controlled ventilator, the leak test is typically included in the device's self-test program, which you should run to confirm circuit integrity. To run a leak test manually, trigger the ventilator to deliver a small volume (200–300 mL for adult ventilators) at low flow into a circuit that is occluded at the patient connector (most circuits provide a cap for this purpose). If the resulting pressure readily exceeds the ventilator's pressure limit or can be held at a static level (at zero flow during a pause), no leakage is present. If you cannot reach the ventilator's pressure limit or hold the pressure during an inspiratory pause, the circuit has a leak. If the ventilator fails the automated or manual leak test, recheck all circuit connections and repeat the test. If a repeat leakage test also fails, replace the circuit.

Incorporating Drug Aerosol Delivery Systems in Ventilator Circuits

Depending on the drug and protocol, you will use either a small-volume nebulizer (SVN) or a metered-dose inhaler (MDI) to deliver aerosolized drugs to patients receiving ventilatory support. In general, MDIs are preferred for this procedure because SVNs add flow and can therefore affect both machine sensitivity and the accuracy of volume and flow measurements.

The following guidelines apply to incorporating drug aerosol delivery systems in ventilator circuits:

1. Because an HME traps aerosol, *you must remove it before aerosol therapy and replace it afterward*.
2. HEPA filters are needed to prevent drug residue from entering the ventilator and affecting its performance.
   a. For dual-limb circuits, be sure that inspiratory and expiratory HEPA filters are in place.
   b. For single-limb circuits, you normally need only an inspiratory HEPA filter; expiratory filtration may be required on patients with disorders requiring droplet or respiratory precautions.
3. Proper positioning is critical to ensure good drug deposition in the lungs.
   a. With dual-limb circuits:
      i. Place the SVN or MDI adaptor in the *inspiratory* limb.
      ii. Position SVNs about 1–1½ feet from the patient.
      iii. With MDIs, place a spacer or holding chamber in line in the ventilator circuit.
   b. With single-limb circuits:
      i. Place the device on the patient side of the exhalation port (closest to the patient).
      ii. Upon completion of the treatment, inspect and remove the exhalation port for any drug residue (it can cause valve sticking). If you find residue, either clean the valve/port or replace the circuit.

PEEP/CPAP Valves

Most ventilators provide PEEP/CPAP. This is accomplished via a PEEP/CPAP valve, which generates a set level of positive pressure against which the patient must exhale. As discussed above, the two most common types of PEEP/CPAP valves are the electromechanical type and the pressurized balloon/diaphragm. You do not normally select a PEEP/CPAP valve, since these devices are built into either the ventilator or the breathing circuit. The exception is the underwater column-type PEEP/CPAP valve, which can be used with any ventilator or circuit that separates out the patient's expired gases. Spring-loaded disk PEEP/CPAP valves may also be chosen to provide positive expiratory pressure when using a bag-valve-mask.

Troubleshooting Ventilator Circuits and Interfaces

As described in Chapter 8, good quality-control procedures can prevent or minimize many of the common problems with ventilators and their circuits. When problems do occur at the bedside, they can be due to the ventilator, the ventilator circuit, or the patient. Because safety considerations demand that you always attend to patient needs first, *when any major problem occurs, you should immediately remove the patient from the ventilator and provide appropriate support using a manual resuscitator connected to an oxygen source.* This action alone eliminates the ventilator/circuit as the potential cause of the problem and usually buys the time needed to properly troubleshoot the entire patient-system. Chapters 13 and 14 describe how you should respond to alarms and changes in the status of patients receiving mechanical ventilation. Here we focus on troubleshooting the ventilator circuit and related equipment.

The most common problems encountered with ventilator circuits in general include leaks, obstructions, expiratory/PEEP valve problems, humidification and temperature regulation problems, and infection/cross-contamination. Specific to NPPV are problems with the patient interface.

Leaks, Obstructions, and Expiratory/PEEP Valve Problems

Table 6-17 summarizes common circuit-leak, obstruction, and expiratory/PEEP valve problems that you may encounter, along with their relevant symptoms/clues and potential solutions.

Circuit leaks are among the most common problems causing loss of ventilator volume and pressure. However, ventilator malfunction can have the same effect. To distinguish a circuit leak from a ventilator malfunction, run a circuit leak test. If the circuit leak test is negative, then the ventilator may

Table 6-17 Troubleshooting Common Ventilator Circuit Problems

Problem	Clue	Solution
Leaks	Low-volume alarm Low-pressure alarm	Check/correct loose circuit connections
Inspiratory obstructions (e.g., kinks, condensate, HME blockage)	Low-volume alarm High-pressure alarm	Find/correct obstruction Drain condensate Replace HME
Expiratory obstructions (e.g., kinks, condensate, blocked exhalation port [patient, bedding])	Low-volume alarm High-pressure alarm	Find/correct obstruction Drain condensate Prevent expiratory port blockage
Expiratory/PEEP valve malfunction	Open or leaking: • Low-volume alarm • Low-PEEP/CPAP alarm Obstructed/sticking • High-pressure alarm • High-PEEP/CPAP • Expiratory flow impeded	Single-limb circuits: • Check expiratory valve line • Replace circuit If double-limb circuit with internal expiratory valve, replace ventilator

not be delivering the preset volume. *To determine whether a ventilator is delivering the preset volume, compare the ventilator setting to that measured at the ventilator outlet using a calibrated volumeter.*

Circuit obstructions are always associated with low-volume and high-pressure alarms. Expiratory obstruction is the more serious of the two since it can result in rebreathing, asphyxia, and/or barotrauma. The most dangerous type of expiratory obstruction occurs when the exhalation port on single-limb circuits is obstructed. To avoid this problem, you must prevent patients from grasping onto the circuit, and make sure that nothing is placed over the exhalation port area (e.g., sheets or bedding).

Humidification and Temperature-Regulation Problems

To avoid humidification or temperature-regulation problems with ventilator circuits in patients with artificial airways, your most important task is to ensure that gas delivered at the patient's airway is carrying *at least* 30 mg/L water vapor. Most current-generation HMEs meet this standard, as long as the minute volumes are not excessive. Heated humidifiers can easily meet and exceed this minimum and are typically set to deliver gas saturated with water vapor (100% room humidity) at proximal airway temperatures between 32 and 35°C. Unfortunately, since few humidification systems actually measure humidity levels, it is difficult to verify that these conditions are being met. *To ensure adequate humidification, always confirm that a few drops of condensation remain at or near the patient connection.*

Heated-wire systems pose a few additional problems. If the temperature of the wires is controlled separately from the humidifier, this can affect the relative humidity delivered to the patient. If the wires heat the gas in the circuit above the temperature at the outlet of the humidifier, then the relative humidity of the gas decreases, which can result in drying of secretions and/or mucous plugging. However, if the wires do not at least maintain the gas temperature at the same levels as at the outlet of the humidifier, cooling and condensation will occur in the delivery tubing.

Last, when heated-wire circuits are used to deliver gas to infants under radiant warmers or in incubators, two temperature zones are created—that of the room and that of the incubator or warmer. This essentially "confuses" the servo-control mechanism. Depending on the circumstances, this can result in either under- or overhumidification of the patient. To avoid this problem in radiant warmers, place the temperature probe and heater wire at the Y-piece and cover them with a light reflective shield to minimize spurious radiant warming. If the infant is in an incubator, the position of the probe/wires varies according to the set temperature:

- If the incubator temperature is set to less than 32°C, the temperature probe and heater wire should be placed at the Y-piece.
- If the incubator temperature is set to greater than 32°C, the temperature probe and heater wire should be placed just outside the incubator, with an unheated extension delivering the gas into the enclosure.

Infection and Cross-Contamination

In heated humidification systems that do not use heated-wire circuits, tubing condensation is a potential source for nosocomial infection. For this reason, you should always apply standard infection control methods when handling any breathing circuit. Specifically, in order to minimize nosocomial infections such as ventilator-associated pneumonia, the AARC recommends that you:

- Avoid regular changing of ventilator circuits—change only when absolutely necessary.
- Avoid unnecessary disconnection of the circuit or its components (e.g., for suctioning [consider in-line/closed suction catheter systems]).
- Avoid excessive accumulation of condensate in the circuit and accidental drainage back into the patient's airway; avoid contamination during circuit disconnection or disposal of condensate.
- As appropriate for the patient, consider HMEs or heated-wire circuits to eliminate condensate and lower infection risk.

NPPV Interface Problems

The last major area of ventilator circuit troubleshooting is that associated with various NPPV patient interfaces. **Table 6-18** summarizes the most common problems with these interfaces and their potential solutions.

Table 6-18 Common Noninvasive Positive Pressure Ventilation (NPPV) Interface Problems

Interface	Problems	Remedy
Nasal masks	Mouth leakage	Use chin strap (see Figure 6-5)
	Discomfort	Refit, adjust strap tension, change mask type
	Nasal bridge redness, pressure sores	Reduce strap tension, use forehead spacer, use nasal pillows, use artificial skin
	Skin rash	Use steroid cream, switch mask type
Oronasal masks	Rebreathing	Use plateau exhalation valve
	Impedes speech/eating	Permit periodic removal if tolerated
	Claustrophobia	Choose a clear mask with minimal bulk
	Aspiration	Exclude patients who cannot protect airway; use nasogastric tubes for nausea/abdominal distention
Nasal pillows	Mouth leakage	Use chin strap
	Discomfort	Proper fit, adjust strap tension, change mask type
	External nares redness, pressure sores	Clean/replace or use different-size pillows; reduce strap tension; temporarily use nasal mask
Oral devices	Dry mouth, throat, lips	Provide supplemental humidification; apply oral lubricant/saliva replacement
	Numb lips	Extend the distance between lips and flange
	Gum discomfort	Try a smaller seal
	Device falls out at night	Tighten the holder/use a larger seal
	Nasal leak	Consider noseplugs
	Sore jaw	Discourage biting down on appliance; device should be allowed to "float" in the mouth
	Excessive salivation	Usually temporary/resolves after initial use

Artificial Airways

An artificial airway is required when the patient's natural airway can no longer perform its proper functions. According to the AARC, conditions requiring management of the airway include airway compromise, respiratory failure, and the need to protect the airway.

General Selection, Use, and Troubleshooting

Table 6-19 outlines the basic indications, key factors in selection and use, and major troubleshooting considerations associated with the airways you use or encounter most frequently.

In addition to these devices, you may encounter four other specialized tracheal airway devices: (1) fenestrated tracheostomy tubes, (2) "speaking" tracheostomy tubes, (3) speaking valves, and (4) tracheostomy buttons. **Table 6-20** (see page 178) outlines the basic indications, key factors in selection and use, and major troubleshooting considerations associated with these specialized airway devices.

Vacuum Systems, Suction, and Pleural Drainage Devices

Suction Systems

Suctioning involves the removal of secretions or other fluids from the large airways using negative pressure. You select suction equipment when this procedure is indicated. According to the AARC, suctioning is indicated when you need to:

- Remove accumulated pulmonary secretions
- Obtain a sputum specimen
- Maintain the patency of an artificial airway
- Stimulate a cough in patients unable to cough effectively

Selection

All suction equipment includes three components: (1) a negative pressure (vacuum) source, (2) a collection system, and (3) a suction device for removing secretions or other fluids.

There are two common sources of negative pressure: (1) portable suction pumps and (2) central piped diameter index safety system (DISS) wall outlets. *You should choose a portable suction pump when a central piped vacuum outlet is unavailable,* as in some ambulatory clinics, for patient transport, and in the home.

Most portable suction pumps are electrically powered, by either line current or battery. Hand-powered portable suction pumps are also available. *You should select a battery- or hand-powered unit for transporting patients who may need suctioning.*

DISS vacuum wall outlets are available at the bedside in most hospital units. The DISS outlet is attached to a central piping system that connects to a large piston-driven suction pump. Negative pressure is adjusted and controlled by a suction regulator that attaches to the DISS outlet. The DISS outlet incorporates a one-way valve that closes the vacuum source off when no regulator is attached.

Table 6-19 Indications, Selection, Use, and Troubleshooting of Selected Artificial Airways

Indications	Selection and Use	Troubleshooting
Oropharyngeal Airways		

1. To prevent tongue from obstructing the upper airway during bag-mask ventilation
2. As a "bite block" in intubated patients
3. Generally contraindicated on conscious patients
	• Proper sizing: measure from the corner of the mouth to the angle of the jaw (see Chapter 10)
	• Proper positioning: airway should curve over and extend past the base of the tongue
		• If airway obstruction due to the tongue is not relieved:
		  • Remove the airway and reinsert/ reposition
		  • Recheck the size of the airway
		• If patient gags or retches, remove the device and maintain airway by positioning the head/neck; consider a nasopharyngeal airway as an alternative

Nasopharyngeal Airways		

1. To prevent upper airway obstruction when an oropharyngeal cannot be placed
2. To minimize trauma associated with repetitive suctioning via the nasal route
3. Contraindicated for infants and small children
	• Proper sizing: for average-sized female select a #6 (24-Fr), for average-sized male select a #7 (28-Fr)
	• When lubricated, the airway should fit through the inferior meatus without force
	• If too large it can cause mucosal trauma, gagging, vomiting, and gastric distention
	• Always insert with the beveled side pointed toward the centerline
	• Use a safety pin to ensure that the airway does not slip into the nose
		• If you cannot pass the airway:
		  • Be sure the airway is lubricated
		  • Try the other nare
		  • Try a smaller airway
		• If a suction catheter will not pass:
		  • Lubricate the catheter
		  • Consider a larger airway

(continues)

175

Table 6-19 Indications, Selection, Use, and Troubleshooting of Selected Artificial Airways (continued)

Indications	Selection and Use	Troubleshooting
Endotracheal Tubes		
1. To establish and protect the airway against aspiration in emergency situations or with unconscious patients 2. To provide short-term positive pressure ventilation (< 7 days) 3. To bypass upper airway obstruction (may require tracheotomy)	• Proper sizing is critical (see Chapter 10) • Inflate cuff to confirm integrity before intubating; deflate fully and lubricate before insertion • Typical adult insertion length from tip to incisors is 19–21 cm for females and 21–23 cm for males • Always check position by breath sounds; confirm with X-ray • Inflate cuff using MOV or MLT technique (see Chapter 10 for details) • See Chapter 10 for details on the procedure for intubation and Chapter 18 for guidance in assisting a physician with intubation	• Tube position (breath sounds) • If breath sounds not equal bilaterally, deflate the cuff, withdraw the tube 1–2 cm (adults), reinflate the cuff, recheck • If breath sounds not heard or the stomach distends, remove the tube/reintubate • Leaks—If a large leak occurs, reinflate the cuff to MOV, recheck for leaks • If leak persists, check the pilot balloon, inflation line, and valve for leaks (bypass by inserting a blunted small-gauge needle with three-way stop cock into the pilot line) • If the inflation line system is leak-free, the cuff is likely blown, requiring reintubation • Obstruction—follow the obstruction algorithm provided in Chapter 10
Laryngeal Mask Airways (LMA)		
1. As an alternative to ET intubation for emergency ventilatory support and airway control in or out of the hospital 2. To provide ventilatory support and/or airway control for patients who are difficult to intubate (high Mallampati classification) 3. Contraindicated in patients at high risk of aspiration	• Proper sizing is critical (infant/small child, 1–1.5; child, 2–3; adolescent/small adult, 3–4; adult, 4–6) • Prior to insertion, be sure to fully deflate mask cuff and lubricate mask (rim and posterior surface) • After proper positioning, inflate mask and confirm effective ventilation; do not exceed recommended maximum volume	• If you need maximum inflation volume to seal, consider a larger mask • Malposition of the airway can cause obstruction or leaks—repositioning the patient's head, readjust the tube's position or adjust the cuff inflation volume • A fiberoptic scope can confirm proper placement

(continues)

Table 6-19 Indications, Selection, Use, and Troubleshooting of Selected Artificial Airways (continued)

Indications	Selection and Use	Troubleshooting
Esophageal-Tracheal Combination Tubes		

1. As an alternative to ET intubation for emergency ventilatory support and airway control in or out of the hospital
2. To provide ventilatory support and/or airway control for patients difficult to intubate due to trauma, bleeding, vomiting, or other factors obscuring the vocal cords
3. Available only for adults; contraindicated in patients with esophageal disease
	• Proper sizing: 41-Fr for patients > 5 ft; 37-Fr for smaller patients
	• Leak test cuffs and then deflate before insertion
	  • proximal cuff (blue/#1): 85 mL
	  • distal cuff (white/#2): 15 mL
	• Insert until the two black marks at the proximal end of the tube are between the tube upper incisors
	• Inflate the distal cuff and ventilate first through the distal connector (#2); good breath sounds confirm tracheal placement
	• If gurgling is heard over the epigastrium while ventilating via the distal connector, the tube is in the esophagus; inflate the proximal cuff to 50–75 mL and ventilate through the proximal connector (#1)
	• ET tubes can provoke a more severe hemodynamic stress response than LMA or Combitube®
		• If you cannot ventilate through either connector the tube likely is inserted too far, causing the large proximal cuff to obstruct the glottis; rectify by withdrawing the tube 2–3 cm at a time while ventilating through connector #1 until breath sounds are heard over the lungs
		• Confirm tube placement via capnography

Tracheostomy Tubes		

1. To provide long-term positive pressure ventilation (> 7 days)
2. To bypass upper airway obstruction (when oral or nasal intubation is not feasible)
3. For patients needing a permanent artificial airway
	• Proper sizing is critical (see Chapter 10)
	• Inflate cuff to confirm integrity before intubating; deflate fully and lubricate before insertion
	• Confirm placement via X-ray
	• Be sure to secure neckplate/flange to avoid extubation; change disposable ties as needed for comfort and cleanliness
	• Inflate cuff using MOV or MLT technique (see Chapter 10)
	• Make sure that a correctly sized spare inner cannula is kept at the bedside
	• See Chapters 10 and 18 for guidance on changing trach tubes and providing tracheostomy care
		• Leaks
		  • If a large leak occurs, reinflate the cuff to MOV, recheck for leaks
		  • If leak persists, check the pilot balloon, inflation line, and valve for leaks (bypass by inserting a blunted small-gauge needle with three-way stop cock into the pilot line)
		  • If the inflation line system is leak-free, the cuff is likely blown, requiring reintubation
		• Obstruction—follow the obstruction algorithm provided in Chapter 10

Table 6-20 Indications, Selection, Use, and Troubleshooting of Specialty Tracheal Airway Devices

Indications	Selection and Use	Troubleshooting
Fenestrated Tracheostomy Tubes		
1. To facilitate weaning from a trach tube 2. To support patients needing intermittent (e.g., nocturnal) ventilatory support	• Sized the same as regular trach tubes (see Chapter 10) • Proper placement confirmed by fiberoptic bronchoscopy • Outer cannula has fenestration (opening) in the posterior wall above cuff • Removal of the inner cannula opens the fenestration • Plugging the tube's outer opening after deflating the cuff allows normal upper airway function • Remove the plug to suction the lower airway • To provide positive pressure or protect the lower airway, reinsert the inner cannula and reinflate the cuff	• ***Never plug the tube with the cuff inflated (attach a warning tag to the plug)*** • If respiratory distress occurs when the tube is plugged, make sure the cuff is fully deflated • If full deflation of the cuff does not relieve the distress, the tube may be improperly positioned between the skin and the stoma or against the back of the trachea; carefully reposition the tube
"Speaking" Tracheostomy Tubes		
1. To allow patients who have inadequate secretion clearance or poor upper airway protective reflexes to vocalize, even when receiving mechanical ventilation 2. For patients not needing a cuff for airway protection, consider a speaking valve instead	• Sized the same as regular trach tubes (see Chapter 10) • Include a separate small line that adds oxygen or air flow to an outlet above the cuff • 4–6 L/min of gas flow provides adequate patient vocalization • A "Y" connector is used to control when flow is applied • *Cuff must be inflated for vocalization*	• Leaks and obstructions are managed the same as a regular trach tube • Separately label the gas supply and cuff inflation lines to avoid accidental mix-up (connecting the cuff inflation line to a flow meter will burst the cuff and may damage the trachea and surrounding structures)
Tracheostomy Buttons		
1. To maintain an open stoma after a trach tube is removed 2. To facilitate weaning from a trach tube 3. To provide long-term access for patients requiring suctioning of the lower airway	• Consists of a short cannula flanged at both ends to help prevent slipping into/out of trachea • Exact insertion length controlled using spacers • Proper placement confirmed by fiberoptic bronchoscopy • A cap seals the button and forces the patient to breathe and cough via the upper airway • Some buttons provide an inner cannula with a standard 15-mm connector to deliver positive pressure ventilation if needed	• Regularly pass a suction catheter through the button to ensure patency • If respiratory distress occurs, the tube likely is protruding too far into the trachea; reposition by changing the number of spacers

(continues)

Table 6-20 Indications, Selection, Use, and Troubleshooting of Specialty Tracheal Airway Devices (continued)

Indications	Selection and Use	Troubleshooting
Speaking Valves		
1. To allow patients with trach tubes or buttons and who have an intact upper airway and good protective reflexes to vocalize, swallow, and cough normally 2. Contraindicated for unconscious patients or for use with HMEs or foam-filled cuffs	• Consists of a one-way valve that allows inspiration through the tube but blocks expiration out the tube • Attaches to trach tubes or buttons via 15-mm connector • ***When used with trach tubes, cuff must be fully deflated*** • Always suction through tube and above cuff before attaching • To provide supplemental O_2, use a trach collar or a speaking valve with a small-bore O_2 adaptor • When used during mechanical ventilation, time- or volume-cycled mode must be used and alarms readjusted to reflect patient expiration via natural airway and not through the breathing circuit	• If patient experiences distress with valve and cuff fully deflated, likely causes are upper airway obstruction, secretions clearance problems, or a trach tube that is too large; remove valve immediately • To prevent sticking due to dried secretions, valve should be cleaned daily in soapy water, rinsed thoroughly, and air dried • Should not be worn during sleep since valve could become clogged and cause obstruction and/or increased work of breathing

Suction regulators can provide either continuous or intermittent vacuum. *For common respiratory care use, you should use continuous vacuum.* Intermittent ("on-demand") suction is used mainly for gastrointestinal applications and surgical drainage.

To select the proper suction device, you need to answer four basic questions:

1. Where do you need to suction?
2. What is the size/age of the patient?
3. What is the condition of the patient?
4. What is (are) the goal(s) of suctioning?

Table 6-21 outlines the key considerations raised by these questions and specifies the appropriate suction device given the circumstances.

Assembly and Use

Most suction systems are preassembled with clear low-compliance tubing connecting the vacuum source (pump or regulator) to the collection bottle to the suction device. These systems also incorporate either a trap or float valve to prevent fluids from being aspirated into the suction pump or regulator. *You should make sure that the collection bottle is not full and the valve is not closed before operating the suction system.* In addition, you should inspect and ensure that all connections are tight, as any leaks will prevent adequate vacuum from being generated.

After checking all components and connections for a tight fit, you should turn the suction ON, either via the ON/OFF switch on electrical units or by adjusting the DISS wall regulator. Then crimp or obstruct the tubing coming from the collection bottle inlet and adjust the suction to the desired level while observing the vacuum gauge.

Negative pressure should be set to the lowest level needed to readily remove the patient's secretions and flush them out of the tubing with water. **Table 6-22** provides guidelines for setting the initial negative pressure levels for suctioning adults, children, and infants using portable and wall suction systems.

Table 6-21 Selection of Suctioning Devices

Question	Considerations	Recommendations
Where to suction	Oral cavity/nasal passages (newborn)	Choose bulb suction
	Oropharynx	Choose Yankauer tip
	Trachea	Select standard suction catheter
	Bronchus (R or L)	Use a Coude (curved) tip catheter
	Nasal route (frequent)	Consider nasopharyngeal airway
Patient size/age	Catheter diameter	Vary; apply formula
	Catheter length	Limit depth with infants
Patient condition	Meconium aspiration	Use meconium aspirator connected to ET tube
	Ventilator/PEEP	Consider closed suction system
	Leakage aspiration	Consider continuous aspiration system
Goals	Airway clearance	Use standard systems
	Sputum collection	Use sputum collection (Lukens) trap

After adjusting the vacuum pressure, connect the selected suction device to the system and implement the procedure. Chapter 11 provides details on procedures used to remove bronchopulmonary secretions, including suctioning. Below are a few additional equipment considerations:

- For routine suctioning of the trachea, select a standard suction kit containing sterile gloves, basin, water, and the proper-size catheter for the patient.
- Any device used to suction the lower airways should be sterile (this excludes Yankauer tips and bulb suction devices).
- To help prevent hypoxemia and atelectasis during suctioning, you will need the appropriate O_2-delivery equipment and a means to hyperinflate the patient. Some ventilators provide these as control functions; for patients not on ventilators you will need an O_2 source, flowmeter, and manual resuscitator with O_2 reservoir; as an alternative consider a double-lumen suction catheter that provides continuous oxygen insufflation.
- In patients for whom interruption of mechanical ventilation could result in reduced functional residual capacity (FRC) or severe hypoxemia (e.g., in cases of ARDS), select a "closed" suction catheter system.
- Patients at high risk for hypoxemia during suctioning should by monitored by pulse oximeter.
- To help minimize trauma to the nasal mucosa in patients requiring frequent suctioning via the nasal route, consider using a nasopharyngeal airway.
- In infants, suction catheters should be inserted only to the tip of the ET tube. This distance equals the tube insertion depth (as marked on the tube) plus the ET adapter length.

Table 6-22 Guidelines for Initial Negative Pressure Levels

Patient Group	Portable Suction Pump	Wall Regulator
Adults	−12 to −15 in Hg	−100 to −120 mm Hg
Children	−7 to −12 in Hg	−80 to −100 mm Hg
Infants	−5 to −7 in Hg	−60 to −80 mm Hg

Closed suction systems are placed directly in line with the ventilator circuit, which allows you to suction without disconnecting the patient from the ventilator. An irrigation port allows instillation of saline solution and flushing of the catheter, while a control valve regulates the application of negative pressure. As with all tracheobronchial suctioning, the patient still should receive a high F_{IO_2} before and after the procedure. Upon completion of closed suctioning of a patient on a ventilator, it is critical that you:

1. Retract the catheter (while firmly holding the T-piece) until its mark is visible in the sleeve
2. Turn off the wall suction regulator
3. Lock the suction thumb control valve in the OFF position by rotating it 180°

Troubleshooting

Most problems with suction systems are identified before beginning the procedure by conducting the equipment check described above. If when crimping or obstructing the tubing coming from the collection bottle you get inadequate suction, perform the following steps to correct the problem:

1. Make sure that the vacuum source is ON
   a. For a portable electrical pump, confirm that it is plugged in to an AC source and that the power switch is ON (if both are true and the pump/compressor still does not run, check the fuse/circuit breaker)
   b. For wall units, make sure that (i) the regulator is a continuous type, (ii) that it is properly fitted to the DISS vacuum outlet, and (iii) that its control switch (if applicable) is set to the ON position
2. Check for/correct leaks (the most common cause of inadequate suction)
   a. Check all tubing connections for tight fit
   b. Check the seal between any bottles or traps with screw-on lids
3. Check for/correct obstructions
   a. Check all tubing for kinks or compression (e.g., bed wheels)
   b. Check to see whether any float valve is blocking the suction source (this occurs normally when the collection bottle is full but can also happen accidentally)

If a leak appears due to the suction device itself (e.g., Yankauer tip, catheter, sputum collection vial, closed suction catheter system) and cannot easily be corrected, replace the device.

Other than leaks, closed suction catheter systems are associated with two other common problems: ET tube displacement/extubation and partial tube obstruction. To avoid ET tube displacement with these systems, *always firmly grasp the T-piece/connector when advancing or withdrawing the catheter*. To prevent partial tube obstruction, upon completing the procedure you must fully retract the catheter until you see its marker.

Pleural Drainage Systems

Pleural drainage systems remove free air and/or fluid from the pleural space via a chest tube. These systems are disposable, presterilized single-patient units that you select according to the patient's age/size (adult, pediatric, or infant). All consist of three key components: (1) a one-way seal, (2) a suction control, and (3) a fluid collection chamber. As depicted in **Figure 6-6**, traditional pleural drainage systems employ a "wet" seal and suction control. Newer units employ a "dry" one-way seal and suction control. Here we focus on the use and troubleshooting of the traditional systems.

Assembly and Use

To assemble a pleural drainage system for evacuation of pleural air or fluid (if the device is being used only to provide a water seal, perform only steps 1–3):

1. Aseptically open the package, being sure not to touch any tube connectors or internal surfaces
2. Position the system *below the patient's chest level*, usually by hanging it on the bed
3. Fill the water seal chamber with sterile water to the desired level (usually 2 cm) via its fill tube or needle diaphragm

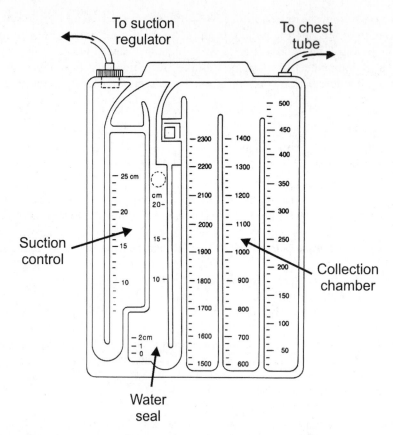

Figure 6-6 Traditional "Wet" Three-Chamber Pleural Drainage System. The suction control chamber water level determines the negative pressure (in cm H_2O) applied to the chest tube. The water seal prevents air from returning to the pleural space. The collection chamber gathers fluid aspirated through the chest tube.

4. Fill the suction control chamber with sterile water through its vent to the desired level, usually 20 cm; be sure that the vent is not obstructed
5. Connect the collection chamber tubing to the chest tube; avoid kinks or loops
6. Connect the suction chamber tubing to the suction outlet
7. Apply negative pressure until bubbling appears in the suction control chamber
8. Check to make sure that the suction control chamber is bubbling and that the water level in the water seal chamber rises and falls with the patient's breathing or the ventilator cycle

Once a pleural drainage system is operating, you should monitor the fluid levels regularly to ensure proper function:

1. If the water seal chamber level is less than 2 cm, refill it
2. If the suction control chamber level is less than the prescribed suction level, refill it
3. If the pleural fluid collection chamber fills, replace the unit with a new one

If you need to transport the patient, make sure the system remains below the patient's chest level and DO NOT clamp the chest tube. This will maintain the water seal and prevent any air from getting into the pleural space.

Troubleshooting

If the unit is set up for suction and there is no bubbling in the suction control chamber:

1. Check the suction control regulator to confirm that it is on
2. Check the suction chamber tubing for leaks (connections) or obstructions/kinking; correct
3. Check atmospheric vent to ensure that it is open and not obstructed

If there is continuous bubbling in the water seal chamber, there is either a leak at the patient *or* a drainage system leak. If the patient has a bronchopleural fistula and is receiving positive pressure, some air leakage is normal. Otherwise, you need to determine the source of the leak and correct it.

To determine the source of a pleural drainage system leak, you should briefly pinch the chest tube near its insertion point into the patient. If bubbling in the water seal chamber stops, the leak is at the insertion point or in the patient; if not, the leak is between the patient and the collection system.

1. If the leak is at the chest tube insertion point, contact the physician immediately. Leaks at the patient are usually due to either an outwardly displaced chest tube or an open insertion wound; use a sterile petroleum jelly gauze pad to temporarily stop insertion point leakage.
2. If leak is in the collection system, check/tighten all tubing connections and apply tape to temporarily seal any tears or holes; prepare a new drainage unit.

If the water level in the water seal chamber does not fluctuate with breathing, the drainage system is obstructed. In these cases:

1. Check the collection chamber tubing compression for kinks or dependent loops; correct if present
2. "Milk" the tubing connected to the chest tube by compressing and releasing it along its length *toward* the collection system (do this regularly to prevent clotting or obstruction)
3. If milking the tubing fails to restore pressure fluctuations in the water seal chamber:
   a. Check the patient for signs of pneumothorax
   b. Immediately notify the physician of the problem

Should the patient exhibit clear signs or symptoms of pneumothorax, be sure to immediately notify the physician and obtain both a thoracentesis kit and a tube thoracotomy tray.

Gas Cylinders, Reducing Valves, Flowmeters, and O$_2$ Blenders

Selection

In most hospitals, oxygen is supplied to all bedsides via a bulk/piped gas system, with compressed air also normally provided via piped outlets to critical care units. These piped gases are provided at the standard pressure of 50 psi for direct application to equipment requiring unrestricted flow, such as most critical care ventilators and oxygen-air blenders. If you need to meter gas flow to the patient, select and attach a *flowmeter* to the 50-psi outlet, using the appropriate DISS connector.

High-pressure gas cylinders are selected whenever a patient needs a therapy gas and a bulk/piped gas supply is not available. Typical settings or situations requiring gas cylinders are in specialized units lacking bulk/piped O$_2$, in the home or some extended care facilities, and during patient transport. In addition, all specialized gases (He, NO, CO, and CO$_2$) are provided in cylinders.

Since all high-pressure gas cylinders store gases at pressures much higher than 50 psi, they cannot be connected directly to any equipment. Instead, you must always use a *pressure-reducing valve* in combination with high-pressure gas cylinder gas. For equipment requiring 50 psi (e.g., ventilators, blenders, Thorpe-tube flowmeters), select a pressure-reducing valve *preset* to that pressure. Variable or *adjustable* pressure-reducing valves are used only in conjunction with a Bourdon-type flowmeter (Bourdon gauge). Technically, the combination of a pressure-reducing valve and a flowmeter is referred to as a gas *regulator*. **Table 6-23** provides guidelines for selecting regulators and reducing valves, connectors, and flowmeters according to setting.

As indicated in Table 6-23, selection of cylinder size is based on two major factors: (1) portability requirements and (2) needed duration of use. If portability is the first consideration (as during

Table 6-23 Guidelines for Selecting Gas Delivery Equipment

Purpose	Setting	Needed Equipment
To provide 50 psi unrestricted flow to ventilators or blenders	Bulk source available (most hospital units)	Connect directly to bulk gas source at 50 psi For precise O_2% use a blender
	Bulk source not available (specialized units, patient transport, specialty gases)	Large gas cylinder (H or K) with preset (50-psi) pressure-reducing valve For air, piston air compressor with reservoir
To deliver a controlled flow of gas to a patient or equipment	Bulk source available (most hospital units)	Connect calibrated Thorpe tube flow meter to bulk gas source at 50 psi
	Bulk source not available (specialized units, patient transport, specialty gases)	Gas cylinder with flow-controlling regulator; cylinder size selected based on portability requirements and needed duration of use For air, portable diaphragm compressor

short patient transports), select a small cylinder, coded as size E through AA. All cylinders in this small size range use a post-type valve stem with indexed pin holes (called a pin-indexed safety system, or PISS) for attaching reducing valves or regulators that use a matching yoke connector.

If you select a small cylinder for transport, you should use a regulator with a flow-metering system that is *unaffected by gravity*. Flow-metering systems unaffected by gravity include Bourdon gauges and fixed pressure-variable orifice (needle valve) regulators such as the Praxair Grab 'n Go™ or Western Medica's Oxytote™. If the patient is receiving O_2 and is being transported for a magnetic resonance imaging study, you must select equipment constructed without iron (e.g., aluminum cylinders and carts and brass and/or aluminum regulators).

If there is no need for portability and/or the duration of use for controlled-flow delivery exceeds an hour, you should select a large cylinder, usually size G, H, or K. All cylinders categorized as "large" have threaded valve outlets (American Standard Safety System [ASSS]) for connecting reducing valves or regulators. In general, these cylinders can store 10 times as much gas as their smaller counterparts.

Although medical-quality air can be provided via cylinder gas, with an unlimited supply freely available, electrically powered air compressors are the preferred source. Air may be piped to the bedside from large-volume compressors or delivered via portable devices at the point of care. Large-volume compressors typically use a piston to pressurize the gas and include a cylinder reservoir to meet unrestricted flow needs under high demand. Most portable compressors use a diaphragm to pressurize the air. This provides much less pressure and flow but is adequate to power small-volume nebulizers.

Assembly and Use of Cylinders, Reducing Valves, and Regulators

Once you have selected the appropriate cylinder and reducing valve or regulator, apply the following guidelines for assembly and use, including transport:

1. Before transporting a cylinder to its point of use:
   a. Check that the label and cylinder colors match. If there is any doubt about the contents, do not use it.
   b. Check the last hydrostatic test date. Do not use a cylinder that has not been appropriately tested.
   c. Make sure the cap used by large cylinders to protect the valve stem is in place.

2. Always use a cart to transport large cylinders (small cylinders used for transport can be placed in the gurney/wheelchair holder on the bed mattress). When moving large cylinders on or off a cart, roll the cylinder rather than lift it.

3. At the point of use, secure the cylinder in a stand, with a chain, or in a cart to prevent it from tipping over; do not chain a cylinder to any movable objects or heat radiators.

4. Remove the protective cap from a large cylinder or the tape seal covering the outlet of a small cylinder. Inspect the outlet for oil, dust, or debris.

5. After orienting the cylinder outlet away from any people in the immediate area and issuing a warning, clear any dust and debris from the valve by rapidly opening and then closing it (referred to as "cracking" the cylinder).

6. Attach the appropriate reducing valve or regulator to the cylinder. Most PISS reducing valves and regulators require a plastic washer to ensure a good seal. To ensure a tight ASSS connection, you will need a cylinder wrench.

7. After attaching the appropriate reducing valve or regulator, attach the needed equipment to the diameter indexed safety system (DISS) outlet (e.g., a flowmeter or 50-psi hose connected to a ventilator or blender; make sure adjustable regulators or flowmeters are OFF).

8. Slowly open the cylinder valve, record the cylinder pressure, and (if required) estimate the duration of flow for the equipment being used (see below). A small cylinder wrench or hand knob may be needed to open the valve of small cylinders.

9. After opening the cylinder valve completely, turn it back a quarter or half turn to prevent it from freezing open.

10. Before equipment is disconnected from a cylinder, the cylinder valve should be closed and the pressure released from any attached devices (e.g., regulators).

To estimate the duration of flow for a high-pressure gas cylinder, you need to know the cylinder factor, cylinder pressure, and flow. **Table 6-24** specifies the factors for commonly used oxygen, air, and helium mixture cylinders.

To compute a cylinder's duration of flow (in minutes), simply multiply the cylinder pressure by the appropriate cylinder and then divide by the flow in L/min.

$$\text{duration of flow (min)} = \frac{\text{pressure (psig)} \times \text{cylinder factor}}{\text{flow (L/min)}}$$

For example, if you need to determine how long an E cylinder of oxygen with a gauge pressure of 1000 psi set to deliver 4 L/min will last (until empty):

Step 1: Determine the cylinder factor for an oxygen E cylinder (Table 6-24), in this case 0.28.

Step 2: Apply the duration of flow equation.

$$\text{duration of flow (min)} = \frac{\text{pressure (psig)} \times \text{cylinder factor}}{\text{flow (L/min)}}$$

Table 6-24 Factors to Calculate Cylinder Duration of Flow (in minutes)

Gas	Cylinder Size			
	D	E	G	H&K
O_2, O_2/N_2, air	0.16	0.28	2.41	3.14
He/O_2	0.14	0.23	1.93	2.50

$$\text{duration of flow (min)} = \frac{1000 \times 0.28}{4} = 70 \text{ minutes (about 1 hour 10 mins)}$$

Note that the above computation is the time until the cylinder is *empty*. Some clinicians suggest changing cylinders when their gauge pressure drops below 500 psi. In these cases, subtract 500 from the cylinder pressure before doing the computation to determine when to change the cylinder.

The following simple rules of thumb for the two most common cylinder sizes used in hospitals can be used as shortcuts to estimate duration of flow:

- A full E oxygen cylinder running at 10 L/min will last about 60 minutes (~ 1 hour).
- A full H/K cylinder at the same flow will last about 10 times longer (~ 10 hours).

For example, a half-full E oxygen cylinder running at 10 L/min will last about 30 minutes (twice the flow, half the time). In contrast, a full H cylinder running at 5 L/min will last over 20 hours (half the flow, twice the time).

Assembly and Use of Oxygen Blenders

Select an oxygen blender in hospital settings when you need to deliver a range of precise O_2 concentrations to either equipment or the patient. All blenders require both unrestricted air and O_2 source gas, normally at standard line pressures of 50 psi. Most blenders output 50 psi at the set O_2%, which can be applied directly to power equipment or metered to control flow going to the patient. To set up a standard O_2 blender:

1. Connect 50-psi hoses from the air source to the air inlet and the O_2 source to the O_2 inlet
2. Check/confirm the pressure alarms by separately disconnecting each gas source; if either alarm fails, replace the device
3. Verify 100% and 21% O_2 settings with a calibrated oxygen analyzer
4. Set the blender to the prescribed O_2%
5. Attach the required delivery device
6. Verify the prescribed O_2% using an O_2 analyzer

Troubleshooting

Cylinders and Regulators

Most problems with cylinders and regulators involve leakage at the valve stem or in the regulator. If a leak occurs when the cylinder valve is opened:

1. Tighten the connection between the regulator and the cylinder valve
2. Recheck the bushing/washer used with PISS connection; leakage will occur if it is missing or an extra one is in place
3. If the regulator is leaking, replace it
4. Check for and correct any leaks between the regulator and any attached equipment

If gas does not flow from the cylinder regulator:

1. Check the pressure gauge for adequate pressure
2. If the gauge indicates cylinder pressure, check the regulator outlet for obstruction
3. If the problem cannot be determined, replace the regulator

Compressors

Well-maintained compressor systems are generally trouble-free. If a problem occurs it is usually with the electrical components or the inlet filters. If the unit fails to operate when the switch is turned on:

1. Check the electrical outlet for power
2. Check the fuse or circuit breaker and replace or reset it (*once only*—take any electrical device out of service if it shorts out a second time)

If during operation the compressor output appears inadequate:

1. Check inlet filter for obstruction
2. Check tubing and connected equipment for obstruction
3. Check tubing and connections for leaks

O_2 Blenders

Blenders function only when provided with adequate air and O_2 source gas pressures. Normally an alarm system warns you if source pressures are inadequate. If a blender pressure alarm sounds when both gas sources are attached:

1. Verify that both gas sources are at the required inlet pressures (usually 35–50 psig)
2. Check for leaks between the gas source and hose and between the hose and blender
3. If these check out, replace the blender

O_2 *blenders do not normally monitor the actual O_2%.* This is why you should always verify the prescribed O_2% using a calibrated oxygen analyzer. If you determine that there is a large discrepancy between blender setting and the actual O_2% using an oxygen analyzer, first recheck the air and O_2 hoses to make sure that they have not been accidently switched. Usually this would be obvious since DISS cheater adaptors would have to be used to make wrong hosing connections. Assuming this is not the case, recheck the O_2% with another analyzer. If you confirm the discrepancy, replace the blender.

Point-of-Care Blood Gas Analyzers

Point-of-care testing (POCT) involves the collection, measurement, and reporting of selected laboratory tests at or near the site of patient care rather than via a central laboratory. Commonly, POCT is indicated for patients in urgent need of assessment for whom central laboratory processing would delay needed therapy. Typically, patients who might need such "real-time" analysis of lab results include those receiving care in the emergency department, critical care units, and operating rooms.

Selection

POCT instruments vary substantially. However, most measure patient blood samples obtained via normal venous or arterial puncture using a small, handheld portable device that employs disposable analysis cartridges specifically designed for each desired battery of tests. The most common POCT tests done by respiratory therapists are for arterial blood gases (ABGs) or combined panels that include ABG measures plus other selected values of importance in managing critically ill patients.

If POCT is ordered for ABG analysis and you are authorized to perform it, you need to obtain the following equipment:

- A complete ABG kit
- A properly charged POCT analyzer
- The appropriate analysis cartridge

Which analysis cartridge you select depends on the tests being ordered. Typically, the simple ABG cartridge provides measures of pH, P_{O_2}, and P_{CO_2}, with calculated values for HCO_3, BE, total CO_2, and O_2 saturation. A variety of combined panel tests provide these measures plus selected electrolyte concentrations (sodium, potassium, chloride, calcium), the anion gap, hematocrit and hemoglobin content, glucose levels, blood lactate, and/or the blood urea nitrogen (BUN).

Assembly and Use

The following outlines the basic procedure for use of the Abbott Laboratories I-STAT POCT instrument. Other devices may employ slightly different procedures.

1. Review the order and obtain the required equipment
2. Use two identifiers to identify the patient
3. Explain the procedure to the patient

4. Follow universal precautions, including gloving
5. Turn the analyzer ON
6. From the menu provided, specify the cartridge type/test panel to be performed
7. Scan or enter the operator and patient IDs*
8. Carefully remove the cartridge from its pouch; avoid touching any contact pads
9. Obtain the sample as usual and analyze it within 3 minutes (do *not* place it in ice)
10. Mix the sample thoroughly and dispense it into the cartridge well to the fill mark
11. Close the sample well cover, insert the cartridge into its port, and confirm placement
12. Enter any requested information—e.g., type of sample, F_{IO_2}, patient temperature
13. View the results shown on the analyzer's display screen
14. Remove the cartridge when indicated by the analyzer
15. Dispose of biohazardous materials according to protocol
16. Communicate test results
17. Turn analyzer OFF
18. Place analyzer in the downloader/recharger

* *Note:* Fingerprints or a smudge on an analyzer's scanner window can cause scanning error. If accessible, clean the scanner window with water or lens cleaner and wipe dry with gauze.

Troubleshooting

POCT analyzers are highly reliable semiautomated computerized devices. Since calibration occurs as part of the test cycle on each cartridge, minimal user intervention is needed. For this reason, assuming that proper quality control procedures are in place (as discussed in Chapter 8), you will seldom need to troubleshoot a POCT analyzer. **Table 6-25** summarizes the few problems that you may encounter in using a POCT analyzer, along with the causes and potential solutions.

Note that you may obtain a POCT result that is *outside the critical range* programmed into the device, such as a pH level less than 7.20 or greater than 7.60. *Such readings are NOT the same as flagged or "outside reportable range" results and should be treated as potentially valid data.* Generally, to validate measures that fall outside the device's critical ranges, you should repeat the analysis using a fresh sample and new cartridge. Some hospital protocols insist that out-of-range POCT results be repeated in the central laboratory. Either way, you should not wait for the repeat results if the findings are life threatening or coincide with the patient's clinical picture. For example, if the POCT result indicates a P_{O_2} less than 40 torr and the patient exhibits signs or symptoms of hypoxemia, increase the F_{IO_2} while awaiting the repeat test results.

Incentive Breathing Devices

According to the AARC, incentive spirometry involves the use of devices to assist patients in performing a sustained maximal inspiration (SMI), or a slow, deep breath followed by a breath hold. Incentive spirometry is indicated for patients predisposed to or diagnosed with atelectasis. The primary contraindication is inability of the patient to cooperate, and the primary hazard is hyperventilation.

Selection

1. Most incentive spirometers are disposable, single patient-use devices that come preassembled from the manufacturer.
2. Most devices are flow oriented, but include a volume accumulator.
   a. A flowmeter with high/low scale helps the patient maintain the desired slow inspiratory flow.
   b. The volume accumulator (usually a simple piston) provides an estimate of the patient's inspired volume and allows you to set a goal for the patient via an adjustable volume indicator.
   c. If there is no volume accumulator, you can estimate the inspiratory volume by multiplying the flow by the inspiratory time. For example, if the patient's sustained flow is 700 cc/sec and the estimated inspiratory time is 3 seconds, then the inspired volume would be: 700 cc/sec × 3 sec = 2100 cc, or about 2100 mL.

Table 6-25 Troubleshooting Common Problems with POCT Analyzers

Problem/Clue	Cause(s)	Solution(s)
Analyzer does not turn ON	Batteries discharged or dead	Check to confirm that the batteries are properly charged; if you cannot properly charge the unit's batteries, replace them.
Analyzer turns ON but fails to display proper startup information	Software startup/boot error	Restart the analyzer (i.e., turn it OFF, wait 10–20 seconds, and then turn it ON again); replace device if second startup fails.
Calibration ERROR message[a]	A problem with the sample, calibrating solutions, sensors, or device electrical or mechanical function	Take the action recommended in the error message and report findings (in some cases this may be a numeric error code that has to be looked up in user's manual); repeat analysis using a fresh sample and new cartridge.
FAILED electrical simulator test[a]	A problem with the device's electrical functions	Report findings and replace the device.
Flagged results	Results outside the analyzer's reportable ranges	Send sample to the central laboratory for analysis.
Results rejected based on quality control criteria	A problem with the sample, calibrating solutions, sensors, or device electrical or mechanical function	Repeat analysis using a fresh sample and new cartridge. If sample integrity is not in question, the results that are not rejected should be reported in the usual manner. If results are rejected twice, send sample to the central laboratory for analysis.

a. ISO International Standard 22870: *Point-of-care testing (POCT)—Requirements for quality and competence* requires that all errors be documented and that a complete audit trail exists for each entry, including resolution of the error or problem.

3. You select an incentive spirometer based on its maximum volume.
   a. Select a device with a maximum volume over 2500 mL for adults.
   b. Select a device with a maximum volume under 2500 mL for pediatric patients (pediatric devices often include colorful, child-oriented labeling to help gain patient compliance).

Assembly

1. Remove the device and its accessories from the packaging.
2. Confirm that the flow indicator and piston move freely by turning the unit upside down.
3. Inspect the connecting tubing, mouthpiece, and spirometer inlet for any obstructions, including loose parts or packaging material.
4. If necessary, attach the flexible tubing to the spirometer inlet and the mouthpiece to the flexible tubing or one-way breathing valve.

Use

Given that incentive spirometry is normally self-administered and performed under limited supervision, good preliminary patient instruction is critical to its success. Details on the use of incentive spirometry are provided in Chapter 12. Below are some key points to consider when incentive breathing is ordered for a patient:

- Patients who are not alert or cannot follow instruction cannot benefit from incentive breathing; consider intermittent positive pressure breathing (IPPB) for these patients.
- If ordered for a surgical patient, this instruction ideally should occur preoperatively.
- Patient instruction should clearly:
  - Establish reasonable volume goals
  - Emphasize the importance of a 5–10 second breath hold
  - Stress the need to repeat the procedure 6–10 times/hr
  - Describe the importance of allowing recovery time between breaths (to prevent hyperventilation)
  - Demonstrate wound splinting and proper cough technique (for surgical patients)
- To confirm patient understanding, always ask the patient to demonstrate the procedure back to you.
- If the need exists to obtain an accurate measure of the patient's inspired volume, attach a one-way breathing valve and calibrated respirometer to the incentive breathing device.

After preliminary patient instruction and confirmation of proper incentive breathing technique, you should arrange for periodic patient visits to monitor therapy compliance and provide additional instruction as necessary. During such visits, you should encourage increasing the inspiratory volume goal and—before leaving—make sure that the device is within the patient's reach.

Troubleshooting

Incentive breathing devices are simple and generally trouble-free. Below are the basic troubleshooting tips:

- Carefully inspect all components before use in order to prevent the potential hazards of device obstruction and/or aspiration of small parts.
- In units with one-way valves, inspect the valve to make sure that it is aligned with direction of flow and functions properly (i.e., inspiration through the device/expiration out to the room).
- If the device doesn't record any inspired flow or volume, check for loose connections or an improperly functioning one-way valve.
- Replace any unit that does not appear to be functioning as expected.

Percussors and Vibrators

You use handheld, externally applied pneumatically or electrically powered percussors and vibrators to aid in secretion clearance during bronchial hygiene therapy. As compared to manual "clapping" and vibration, these devices deliver consistent rates, rhythms, and impact force and do not cause fatigue. There are also useful when home caregivers can't or won't perform manual percussion/vibration and are often preferred by patients over manual methods. In selecting a mechanical percussor or vibrator, however, note that these devices generally are no more effective in facilitating secretion clearance than manual methods.

An alternative to handheld mechanical percussor or vibrator is a high-frequency chest wall oscillation (HFCWO) vest system. These systems consist of a fitted inflatable vest and an air-pulse generator, connected via two large-bore tubes. A rotary valve in the air-pulse generator produces alternating high-frequency positive pressure bursts. You can adjust both the magnitude and the frequency of these positive pressure pulses. Pulse magnitude is scaled in relative units from 1 to 10, while the frequency can be adjusted from 5 to 20 Hz. Typically these devices are used in the home by patients with chronic conditions causing retained secretions, such as cystic fibrosis.

Mechanical oscillations also can be applied *internally* via a technique called intrapulmonary percussive ventilation (IPV). IPV combines high-frequency (100–1800/min) percussive bursts of gas and positive expiratory pressure (PEP) with aerosol therapy.

Selection

- For hospitalized adults or large children receiving postural drainage, percussion, and vibration (PDPV), either an electrically or pneumatically powered percussor or vibrator can be used instead of manual methods.
- For infants or small children, use appropriately sized percussion cups or a percussion "wand" (if percussion cups are not available, you can use a round infant oronasal mask).
- For hospitalized adults or large children requiring percussion or vibration in combination with aerosol drug therapy, consider an IPV device, either pneumatically or electrically (compressor) powered.
- For care of adults or large children requiring PDPV in the home who have caregiver support, choose an electrically powered unit.
- For care of adults requiring PDPV in the home who *do not* have caregiver support, consider a HFCWO vest system or electrically powered IPV device.

Assembly and Use

Handheld percussors and vibrators require little or no assembly. To use:

1. Connect to the needed power source
   a. Connect pneumatically powered devices directly to a 50-psi wall via high pressure DISS tubing (no flowmeter).
   b. Connect electrically powered devices to standard 110/120-volt AC electrical outlets. As with all electrically powered devices used in the hospital, these devices must be either properly grounded or enclosed within a double-insulated case and be used in compliance with OSHA standards (Standard 1910 Subpart S—Electrical—General).
2. If provided, attach a disposable pad for each treatment application
3. To provide percussion, adjust the force to achieve the desired impact (mimicking the typical hollow sound heard with manual cupping), according to patient comfort
4. To provide vibration, use the higher available frequencies (20–30 Hz) and apply during exhalation only
5. Implement your regular bronchial hygiene therapy procedure or protocol, to include directed coughing and (if required) suctioning

To assemble and use an HFCWO vest system:

1. Fit the vest on the patient (fasten it close to the body during a deep inhalation)
2. Connect the air hoses to the air-pulse generator and vest
3. Connect the remote control (on/off switch) to the air-pulse generator
4. Plug the air-pulse generator's power cord into a grounded electrical outlet
5. To initiate therapy, select the mode, frequency, pressure, and treatment time and activate the unit with the remote
6. Implement your regular bronchial hygiene therapy procedure or protocol, to include directed coughing and (if required) suctioning

To assemble and use an IPV device:

1. Connect each of the four color-coded tubes to the breathing head assembly (matching color orifice) and to their corresponding color-coded sockets on the IPV unit.
2. Place the prescribed medication in the nebulizer bowl and dilute with 20 mL sterile water or normal saline; twist-lock the nebulizer bowl back on the nebulizer housing
3. Rotate the percussion control knob arrow to the 12:00 (top) position
4. Attach the IPV unit to 35–60-psig source of medical air or oxygen
5. Set an operating pressure of 35 psig on the line pressure regulator

6. Confirm the function of the IPV unit
   a. Observe mouthpiece or mask for a dense aerosol mist
   b. Hold percussion button down and observe a cyclic percussive function
   c. Rotate the percussion control knob arrow full travel in both directions, and observe a change in percussive impaction rates
   d. Release percussion button and rotate percussion control knob arrow (full counterclockwise) to the EASY position
7. Start IPV therapy by having the patient breathe the aerosol for about a minute
8. Have the patient seal his or her lips tightly around the mouthpiece and activate the percussion button down to apply continuous percussion while breathing
9. Adjust percussion control to ensure visible/palpable chest wall vibrations during application
10. Have the patient release the percussion button to pause therapy or cough
11. Continue therapy for 15–20 minutes; implement your regular bronchial hygiene therapy procedure or protocol, to include directed coughing and (if required) suctioning
12. Process equipment in the same manner as for small-volume nebulizers or IPPB circuits

Troubleshooting

- Failure of a percussor or vibrator to function at all is usually due to lack of source power. Check and confirm proper connections to the pneumatic or electrical power source. If the device is electrically powered, also check for a burned-out fuse or tripped circuit breaker and replace or reset it. For pneumatically powered devices, make sure the source is not flow restricted.
- If an HFCWO vest system fails to oscillate, make sure that the remote is connected and in the activated position; if oscillation is inadequate after adjustment, check all tubing connections and make sure the vest is properly fitted.
- Failure of an IPV device to function properly is usually due to either inadequate source pressure or a loose tubing connection. Make sure that the source gas pressure is at or above 35 psig and check/tighten all connections between the breathing head assembly (matching color orifice) and their sockets on the IPV unit.

Positive Expiratory Pressure Devices

A positive expiratory pressure (PEP) device generates positive pressure during expiration. According to the AARC, positive expiratory pressure devices are indicated to:

- Reduce air trapping in asthma and COPD
- Help mobilize retained secretions
- Prevent or reverse atelectasis
- Optimize delivery of bronchodilators

Due to the increased airway pressures generated by these devices, they are generally contraindicated for patients who cannot tolerate any increased work of breathing, are hemodynamically unstable, or suffer from bullous emphysema, high intracranial pressures (ICP), untreated pneumothorax, sinusitis, epistaxis, or middle ear problems.

Selection

There are three types of PEP devices, summarized in **Table 6-26**. All devices can typically generate between 6 and 25 cm H_2O pressure during passive exhalation and allow unrestricted inspiration.

In general, if the goal is to reduce air trapping in asthma and COPD or to prevent or reverse atelectasis, you can select either a flow or threshold resistor PEP device. Based on your assessment, you may need to choose the best model to match the patient's flow capabilities. For example, the Acapella® device comes in two models: one for patients who can sustain expiratory flows of 15 L/min or higher, and one for those with sustained flows less than 15 L/min. At very low flows (< 5 L/min), oscillations produced by the Flutter valve® become irregular in both frequency and amplitude, suggesting that it may be less effective when used under these conditions.

If concurrent bronchodilator aerosol therapy is indicated, all devices except the Flutter valve® and Threshold™ PEP device provide adaptors for attaching a small-volume nebulizer. If the goal is

Table 6-26 Positive Expiratory Pressure (PEP) Devices

Type of PEP Device	Mechanism to Generate PEP	Example
Flow resistor	Patient exhales against a fixed orifice (size based on patient age and expiratory flow)	TheraPEP® system
Threshold resistor	Patient exhales against an adjustable counterweight, spring-loaded valve, or reverse Venturi	EZPap®a Threshold™ PEP device
Vibratory PEP	Patient exhales against a threshold resistor with an expiratory valve that oscillates at high frequency (10–30 Hz)	Flutter valve® Quake®b Acapella®

a. The EZPap® device also provides positive pressure on inspiration.

b. To generate pressure oscillations, patients using the Quake® device must rotate a crank to open and close the expiratory orifice (frequency determined by the rate of rotation).

to help mobilize retained secretions, then a vibratory PEP device is the best choice. **Figure 6-7** depicts the two most common vibratory PEP devices, the Flutter valve® and Acapella®.

Current evidence indicates that PEP therapy is no more effective than other methods of bronchial hygiene, such as chest percussion and vibration. However, since many patients prefer PEP to these other methods, your selection of this therapy and the device used should take into account the patient's preference.

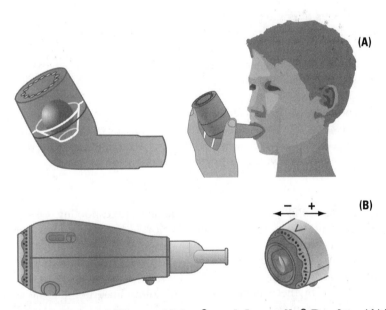

Figure 6-7 The Pipe-Shaped Flutter Valve® and Acapella® Device. (A) The pipe-shaped flutter valve contains a heavy steel ball that sits atop a cone-shaped orifice covered by a perforated cap. When a patient exhales through the mouthpiece, the weight of the ball creates expiratory pressures between 10 cm to 25 cm H_2O. Due to the angle of orifice, the ball rapidly rises and falls, which creates the pressure oscillations. Flutter valve® PEP levels increase when the device is raised above horizontal and with higher expiratory flows. (B) The Acapella® device uses a counterweighted lever and magnet to produce PEP and airflow oscillations. As exhaled gases pass through the device, flow is intermittently blocked by a plug attached to the lever, producing the vibratory oscillations. PEP levels are adjusted using an uncalibrated knob located at the distal end of the device. To increase PEP levels, you turn this knob clockwise.

Assembly and Use

Most PEP devices come preassembled and include a mouthpiece as the patient interface. Depending on the patient, you may need to consider using a mask instead. With most PEP devices, you also will need a manometer and connecting tubing to calibrate/monitor the patient's expiratory airway pressure.

Below are the key considerations in applying PEP therapy:

1. The patient should be seated upright (required for the Flutter valve®) or in a semi-Fowler's position, with the abdomen unrestricted
2. For initial application, you should set PEP to its lowest level:
   a. Largest resistor on the TheraPEP®
   b. Lowest spring tension (< 5) on the Threshold™ PEP
   c. Lowest input flow (~ 5 L/min) on the EZPap®
   d. Horizontal position of the Flutter valve®
   e. Full counterclockwise position of the Acapella® knob
3. Slowly increase the PEP level to between 10 and 20 cm H_2O as tolerated:
   a. Apply a smaller resistor on the TheraPEP®
   b. Increase spring tension (> 5) on the Threshold™ PEP
   c. Increase input flow (> 5 L/min) on the EZPap®
   d. Raise the angle of the Flutter valve® above horizontal
   e. Turn the Acapella® knob clockwise
4. Encourage patient to maintain proper breathing pattern:
   a. Slow, deep inspirations with a 2–3 second breath hold
   b. Active (but not forced) exhalation lasting 3–4 seconds
   c. Overall I:E ratio between 1:3 and 1:4
5. If vibratory PEP is being applied, you should be able to palpate chest wall vibrations over the central airways during exhalation
6. Once you establish a proper breathing pattern, have the patient perform sets of 10–20 breaths
7. If the goal is to help mobilize secretions, implement your regular bronchial hygiene therapy procedure or protocol, to include directed coughing
8. Repeat these steps as needed while monitoring the patient's response

Home-care patients should be instructed to follow these same steps. In addition, you should teach these patients how to disassemble, clear, and maintain the PEP device. Most of these devices can be cleaned in warm, soapy (detergent) water, followed by a good rise and complete drying. Some of these devices can be processed in a dishwasher if properly disassembled.

Troubleshooting

Based on their simple design, PEP devices require minimal troubleshooting. Obviously, if the device fails to generate pressure during patient expiration, the most likely problem is a leak, either in the device itself or in the system connecting it to a pressure manometer. In these cases, you should recheck and tighten all connections. Also, if a Flutter valve® is incorrectly positioned upside down, no expiratory pressure will generated. Too high a pressure can occur in any of these devices if the outlet port is obstructed—for example, by the patient's hand or bedding. Ensuring that the outlet port remains open will overcome this problem.

Manometers

Selection

A manometer is a device that measures pressure. There are three primary types of pressure-measuring devices used in respiratory and critical care: fluid columns, aneroid manometers, and electronic pressure transducers. **Table 6-27** briefly describes each of these devices, along with their common applications and usage considerations.

Table 6-27 Types of Manometers and Their Clinical Applications

Device Description	Common Applications	Considerations
Fluid columns		
Measure pressure as the height of a column of fluid with known density (i.e., water or mercury)	To measure atmospheric pressure (barometer) To measure static or slowing changing pressures (e.g., CVP) To measure systolic/diastolic blood pressures (occlusion method) To calibrate other pressure-measuring devices	Most accurate measure of static pressures Not suited for measuring rapidly changing pressures Accuracy depends on position (must be vertical) Can be messy or hazardous (mercury)
Aneroid (liquid-free) manometers		
Measure pressure in a metal chamber that expands and contracts with applied pressure changes; chamber motion activates a geared pointer, which provides a scale reading analogous to pressure	To measure systolic/diastolic blood pressures (noninvasive occlusion method) To measure airway pressure on ventilators or MIP/MEP on spontaneously breathing patients To measure tracheal tube cuff pressures To measure pressures in gas cylinders To measure vacuum (negative pressure) on wall and portable suction units	Avoid the mess and hazards associated with fluid columns Can display rapidly changing pressures Not useful if measurements need to be stored or analyzed Require calibration to ensure accuracy
Electronic pressure transducers		
Most common design (strain gauge) measures pressure via expansion and contraction of a flexible metal diaphragm connected to electrical wires; bending of the diaphragm changes the current flow through it, which is proportional to the pressure changes	To continuously measure/monitor rapidly changing pressures (e.g., arterial blood pressure, CVP, airway pressures), including those measured during selected PFT test procedures like body plethysmography	Good at displaying rapidly changing pressures Can be connected to a graphics display or paper recorder Output can be digitized and stored for computer analysis Require physical and electrical calibration

So which pressure measurement device do you select? Most of the time you have no choice—the device is already connected to the system being checked or monitored. However, a few key pointers can be helpful when given a specific task involving pressure measurement:

- To measure atmospheric pressure when calibrating a blood gas analyzer, use a barometer.
- To measure static pressures in compressed gas cylinders, use an aneroid gauge calibrated for high pressures.
- To measure low relative pressures intermittently (NIF, cuff pressures), use a low-pressure aneroid manometer calibrated in the units being measured or reported.
- To measure and display rapidly changing pressures continuously, use a calibrated electronic pressure transducer.
- If pressure data need to be recorded, stored, or analyzed, use an electronic pressure transducer (and computer system).
- To calibrate either a low-pressure aneroid manometer or electronic pressure transducer, use a U-tube fluid column (Hg or H_2O).

Use

To obtain a pressure reading from an aneroid gauge or digital display, simply read the device's indicator pointer/needle. Getting an accurate pressure reading from a fluid column is a bit different. Generally, the pressure for a fluid column is equivalent to the height of the column, with the units based on the column scale and fluid used. For example, when using a mercury barometer or sphygmomanometer, the pressure is equivalent to the height of the mercury column, with the units being mm Hg. Likewise, for a CVP manometer, the pressure is equivalent to the height of the water column, with the units being cm H_2O.

The U-tube fluid manometer represents a special case (**Figure 6-8**). These devices are typically used to measure small static gas pressure differences. Its most common application is as a calibration standard for mechanical manometers or electronic pressure transducers. As shown in Figure 6-8, you read the pressure as the difference in height between the two liquid levels.

Depending on their application, manometers may be calibrated in cm H_2O (ventilators, airway pressure, cuff pressure), mm Hg (wall suction, sphygmomanometers), or pounds per square inch/psi (cylinder regulators). Some manometers even use SI units (kilopascals). Respiratory therapists must be able to convert among these various units. **Table 6-28** provides the factors needed to convert one pressure measurement unit to another.

Troubleshooting

The primary problem in measuring pressure is inaccurate readings. To obtain accurate pressure measurements, you must make sure that the manometer you use is properly calibrated. As a first step for any device that measures pressure *relative* to atmospheric pressure, check and confirm that it reads zero pressure units when open to the atmosphere. If not, either reset the device to zero or replace it. Some aneroid manometers have a calibrating screw that you can use to set a zero pressure reading. Pressure transducers typically include an electronic zeroing mechanism. Unfortunately, zeroing a pressure manometer does not always ensure accurate readings of pressures above or below atmospheric pressure. To ensure accurate readings of pressures above or below atmospheric pressure, the device

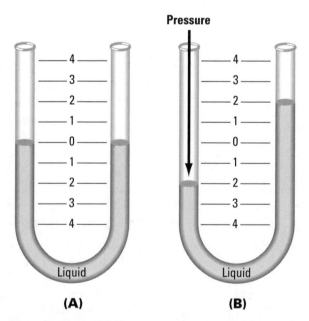

Figure 6-8 U-Tube Manometer. (A) At zero pressure relative to atmospheric, the liquid levels on the two sides of the U-tube are equal. (B) When pressure is applied to one side of the manometer, the liquid is displace down on that side and up on the opposite side. You read the pressure as the difference in height between the two liquid levels. In this example the difference in height is +2 − (−2) = 4 units. If the liquid is water and the scale is in centimeters, the reading would be 4 cm H_2O.

Table 6-28 Pressure Conversion Factors

Conventional Unit	Alternate Unit	Factor[a]
cm H_2O	kilopascal (kPa)	0.0981
mm Hg (torr)	kPa	0.1333
mm Hg (torr)	cm H_2O	1.363
lbs/in2 (psi)	kPa	6.895
psi	cm H_2O	70.31
a. To convert from conventional to alternate unit, *multiply* conventional unit by factor. To convert from alternate unit back to conventional unit, *divide* alternate unit by factor. Examples: 10 mm Hg (torr) = 10 × 1.363 cm H_2O = 13.6 cm H_2O; 25 cm H_2O = 25/1.363 = 18.3 mm Hg		

must undergo calibration. For a simple aneroid manometer this may simply mean comparing its readings to either a fluid column manometer or a precision laboratory instrument verified for calibration measurements. Calibrating electronic transducers is a more complicated process usually performed by biomedical engineers.

The measurement system must be leak-free in order to obtain accurate pressure readings. When you assemble any pressure measurement system, you need to check and confirm that all connections are tight and leak-free.

In addition, when measuring vascular pressures via liquid-filled lines, any partial obstruction, such as that caused by air bubbles or small clots, can reduce the amplitude of the pressure fluctuations, a phenomenon called *damping*. **Figure 6-9** portrays damping of a pulmonary artery pressure waveform and its correction by flushing the catheter line.

When measuring vascular pressure such as central venous, pulmonary artery, or capillary wedge pressures, it is also essential to ensure that the base of the fluid column or pressure transducer is positioned at a level equal to the point of measurement—i.e., the right atrium (also called the *phlebostatic axis*). Otherwise, the system will behave like a U-tube manometer and overestimate pressures if placed too low, or underestimate pressures if placed too high. Note that any change in the patient's position will have the same effect and will require readjusting the location of the fluid column or pressure transducer.

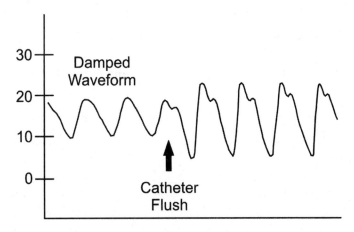

Figure 6-9 Damping of Pulmonary Artery Pressure Measurement Due to Partial Obstruction of the Fluid Line (Due to Bubbles and/or Small Clots). Flushing the catheter eliminates the damping and restores the normal pulse-pressure waveform.

Bedside Pulmonary Function Devices

Selection

Devices used to measure pulmonary function at the bedside include respirometers and portable electronic spirometers. Portable spirometers, most of which incorporate a pneumotachometer, are used to obtain pulmonary function measures equivalent to those assessed in a pulmonary lab, but at the bedside in an office or clinic. As indicated in **Table 6-29,** which type of device you select depends on what you plan to measure.

Mechanical Respirometers

Mechanical respirometers like the Wright and Haloscale measure gas volume via a turbine-like design in which flow rotates a foil vane (flow measurement is unidirectional). A gear mechanism translates these vane rotations into movement of indicator hands on a watch-like analog dial. The dial has two separate scales, a larger outer scale and a smaller inner scale, each divided in units of volume. One scale indicates liters (for minute tidal volume), while the other indicates fractions of a liter (for tidal volume). An ON/OFF switch unlocks/locks the gear mechanism, while a rest button zeros the indicator hands.

The adult Wright respirometer is accurate within 2% at 16 L/min. A pediatric (infant/small child) model is available that is accurate within 5% when measuring volumes between 15 and 200 mL. As with most turbine systems, these devices tend to over-read at high flows and under-read at low flows. Because the adult Wright can be damaged by flows greater than 60 L/min, *it should not be used to measure forced inspiratory or expiratory volumes.* The recommended maximum flow through the pediatric version is 30 L/min.

Use. Before each use, you should check the respirometer for proper function. To do so:

1. Inspect the inlet and outlet of the device to make sure they are clean, free from deposits, and dry
2. Check the foil vane. If it is bent or damaged, the respirometer must be repaired
3. Check the turbine/gear mechanism:
   a. Reset the pointers to zero and ensure that the unit is ON
   b. Cup the device in the palm of one hand, with the inlet facing the base of your thumb
   c. Blow gently into the palm of the hand; the indicator hands should rotate smoothly and slowly and the mechanism should operate silently at this low flow
4. Check the ON/OFF control while the pointers are rotating
5. Press the RESET button to return the pointers to zero

Once you confirm proper operation, you should set up the device for expired volume measurements, as described in **Figure 6-10**. As assembled, this setup can be attached directly to an ET or tracheostomy tube. A mask or mouthpiece and noseclips will be needed for patients with intact upper airways.

Table 6-29 Selection of Devices to Measure Volumes and Flows at the Bedside or in the Clinic

Desired Measures	Type of Device	Examples
Tidal volume, minute volume, inspiratory capacity, slow vital capacity	Mechanical turbine-type volumetric meter	Wright respirometer Haloscale respirometer
Forced vital capacity and related measures (e.g., peak flow, FEV_t, $FEF_{25-75\%}$)	Pneumotachometer with computerized integrator	Variety of portable electronic spirometers, provided by various manufacturers (e.g., Puritan-Bennett, Vitalograph, Viasys, Jones Medical, QRS Diagnostics, SDI Diagnostics)

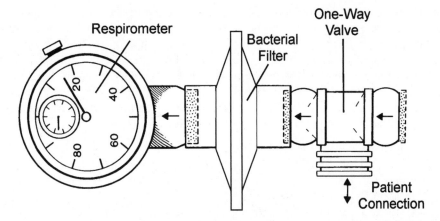

Figure 6-10 Basic Equipment Setup of Wright Respirometer for Beside Volume Measures. A one-way breathing valve with a 22/15 mm patient connector separates out the inspired and expired volume. A bacterial filter protects the patient and respirometer from contamination. Replacement of the valve and filter allows the respirometer to be used on multiple patients. Here the respirometer is placed to measure expired volumes (its normal use). By placing the respirometer and filter on the inspiratory side of the valve, you can measure inspiratory capacity.

Adapted from: Kacmarek, R. M., Foley K., Cheever, P., & Romagnoli, D. (1991). Determination of ventilatory reserve in mechanically ventilated patients: A comparison of techniques. *Respiratory Care, 36*, 1085–1092.

To use a respirometer to obtain volume measurements at the bedside:

1. Instruct the patient in the desired maneuver (slow vital capacity, minute volume)
2. Attach the equipment to the patient by the one-way valve connector
3. Move the ON/OFF switch to the ON position during patient inhalation
4. Have the patient perform the desired maneuver (timed for minute volume)
5. When the maneuver is completed, move the ON/OFF switch to the OFF position
6. Record (compute) the desired measures*
7. For multiple measures on the same patient, retain the valve and filter assembly at the bedside

*If measuring minute volume, count the breath frequency over the one-minute collection interval and read the accumulated value from the respirometer dial. Then compute the tidal volume by dividing the minute volume by the breath frequency, i.e., $V_T = \dot{V}_E \div f$.

Generally, proper use of the one-way valve and bacterial filter will prevent gross contamination of the respirometer. Should a Wright respirometer become contaminated, it should be gas sterilized with ethylene oxide and properly aerated (24 hours in room air).

Troubleshooting. Mechanical respirometers are simple-to-use but very delicate instruments that can be easily damaged. Damage can occur when the device is dropped or when it is exposed to excessive flows. You can avoid dropping these devices by always using the accessory neck strap. You can avoid damage due to excessive flows by never using these devices to measure forced breathing maneuvers. If the device fails to operate after checking it for proper function:

1. Check the position of the ON/OFF switch
2. If measuring expiratory volumes, be sure that the valve/filter assembly (Figure 6-10) is attached to the respirometer inlet, not the outlet

Portable Electronic Spirometers

These devices combine a flow-sensing pneumotachometer with a computer module. The spirometer computer module stores reference equations, provides input keys to select test options and specify essential patient information, converts the flow signal into volume via electronic integration, and provides test output data via a screen and/or printer. Depending on the manufacturer, the pneumotachometer used by these devices may sense flow either directly (via a turbine, hot wire, or Doppler method) or by measuring the "back pressure" created as gas flows through a restriction. **Figure 6-11** depicts a pneumotachometer that senses flow by measuring pressure differences across a resistive element.

You select a portable electronic spirometer when you need to measure forced vital capacity and related measures (e.g., peak flow, FEV_t, $FEF_{25-75\%}$) at the bedside or in the clinic. In selecting a portable spirometer for use at the bedside or clinic, you should make sure that it:

- Meets American Thoracic Society standards for diagnostic spirometry (1994 update):
  - Volume range 0.5–8.0 L with accuracy of ± 3% or 0.05 L, whichever is greater
  - Flow range ± 14 L/sec with accuracy of ± 5% or 0.20 L/sec, whichever is greater
- Allows selection of various common reference equations:
  - Adults: Morris, Knudson, Crapo, NHANES III
  - Children: Hsu, Polgar, Dockerty, NHANES III
- Adjusts normal values for gender, height, age, and ethnicity
- Provides automated validity checks on maneuver, including:
  - Back extrapolated volume
  - Time to peak expiratory flow
  - End-of-test volume
- Provides appropriate corrective prompts based on maneuver validity checks
- Provides, stores, and compares the results of multiple/repeat testing on patients
- Prints both tabular data and applicable graphs (FEV vs. time; flow × volume)

Use. Proper use of portable spirometers involves (1) regular calibration and (2) proper application of the measurement procedure. Calibration of pulmonary function equipment in general, and portable spirometers in particular, is covered in Chapter 8. Here we focus on proper application of the procedure.

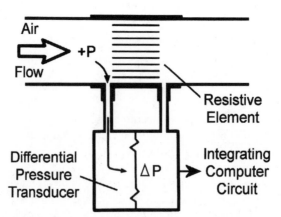

Figure 6-11 Differential Pressure (Fleisch) Pneumotachometer. Air flowing through a resistive element (parallel metal or ceramic tubes) creates a pressure difference across the element, which is directly proportional to flow. These pressure changes are measured by an electronic pressure transducer that sends its output signal to a computerized circuit. The computerized circuit converts the flow measurements to volume via electronic integration. For continuous use, the pneumotachometer typically is heated to maintain a constant temperature and prevent condensation.

Adapted from: Sullivan, W. J, Peters, G. M., & Enright, P. L. (1984). Pneumotachography: Theory and clinical application. *Respiratory Care, 29,* 736–749.

Unlike many physiologic measurements, forced expiratory measures are very dependent on the patient properly performing the procedure, as instructed and coached by the clinician. Key points that help ensure accurate and reproducible results include the following:

1. Make sure the spirometer is turned on and insert a new mouthpiece or sensor. Portable spirometers use either disposable or nondisposable pneumotachometers. Some disposable sensors include individual calibration information that must be inputted or scanned into the computer module before testing.
2. Be sure to accurately input all requested patient data, typically including age, gender, height, ethnicity, and smoking history; patient height should be measured in stocking feet.
3. Remove candy, gum, and/or dentures from the patient's mouth and loosen any tight clothing.
4. Patient may sit or stand, but be consistent by recording the patient's position.
5. Demonstrate the procedure using your own mouthpiece/sensor, being sure to show:
   a. How to hold the sensor steady/avoid jerky motions (can cause flow errors)
   b. How deeply to inhale
   c. How to correctly place the mouthpiece on top of the tongue
   d. How fast and long to exhale (at least 6 sec)
6. Use nose clips to prevent patient leaks.
7. Have the patient perform the maneuver while you carefully observe test performance.
   a. Ensure that the patient breathes in as deeply as possible (full inspiratory capacity)
   b. Have the patient forcibly *blast* the breath out, as fast and as long as possible
   c. Loudly prompt *more, more, more, more* until the subject has exhaled *for at least 6 seconds* (patients with severe COPD may take up to 15 seconds to fully exhale)
   d. Carefully observe the patient for poor technique and correct as needed
8. Repeat the procedure until you have three acceptable maneuvers (may require four to eight efforts).
9. Print and review the results.

Troubleshooting. Problems with portable spirometry may be due to procedural errors or device malfunction. The most common problems involve poor procedural technique, which can result in erroneous measurements. The most common technique-related problems include:

- Incomplete inhalation (< inspiratory capacity)
- Inadequate expiratory force
- Breathing during maneuver
- Lips not tight around the mouthpiece
- Too slow a start to forced exhalation
- Stopping exhalation before all gas expelled
- Some exhalation through the nose
- Coughing during the maneuver

Devices that incorporate automated validity checks can detect many of these errors, including incomplete inhalation, inadequate expiratory force, too slow a start to forced exhalation, and stopping exhalation before all gas expelled. To detect and correct these problems, the National Lung Health Education Program (NLHEP) recommends several validity checks and corrective prompts, as specified in **Table 6-30**.

If using a device that does not provide automated validity checks, you will need to detect these errors by carefully observing the patient throughout the maneuver and examining the graphic results. Chapter 8 provides details on how to manually detect patient-related errors that affect the validity of the forced vital capacity measurement.

When used and maintained in accordance with the manufacturer's instructions, modern portable spirometers are generally trouble-free. As outlined in **Table 6-31**, malfunctions that do occur usually involve power source problems, computer software or hardware errors, incorrect calibration, or misassembly or damage to the sensor.

Table 6-30 NLHEP Recommended Validity Checks and Device Corrective Prompts for Portable Spirometers

Validity Checks	Device Corrective Prompts
Back extrapolated volume > 150 mL	"Don't hesitate"
Time to peak expiratory flow > 120 msec[a]	"Blast out faster"
Forced expiratory time < 6.0 sec *and* end-of-test volume[b] > 100 mL	"Blow out longer"
Repeat FEV_6 values do not match within 150 mL	"Take deeper breath"

a. > 160 msec for school-age children and adolescents.

b. End-of-test volume = change in exhaled volume during the last 0.5 sec of the maneuver.

Table 6-31 Troubleshooting Common Problems with Portable Spirometers

Problem/Clue	Cause(s)	Solution(s)
Device does not turn ON	Device lacks electrical power	If AC powered, confirm connection to working line power outlet If battery powered, check/replace batteries
Device turns ON, but does not complete or fails power-on self-test (POST)	Failure of boot/startup program or central processing unit (CPU) failure	Record error message Turn device OFF, wait 20 seconds, then turn it back ON Replace device if repeat failure
Sensor will not zero	Sensor is moving during zeroing	Place sensor on table top and repeat
Device fails volume calibration (± 3%)	Incorrect temperature or pressure/altitude input[a]	Recalibrate device, being sure to enter proper temperature and pressure/altitude
	Loose connections or leaks in spirometer system	Tighten connections and correct leaks
	Flow sensor misassembled or damaged	Reassemble or replace flow sensor
	Flow sensor obstructed with foreign matter	Clean or replace flow sensor
Test begins/volume accumulates before patient exhales	Sensor and/or tubing is not stationary at the start of test	Have the patient hold the sensor assembly steady until prompted to begin maneuver
Flow measures appear to be reversed (differential pressure sensors only)	Flow sensor inlet and outlet pressure tubing connections reversed	Check/correct and confirm proper tubing connections
Device does not sense beginning of exhalation	Sensor pressure tubing not connected	Check/correct and confirm proper tubing connections
	Flow sensor misassembled or damaged	Reassemble or replace flow sensor
False high or low volume or flow readings suspected	Device out of calibration Incorrect temperature or pressure/altitude input	Recalibrate device, being sure to enter proper temperature and pressure/altitude

(continues)

Table 6-31 Troubleshooting Common Problems with Portable Spirometers (continued)

Problem/Clue	Cause(s)	Solution(s)
	Incorrect temperature or pressure/altitude input	Recalibrate device, being sure to enter proper temperature and pressure/altitude
	Flow sensor misassembled or damaged	Reassemble or replace flow sensor
	Leaks in patient or spirometer system (low readings only)	Correct leaks Use nose clips Ensure proper lip seal
	Teeth, lips, or tongue obstructing mouthpiece (low readings only)	Correct patient technique
False high or low % normal computations suspected	Incorrect patient data entry (e.g., age, height, gender)	Verify/reenter correct patient data
a. Overestimation of room temperature will result in lower than actual volume/flow reading; incorrectly entering an altitude above sea level will result in higher than actual volume/flow reading.		

O_2, He, CO, and Specialty Gas Analyzers

Most respiratory therapists are skilled in monitoring FiO_2s using portable oxygen analyzers. Details on the use and troubleshooting of these devices are provided in Chapter 8. New to the NBRC exam for 2009 is the expectation that you are familiar with other specialty gas analyzers. To that end, **Table 6-32** outlines the analysis method employed, common clinical usage, performance standards, and calibration considerations for all gas analyzers that you may encounter in clinical practice.

Other than what gas needs to be analyzed, the key consideration in selecting a gas analyzer is its response time. If real-time analysis is needed during breathing, the analyzer must have a rapid response time, in general less than 500 msec. Also note that although usage and performance standards vary greatly, essentially all gas analyzers should undergo a two-point calibration before each use.

ECG Monitors and 12-Lead ECG Machines

ECG Monitors

Bedside monitors typically provide continuous monitoring of multiple patient parameters. Most can display (1) the ECG, (2) respirations/impedance pneumography (via the ECG leads), (3) blood pressure (continuous invasive or intermittent noninvasive), and (4) oxyhemoglobin saturation (SpO_2).

When to Recommend and Use

ECG monitors are designed to identify and warn clinicians of abnormal changes in a patient's heart rate or rhythm, and to provide data essential in arrhythmia management. Continuous bedside monitoring of the ECG is a standard of care for critically ill and/or unstable patients. This would normally include any patients in special care units and those admitted to the emergency department who are hemodynamically unstable, are unconscious, or have chest pain. For critically ill and/or unstable patients who must be transported, you should select a portable (battery-powered) patient monitor.

Setup and Troubleshooting

The key to proper ECG monitoring is proper placement of the leads and electrodes. In addition, you need to know how to ensure a good signal, properly set the alarms, and recognize poor signal quality and its causes.

Table 6-32 Therapy and Diagnostic Gas Analysis

Gas	Analysis Method(s)	Usage	Performance Standards and Calibration Considerations

O_2	• Paramagnetic
	• Electrochemical:
	  • Galvanic cell
	  • Polarographic
	  • ZrO_2
		• Bedside F_{IO_2} monitoring
		• Metabolic analysis (O_2 consumption)
			• For bedside monitoring (primarily Galvanic cell or polarographic sensors):
			  • Accuracy ± 2% for bedside monitoring
			  • Response time 90% of scale range in ≤ 20 sec
			• For metabolic analysis (primarily ZrO_2 sensors):
			  • Accuracy 1.0%
			  • Precision 0.01%
			  • Response time < 100 msec
			• Two-point calibration (21% and 100%) should be done just prior to each test

N_2	• Emission spectroscopy
	• Mass spectrometry
		• FRC determination (nitrogen washout)	• For real-time (breath) analysis:
			  • Accuracy ± 0.2% over the entire range N_2% (0–80%)
			  • 95% response time 30–60 msec to a 10% step change in N_2%
			• Two-point calibration (100% O_2 and room air) should be done just prior to each test
			• Linearity should be checked every 6 months with a 40% N_2 calibration gas mixture

He	• Thermal-conductivity	• FRC determination (helium dilution)
		• Single-breath D_{LCO} (as tracer gas)
			• For FRC or D_{LCO}:
			  • Measurement range 0–10%
			  • Resolution 0.01%
			  • 95% response time of 15 sec to a 2% step change in He%
			  • Stability ±0.5% full scale, confirmed weekly (drift ≤ 0.02% in 10 mins)
			• Two-point calibration (zero and full scale) should be done just prior to each test
			• CO_2 and water must be removed before the sample is analyzed; CO_2 first (since its absorption creates water vapor) followed by removal of water vapor

(continues)

Table 6-32 Therapy and Diagnostic Gas Analysis (continued)

Gas	Analysis Method(s)	Usage	Performance Standards and Calibration Considerations
CO	• Infrared absorption • Electrochemical	• Single-breath DLCO • Assessment of smoking status	• Accuracy less important than linearity and stability (DLCO is based on relative changes in CO%) • Linearity within ± 0.5% from zero to full span (checked every 3 months) • Stability ±0.001% absolute CO% • Two-point calibration (zero and full scale) should be done just prior to each test
NO, NO$_2$	• Chemiluminescence • Electrochemical	• Nitric oxide therapy • Monitoring airway inflammation (expired NO)	• For nitric oxide: • Resolution 1 ppm • Accuracy between 1 and 20 ppm: ± (0.5 ppm + 20% actual concentration) • Accuracy above 20 ppm: ± (0.5 ppm + 10% actual concentration) • Response time for breath-by breath analysis of < 500 msec • Response time for monitor/alarm of 0–90% rise time in ≤ 30 seconds • drift < 1% of full scale/24 hours • For NO$_2$: • Accuracy ± 20% of the actual %, or 0.5 ppm, whichever is greater • Daily 1-point automated "zero" calibration (room air) while on patient • Monthly two-point high range using 45 ppm NO/10 ppm NO$_2$ calibrating gases

Bedside ECG monitors use a three-lead system to acquire the ECG signal, with lead placement as described in **Figure 6-12**. ECG electrodes are disposable self-adhesive systems that come prefilled with electrolyte gel to ensure good signal pickup. In most cases, you need only clean the skin site with an alcohol swab (to remove skin oils) before placement. In some cases the skin over the electrode area may need to be shaved and/or gently abraded with emery tape in order to get good contact and a satisfactory signal.

Once all three electrodes are positioned, you select among leads I, II, or III using a switch or button on the monitor. Limb lead II is the most common monitoring lead configuration, because it normally produces the largest positive R wave. Getting a large positive R wave is important with a bedside ECG monitor, because the R-R interval is used to compute the ECG heart rate.

Once you obtain a satisfactory signal, you should set the high and low rate alarms. As with ventilator alarms, you want to be sure not to set the ECG monitor alarms too close to the patient's actual rate, as this will cause frequent false alarms. Instead, apply the protocol used in the unit to which the patient was admitted.

On ECG monitors that include both ECG rate and pulse oximeter rate displays, the two measures can often be very different—with one alarming and one indicating normal. A discrepancy like this indicates either (1) pulseless electrical activity (ECG OK, but low or no pulse oximeter rate) or (2) an error in one of the monitored parameters. Check both the ECG leads *and* the pulse oximetry sensor for proper position and good contact.

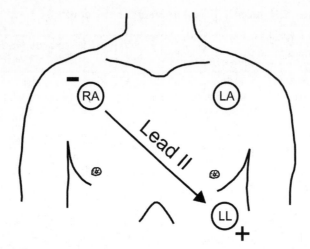

Figure 6-12 ECG Monitor Lead Placement. Place the RA/White electrode below the right clavicle, the LA/Black below the left clavicle, and the LL/Red just below the left pectoral muscle. When set to Lead II, the RA electrode is the negative pole, the LL electrode is the positive pole and the LA electrode serves as the ground lead. Due to the electrical axis of the normal heart, this configuration usually produces the largest positive R wave.

12-Lead Electrocardiogram

A modern 12-lead electrocardiogram (ECG) machine is a computer data acquisition and storage system. ECG information is obtained using 10 sensors or leads, which provide 12 separate electrical views of the heart's electrical activity. Once obtained, the 12-lead electrocardiogram can be stored as digital data in the computer's memory, printed as a "hard copy" for manual reading, or electronically transmitted to a remote location for interpretation. Physicians and other health personnel use the data obtained from a 12-lead ECG to assess rhythm disturbances, determine the heart's electrical axis, and identify the site and extent of myocardial ischemia or damage.

When to Recommend or Use

You should recommend a 12-lead ECG to:

- Screen for heart disease (e.g., CAD, LVH)
- Rule out heart disease in surgical patients
- Evaluate patients with chest pain
- Follow the progression of patients with CAD
- Evaluate heart rhythm disorders

Device Calibration

As with most clinical measurement instruments, ECG machines should be regularly calibrated to ensure that they can obtain accurate data. Typically, ECG machine calibration is performed by your biomedical engineering department using a 12-lead ECG simulator. The simulator provides standardized electrical signals to each lead, which allows the tester to check and confirm that the device can produce good-quality, artifact-free ECG waveforms. Simulator calibration also allows testing of the machine's computerized self-diagnostics and alarm/warning systems, including the ability to sense a poor signal or a missing lead.

Setup and Troubleshooting

In addition to the ECG machine, you need the following equipment to obtain a 12-lead ECG:

- Lead wire set
- Electrodes/sensors
- ECG paper
- Alcohol and gauze pads (to prepare site)
- CDC barrier precautions (as needed)

Figure 6-13 shows the proper lead placement for obtaining a 12-lead ECG. Note that there are only 10 actual leads to place, not 12. One (the right leg) doesn't really count, since it is just a ground lead. The difference is the three augmented limb leads (aVR, aVL, and aVF), which use the RA, LA, and LL electrodes to obtain their data.

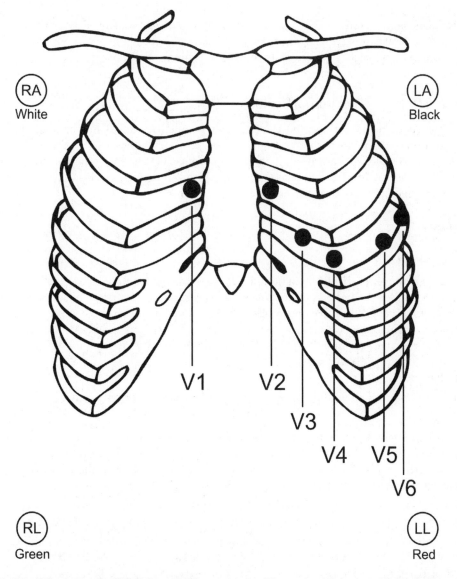

Figure 6-13 Diagnostic ECG Lead Placement. Place the RL/green lead on the right leg, LL/red lead on the left leg, RA/white lead on right arm, and LA/black lead on the left arm. Then place the 6 chest leads as follows: V1—4th intercostal space, right sternal border; V2—4th intercostal space, left sternal border; V3—between V2 and V4; V4—5th intercostal space, midclavicular line; V5—5th intercostal space, anterior axillary line; and V6—5th intercostal space, midaxillary line.

Once all sensors are properly positioned, you should verify that the device is receiving a good-quality, artifact-free ECG signal. Fortunately, most newer units automatically detect common problems and will not begin recording until a good signal can be obtained. The two most common problems are absent or "noisy" signals. Failure to obtain a signal is usually due to a loose, missing, or defective lead. A noisy ECG signal may be caused by a poor electrical connection, motion artifact, or improper filtering of extraneous electrical activity. In either case you should:

1. Verify that the ECG snaps and connectors are clean and corrosion-free.
2. Verify that the lead electrodes are connected properly to the patient.
3. Verify that the electrode gel is not dry; replace any suspect electrodes.
4. Check the ECG main cable for continuity; replace if damaged.
5. Confirm that the patient is motionless; if necessary, support the patient's limbs.
6. Verify that the device's filter settings (if available) are properly set.

Other possible errors include setting the wrong paper speed and sensitivity. Normal paper speed is 25 mm/sec, and there are few reasons to change it. Normal sensitivity is 10 mm per millivolt, as confirmed by a calibration spike of two large 5-mm boxes. Settings other than these can result in misinterpretation of the electrocardiogram.

Noninvasive Oximetry Monitoring Devices

The noninvasive oximetry monitoring devices you should be most familiar with include pulse oximeters and transcutaneous monitors. You select a pulse oximeter to spot check, monitor, or obtain trend data on a patient's oxygen saturation (SpO_2). You select a transcutaneous monitor to provide continuous estimates of arterial blood gases (PO_2 and PCO_2) in infants. Details on assessing and interpreting noninvasive oximetry data are provided in Chapter 13.

Pulse Oximeters

Setup and Assembly

Although pulse oximeters vary widely in design, the steps involved in their setup and assembly are similar. **Table 6-33** outlines the basic steps, including key considerations for obtaining good saturation data.

For monitoring critically ill patients, pulse oximetry readings should be compared to a simultaneous measure of actual arterial O_2 saturation, as measured by laboratory oximetry. You can then use the difference between the SaO_2 and SpO_2 to "calibrate" the pulse oximetry reading.

Troubleshooting

The most common problem with pulse oximeters is an unstable or poor-quality signal. In these cases you should:

- Recheck the site and clean it and the probe (if multi-use) with alcohol.
- Reposition the probe to ensure that the transmitted light is directly opposite the detector.
- Remove any fingernail polish or "fake" nails (in emergencies, rotate the probe 90°).
- Try a different site, particularly if the probe has been in place for several hours.
- Replace the probe (if disposable) or try a different type of probe.

If an oximeter displays an error message indicating that the probe is OFF or disconnected, check the probe's connection to the oximeter and whether it is malpositioned on the patient. Reconnect or reposition the probe as needed. Last, if bright ambient light appears to be interfering with the reading, shield or cover the probe or reposition it to an unaffected area.

Table 6-33 Key Considerations in the Setup of Pulse Oximeters

Setup Steps	Key Considerations
1. If AC powered, connect the power cord to an appropriate power source.	• Most oximeters incorporate a battery that provides power if an electrical outlet is not available.
2. Connect the appropriate probe to the oximeter.	• There are special probes for neonates and pediatrics patients. • Proper probe size is essential for accurate readings.
3. Turn ON the power.	• Most oximeters perform an internal power-on self-test (POST) before reading the SpO_2. • Always verify that the unit has passed the POST.
4. Attach the probe to the patient.	• For continuous monitoring, disposable probes with adhesive strips are more stable and comfortable. • For spot checks a nondisposable, multi-patient probe is satisfactory. • Always disinfect a multi-use probe with alcohol before applying it to a patient. • Tightly applying either disposable or multi-patient probes may result in inaccurate readings or cause skin damage.
5. Verify a good signal.	• If displayed, observe the waveform to verify a good pulse signal. • Alternatively, use the oximeter's pulse strength/rate indicator lights to verify a good signal. • Always check the oximeter's displayed rate against an ECG monitor or count the actual pulse rate.
6. For continuous monitoring, set the alarm limits.	• Set the low alarm according to your institution's protocol, usually between 92% and 94%.
7. For overnight oximetry, adjust the devices for TREND recording.	• Select the planned period (e.g., 8 hr, 12 hr). • If settable, adjust the capture rate/response time to the fastest allowable (usually 2–6 sec). • Confirm that there is sufficient memory to make the recording for the specified period/capture rate. • If needed or appropriate, turn alarms off.

Transcutaneous Monitors

Transcutaneous blood gas monitoring provides continuous, noninvasive estimates of arterial PO_2 and PCO_2 via a sensor placed on the skin. The sensor includes electrochemical PO_2 and PCO_2 electrodes similar to those found in bench-top blood gas analyzers and a heating element. The heating element "arterializes" the blood by dilating the underlying capillary bed and increasing its blood flow. Oxygen and carbon dioxide diffuse from the capillaries through the skin and into the sensor's contact gel, where their pressures are measured by the PO_2 and PCO_2 electrodes. These pressures are referred to as transcutaneous (tc) partial pressures (i.e., $PtcO_2$ and $PtccO_2$).

Transcutaneous blood gas monitoring is used primarily in infants when the need exists to:

• Continuously monitor arterial oxygenation and/or ventilation
• Continuously monitor for excessive arterial oxygenation (hyperoxia)
• Quantify real-time changes in ventilation and oxygenation due to diagnostic or therapeutic interventions
• Assess functional shunts or determine the response to an O_2 challenge in infants with congenital heart disease

You should avoid using a transcutaneous monitor on patients with poor skin integrity or those with an adhesive allergy. Since accurate $Ptco_2$ and $Ptcco_2$ values generally require that the patient be hemodynamically stable, you should not use these devices on patients in shock or with poor peripheral circulation. Lengthy setup and stabilization time (10–20 minutes) also makes the transcutaneous monitor a poor choice for assessing gas exchange in emergency situations.

Setup and Assembly

Although transcutaneous monitors vary widely in design, the steps involved in their setup and assembly are similar, as outlined below:

1. Plug the unit into an appropriate grounded or double-insulated electrical outlet.
2. Attach the cable from the electrode to the appropriate jack on the monitor.
3. Membrane the sensor and calibrate the device according to the manufacturer's instructions.
4. Adjust the temperature to the desired range (usually 42–45°C).
5. Choose a site that has low fat density and good circulation (e.g., the side of chest, the abdomen, inner thigh, inner arm, or buttocks); avoid an infant's back, or thick or hairy skin.
6. Clean the selected site with alcohol. For larger children, rub to remove the outer layer of the epidermis.
7. Apply a ring of double-sided adhesive to the sensor.
8. Place a small amount of contact gel on the sensor face and apply to the prepared site using an adhesive ring. Be sure the edges are sealed and the sensor lies flat on the skin.
9. Allow 10–20 minutes for the reading to stabilize.
10. To avoid burns and other skin damage, change the sensor site frequently (every 2–6 hours, depending on the sensor temperature and manufacturer recommendation).

Calibration and Validation

Like bench-top blood gas analyzers, transcutaneous Po_2/Pco_2 monitors require two-point calibration using precision gas mixtures. Most manufacturers provide a precision gas calibration system with their monitors, and a semiautomated software routine prompts you through the steps involved. Failure to calibrate is usually due to a defective or leaking membrane, or excessive trapped air under the membrane. In both cases, the calibrating Pco_2 values will be lower than expected, as will the high calibrating Po_2 measure. If a transcutaneous monitor fails to calibrate, you should re-membrane the sensor.

In order to validate the transcutaneous readings, the $Ptco_2$ and $Ptcco_2$ values should be compared with concurrently obtained arterial blood gas measurements. For an infant with an anatomic shunt, both the transcutaneous and arterial values must be obtained on the same side. If the transcutaneous and arterial values differ significantly, the patient may be hemodynamically unstable or have poor peripheral circulation. If the patient has good peripheral circulation, try an alternate sensor site. If an alternate sensor site does not provide valid data, re-membrane and recalibrate the sensor. If the transcutaneous and arterial values still differ significantly, consider another mode of monitoring, such as pulse oximetry or serial blood gas analysis.

Troubleshooting

Aside from difficulty validating the $Ptco_2$ and $Ptcco_2$ against the patient's arterial values, the most common problem with transcutaneous monitoring is air leaking around the adhesive ring. Air leaks always cause a dramatic fall in $Ptcco_2$. If the leak is large, the $Ptco_2$ and $Ptcco_2$ values will mimic those of room air (Po_2 ~ 150 torr/ Pco_2 ~ 0 torr). In these cases, reapply the sensor using a new adhesive ring.

Aerosol Drug Delivery Systems

You use aerosol drug delivery systems to administer selected drug agents to patients via the lungs by inhalation. The selection and administration of aerosolized drugs is covered in Chapter 12. Here we focus on the selection, use, and troubleshooting of the devices used, including small-volume nebulizers (SVNs), metered-dose inhalers (MDIs), and dry powder inhalers (DPIs).

Selection

Figure 6-14 outlines a general algorithm for selecting an aerosol drug delivery system. As indicated in this figure, your first must determine the available formulations for the prescribed drug. Given that some drugs are available only in a single formulation (such as for DPI administration only), your choice in these cases will be limited to that delivery system. However, if the drug is available in multiple formulations, you should assess the patient to determine the best delivery system. In general, SVN administration should be reserved for acutely ill adults who cannot use either a DPI or an MDI. Most infants and small children should receive aerosolized drugs via an MDI with a valved holding chamber and mask (an SVN is an alternative if tolerated by the patient). If an adult who is not acutely ill has

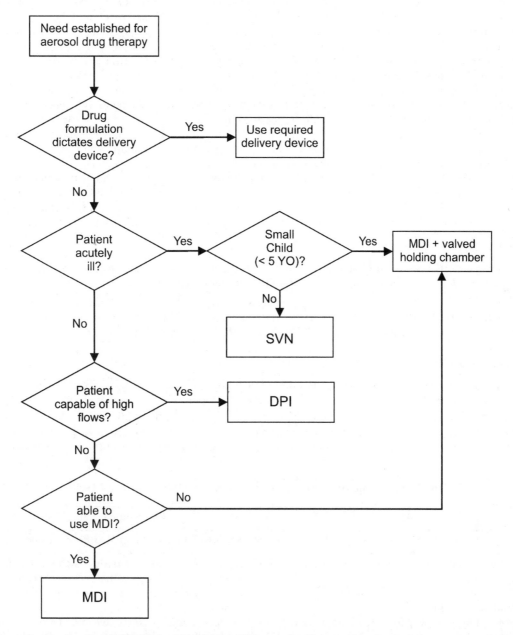

Figure 6-14 Basic Selection of Aerosol Drug Delivery Devices. In many cases, the drug formulation will dictate the choice. Otherwise, assessment of the patient's acuity, age, inspiratory flows, and ability to properly use an MDI will determine the best device to use on a patient. If several different devices qualify, patient preference should be the deciding factor.

Table 6-34 Assembly and Operational Check of Aerosol Delivery Devices

Metered-Dose Inhaler (MDI)	Dry Powder Inhaler (DPI)	Small-Volume Nebulizer (SVN)
• Check the expiration date on the canister; discard if expired • Inspect the canister outlet and its boot for any particulate matter or foreign objects • If needed, rinse the canister outlet and boot in warm, running water; air dry • Warm the canister to hand or body temperature, then shake vigorously • Fit the canister firmly in its boot, and remove the boot cap • If the canister is new or hasn't been used for several days, test spray it into the air • Confirm proper patient technique • After administration, disassemble apparatus and recap mouthpiece	• Check the expiration date on the canister; discard if expired • Confirm sufficient remaining doses (multi-dose systems only) • Inspect the outlet for any dirt or caked powder—use dry cloth or small brush to wipe away; *never use water* • Remove any mouthpiece cap • Load the dose of medicine (usually by moving a lever or twisting a knob until it clicks) • Keep mouthpiece in horizontal position to avoid loss of drug • Confirm proper patient technique • After administration, recap mouthpiece and store at room temperature in a dry place	• Select mask or mouthpiece (use a mask for patients who cannot use a mouthpiece) • Aseptically remove components from package • Connect the SVN to mask or T-tube • If T-tube, connect mouthpiece and reservoir tube • Connect gas delivery tubing to nebulizer input • Connect gas delivery tubing to flow meter/compressor • Aseptically place drug and diluent in SVN reservoir (4 mL fill volume is ideal) • Turn flow meter/compressor on • Confirm adequate aerosol production • After administration, rinse SVN with sterile water, blow dry with gas source, and store aseptically in plastic bag

difficulty properly coordinating MDI actuation with breathing, you should also consider using a holding chamber. A breath-actuated MDI is an alternative for such patients. Patients prescribed steroids by MDI should use either a spacer or a holding chamber in order to minimize pharyngeal deposition. DPIs are ideal for maintenance therapy in outpatient adults, larger children, and adolescents who can generate sufficient inspiratory flow to carry the powder into the lungs.

Assembly and Use

Most aerosol delivery devices come preassembled or require minimal assembly. **Table 6-34** highlights what you need to do when assembling and checking the operation of these devices.

Aerosol drug delivery is both patient- and device-dependent. **Table 6-35** outlines the optimal technique and key therapeutic issues involved in using common aerosol delivery devices, as specified by the National Heart, Lung, and Blood Institute's National Asthma Education and Prevention Program.

Table 6-35 Optimal Technique and Therapeutic Issues in Using Aerosol Delivery Devices

Optimal Technique	Therapeutic Issues
Metered-dose inhaler (MDI) for beta$_2$-agonists, steroids, cromolyn sodium, anticholinergics	
• Patient should open mouth wide and keep tongue down • Actuate during 3–5 sec deep inhalation, followed by 10-sec breath hold • Holding MDI 2″ away from open mouth may enhance lung deposition • Use closed mouth method only if (a) patient cannot use open-mouth technique, (b) a spacer is not available, and (c) the drug is *not* a steroid	• Young children and the elderly may have difficulty coordinating inhalation with device actuation • Patients may incorrectly stop inhalation at actuation • To reduce amount of drug swallowed and absorbed systemically, patients should rinse mouth with water

(continues)

Table 6-35 Optimal Technique and Therapeutic Issues in Using Aerosol Delivery Devices (continued)

Optimal Technique	Therapeutic Issues
Spacer or valved holding chamber (VHC) for use with MDIs	
• Slow (30 L/min or 3–5 sec) deep inhalation, followed by 10-sec breath hold immediately following actuation • Actuate only once into spacer/VHC per inhalation • Face mask (if used) should fit snugly and allow 3–5 breaths/actuation • Rinse plastic VHCs once a month in water with diluted dishwashing detergent (1–2 drops per cup of water) and let drip dry	• Indicated for patients who have difficulty performing adequate MDI technique • Simple spacers still require coordinating actuation with inhalation; VHCs are preferred • Face mask allows MDIs to be used with small children but reduce lung deposition by 50% • Because spacers and VHCs decrease oropharyngeal deposition, their use with MDI steroids can help reduce the risk of topical side effects such as thrush • Use antistatic VHCs or rinse plastic nonantistatic VHCs with dilute household detergents to enhance efficacy and delivery to lungs
Breath-actuated MDI for beta$_2$-agonists	
• Tight seal around mouthpiece and slightly more rapid inhalation than standard MDI, followed by 10-sec breath hold	• Useful for patients who cannot coordinate inhalation with actuation, such as the elderly • Patients may incorrectly stop inhalation at actuation • Cannot be used with spacers or VHCs
Dry powder inhaler (DPI) for beta$_2$-agonists, steroids, anticholinergics	
• Do NOT use with a spacer or VHC • Lips must be tightly sealed around the mouthpiece to avoid loss of drug • After loading, most DPIs must be held horizontal to avoid loss of drug • Requires rapid (60 L/min or 1–2 sec), deep inhalation • Patient must exhale to room (not back into device) • Children < 4 years old may not generate sufficient flow to use	• Dose is lost if patient exhales into the device after loading • Exhaling into device may cause clogging due to moisture caking any powder residue • Rapid inhalation increases deposition in large airways • To reduce amount of drug absorbed systemically, patient should rinse mouth with water • The device should never be washed or rinsed in water • Between uses the device should always be stored with the cap on in a dry place
Small-volume nebulizer (SVN) for beta$_2$-agonists, steroids, cromolyn sodium, anticholinergics	
• Slow tidal breathing with occasional deep breaths • Use a tightly fitting face mask for those unable to use a mouthpiece • Avoid using the "blow by" technique (i.e., holding the mask or open tube near the infant's nose and mouth)	• Less dependent on patient's coordination and cooperation • As effective as MDI + VHC for delivering bronchodilators to patients with mild to moderate exacerbations of asthma • Delivery method of choice for cromolyn in young children • More expensive and time consuming than other methods • Output depends on device and operating parameters—e.g., fill volume, driving gas flow • Use of a face mask reduces lung deposition by 50% • Bacterial infections can occur if not cleaned properly

Adapted from: National Heart, Lung, and Blood Institute National Asthma Education and Prevention Program. (2007). Expert panel report 3 (EPR3): Guidelines for the diagnosis and management of asthma. Washington, DC: U.S. Department of Health and Human Services.

Troubleshooting

Most problems with MDIs and DPIs involve poor patient technique. With SVNs, the most common problem is inadequate aerosol production. **Table 6-36** summarizes the problems you are likely to encounter with aerosol delivery devices and their solutions.

Bronchoscopes

As discussed in Chapter 18, as a respiratory therapist you often may serve as bronchoscopic assistant to a physician. Key equipment involved in bronchoscopy includes the bronchoscope itself (described in more detail in Chapter 18), its disposable suction and biopsy valves, the portable light source, assorted bronchoscopic instruments (e.g., brushes, forceps, aspiration needles), an oral insertion guide/ bite block, specimen-collection devices, a regulated vacuum source and suction supplies, syringes, pulse oximeter, O_2-delivery equipment, and a BVM resuscitator. Troubleshooting of vacuum/suction systems, pulse oximeters, O_2-delivery equipment, and BVM resuscitators is covered separately in other sections of this chapter. Here we focus on the care of the bronchoscope during use and its subsequent cleaning, disinfection, and proper storage.

In terms of equipment care and use, it is important to understand that a fiberoptic bronchoscope is a very delicate instrument. In particular, the outer sheath of the scope, filaments in the viewing channel, and objective (distal) lens are very easily damaged. In addition, the working channel lining can easily be ruptured by rigid or sharp instruments.

When damage occurs to the fiberoptic filaments due to coiling, overzealous bending, or twisting of the insertion tube, numerous black dots begin appearing in the eyepiece. Damage to the outer sheath or working channel lining can allow fluid invasion of the scope, which can cause the image to appear foggy. The possibility of fluid invasion is confirmed by leak testing the scope during cleaning and disinfection.

To avoid damage to the scope during use, you must ensure proper handling of the device. Key points in this regard are to:

- Avoid letting the distal end strike any hard surface (damages the distal objective lens).
- Avoid forced angulation of the insertion tube (damages the fiberoptic filaments).
- Avoid direct axial twisting of the of the insertion tube (damages the fiberoptic filaments).
- Use only instruments with external diameters properly sized for internal diameter of the working channel.
- Keep the proximal portion of scope as straight as possible during instrument insertion.
- Avoid use of force when inserting instruments into the working channel.
- Avoid using petroleum-based lubricants for insertion (damage the scope's outer sheath).
- Always replace (don't repair) bronchoscope instruments.
- Always use a bite block whenever the tube is inserted via the mouth or oral ET tube.

Table 6-36 Troubleshooting Aerosol Delivery Devices

Metered-Dose Inhaler (MDI)	Dry Powder Inhaler (DPI)	Small-Volume Nebulizer (SVN)

• Poor patient response: check and correct patient technique
• Empty canister (floats horizontally in water): replace with new
• Cold canister: hand warm
• Loose fitting in boot: reset
• Failure to detach cap: remove
• Obstructed outflow: remove foreign material or clean canister outlet and boot
	• Poor patient response: check and correct patient technique
	• Caked powder residue in outlet: clean with dry cloth or use small brush provided with unit; make sure device always stored with cap on in a dry place
	• Patient observes powder in air during use: make sure proper technique is used, especially DPI position (horizontal), tight lip seal, and exhalation to room (*not* back into device)
		• Inadequate aerosol production caused by:
		  • Inadequate pressure/flow: make sure the source gas is turned on and properly set
		  • Leaks in delivery system: confirm that all connections are tight
		  • Inadequate fill volume: fill SVN to 4 mL
		  • Nebulizer malpositioned: reposition vertically
		  • Obstructed jet: replace SVN

In addition, to avoid endobronchial ignition/fire during Nd-YAG laser bronchoscopy, you should ensure that:

- The laser tip is as far away from the ET tube as possible when fired.
- The laser tip is at least 5 mm away from scope outlet when fired.
- The oxygen concentration is kept below 40% (if possible).
- Alcohol is NOT used to clear the laser tip after use.

If during the procedure suction appears inadequate, first check the vacuum regulator setting and all connections to the scope. If the problem persists, remove and clean or replace the scope's suction valve.

Because fiberoptic bronchoscopes are a proven source for the spread of infection, it is essential that you properly clean, disinfect, and store this equipment after completion of the procedure. The accompanying box outlines the key elements involved in processing bronchoscopes after use, as recommended by the American College of Chest Physicians.

Processing of Bronchoscopes After Use

Cleaning

1. While still at the bedside, flush water or saline through the scope's working channel for 20 seconds
2. To avoid drying of organic material, immediately transport the scope in a sealed contaminated equipment bag to a processing area
3. Mechanically clean (e.g., by ultrasonics) all reusable accessory instruments and send for autoclave processing
4. Remove all disposable parts (suction/biopsy valve), cap and seal all light/electrical connectors, and place the scope in a cleaning basin
5. Following the manufacturer's protocol, perform a leak test on the scope; any instrument that fails the leak test must be removed from service until repaired
6. Add enzymatic cleaner to the water and soak the scope for 5 minutes
7. Using the enzymatic solution, wipe external surfaces with wet gauze and flush the suction channel
8. Insert an appropriate-size cleaning brush through the working channel of the scope and brush all ports until there is no more visible debris being removed
9. Flush the channel again to remove all loosened material
10. Drain the enzymatic solution from the basin
11. Rinse all internal and external surfaces with water to prepare the scope for disinfection

High-Level Disinfection

1. Place the bronchoscope in either an automatic endoscope reprocessor (AER) or a basin used for manual disinfection
2. Use only FDA-cleared disinfectants that are compatible with the scope; minimum effective concentration of the disinfectant must be checked with each process
3. Fully immerse the scope in the disinfectant, exposing all surfaces for the proper time (at least 20 minutes for glutaraldehyde); if manually disinfecting, be sure to fill the channel with the disinfectant using a syringe

Postprocessing

1. After proper immersion time, rinse the scope and its working channel with either sterile or filtered tap water according to the recommendations of the disinfectant supplier
2. Dry the working channel with 70% alcohol, purged with compressed air
3. Remove the watertight caps from the scope and hang it vertically in a storage cabinet without attaching any valve
4. Document the disinfection process (patient ID, date of the procedure, bronchoscopist, model and the serial number of the scope, and the date of reprocessing)

Adapted from: Mehta, A. C., Prakash, U. B., Garland, R., et al. (2005). Consensus statement: Prevention of flexible bronchoscopy-associated infection. *Chest, 128*, 1742–1755.

COMMON ERRORS TO AVOID

You can improve your score by avoiding these mistakes:

- Never use a Thorpe tube to meter O_2 during patient transport; instead, use a gravity-independent device such as a Bourdon gauge.
- Avoid selecting or using an air-entrainment device when the patient needs a high F_{IO_2}; use a nonrebreathing mask or blended high-flow system instead.
- Never heat the gas used to deliver bland aerosols into pediatric mist tents; these systems must always run cool.
- Never use a gas-powered resuscitator on an infant or child.
- Avoid regular changing of ventilator circuits; change them only when absolutely necessary.
- Never cover a heated-wire ventilator circuit with towels, drapes, or linens.
- Avoid using oronasal (full-face) masks as the noninvasive interface for ventilating patients with hypercapnic respiratory failure.
- Avoid using oropharyngeal airways in conscious patients.
- Never plug a fenestrated tracheostomy tube with the cuff inflated.
- Never clamp a patient's chest tube during transport; the one-way seal must be maintained.
- Never use a mechanical vane-type respirometer to measure forced expiratory volumes; use a portable electronic spirometer instead.
- Never accept an FEV maneuver obtained during bedside spirometer that lasts for less than 6 seconds.
- Avoid using transcutaneous O_2/CO_2 monitors in emergency situations or on patients in shock or with poor peripheral circulation.
- Never wash or rinse a dry powder inhaler in water.
- Never forcefully bend or twist the insertion tube portion of a fiberoptic bronchoscope.
- Avoid using petroleum-based lubricants for bronchoscope insertion.

SURE BETS

In some situations you can always be sure of the right approach to a clinical problem or scenario:

- Although estimated F_{IO_2}s are important, always rely on evaluating the patient's actual response to O_2 therapy, ideally by ABGs or pulse oximetry.
- Always deliver the highest possible F_{IO_2} (via nonrebreathing mask or high-flow cannula) to patients in emergency settings suspected of being hypoxemic.
- Always have home-care patients who experience problems with an O_2-conserving device switch to a nasal cannula at an equivalent liter flow (2–3x).
- Always ensure a neutral thermal environment when delivering O_2 to infants.
- To avoid overinflation, always select the appropriate manual resuscitator with the correct stroke volume and mask size.
- Whenever any major problem occurs during mechanical ventilation, always remove the patient from the ventilator and provide appropriate support using a manual resuscitator connected to an O_2 source.
- Always treat a combined low-volume and high-pressure alarm condition during mechanical ventilation as signaling an obstruction.
- To ensure adequate humidification in a ventilator circuit, always confirm that a few drops of condensation remain at or near the patient connection.
- If using an active humidification system in a ventilator circuit, always be sure that the HEPA filter is positioned proximal to or upstream from the humidifier.
- When providing aerosol drug therapy through a ventilator circuit, always remove the HME before the procedure and replace it afterward.
- Always check the position of an endotracheal tube by breath sounds—but always *confirm* with a chest X-ray.
- To positively identify the contents of a medical gas cylinder, always read the cylinder label.

- Always verify the prescribed O_2% provided by a blender using a calibrated oxygen analyzer.
- Before using any computerized electronic device, always verify that it passes its power-on self test.
- Always send flagged point-of-care test results to the central laboratory for analysis.
- Always check a pulse oximeter's displayed rate against an ECG monitor or count the actual pulse rate.
- Always use a bite block when inserting a fiberoptic bronchoscope via the mouth or through an oral ET tube.

PRE-TEST ANSWERS AND EXPLANATIONS

Below are this chapter's pre-test answers and explanations. Be sure to review each answer's explanation thoroughly to help you understand why it is correct. If the explanation is still unclear to you, review the chapter contents or the references and/or refer to this chapter's supplemental resources on the CD.

6-1. **Correct answer: C.** Check the entrainment ports. Because air-entrainment masks mix air and oxygen at a constant ratio, an alteration in the delivered oxygen concentration could result only from an alteration in the mixing ratio. Since jet size (for a given adapter) is fixed, the problem must be with the entrainment ports. Obstruction of the entrainment ports will decrease air entrainment and raise the delivered oxygen concentration.

6-2. **Correct answer: B.** 48 L/min. To compute the total output flow delivered by an air-entrainment device, multiply the sum of its ratio parts by the input flow. A 35% air-entrainment mask mixes air an oxygen at a fixed 5:1 ratio; thus $(5 + 1) \times 8 = 48$ L/min.

6-3. **Correct answer: C.** Check the mask for a snug fit. If a nonrebreathing mask reservoir bag does not deflate at all when the patient inspires, either the flow is higher than needed, there are large inspiratory air leaks (around the mask or through the exhalation valves), or the inspiratory valve is jammed. The most common cause is large air leakage, which can easily be corrected by making sure that the mask is fit comfortably tight to the patient's face.

6-4. **Correct answer: D.** A clogged capillary tube in the nebulizer. Since most croup tents use large-volume jet nebulizers to generate mist, insufficient mist indicates malfunction of the nebulizer. The most common cause of nebulizer malfunction is clogging of the capillary tube that feeds liquid water to the jet.

6-5. **Correct answer: B.** Large-reservoir heated jet nebulizer. The large-reservoir air-entrainment jet nebulizer is the primary gas-powered aerosol generator used to provide humidification to the respiratory tract.

6-6. **Correct answer: B.** Increasing O_2 flow to the bag. Think of the reservoir bag of a bag-valve manual resuscitator as equivalent to the bag on a reservoir mask. If the reservoir bag collapses during the resuscitator's refill phase (equivalent to patient inspiration), the flow is inadequate and should be increased until the bag does not empty.

6-7. **Correct answer: A.** Absence of the inlet valve. If a bag-valve resuscitator fills rapidly but collapses on minimal pressure and delivers little volume, the likely problem is a missing, torn, or malpositioned inlet valve. In this case, when you squeeze the bag, gas follows the path of least resistance and escapes out the inlet port (instead of going to the patient). This problem could have been avoided by performing an operational check on the bag before applying it to the patient. If discovered after application, you should quickly secure a working replacement bag.

6-8. **Correct answer: B.** Variable flow control and adjustable I:E ratios. Of the functions listed, the most important capability when selecting a ventilator for an intubated adult patient with severe expiratory airway obstruction would be variable flow control and adjustable I:E ratios. This will allow clinicians to make sure the expiratory time is sufficiently long to prevent air trapping/auto-PEEP.

6-9. **Correct answer: B.** Single-limb circuit with expiratory balloon valve. Most home-care ventilators use a single-limb circuit with expiratory balloon valve. Single-limb circuits have a separate pneumatic line running from the ventilator to the expiratory valve that pressurizes the expiratory valve during inspiration in order to block gas outflow during the application of positive pressure. An expiratory valve can also be used to control or retard expiratory flow or provide CPAP/PEEP. The mechanical deadspace in these circuits is that between the built-in expiratory valve and patient airway.

6-10. **Correct answer: C.** Bleed supplemental O_2 from a flowmeter into the circuit. Most NPPV ventilators and BiPAP™ devices use a simple air blower to generate pressure. In order to provide supplemental oxygen with these devices, you place a small-bore tubing adapter at either the patient interface or machine outlet. After connecting this adapter to a flowmeter via O_2 delivery tubing, you bleed O_2 into the circuit until the desired level is confirmed by O_2 analysis. Note that high supplemental O_2 flows can interfere with the proper triggering or cycling of some NPPV ventilators. For this reason, you should always follow the manufacturer's recommendations when considering how best to increase the F_{IO_2} of these devices.

6-11. **Correct answer: D.** Low volume + low pressure. When delivering volume-oriented ventilatory support, potential system leaks are indicated by a low-volume and low-pressure alarm condition. In such cases you should quickly check for and correct any loose circuit connections.

6-12. **Correct answer: B.** Fenestrated tracheostomy tube. A fenestrated tracheostomy tube is the best choice to support patients needing intermittent (e.g., nocturnal) ventilatory support. For positive pressure ventilation, the inner cannula is inserted to close the fenestration and the cuff inflated to provide a seal. When the patient is not on the ventilator, the inner cannula is removed (to open the fenestration), the cuff is deflated, and the tube is plugged. This allows normal use of the upper airway.

6-13. **Correct answer: A.** I and III only. An obstruction in the ET tube of a patient who is being mechanically ventilated increases flow resistance and thus the peak pressure needed by a volume-cycled ventilator to deliver its preset volume. In addition, you could detect the obstruction by trying to pass a suction catheter through the ET tube. Failure to pass a suction catheter through a tracheal airway indicates tube obstruction.

6-14. **Correct answer: C.** Replace the endotracheal tube. A cuff that fails to inflate when injected with air has a large leak. The faulty ET tube should be replaced and the new tube tested in the same manner.

6-15. **Correct answer: B.** Use a 10-Fr catheter. The catheter is too large for the ET tube. In general, the outside diameter of a suction catheter should not be more than about 1/2 as large as the inside diameter of the airway through which it passes. To quickly estimate the correct catheter size in French units (Fr), simply multiply the internal diameter (ID) of the tracheal tube (in mm) by 2 and select the next smallest catheter size. In this example, to suction a patient with a 6.0-mm tube, 2 × 6 = 12. Next smallest catheter size = 10 Fr. Thus a 10-Fr catheter is the best size to use on this patient.

6-16. **Correct answer: B.** Clearance of secretions. Conditions that could cause suctioning to stop suddenly during tracheobronchial aspiration include (1) disconnected tubing (leak; loss of vacuum), (2) a full suction reservoir (ball-valve shutoff), and (3) plugging of the catheter (system obstruction). Normal clearance of secretions would not cause loss of suction pressure.

6-17. **Correct answer: C.** 7.2 hours. Duration of flow = (cylinder factor × psig) ÷ flow. The factor for an H cylinder is 3.14. Thus duration of flow = (3.14 × 1100) ÷ 8 = 432 minutes = 7.2 hours.

6-18. **Correct answer: C.** I and III only. Yoke connectors for cylinders A–E use a hand screw to hold the yoke on the valve stem. If not tightened properly, a leak could result. In addition, the small receiving nipple on the yoke is normally sealed to the gas outlet with a nylon bushing. A missing or damaged bushing could also cause a leak. Missing DISS pins would not in themselves cause a leak.

6-19. **Correct answer: B.** Place the sample in an ice slush. When obtaining an arterial sample for analysis using a point-of-care analyzer, the equipment used and procedure performed are essentially the same as when preparing the sample for central lab analysis. The exceptions are (1) the sample should be analyzed within 3 minutes; and (2) the sample should NOT be placed in ice.

6-20. **Correct answer: B.** Incentive breathing therapy. Incentive spirometry is the first choice for treating suspected or confirmed atelectasis in an alert patient who does not have evidence of bronchospasm or secretion clearance problems.

6-21. **Correct answer: A.** Highest; exhalation. To provide vibration with a mechanical percussor, you should use the higher available frequencies (20–30 Hz) and apply during exhalation only.

6-22. **Correct answer: B.** Recheck and tighten all connections. If a PEP device fails to generate pressure during patient expiration, the most likely problem is a leak, either in the device itself or in the connecting tubing (including any connection to a pressure manometer. In these cases, you should recheck and tighten all connections.

6-23. **Correct answer: D.** To measure rapid pressure changes. Fluid column pressure manometers are to used to measure (1) atmospheric pressure (barometer); (2) static or slowing changing pressures—e.g., CVP; (3) systolic/diastolic blood pressures (occlusion method); and also to calibrate other pressure measuring devices. They are not suited for measuring rapidly changing pressures, their accuracy depends on position, and they can be messy or hazardous (if mercury is used).

6-24. **Correct answer: A.** A computerized electronic spirometer with flow sensor. If you need to measure a patient's forced vital capacity or related measures (e.g., peak flow, FEV_t, $FEF_{25-75\%}$) at the bedside, you should choose a portable electronic spirometer that incorporates a flow sensor (pneumotachometer) and computer analysis module. Mechanical turbine-type volumeters like the Wright respirometer are used to measure tidal volume, minute volume, inspiratory capacity, and slow vital capacity. Because the Wright respirometer can be damaged by flows greater than 60 L/min, it should not be used to measure forced inspiratory or expiratory volumes.

6-25. **Correct answer: A.** "Don't hesitate." In adults, a back extrapolated volume greater than 150 mL indicates patient hesitation at the beginning of the breath, which will invalidate the results. In these cases, you need to make sure the patient does not hesitate when beginning the forced exhalation.

6-26. **Correct answer: C.** Turning off filtering of extraneous electrical activity. The two most common problems in obtaining a good 12-lead ECG recording are absent or "noisy" signals. In either case you should check and confirm that: (1) the ECG snaps and connectors are clean and corrosion-free; (2) the lead electrodes are connected properly to the patient; (3); the electrode gel is not dry (replace any suspect electrodes); (4) the main lead cable is undamaged; (5) the patient is motionless; and (6) the device's filter settings (if available) are properly set to eliminate extraneous electrical activity.

6-27. **Correct answer: D.** Pulse oximeter. If you need to spot check, monitor, or obtain trend data on a patient's oxygen saturation (SpO_2), you should select a pulse oximeter. You would select a laboratory hemoximeter if you needed precise measures of both normal and abnormal hemoglobin saturations. A transcutaneous monitor would be your best choice to continuously and noninvasively monitor arterial blood gases (PO_2 and PCO_2) in infants.

6-28. **Correct answer: D.** Air leakage around the sensor's adhesive ring. The most common problem with transcutaneous monitoring is air leaks around the adhesive ring. Air leaks always cause a dramatic fall in Ptcco$_2$. If the leak is large, the Ptco$_2$ and Ptcco$_2$ values will mimic those in room air (Po$_2$ ~ 150 torr/ Pco$_2$ ~ 0 torr). In these cases, reapply the sensor using a new adhesive ring.

6-29. **Correct answer: C.** MDI with holding chamber and a mask. Most infants and small children should receive aerosolized drugs via an MDI with a valved holding chamber and a mask. If tolerated by the patient, an SVN with a mask could be considered as an alternative. Avoid using the "blow by" technique (i.e., holding the mask or open tube near the infant's nose and mouth) with small-volume nebulizers.

6-30. **Correct answer: B.** Small-volume nebulizer. A small-volume nebulizer (SVN) is the method of choice for administering cromolyn sodium to young children. You should use a tightly fitting face mask for any child unable to use a mouthpiece.

POST-TEST

A post-test for this chapter that includes automated scoring and feedback is available on the accompanying CD. Be sure to complete this additional assessment to confirm your mastery of this chapter's objectives.

REFERENCES

American Association for Respiratory Care. (1991). Clinical practice guideline. Incentive spirometry. *Respiratory care, 36*, 1402–1405.

American Association for Respiratory Care. (1992). Clinical practice guideline. Humidification during mechanical ventilation. *Respiratory care, 37*, 887–890.

American Association for Respiratory Care. (1992). Clinical practice guideline. Pulse oximetry. *Respiratory care, 37*, 891–897.

American Association for Respiratory Care. (1993). Clinical practice guideline. Endotracheal suctioning of mechanically ventilated adults and children with artificial airways. *Respiratory care, 38*, 500–504.

American Association for Respiratory Care. (1993). Clinical practice guideline. Use of positive airway pressure adjuncts to bronchial hygiene therapy. *Respiratory care, 38*, 516–521.

American Association for Respiratory Care. (1995). Clinical practice guideline. Management of airway emergencies. *Respiratory care, 40*, 749–760.

American Association for Respiratory Care. (1996). Clinical practice guideline. Selection of a device for delivery of aerosol to the lung parenchyma. *Respiratory care, 41*, 647–653.

American Association for Respiratory Care. (2002). Clinical practice guideline. Oxygen therapy for adults in the acute care facility. 2002 revision and update. *Respiratory care, 47*, 717–720.

American Association for Respiratory Care. (2003). Clinical practice guideline. Care of the ventilator circuit and its relation to ventilator-associated pneumonia. *Respiratory care, 48*, 869–879.

American Association for Respiratory Care. (2004). Clinical practice guideline. Transcutaneous blood gas monitoring for neonatal and pediatric patients. 2004 revision and update. *Respiratory care, 49*, 1070–1072.

American Thoracic Society. (1995). Standardization of spirometry. 1994 update. *American journal of respiratory and critical care medicine, 152*, 1107–1136.

Blazer, C. (1994). *Quick reference to respiratory therapy equipment assembly and troubleshooting.* St. Louis: Mosby, 1994.

Branson, R. D., Hess, D., & Chatburn, R. L. (1998). *Respiratory care equipment* (2nd ed.). Philadelphia: Lippincott.

Cairo, J. M., & Pilbeam, S. P. (2004). *Mosby's respiratory care equipment* (7th ed.). St. Louis: Mosby.

Dolovich, M. B., Ahrens, R. C., Hess, D. R., et al. (2005). Device selection and outcomes of aerosol therapy: Evidence-based guidelines, *Chest, 127*, 335–371.

Ferguson, G. T., Enright, P. L., Buist, A. S., & Higgins, M. W. (2000). Office spirometry for lung health assessment in adults: A consensus statement from the National Lung Health Education Program. *Chest, 117*, 1146–1161.

Fink, J. B., & Hunt, G. E. (1999). *Clinical practice in respiratory care.* Philadelphia: Raven-Lippincott.

Hess, D. R., & MacIntyre, N. R. (Eds.). (2002). *Respiratory care: Principles and practices.* Philadelphia: W. B. Saunders.

McCoy, R. (2000). Oxygen-conserving techniques and devices. *Respiratory Care, 45,* 95–103.

Mehta, A. C., Prakash, U. B., Garland, R., et al. (2005). Consensus statement: Prevention of flexible bronchoscopy-associated infection. *Chest, 128,* 1742–1755.

White, G. C. (1999). *Equipment theory for respiratory care* (3rd ed.). Albany, NY: Delmar

Wilkins, R. L., Stoller, J. K., & Kacmarek, R. M. (Eds.). (2009). *Egan's fundamentals of respiratory care.* (9th ed.). St. Louis: Mosby.

Ensure Infection Control

Craig L. Scanlan

INTRODUCTION

Infection control is a small part of the NBRC CRT exam, but it is a big part of your job. Most students and clinicians are familiar with the basics, such as hand hygiene and isolation procedures. However, the CRT exam includes some areas of infection control that you may not be regularly involved in, such as equipment disinfection. In addition, if you have been out of school for more than a few years, there may have been changes in infection control guidelines that were not covered in your classes or clinical rotations. Moreover, new protocols recently have been promoted to decrease the incidence of ventilator-associated pneumonia (VAP) and to combat the spread of emerging infections such as severe acute respiratory syndrome (SARS). For these reasons, you should spend a reasonable portion of your exam preparation time on this topic, with an emphasis on the areas that you are not regularly involved in or for which newer guidelines or protocols might apply.

OBJECTIVES

After completion of this chapter, you should demonstrate the knowledge needed to:

1. Ensure cleanliness of equipment by
   a. Selecting or determining appropriate agent and technique for disinfection and/or sterilization
   b. Performing procedures for disinfection and/or sterilization
   c. Monitoring effectiveness of sterilization procedures
2. Ensure proper handling of biohazardous materials
3. Adhere to infection control policies and procedures
4. Incorporate ventilator-associated pneumonia protocol
5. Implement infectious disease protocols, e.g.,
   a. Avian flu
   b. SARS
   c. Transmission prevention

WHAT TO EXPECT ON THIS CATEGORY OF THE CRT EXAM

Number of questions: 3
Level of questions: 2/3 application and 1/3 analysis

WHAT'S NEW FOR 2009

As of July 2009, this section of the NBRC CRT examination includes the following *new infection control topics*:

- Incorporate ventilator-associated pneumonia (VAP) protocol
- Implement infectious disease protocols (e.g., for avian flu, SARS, and transmission prevention)

Adhering to infection control policies and procedures (such as by taking standard precautions) is not new to the CRT exam, but as of July 2009 appears in this category of questions.

PRE-TEST

Carefully respond to each of the following questions. After completing the pre-test, compare your answers with those provided at the end of this chapter. Then thoroughly review each answer's explanation to help understand why it is correct.

7-1. The first step in processing reusable equipment is:
   A. Pasteurization
   B. Cleaning
   C. Disinfection
   D. Sterilization

7-2. The label of a disinfectant indicates that it does NOT inactivate or kill either *Mycobacterium tuberculosis* or bacterial spores. What class of disinfectant is this?
   A. Surface active
   B. Low-level
   C. Intermediate-level
   D. High-level

7-3. A patient with pneumonia has her noninvasive ventilatory support discontinued. Which of the following should be used to disinfect the device's nondisposable breathing circuit before it is placed back into service?
   A. Pasteurization
   B. Isopropyl alcohol
   C. Acetic acid
   D. Hydrogen peroxide

7-4. For patients receiving bronchodilator therapy via small-volume nebulizer (SVN), which of the following precautions would be beneficial in preventing nosocomial infection?
   I. Use a different SVN for each patient
   II. Change the nebulizer and tubing every 24 hours
   III. Perform thorough handwashing prior to each therapy session
   A. I only
   B. II only
   C. I and III only
   D. I, II, and III

7-5. A patient who was hospitalized with ARDS of unknown etiology recently traveled to an area with a documented outbreak of severe acute respiratory syndrome (SARS). Which of the following infection control precautions should you recommend for this patient?
   I. Airborne precautions
   II. Contact precautions
   III. Droplet precautions
   A. I and II only
   B. I, II, and III
   C. I and III only
   D. II and III only

7-6. ALL of the following help minimize the risk of cross-contamination during suctioning *except*:
  A. Using a fresh sterile single-use catheter on each patient
  B. Using only sterile fluid to remove secretions from the catheter
  C. Instilling 10 mL sterile saline before the suctioning attempt
  D. Performing proper handwashing and gloving before suctioning

7-7. If sterilization is not feasible, which of the following are acceptable alternatives for processing a specialized reusable plastic airway?
  I. Exposure to a high-level chemical disinfectant
  II. Surface disinfection with 70% ethyl alcohol
  III. Pasteurization at 63°C for 30 minutes
  A. I and II only
  B. II and III only
  C. I and III only
  D. I, II, and III

7-8. What is the primary reason for using chemical indicators in equipment sterilization processing?
  A. To warn the user about the presence of toxic residues
  B. To show that a package has been through a sterilizing process
  C. To indicate the remaining safe shelf-life of the equipment
  D. To verify that the sterilization process has worked

7-9. Cultures taken from a respirometer that has been used in the surgical intensive care unit to monitor several patients indicate that it is contaminated. The most practical way to prevent cross-contamination is to:
  A. Provide a new respirometer for each patient
  B. Sterilize the respirometer after each use
  C. Replace the respirometer with a water-sealed spirometer
  D. Use a disposable HEPA filter and one-way valve for each patient

7-10. All of the following will reduce the incidence of ventilator-acquired pneumonia (VAP) on your patients *except*:
  A. Elevating the head of the bed at least 30°
  B. Implementing daily spontaneous breathing trials
  C. Continuously aspirating subglottic secretions
  D. Changing ventilator circuits every 48 hours

WHAT YOU NEED TO KNOW: ESSENTIAL CONTENT

Key Terms and Definitions

Basic to your understanding of infection control are some key terms and definitions, summarized in **Table 7-1**.

Ensuring Equipment Cleanliness

Most of the key information on the processing and maintenance of equipment and devices derives from governmental guidelines, primarily those developed by the Centers for Disease Control and Prevention (CDC).

Selecting Appropriate Methods to Ensure Equipment Cleanliness

To help you select the best method to ensure equipment cleanliness, the CDC defines three levels of infection risk, as delineated in **Table 7-2** (see page 226).

Note that some of the same liquid chemical solutions (e.g., glutaraldehyde [Cidex] and ortho-phthalaldehyde [OPA]) can be used to either sterilize or provide high-level disinfection of equipment and are commonly used for heat-sensitive items. The differences in level of activity of these solutions

Table 7-1 Key Terms Used in Infection Control

Term	Meaning
Antiseptic	A chemical that kills microorganisms on living skin or mucous membranes
Bacteriostatic	A descriptive term for chemical agents that inhibit the growth of bacteria but do not necessarily kill them
Cleaning	The physical removal of foreign material (e.g., dirt or organic material, usually with water, detergents, and mechanical action [washing]); cleaning generally removes rather than kills microorganisms
Decontamination	The removal of disease-producing microorganisms to leave an item safe for further handling
Disinfection	A general term for the inactivation of disease-producing microorganisms on inanimate objects, usually specified by level
Disinfection, high-level	The destruction of vegetative bacteria, mycobacteria, fungi, and viruses, but not necessarily bacterial spores; some high-level disinfectants ("chemical sterilants") are capable of sterilization with adequate contact time
Disinfection, intermediate-level	The destruction of vegetative bacteria, mycobacteria, most viruses, and most fungi, but not resistant bacterial spores
Disinfection, low-level	The destruction of most vegetative bacteria, some fungi as well as some viruses (e.g., hepatitis B/C, HIV), but not mycobacteria or bacterial spores; low-level disinfectants are typically used to clean environmental surfaces
Germicidal	A general descriptive term for chemical agents capable of killing microorganisms; *bactericidal, virucidal, fungicidal,* or *sporicidal* are related terms for chemicals capable of killing these specific categories of microorganisms
Sanitation	A process that reduces microorganisms on environmental surfaces to minimize any infectious hazard (e.g., on furniture, floors)
Sterilization	The destruction of all forms of microbial life including bacteria, viruses, spores, and fungi

are time and temperature. For example, high-level disinfection with Cidex can be achieved in 20 minutes at room temperature. However, true sterilization requires a full 10 hours.

Disinfecting, Sterilizing, and Maintaining Equipment

The CDC recommends the following general measures for sterilization or disinfection and maintenance of equipment and devices:

1. Disassemble and thoroughly clean all equipment before it is sterilized or disinfected.
2. Consider all reusable breathing circuit components (including tubing, valves, nebulizers, and humidifiers) to be semicritical items.
3. Whenever possible, use steam sterilization (autoclaving) or high-level disinfection for reprocessing semicritical equipment or devices that are not sensitive to heat and moisture.
4. Use low-temperature sterilization methods (gas, vapor, plasma, or immersion in a liquid chemical sterilant) for equipment or devices that are heat- or moisture-sensitive. After disinfection, protect these items with appropriate rinsing, drying, and packaging, taking care not to contaminate the disinfected items in the process.

Table 7-2 Infection Risk Categories of Equipment

Category	Description	Example	Processing
Critical items	Devices introduced into blood stream or other parts of the body	• Surgical devices • Intravascular catheters • Implants • Heart–lung bypass components • Dialysis components • Bronchoscope forceps/brushes	Sterilization *For heat-tolerant items:* • Steam under pressure (autoclaving) *For heat-sensitive items:* • Gas or ionized vapor (ethylene oxide, hydrogen peroxide) • Immersion in liquid chemical sterilant (e.g., glutaraldehyde, ortho-phthaladehyde)
Semi-critical items	Devices that contact intact mucous membranes	• Endoscopes/bronchoscopes • Oral, nasal, tracheal airways • Ventilator circuits/humidifiers • PFT mouthpieces/tubing • Nebulizers • Laryngoscope blades • Nondisposable resuscitation bags • Pressure, gas, or temp probes	Sterilization *or* high-level disinfection via either: • Immersion in liquid high-level disinfectant (e.g., glutaraldehyde, ortho-phthalaldehyde) • Pasteurization (immersion in hot water at > 158°F/70°C) for 30 minutes)
Non-critical items	Devices that touch only intact skin or do not contact patient	• Face masks (external) • Blood pressure cuffs • Ventilators	Detergent washing or exposure to low- or intermediate-level disinfection

5. When rinsing reusable semicritical respiratory equipment after they have been immersed in a liquid disinfectant, use sterile water. If this is not feasible, rinse the device with filtered water or tap water, and then rinse with isopropyl alcohol and dry with forced air or in a drying cabinet.

6. Do not reprocess equipment designed for single use only (unless data show that reprocessing the equipment does not change the structural integrity or function of the equipment or device).

Regarding sterilization, disinfection, and maintenance of *specific* respiratory care equipment and devices, the CDC recommends the following.

- Ventilators
  ○ Do not routinely sterilize or disinfect the internal machinery of ventilators.
  ○ Do not routinely change in-use ventilator circuits, attached humidifiers, or closed suction systems. Change these components only if visibly soiled or malfunctioning.
  ○ Sterilize or high-level disinfect nondisposable ventilator circuit volume/flow-measuring devices, oxygen sensors, and thermometers between patients.
  ○ Periodically drain and discard any condensate that collects in ventilator circuits. Be sure to avoid letting condensate drain toward the patient. Wear gloves to drain and handle circuit condensate and decontaminate hands after the procedure.
  ○ Use sterile water to fill bubble humidifiers.

- ○ Do not place bacterial filters distal to humidifier reservoirs.
- ○ Change in-use heat and moisture exchangers (HMEs) if they malfunction or become visibly soiled; do not routinely change HMEs more frequently than every 48 hours.
- ○ Do not routinely change ventilator circuit with HMEs unless they are grossly contaminated or malfunctioning.
- Oxygen "wall" humidifiers
  - ○ Follow manufacturers' instructions for use of oxygen humidifiers.
  - ○ Change any in-use humidifier tubing and/or the cannula or mask when it malfunctions or becomes visibly contaminated.
- Large-volume nebulizers (e.g., with aerosol masks, T-tubes)
  - ○ Whenever possible use prefilled, sterile disposable nebulizers.
  - ○ If not prefilled, fill reservoirs with sterile water just before use.
  - ○ If not prefilled, discard old water before refilling.
  - ○ Do not drain condensate back into reservoir or allow it to flow into airway.
  - ○ Do not handle the internal parts of large-volume nebulizers; replace if malfunctioning.
  - ○ Replace large-volume nebulizers with sterile or high-level disinfected equipment every 24 hours.
- Small-volume medication nebulizers
  - ○ Use only sterile fluid for nebulization; dispense fluids aseptically.
  - ○ Whenever possible, use single-dose aerosolized medications. If multidose vials are used, follow manufacturers' instructions for handling and storing.
  - ○ Between treatments on the same patient, medication nebulizers should be cleaned, disinfected, rinsed with sterile water (if rinsing is needed), and dried.
- Room-air humidifiers
  - ○ Do not use large-volume room-air humidifiers that create aerosols unless they can be sterilized or high-level disinfected at least daily and filled only with sterile water.
- Resuscitation bags
  - ○ Between their uses on different patients, sterilize or high-level disinfect reusable hand-powered resuscitation bags.
- Suctioning equipment
  - ○ When using an open-suction system, use a sterile single-use catheter for each incident.
  - ○ Use only sterile fluid to remove secretions from the suction catheter.
  - ○ Change suction collection tubing (up to the canister) between patients.
  - ○ Change suction collection canisters between patients except in short-term care units.
- Mist tents
  - ○ Between uses on different patients, replace all mist tent components with those that have been sterilized or high-level disinfected.
  - ○ Subject mist-tent nebulizers, reservoirs, and tubings that are used on the same patient to daily low-level disinfection (e.g., with 2% acetic acid) or pasteurization followed by air drying.
- Pulmonary-function equipment (lab and bedside)
  - ○ Do not routinely sterilize or disinfect the internal workings of laboratory spirometers between uses on different patients; instead, change the mouthpiece and filter between patients.
  - ○ Bedside pulmonary function equipment (e.g., respirometers, peak flow meters) used on multiple patients should not directly touch any part of a ventilator circuit or a patient's mucous membranes. Rather, disposable extension pieces/valves and low-resistance HEPA filters should be used to isolate these devices. If these devices cannot be isolated from the patient or circuit, they must be sterilized or undergo high-level disinfection between use on different patients.

Monitoring the Effectiveness of Sterilization Procedures

Mechanical, chemical, and biological techniques are used to determine whether sterilization procedures actually work. Generally all three methods are used together, with good records kept to document all monitoring activity. **Table 7-3** summarizes these monitoring methods, as described by the CDC.

Table 7-3 Methods to Monitor Sterilization Procedures

Method	Description	Comments
Mechanical methods	Assess the cycle time, temperature, and pressure of sterilization equipment.	Correct readings do not ensure sterilization, but incorrect readings might indicate a problem.
Chemical indicators	Assess physical conditions occurring inside sterilizers via chemical reactions that change the color of the indicator when the proper conditions are achieved (e.g., the correct temperature or gas concentration). Internal chemical indicators should be placed in every package to ensure that the sterilization agent has reached the instruments inside. An external indicator (typically color-changing tape) should be used when internal indicator cannot be seen from outside the package.	Chemical indicator changes are visible immediately after sterilization and thus can warn of problems with the process. If a chemical indicator does not change color as expected, the affected item(s) should not be used.
Biological indicators	Assess whether sterilization process actually kills bacterial spores that are impregnated on paper strips that are exposed to growth media and incubated after processing. Included in every cycle that includes critical items; otherwise should be used at least once a week for each sterilizer.	Most valid method for verifying that sterilization has occurred; indicators must be placed in sterilizers as per manufacturer's recommendations. Incubation period requires holding processed equipment until negative results are confirmed and compared to a control strip (which should test positive for bacterial growth). If proper mechanical readings and chemical indicator changes are obtained, a single positive result from a biological test strip should require recall of critical items only, with repeat testing to determine whether a true processing problem exists.

Properly Handle Biohazardous Materials

Biohazardous materials include noninfectious agents (e.g., poisons, radioactive substances, flammable or explosive chemicals) and infectious items such as isolation or contaminated wastes, blood and blood products, and contaminated sharps. The biohazardous materials of most importance to respiratory therapists are infectious waste items. Key recommendations for the proper handling of infectious waste that have been developed by the CDC's Healthcare Infection Control Practices Advisory Committee and the National Institute for Occupational Safety and Health (NIOSH) are summarized below.

- You should separate infectious and noninfectious wastes at the point of generation; manage medical wastes generated in isolation areas using the same methods as for medical wastes from other patient-care areas.

- You should discard and contain all solid infectious waste except contaminated sharps at their point of origin in clearly identifiable (red or orange) containers or plastic bags that are leak-proof and tear/puncture-resistant and marked with the universal symbol for biological hazards.
- You should prevent biohazard bags from coming into contact with sharp external objects.
- If the surface of a biohazard bag gets contaminated or punctured, place it inside a second bag ("double bagging").
- To properly handle contaminated sharps:
  ○ Never recap used needles, handle them using both hands, or point a needle toward any part of the body; rather, use either a one-handed "scoop" technique or a mechanical device designed for holding the needle sheath.
  ○ Do not remove used needles from disposable syringes by hand, and do not bend, break, or otherwise manipulate used needles by hand.
  ○ Place all used sharps in an impervious rigid, puncture-resistant container made for this purpose.
- Most liquid wastes (e.g., blood, suction fluids) can be either inactivated in accordance with state-approved treatment technologies or carefully poured down a utility sink drain or toilet. If transported, liquid wastes should be placed in capped or tightly stoppered bottles or flasks. Large quantities of liquid wastes may be placed in containment tanks.
- When transporting bagged waste and containers of sharps and liquids away from the point of origin, place them within a rigid or semi-rigid container such as a bucket, box, or carton lined with plastic bags.
- Medical wastes requiring storage should be kept in labeled, leak-proof, puncture-resistant containers under conditions that minimize or prevent foul odors; the storage area should be well ventilated and inaccessible to pests.
- After each use, disinfect carts and recyclable containers that are used repeatedly for transport and treatment of bagged waste. Single-use containers should be destroyed as part of the treatment process.
- Should a spill of liquid infectious waste occur (e.g., blood or body fluids):
  ○ Use gloves and other protective personal protective equipment (PPE) appropriate for the task.
  ○ If the spill contains large amounts of blood or body fluids, clean the visible matter with disposable absorbent material; discard as infectious waste.
  ○ Swab the area with a cloth or paper towels moderately wetted with an Environmental Protection Agency (EPA)–registered hospital disinfectant labeled tuberculocidal or with registered germicides with specific label claims for HIV or hepatitis B virus and allow the surface to dry.
  ○ If an EPA-registered disinfectant or germicide is not available, household bleach (1:100 dilution) can be used to decontaminate nonporous surfaces after cleaning; use a more concentrated solution (1:10) for spills involving large amounts of blood or body fluid.

Interestingly, recent research indicates that medical wastes are no more infective than wastes coming from the home. Moreover, although items that have contact with blood or body fluids are potentially infective, treating all such wastes as infective is not practical or necessary. For this reason, the CDC now suggests that waste handling and disposal precautions be based on judgment about the relative risk of disease transmission, in accord with local and/or state regulations.

Final disposition of infectious wastes usually involves treatment by either sterilization or incineration, with the solid waste products or their ashes either buried in a sanitary landfill (in compliance with state, federal, and local laws) and liquid or ground-up waste discharged into a sanitary sewer system.

Adhere to Infection Control Policies and Procedures

CDC Standard Precautions

Standard precautions are based on the assumption that every patient is potentially infected with an organism that could be transmitted to others. The components of standard precautions include hand hygiene, personal protective equipment or PPE (including gloves, gowns, and masks/eye protection), patient-care equipment procedures, needles and sharps handling, patient resuscitation, and respiratory hygiene/cough etiquette. **Table 7-4** specifies the CDC's recommendations for each major component of standard precautions.

Given that most hospital-acquired infections occur due to direct or indirect contact between patients and health care workers, good hand hygiene is the single most important measure to help prevent transmission of disease-causing microorganisms in hospitals. Good hand hygiene is also a component of the new respiratory hygiene/cough etiquette guideline, which also applies to health care workers. When examining and caring for patients with signs and symptoms of a respiratory infection, you should wear a mask and maintain good hand hygiene. If you have a respiratory infection, you should avoid direct patient contact, especially with any high-risk patients. If this is not possible, then you should wear a mask while providing care.

Table 7-4 Centers for Disease Control and Prevention's Standard Precautions Recommendations

Component	Recommendations
Hand hygiene	• Perform after touching blood, body fluids, secretions, excretions, contaminated items • Perform immediately after removing gloves • Perform between patient contacts
Gloves	• Use for touching blood, body fluids, secretions, excretions, contaminated items • Use for touching mucous membranes and non-intact skin
Gown	• Use during procedures and patient-care activities when contact of clothing/exposed skin with blood/body fluids, secretions, and excretions is anticipated
Mask, eye protection (goggles, face shield)[a]	• Use during procedures and patient-care activities likely to generate splashes or sprays of blood, body fluids, secretions, *especially suctioning and endotracheal intubation*
Soiled patient-care equipment	• Handle in a manner that prevents transfer of microorganisms to others and to the environment • Wear gloves if equipment visibly contaminated • Perform hand hygiene after handling
Needles and other sharps	• Do not recap, bend, break, or hand-manipulate used needles • If recapping is required, use a one-handed scoop technique • Use safety features when available • Place used sharps in puncture-resistant container
Patient resuscitation	• Use mouthpiece, resuscitation bag, other ventilation devices to prevent contact with mouth and oral secretions
Patient placement	• Single-patient room if patient is at increased risk of transmission, is likely to contaminate the environment, does not maintain appropriate hygiene, or is at increased risk of acquiring infection or developing adverse outcome following infection
Respiratory hygiene/ cough etiquette	• Patients/visitors who are sneezing or coughing should be instructed to: • Cover the mouth/nose when sneezing/coughing • Use tissues and dispose in no-touch receptacle • Observe hand hygiene after soiling of hands with respiratory secretions • In common waiting areas wear surgical mask if tolerated or maintain spatial separation, > 3 feet if possible.

a. During aerosol-generating procedures on patients with suspected or proven infections transmitted by respiratory aerosols (e.g., SARS), wear a fit-tested N95 or higher respirator in addition to gloves, gown, and face/eye protection.

Which PPE you use in a particular situation depends on the transmission category under which your patient is categorized (discussed in the next section.) In general, PPE should be applied and removed in the following sequence:

Order of Applying PPE	Order of Removing PPE
1. Hair and foot coverings	1. Head and foot coverings
2. Gown	2. Goggles or face shield
3. Mask	3. Mask
4. Goggles or face shield	4. Gloves (remove by pulling gloves down from wrist and turning them inside out)
5. Gloves	5. Gown (remove from the inside out)

Transmission-Based Precautions

Transmission-based precautions represent additional measures designed to prevent the spread of infection by microorganisms that are transmitted via particular routes. *Transmission-based precautions are always used in combination with standard precautions.* The three routes of transmission addressed by these extra precautions include:

- *Contact transmission:* the spread of microorganisms by direct or indirect contact with the patient or the patient's environment, including contaminated equipment
- *Droplet transmission:* the spread of microorganisms in the air via large droplets (larger than 5 μm)
- *Airborne transmission:* the spread of microorganisms in the air via small droplet nuclei (5 μm or smaller)

Most NBRC candidates understand that respiratory therapy equipment can be a vehicle for (indirect) contact transmission between patients and that aerosol therapy devices can spread microorganisms via either the droplet or airborne routes. However, the difference between the droplet and airborne routes is not always well understood. Because large droplets tend to fall out of suspension quickly, they tend to travel only short distances. Thus *droplet transmission requires close contact*, generally three feet or less. In contrast, the smaller droplets generated when talking, coughing, or sneezing and during procedures such as suctioning or intubation are very stable and can be transmitted in the air over long distances, such as between patient rooms. **Table 7-5** summarizes the CDC's precautions designed to thwart each of these types of disease transmission, including the most common infections to which they apply.

Incorporate Ventilator-Associated Pneumonia Protocol

The CDC defines ventilator-associated pneumonia (VAP) as pneumonia occurring in patients who have received mechanical ventilation for more than 48 hours. VAP is the leading cause of death among patients with hospital-acquired infections. Even among those patients who survive, VAP increases ventilator days and prolongs both the time spent in intensive care and the overall length of hospital stay. To decrease the human and economic costs of this significant problem, the CDC has developed what is commonly referred to as the "VAP bundle" of preventive strategies. The four key components included in the VAP bundle are:

- Elevating the head of the bed 30° or more (unless contraindicated)
- Implementing a daily "sedation vacation" and weaning assessment
- Providing peptic ulcer disease prophylaxis
- Providing deep venous thrombosis prophylaxis

VAP is associated with gastric reflux aspiration. Elevating the head of the bed helps prevent gastric reflux aspiration, as does prophylaxis against peptic ulcer disease. Elevating the head of the bed also improves the distribution of ventilation and the efficiency of diaphragmatic action and may help prevent atelectasis. In addition to elevating the head of the bed, regular turning, as provided by kinetic bed therapy, may also reduce the incidence of VAP.

Table 7-5 Centers for Disease Control and Prevention's Transmission-Based Precautions Recommendations

Category	Used for	Precautions
Contact precautions	Gastrointestinal infections (including diarrhea of unknown origin), wound and skin infections, multi- drug-resistant infection or colonization (e.g., MRSA, SARS, avian flu, smallpox)	• Apply standard precautions • Place the patient in a private room • Wear clean gloves and gown when entering the room • Change gloves after having contact with any infectious material • Remove gloves and gown before leaving the room and wash hands immediately with an alcohol-based rub
Droplet precautions	Bacterial meningitis, whooping cough (*Bordetella pertussis*), influenza, mumps, rubella, diphtheria, pneumonic plague, Group A *Streptococcus pneumoniae* infections, SARS, *Mycoplasma pneumoniae*, and epiglottitis (due to *Haemophilus influenzae*)	• Apply standard precautions • Place the patient in a private room (special air handling and ventilation are not necessary and the door can stay open) • Wear a surgical mask when within 3 feet of the patient (some facilities may require donning a mask to enter the room) • Use eye/face protection if aerosol-generating procedure performed or contact with respiratory secretions anticipated • Patients who must be transported outside their rooms should wear a mask and follow respiratory hygiene/cough etiquette
Airborne precautions	TB, measles (rubeola), chickenpox, (varicella-zoster), *Aspergillus* infections, SARS, smallpox (variola)	• Apply standard precautions • Place the patient in a private negative-pressure airborne infection isolation room (AIIR) with the door closed • Wear a fit-tested[a] NIOSH-certified N95 or higher level respirator when entering the room • Use eye/face protection if aerosol-generating procedure performed or contact with respiratory secretions anticipated • Whenever possible, nonimmune health care workers should not care for patients with vaccine-preventable airborne diseases (e.g., measles, chickenpox, smallpox) • In settings where airborne precautions cannot be implemented, apply droplet precautions (e.g., placing the patient in a private room with the door closed, masking the patient) • Patients who must be transported outside their rooms should wear a mask and follow respiratory hygiene/cough etiquette

a. In addition to being fit-tested for a respirator, you need to perform a user-seal check each time you use it (according to the manufacturer's specifications).

Daily cessation of sedative drugs has been shown to decrease the duration of mechanical ventilation in critically ill patients. In conjunction with this sedation vacation, patients should undergo regular spontaneous breathing trials to assess their readiness for weaning from the ventilator. In general, the sooner a patient can be extubated, the lower the chances of developing VAP. The primary contraindication against implementing a daily sedation vacation/weaning assessment is the need for neuromuscular blockade. The primary hazard when decreasing sedation is accidental (self-) extubation.

To minimize this risk, ensure that the patient is adequately supervised and that appropriate hand or arm restraints are used as needed. More details on weaning procedures and protocols are provided in Chapters 12, 14, and 15.

Other nursing and respiratory care strategies potentially helpful in preventing VAP include general infection control procedures, airway management techniques, equipment maintenance, and oral care.

In terms of *general infection control* procedures, you should always implement both standard precautions *and* any needed transmission-based precautions on your ventilator patients. This must include rigorous hand hygiene before and after contact with a patient's mucous membranes, respiratory secretions, or related equipment (e.g., ventilator circuit, suction apparatus, ET tube).

Airway management techniques that can help decrease the incidence of VAP include the following:

- Avoid intubation when possible (use noninvasive ventilation instead).
- Intubate via the oral (as opposed to nasal) route.
- Maintain proper ET tube cuff pressures.
- Aspirate subglottic secretions.
- Use only sterile water or saline to flush suction catheters.

Since endotracheal intubation is a prime factor associated with VAP, avoiding invasive ventilation altogether is a good preventive strategy, if feasible. If intubation is necessary, the oral route is preferred since nasotracheal tubes are associated with a high incidence of sinus infection. Because low ET tube cuff pressures allow "leakage-type" aspiration, proper cuff management is critical. *Current research suggests that the commonly used minimal leak technique may be a contributing factor and should be discouraged.* Instead, the Institute for Clinical Systems Improvement recommends that you maintain cuff pressures at 20–25 cm H_2O. When the cuff is properly inflated, secretions tend to pool above the cuff and present an aspiration risk. To prevent aspiration of these subglottic secretions, the American Thoracic Society and CDC both recommend that they be continuously aspirated using a specially designed endotracheal tube that includes a suction lumen above the cuff. Use of these CASS (Continuous Aspiration of Subglottic Secretions) tubes is discussed in more detail in Chapter 11. Last, PRN (as needed) endotracheal suctioning must be performed on all intubated patients. The CDC recommends that you always use sterile fluids to flush the suction catheter between repeated attempts to aspirate secretions through the ET tube. Regarding suction apparatus, current evidence does not indicate that closed, in-line suctioning systems are any better than standard suctioning at preventing VAP. Closed suction systems, however, are better at preventing hypoxemia during suctioning and for this reason should be considered in patients susceptible to desaturation, such as those with ARDS.

In regard to *equipment maintenance*, the CDC recommends *against* routine changing of ventilator circuits. Instead, you should change the circuit only when it is visibly soiled or malfunctioning. Regarding humidification equipment, current evidence indicates no difference in the incidence of VAP between patients supported with heated humidifiers versus those with heat and moisture exchangers (HMEs). However, when using heated humidification, the CDC recommends that you regularly drain any condensate that collects in the ventilator circuit *away from the patient* and properly discard it.

Oral care is the last supplemental strategy potentially helpful in preventing VAP. Good oral care involves (1) assessment of the oral cavity every 8 hours and as needed for hydration, lesions, or infections; (2) the provision of oral care every 2–4 hours and as needed, using a non-alcohol-based antiseptic solution like chlorhexidine; (3) regular brushing of the teeth every 8–12 hours (using chlorhexidine gel or toothpaste with a bicarbonate base); and (4) application of a water-soluble mouth moisturizer and/or lip balm after oral care.

Implement Specific Infectious Disease Protocols

Over the past decade, several new infectious disorders have emerged and are raising concern in the health care community. These infections are difficult to diagnose and treat and have the potential to cause serious epidemics. Here we focus on the two most recent of these emerging infections, avian or bird influenza and severe acute respiratory syndrome (SARS). Both are identified by the NBRC as potential areas for testing.

Avian (Bird) Influenza

Avian, or bird, influenza refers to infection in humans by an influenza A–type virus found chiefly in birds. Currently, the risk of contracting avian influenza is low because the virus does not normally infect humans or spread easily among them. Most avian influenza cases have been attributed to contact with infected poultry and have occurred mainly in Asia. When infection does occur, symptoms are similar to those of human influenza (i.e., fever, cough, sore throat, and severe muscle aches). However, the avian influenza virus can be much more virulent than the human version and can quickly progress to an acute and life-threatening pneumonia, even in otherwise healthy individuals.

For these reasons, all patients who present to a health care setting with flu-like symptoms should follow the respiratory hygiene and cough etiquette protocol *and* be questioned regarding their recent travel history and contact with other sick individuals. If a patient is suspected of or confirmed as having avian influenza, the CDC currently recommends the following protocol to help prevent the spread of this dangerous infection:

- Standard precautions:
  - Pay careful attention to hand hygiene before and after all patient contact or contact with items potentially contaminated with respiratory secretions.
- Contact precautions:
  - Use gloves and gown for all patient contact.
  - Use dedicated equipment such as stethoscopes, disposable blood pressure cuffs, and disposable thermometers.
- Eye protection (i.e., goggles, face shields):
  - Wear when within 3 feet of the patient.
- Airborne precautions:
  - Place the patient in an airborne infection isolation room (AIIR).
  - If an AIIR is unavailable, use portable HEPA filtration.
  - Use a fit-tested, NIOSH-approved N-95 respirator when entering the room.

The CDC recommends that these precautions be continued for 14 days after onset of symptoms or until laboratory testing indicates that the patient is not infected with the avian influenza virus.

Severe Acute Respiratory Syndrome (SARS)

Severe acute respiratory syndrome (SARS) is a respiratory infection caused by a coronavirus (SARS-CoV). SARS cases first occurred in Asia in 2003, with the infection that year spreading to dozens of countries on all major populated continents except Australia. The route of transmission for SARS is thought to be via contact (direct or indirect) and/or respiratory droplets.

Public health efforts have focused on the early detection and isolation of patients who may be infected with SARS-CoV. For this reason, the CDC recommends that patients who require hospitalization for X-ray-confirmed pneumonia or ARDS of unknown etiology and who within 10 days have either (1) traveled to an area with documented SARS infections or (2) had direct contact with a patient suspected of having SARS be placed on droplet precautions until it is determined that the cause of the pneumonia is not contagious.

If either the suspicion of SARS is strong or laboratory evidence confirms a SARS-CoV infection, *the CDC recommends a combination of standard, contact, and strict airborne precautions.* Given the highly infectious nature of the virus, the CDC recommends the following additional measures to prevent transmission to and from patients, health care workers, and visitors:

- Patient placement:
  - Place the patient in an airborne infection isolation room (AIIR).
  - Designate "clean" and "dirty" areas for isolation materials.
  - Maintain a stock of clean patient care and PPE supplies outside the patient's room.
  - Locate dirty receptacles close to the point of use and separate from the clean supplies.
  - Designate the location where reusable PPE will be placed for cleaning and disinfection before reuse.

- Provide each patient with patient-dedicated equipment (e.g., thermometer, blood pressure cuff, stethoscope).
- Limit staff to the number sufficient to meet patient-care needs.
- Patient transport:
  - Limit patient movement and transport outside the AIIR to medically necessary purposes. Whenever possible, use portable equipment to perform X-rays and other procedures in the patient's room.
  - If transport or movement is necessary, ensure that the patient wears a surgical mask, puts on a clean patient gown, and performs hand hygiene before leaving the room.
  - Limit contact between SARS patients and others by using less-traveled hallways and elevators when possible.
- Visitors:
  - Limit visits to persons who are necessary for the patient's emotional well-being and care.
  - Visitors who have been in contact with the patient are a possible source of SARS. Therefore, they should be screened for SARS and instructed on the use of PPE and other precautions while in the patient's room.
- Hand hygiene:
  - Perform proper hand hygiene after contact with the patient or the patient's environment.
- Personal protective equipment (PPE):
  - Gowns and gloves
    - Wear a standard isolation gown and pair of nonsterile patient-care gloves for all patient contact.
    - Don gloves, gown, respiratory protection, and eye protection (as needed) before entering the room.
    - Gloves should cover the cuffs of the gown.
  - Respiratory protection
    - Wear a fit-tested NIOSH-certified N-95 respirator when entering the room.
    - Discard disposable respirators upon leaving the patient room or area.
  - Eye and face protection
    - Routinely wear eye protection when within 3 feet of the patient.
    - If splash or spray of respiratory secretions or other body fluids is likely, protect the eyes with goggles or a face shield.
  - Safe practices when wearing PPE
    - Avoid touching the face with contaminated gloves.
    - Avoid unnecessary touching of surfaces and objects with contaminated gloves.
  - Removing PPE in a manner that prevents contamination of clothing and skin is a priority.
- Medical waste:
  - Contain and dispose of SARS-CoV-contaminated medical waste, including used needles and other sharps, according to facility-specific procedures and/or local or state regulations.
  - Discard as routine waste used patient-care supplies that are not likely to be contaminated (e.g., paper wrappers).
  - Wear disposable gloves when handling waste. Perform hand hygiene after removal of gloves.
- Patient-care equipment:
  - Follow standard practices for handling and reprocessing used patient-care equipment, including medical devices.
  - Wear gloves when handling and transporting used patient-care equipment.
  - Wipe heavily soiled equipment with an EPA-approved hospital disinfectant before removing it from the patient's room.
  - Follow current recommendations for cleaning and disinfection or sterilization of reusable patient-care equipment.
  - Wipe external surfaces of portable equipment for performing X-rays and other procedures in the patient's room with an EPA-approved hospital disinfectant upon removal from the patient's room.

- Aerosol-generating procedures (e.g., aerosol drug delivery, sputum induction, bronchoscopy, suctioning, intubation, and noninvasive and high-frequency oscillatory ventilation):
  - Perform only those aerosol-generating procedures that medically necessary.
  - Perform aerosol-generating procedures in an AIIR; keep doors closed and minimize entry and exit during the procedure.
  - Allow only essential personnel in the room during any aerosol-generating procedure.
  - Use HEPA filtration on the expiratory limb of mechanical ventilators, especially during high-frequency oscillatory ventilation.
  - Consider appropriate sedation during intubation and bronchoscopy to minimize coughing.
  - PPE for aerosol-generating procedures:
    - PPE should cover the torso, arms, and hands as well as the eyes, nose, and mouth.
    - Consider using disposable full-body isolation suits to afford greater protection, especially around the neck.
    - Consider using a surgical hood with an N-95 respirator (to fully cover the head, neck, and face).
    - Consider using a powered air-purifying respirator (PAPR) for higher levels of protection.
    - If PAPR system is not available, consider using head gear with a full face shield.

Note that the protocols developed to combat the spread of both avian influenza and SARS are based on suspected *multiple routes of transmission*. Given this perspective, any newly discovered respiratory infections will likely also be presumed to spread via both contact and through the air. For this reason, the protocols described for avian influenza and SARS should serve as good examples for future emerging respiratory infections that pose health risks, as well as for NBRC questions about how to manage them.

COMMON ERRORS TO AVOID

You can improve your score by avoiding these mistakes:

- Don't pasteurize or immerse any electrically powered equipment in liquid disinfectants; use gas sterilization instead.
- Don't confuse sterilization (which kills *all* microorganisms, including bacterial spores) with high-level disinfection (which kills all microorganisms *except* bacterial spores).
- Don't select steam autoclaving for any heat-sensitive items needing sterilization.
- Never drain tubing condensate back into humidifier or nebulizer reservoirs.
- Don't routinely change ventilator circuits; change these components only if visibly soiled or malfunctioning.
- Don't recap, bend, break, or otherwise manipulate used needles with your hands.
- Don't intubate a patient if noninvasive ventilation will suffice; this will minimize ventilator-associated pneumonia.
- When wearing PPE, avoid touching surfaces, objects, and your face with contaminated gloves.

SURE BETS

In some situations you can always be sure of the right approach to a clinical problem or scenario:

- Always disassemble and inspect nondisposable equipment before cleaning.
- Always ensure that all equipment that has been cleaned via washing is dried properly before further processing.
- Always ensure that all nondisposable critical items (devices introduced into the blood stream or other parts of the body) are sterilized before reuse.
- Always treat any nondisposable equipment that comes in contact with a patient's airway as semicritical and in need of either high-level disinfection or pasteurization before reuse.
- Always recognize that among semicritical respiratory therapy equipment, nebulizers and aerosol generators pose the greatest infection risk.
- Always use sterile solutions to fill nebulizers and aerosol generators.

- Always used low-resistance HEPA filters to isolate bedside and laboratory pulmonary function equipment from the patient.
- Always wear a mask and maintain good hand hygiene when examining or caring for patients with signs and symptoms of a respiratory infection.
- Always perform a user-seal check each time you use an N-95 respirator for airborne precautions.

PRE-TEST ANSWERS AND EXPLANATIONS

Below are this chapter's pre-test answers and explanations. Be sure to review each answer's explanation thoroughly to help you understand why it is correct. If the explanation is still unclear to you, review the chapter contents or the references and/or refer to this chapter's supplemental resources on the CD.

7-1. **Correct Answer: B.** Cleaning. The first step in equipment processing is cleaning. Equipment is cleaned by removing dirt and organic material from its surfaces, usually by washing. If equipment is improperly cleaned, subsequent processing efforts may be ineffective.

7-2. **Correct Answer: B.** Low-level. A low-level disinfectant inactivates most bacteria, some viruses, and fungi but cannot destroy resistant microorganisms such as *Mycobacterium tuberculosis* or bacterial spores.

7-3. **Correct Answer: A.** Pasteurization. Reusable breathing circuits are semicritical items. According to CDC recommendations, reusable semicritical equipment should be sterilized or undergo high-level disinfection. Of the available options, only pasteurization meets this standard.

7-4. **Correct Answer: D.** I, II, and III. To minimize the likelihood of infection in patients receiving bronchodilator therapy via SVN, you should (1) use a different SVN for each patient, (2) change the SVN and tubing every 24 hours, and (3) perform thorough handwashing prior to each therapy session. It is also recommended that the nebulizer *not* be rinsed with tap water but rather rinsed with sterile water and blown dry between uses.

7-5. **Correct Answer: B.** I, II, and III. If either the suspicion of SARS is strong or laboratory evidence confirms a SARS-CoV infection, the CDC recommends a combination of standard, contact, and strict airborne precautions to manage these patients.

7-6. **Correct Answer: C.** Instilling 10 mL sterile saline before the suctioning attempt. To decrease the risk of patient contamination during suctioning, you should use a fresh sterile single-use catheter on each patient and use only sterile water or saline to clear the catheter. In addition, both the suction collection tubing and collection canister should be changed between patients, except in short-term care units (where only the collection tubing should be changed)

7-7. **Correct Answer: C.** I and III only. Because it directly comes in contact with mucous membranes, a reusable airway is categorized as semicritical equipment. If sterilization of a semicritical item is not feasible, the alternatives are high-level disinfection or pasteurization.

7-8. **Correct Answer: B.** To show that a package has been through a sterilizing process. Chemical indicators are usually impregnated on packaging tape. These indicators change color when exposed to specific conditions, telling the user that the package has been processed via an appropriate sterilizer cycle. Chemical indicators cannot ensure that the contents are actually sterile. Only biological indicators can provide that information.

7-9. **Correct Answer: D.** Use a disposable HEPA filter and one-way valve for each patient. The best way to prevent the contamination of a Wright respirometer used on several different patients is to use a one-way valving system, preferably with an in-line HEPA filter. Such an approach can ensure that patients only breathe out through the device, thus preventing cross-contamination.

7-10. **Correct Answer: D.** Changing ventilator circuits every 48 hours. The key components recommended by the CDC to reduce the incidence of VAP include elevating the head of the bed at least 30°, implementing a daily "sedation vacation" and spontaneous breathing trial, and providing peptic ulcer and deep venous thrombosis disease prophylaxis. Airway management techniques that can help decrease the incidence of VAP include: (1) avoiding intubation when possible (using noninvasive ventilation instead); (2) intubating via the oral (as opposed to nasal) route; (3) maintaining proper ET tube cuff pressures; (4) aspirating subglottic secretions; and (5) using only sterile water or saline to flush suction catheters. *Ventilator circuits should be changed only when visibly soiled or malfunctioning.*

POST-TEST

A post-test for this chapter that includes automated scoring and feedback is available on the accompanying CD. Be sure to complete this additional assessment to confirm your mastery of this chapter's objectives.

REFERENCES

American Association for Respiratory Care. (2003). Clinical practice guideline. Care of the ventilator circuit and its relation to ventilator-associated pneumonia. *Respiratory care, 48,* 869–879.

Centers for Disease Control and Prevention. (2002). Guideline for hand hygiene in health-care settings. Recommendations of the Healthcare Infection Control Practices Advisory Committee and the HICPAC/SHEA/APIC/IDSA Hand Hygiene Task Force. *Morbidity and mortality weekly report, 51(RR16),* 1–44.

Centers for Disease Control and Prevention. (2003). Guidelines for environmental infection control in health-care facilities: Recommendations of CDC and the Healthcare Infection Control Practices Advisory Committee. *Morbidity and mortality weekly report, 52(RR-10),* 1–48.

Centers for Disease Control and Prevention. (2004). Guidelines for preventing health-care-associated pneumonia, 2003. Recommendations of CDC and the Healthcare Infection Control Practices Advisory Committee. *Morbidity and mortality weekly report, 53(RR03),* 1–36.

Centers for Disease Control and Prevention. (2004). Interim recommendations for infection control in health-care facilities caring for patients with known or suspected avian influenza.

Centers for Disease Control and Prevention. (2004). Public health guidance for community-level preparedness and response to Severe Acute Respiratory Syndrome (SARS) Version 2, Supplement I: Infection control in healthcare, home, and community settings.

Institute for Clinical Systems Improvement. (2007). *Prevention of ventilator-associated pneumonia.* (3rd ed.). Bloomington, MN: Author.

Siegel, J. D., Rhinehart, E., Jackson, M., Chiarello, L., and the Healthcare Infection Control Practices Advisory Committee. (2007). *2007 Guideline for isolation precautions: Preventing transmission of infectious agents in healthcare settings.* Atlanta, GA: Centers for Disease Control and Prevention.

Perform Quality Control Procedures

John A. Rutkowski
Craig L. Scanlan

CHAPTER

8

INTRODUCTION

The quality of care you provide depends in part on the proper performance of the equipment you use to diagnose or treat your patients. Quality control (QC) is a process designed to ensure that the devices you use on patients regularly perform as expected. For diagnostic equipment, QC processes ensure consistently accurate measurements. For therapeutic equipment, QC processes ensure proper device function and patient safety.

Unfortunately, unless you work in the blood gas or PFT lab, or are responsible for collaborating directly with your biomedical engineering department, you likely do not regularly engage in most QC processes. The NBRC, however, expects every CRT candidate to be familiar with the basics of QC as applied to the common medical devices used in respiratory care. For this reason, you should plan on spending a reasonable portion of your exam preparation time on this topic.

OBJECTIVES

After completion of this chapter, you should demonstrate the knowledge needed to:

1. Perform quality control procedures for:
   a. Blood gas analyzers and CO-oximeters
   b. Point-of-care analyzers
   c. Pulmonary function equipment
   d. Mechanical ventilators
   e. Oxygen and specialty gas analyzers
   f. Noninvasive monitors
   g. Gas metering devices
2. Record and monitor QC data using accepted statistical methods

WHAT TO EXPECT ON THIS CATEGORY OF THE CRT EXAM

Number of questions: 4
Level of questions: about 25% recall, 75% application

WHAT'S NEW FOR 2009

As of July 2009, this section of the NBRC CRT examination includes the following *new topics*:

- Quality control of:
  - Gas analyzers
  - Point-of-care analyzers
  - Pulmonary function equipment
  - Noninvasive monitors
- Recording and monitoring QC data using accepted statistical methods

PRE-TEST

Carefully respond to each of the following questions. After completing the pre-test, compare your answers with those provided at the end of this chapter. Then thoroughly review each answer's explanation to help understand why it is correct.

8-1. To avoid the preanalytical errors that are associated with air contamination of a blood gas sample, all of the following are appropriate *except*:
- **A.** Removing of all air bubbles
- **B.** Mixing only after air has been completely removed
- **C.** Capping syringe quickly
- **D.** Using the minimum amount of heparin

8-2. The best way to avoid arterial blood gas analysis errors associated with blood metabolism is to:
- **A.** Analyze the sample immediately
- **B.** Place the sample in an ice slush
- **C.** Keep the sample at body temperature
- **D.** Use dry (lithium) heparin

8-3. How often should a $Ptco_2$ electrode be relocated in a neonate?
- **A.** Every 2 hours
- **B.** Every 8 hours
- **C.** Once a day
- **D.** There is no need to change the site

8-4. Under ideal conditions, electrochemical oxygen analyzers have an accuracy of:
- **A.** ± 1%
- **B.** ± 2%
- **C.** ± 5%
- **D.** ± 10%

8-5. Which of the following hemoximeter measurements are affected by air contamination?
- **A.** HbCO levels
- **B.** metHb levels
- **C.** HbO_2 levels
- **D.** Total Hb levels

8-6. Which of the following devices would you select to assess the output accuracy of a Bourdon gauge regulator used for O_2 transport?
- **A.** Mercury manometer
- **B.** Clark electrode
- **C.** Paramagnetic oxygen analyzer
- **D.** Precision flowmeter

8-7. To periodically confirm the validity of blood gas analyzer results, you would perform:
- **A.** External statistical quality control
- **B.** Instrument performance validation
- **C.** Regular preventive maintenance
- **D.** Control media calibration verification

8-8. According to ATS recommendations, diagnostic spirometers should be calibrated to within:
- **A.** ± 1.5 cm H_2O/L/sec resistance
- **B.** ± 3% or 50 mL, whichever is greater, using a 3-liter syringe
- **C.** ± 5% or 100 mL, whichever is greater, using a 3-liter syringe
- **D.** ± 10% or 500 mL, whichever is greater, using a 5-liter syringe

8-9. How often should ventilators be tested to verify their performance?
- **A.** Daily
- **B.** Between patient uses
- **C.** Once a week
- **D.** Once a year

8-10. A fuel cell oxygen analyzer is reading 18% when exposed to ambient air. The initial corrective action should be to:

A. Calibrate the sensor
B. Check the batteries
C. Replace the fuel cell
D. Replace the display

WHAT YOU NEED TO KNOW: ESSENTIAL CONTENT

Key Terms and Definitions

Basic to your understanding of quality control are some key terms and definitions, summarized in **Table 8-1**.

Laboratory Blood Gas and Hemoximetry Analyzers

Most of the quality control specifications for the collection, analysis, and reporting of laboratory tests are based on governmental guidelines promulgated by the Centers for Medicare and Medicaid (CMMS) and implemented through the Clinical Laboratory Improvement Act (CLIA) program. The goal of CLIA regulations is to ensure quality laboratory testing performed on humans.

As with most laboratory tests, quality control processes for blood gas and hemoximetry analyses focus on eliminating errors in sample collection (the pre-analytical phase), sample measurement (the analytical phase), and reporting (the post-analytical phase). Here we focus primarily on the pre-analytical and analytical phases of blood gas and hemoximetry QC.

Pre-Analytical Phase

The pre-analytical phase involves all blood collection and handling procedures conducted prior to actual sample analysis. Depending on the indication for the test and the availability of collection sites, you obtain blood samples from various locations. Sampling from the various sites may require different equipment and procedures. For this reason, you must be proficient with the techniques involved (see Chapter 13 for details). Also important is your strict compliance with applicable infection control procedures whenever sampling blood (discussed in Chapter 7). Last, to avoid interpretation errors during the analytical phase, for each sample you obtain you must document the patient's F_{IO_2}, oxygen delivery device, mode of ventilation, and the results of any related assessments made at the time of sampling.

The most common pre-analytical errors that affect blood gas and hemoximetry measurements are air contamination, venous admixture, excess anticoagulant, and continued blood metabolism. As indicated in **Table 8-2** (see page 243), these errors can have a significant effect on the validity of these measurements. Obviously, such errors can result in incorrect therapeutic decisions and potentially bring harm to patients. For this reason, you must always strive to ensure that the blood sample being analyzed is free of these common errors.

Analytical Phase

The analytical phase of blood gas and hemoximetry measurement involves four key elements: (1) analyzer calibration and calibration verification, (2) actual sample testing, (3) interpretation of the results, and (4) ongoing review of quality control and proficiency testing results.

Analyzer Calibration

Calibration is the process whereby the response of an instrument is compared and adjusted to a known standard. The standards used to calibrate blood gas analyzers are precision gases and buffer solutions with known values for pH, P_{CO_2}, and P_{O_2}. Similarly, hemoximeter calibration involves measurement of standard solutions with known values for total Hb, HbO_2, carboxyhemoglobin (COHb), and methemoglobin (MetHb).

As depicted in **Figure 8-1**, calibration involves adjusting the analyzer to ensure that its response is accurate and linear—i.e., that the measured value (response) equals the known value. In this example, the precalibrated response of the analyzer is linear, but positively biased. For example, at a known value of 0 the analyzer response is 20, and at a known value of 40 the response is about 85—both

Table 8-1 Key Terms Used in Quality Control

Term	Meaning
Calibration	A known relationship between the response generated by the measurement and the value of the substance being measured.
Two-point calibration	Two gas mixtures containing known concentrations of O_2 and CO_2, and/or two solutions with precisely known pH values, are used to generate low and high expected values for calibration of the analyzer.
One-point calibration	One gas mixture containing known concentrations of O_2 and CO_2, and/or a solution with a precisely known pH value, are used to generate an expected value to adjust for sensor drift of the analyzer.
Drift	The difference between successive calibrations.
Calibration verification	Analyzing of control media (in the same manner as patient samples) to confirm that the calibration of the instrument has remained stable throughout the lab's reportable range.
Statistical quality control	The application of statistical analysis and other procedures as a tool to detect problems that could invalidate patient results.
Mean	Determined by adding a group of measurements and then dividing by the number of measurements.
Standard deviation	A statistical measure of the degree to which an individual value in a probability distribution tends to vary from the mean of the distribution. It is used to determine the variability of a series of measurements.
Coefficient of variation (CV)	Standard deviation as a percent of the mean. The CV is useful in gauging precision.
Control charts	A record of the measurements of standard samples from each electrode. Used for statistical evaluation of electrode performance. May be referred to as a Levy-Jennings chart.
Point-of-care testing	Analysis of samples at the location at which a procedure is being performed or the patient is located.
Analytical errors	Results errors due to mistakes made during the analysis.
Pre-analytical errors	Results errors due to mistakes in collection, or handling and storage, of samples prior to analysis.
Post-analytical errors	Results errors due to mistakes made in data handling and results reporting.
Precision	An instrument's ability to measure a known value repeatedly. Sometimes referred to as reproducibility of results.
Accuracy	An instrument's ability to produce measurements that are close to true value.
Proficiency testing	The application of external methods for quality control. Required by the Clinical Laboratory Improvement Act (CLIA) of 1967 and updated in 1988. Test samples with unknown values are received from an agency, analyzed, and returned to the agency for evaluation. Allows for interlaboratory comparisons.
Interinstrumental comparison	Laboratories operating more than one analyzer must demonstrate little variation in results from two or more analyzers.
Tonometer	A device in which a liquid (blood/control media) comes into contact with and equilibrates with a gas that has known P_{CO_2} and P_{O_2} values.
Reportable range	Results values over which the laboratory can verify the accuracy of the instrument.

Table 8-2 Common Pre-Analytical Errors in pH/Blood Gas Analysis and Hemoximetry

Error	Effect	Recognition	Avoidance
Air contamination	Decreases P_{CO_2} Increases pH Increases P_{O_2}	• Visible bubbles • Results not consistent with patient's condition	• Expel bubbles • Do not mix samples with air bubbles • Cap syringe, seal capillary tubes quickly
Venous admixture	Increases P_{CO_2} Raises pH Decreases P_{O_2}	• No pulsations as syringe fills • Results not consistent with patient's condition	• Do not aspirate sample • Avoid brachial/femoral sites • Use short-bevel needles
Excess anticoagulant	Decreases P_{CO_2} Decreases pH Increases P_{O_2}	• Liquid heparin remains in syringe prior to sampling	• Eject liquid heparin until only "deadspace" is filled • Use "dry" heparin • Collect > 2 mL from adults and > 0.6 mL from infants
Continued metabolism	Increases P_{CO_2} Decreases pH Decreases P_{O_2}	• Time lag between collection and analysis of sample • Results not consistent with patient's condition	• Analyze quickly • 15 minutes for syringes • 3 minutes for capillary tubes

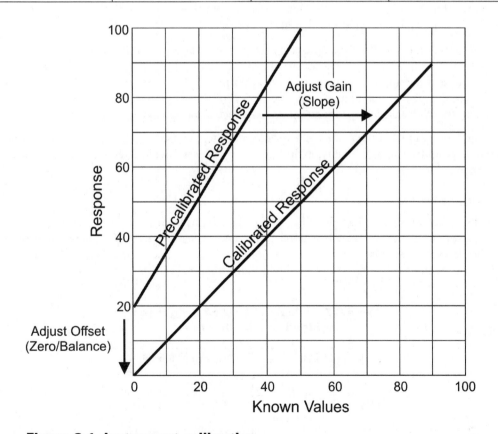

Figure 8-1 Instrument calibration.

clearly inaccurate measurements. Calibration requires adjusting both the offset ("balancing" or "zeroing" the analyzer) and the gain or slope of the instrument. Only after these two adjustments are made can we say that the analyzer is properly calibrated.

The calibration method depicted in Figure 8-1 requires a "two-point calibration," in which two different known values are used. **Table 8-3** provides the typical ranges used for two-point calibration of blood gas analyzers. Only by performing a two-point calibration can you properly adjust both the offset and gain (slope) of the instrument.

Single or one-point calibration can also be performed. However, when you measure only one known value, you can adjust only the gain of the instrument. In this case, measurement errors will still occur if the instrument is not properly zeroed.

Modern microprocessor-based blood analyzers include automated calibration routines that take place in the background at regularly scheduled intervals. However, to ensure that the analyzers you use are providing valid measurements, you must perform *calibration verification*. Calibration verification involves analysis of pre-prepared *control media*. Control media are analytes that are independently certified to provide a known measurement value when tested. Typically, calibration verification involves analysis of at least *three* different levels of control media spanning the full range of expected results and is conducted at least once every 24 hours. In addition, calibration verification should be conducted after any instrument maintenance and whenever there is a question regarding instrument performance.

For blood gas analyzer calibration verification, commercial control media generally suffice. However, both the AARC and Clinical and Laboratory Standards Institute recommend tonometry as the best reference standard for assessing PO_2 and PCO_2 measurements, especially when issues of accuracy arise.

Sample Testing

Testing should always be performed by individuals who meet the specific competency requirements for the applicable procedures, as documented at least annually. Sample testing must follow an established protocol that conforms to the recommendations of the instrument manufacturer. If you are responsible for performing the analysis, you always must:

- Confirm that the specimen was properly labeled and stored prior to analysis.
- Assess the sample for any obvious pre-analytical errors—e.g., air bubbles or clots.
- Confirm that the applicable analyzer calibration procedures were completed prior to analysis.
- Analyze the sample within an acceptable period of time.
- Ensure that the sample is properly aspirated/injected into analyzer.

Whenever you report the results of any laboratory test you conduct, you also should provide a brief statement addressing test quality, including any problems encountered with the specimen or its measurement.

Interpretation of Results

Test results always should be interpreted by the ordering physician and must consider the rationale for the measurement and the related patient information. Ideally, specific physician alert or "panic" values should be pre-established for manual or computerized notification and follow-up. Last, proper interpretation requires active review of quality control and proficiency testing results.

Table 8-3 Typical Calibration Ranges for Blood Gas Analyzers

Analyte	Calibration Range
pH	6.840–7.384
PO_2	80–150 mm Hg
PCO_2	40–80 mm Hg

Review of Quality Control and Proficiency Testing Results

To conduct comprehensive quality control, you need to record and continuously monitor data using accepted statistical methods. To do so, you plot the results of control media analyses on graphs, with a separate chart for each level of control and each analyte reported. The most common plotting format used for statistical QC is the Levy-Jennings chart. As depicted in **Figure 8-2**, a Levy-Jennings chart plots individual values for control media analyses over multiple measurement and compares these individual values with the mean and standard deviation (SD) of the data. Typically, bounding limits are set to within 2 or 3 SDs. Control measurements that consistently fall within these limits indicate that the analyzer is "in control" and ready for patient measurement. For example, Figure 8-2 depicts *normal variation* in the measurement of a P_{CO_2} control value standardized to 40 torr (mm Hg). The variation is considered normal because it consistently falls within 2+ SD of the mean for this measure.

Control measurements that fall outside the statistical bounding limits indicate *analytical error*. **Figure 8-3** depicts this situation, with the sixth observation falling above the +2 SD bounding limit. Single aberrant values like these are relatively common (occurring on average once in every 20 analyses) and are due to *random errors* of measurement that occur with any laboratory instrument. As long as subsequent measures are in control, no remedial action is needed. In contrast, frequent random errors like this one would indicate a lack of precision—i.e., poor repeatability of measurement. Any instrument that demonstrates poor repeatability over time is deemed "out of control." In such cases, you would have to identify the problem, take appropriate corrective action, and confirm that the analyzer is back in control prior to reporting the results for any patient sample.

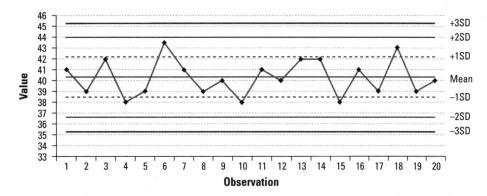

Figure 8-2 Levy-Jennings Chart for P_{CO_2} Control Value of 40 Torr Showing Analyzer in Control.

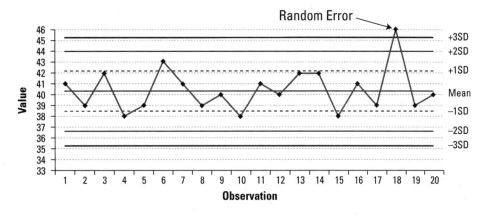

Figure 8-3 Levy-Jennings Chart for P_{CO_2} Control Value of 40 Torr Showing a Single Random Error. As long as subsequent measures are in control, no remedial action is needed.

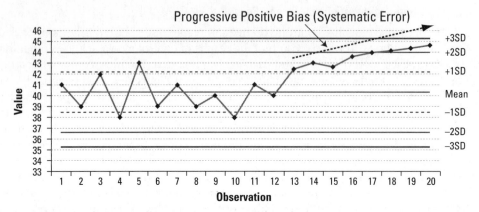

Figure 8-4 Levy-Jennings Chart for Pco₂ Control Value of 40 Torr Showing Developing Positive Bias Error. Bias errors usually indicate faulty procedure or failure of an instrument component. In this example, no patient samples should be analyzed until the problem is found and corrected.

Figure 8-4 demonstrates a different type of error, called *systematic error* or *bias*. Note that beginning with observation 13 and continuing through observation 20 there is an upward trend in the reported values for the 40-torr Pco₂ control. Over time, this particular trend is shifting the mean above the control value, causing a positive bias in measurement. Although generally less common than random errors, bias errors like these are usually more serious, indicating either incorrect procedure or instrument component failure. As with random errors, any time systematic errors take an instrument out of control, no patient samples should be analyzed until the problem is corrected. **Table 8-4** compares and contrasts these two types of analytical errors in terms of common contributing factors and appropriate corrective actions.

Supplementing "in-house" quality control procedures is a process called *proficiency testing*, required for most analytic laboratories by specific CLIA provisions. Under proficiency testing requirements, laboratories receive unknown samples from an outside agency on a regular schedule.

Table 8-4 Comparison of Instrument Analytical Errors and Their Correction

Type of Error	Contributing Factor(s)	Corrective Actions
Random errors	• Statistical probability • Contamination of sample • Improper handling of sample	• Reanalyze control sample after performing a two-point calibration • If repeat quality control analysis is "in control," no further action is needed • If repeat quality control analysis is "out of control," continue corrective actions according to manufacturer recommendations.
Bias errors	• Contaminated buffer solutions • Incorrect gas concentrations • Component degradation/failure • Incorrect procedure	• Troubleshoot suspected problem(s) • Repair or replace problematic components • Corrective action(s) continue until an acceptable two-point calibration is achieved and quality control sample values are within 2 SD of the mean value

The samples are analyzed and the results reported back to the agency. The agency compares the results against its own and those of other laboratories using similar instrumentation. Discrepancies must be addressed and remediated in order for any laboratory to maintain CLIA certification, which is a prerequisite for Medicare/Medicaid reimbursement.

Point-of-Care Analyzers

As described in Chapter 6, point-of-care testing (POCT) involves the collection, measurement, and reporting of selected laboratory tests at or near the site of patient care, rather than via a central laboratory. Instruments used for POCT vary substantially. The most common POCT tests that you are likely to perform are for arterial blood gases (ABGs) or combined panels that include ABG measures plus other selected values of importance in managing critically ill patients.

As with measurements made in a central lab, POCT quality assurance requires that all individuals performing these tests demonstrate current competency with the applicable equipment and procedures. In addition, as a component of quality control, *all POCT results must be auditable*. This means that the test results must be traceable to the patient tested, the instrument operator, the date and time of the test, and the instrument and process used. In addition, as with centralized lab testing, QC logs and records of instrument maintenance must be maintained.

In terms of instrument calibration, most of the POCT analyzers use self-contained cartridges for each analysis performed. Typically, these cartridges include aqueous buffer solutions that provide automated calibration just prior to sample analysis. Other POCT analyzers employ a computer chip to calibrate each new set of test cartridges or strips. When these devices fail to properly calibrate, sample analysis usually stops. For cartridge-based instruments, the first step in such cases is usually to rerun the test with a new cartridge. If a second attempt fails, you should remove the device from service and either obtain a replacement or send the sample to the central lab for analysis.

As a component of their quality assurance program, most facilities also require that the performance of POCT analyzers regularly be compared with a calibrated bench-top analyzer. This is done by performing dual analysis of the same sample at the same time on both instruments. Based on accumulated data and statistical rules for these between-instrument comparisons, one can then determine if the POCT results meet the same standards for accuracy and precision as required for regular lab testing. In addition, most facilities use external proficiency to help further ensure the quality of their POCT test programs.

Pulmonary Function Equipment

Pulmonary function testing (PFT) is a critical component in the assessment of lung disease. As with laboratory assessment of blood specimens, erroneous PFT results can lead to inappropriate clinical decisions. For these reasons, an effective quality assurance program is required to make certain that PFT data is both accurate and reproducible.

Key organizations contributing to this effort include the American Thoracic Society (ATS), the American Association for Respiratory Care (AARC), and the National Institute for Occupational Safety and Health (NIOSH). What follows here is based heavily on the guidelines and standards promulgated by these organizations. In general, all these organizations agree that an effective PFT quality assurance program must include at least the following elements:

- Proper technician training and review
- Accurate spirometry equipment
- Daily spirometer checks
- Individual maneuver validity checks
- Monthly spirometry quality reports
- Documentation of equipment maintenance

Proper training of those involved in testing, with annual reviews of competency, are always key components of any quality process, as is ongoing documentation of both QC testing and equipment maintenance. Here we focus on ensuring the accuracy of the equipment and obtaining valid test results.

Accuracy of PFT Equipment

To ensure the accuracy of PFT equipment, you need to confirm absolute volume and flow values, check volume and flow linearity, assess system leakage, and validate time measurements. **Table 8-5** summarizes the quality control tests used to confirm these measurements, as recommended by the ATS and the European Respiratory Society.

Because volumetric spirometers (bell or bellows systems) are prone to leaks, you should check for leaks every day before the volume calibration check. You should also perform a leak test after cleaning and reassembly of the spirometer components. To leak test a volumetric spirometer, follow these steps:

1. Inject about 3 L of room air into the spirometer
2. Occlude the breathing circuit at the patient interface
3. Use the manufacturer's recommended method to pressurize the system to 3 cm H_2O
4. Observe for any change in volume over one minute

Depending on the device and the manufacturer's recommendations, a metal weight, spring, or rubber band can be used to pressurize the system. When pressurized, the system should lose no more than 10 mL during the one-minute observation interval. Any larger volume loss indicates a leak, which must be corrected before any patient testing. Common sources for spirometer leaks include loose connections, cracked circuit tubing, and missing or damaged seals.

Volume calibration requires a large-volume (3.0 L) calibration syringe. The ATS volume accuracy standard for diagnostic spirometers is ± 3% or ± 50 mL, whichever is larger. On computerized PFT systems, you may need to enter the ambient temperature and altitude or barometric pressure prior to calibration. You also may need to make sure that the BTPS (body temperature pressure, saturated) correction is turned off, otherwise the calibrating volume measurement will be about 10% higher than actual. If the device uses a differential pressure transducer to measure flow, you also will have to zero this sensor before volume or flow calibration. **Figure 8-5** depicts a normal volume calibration graph, showing a percent error computation that falls within the ATS accuracy standard for a 3.0-L calibrating syringe (between 2.91 and 3.09 L).

If you obtain a low volume (< 2.91 L), first repeat the leak check. If you obtain a high volume (> 3.09 L), recheck the volume/flow zeroing, make sure that BTPS correction is off, and confirm that the temperatures of the syringe and spirometer are the same. Do not proceed with patient testing unless you (1) can identify the cause of the inaccurate reading and (2) obtain an accurate volume calibration upon repeat measurement.

Table 8-5 PFT Equipment Quality Control

Test	Minimum Interval	Action
Leaks	Daily	3 cm H_2O constant pressure for 1 minute (< 10 mL)
Volume	Daily	Calibration check with a 3-L syringe check
Volume linearity	Quarterly	1-L increments with a calibrating syringe over entire volume range
Flow linearity	Weekly	Test at least three different flow ranges
Time	Quarterly	Mechanical recorder check with stopwatch
Software	New versions	Log installation date and perform test using "known" subject

From: Miller, M. R., Hankinson, J., Brusasco, V., et al. (2005). Standardisation of spirometry. *European Respiratory Journal, 26,* 319–338. Reproduced with permission from the European Respiratory Society. This book has not been reviewed by the European Respiratory Society prior to its release; therefore, the European Respiratory Society may not be responsible for any errors, omissions, or inaccuracies, or for any consequences arising there from, in the content.

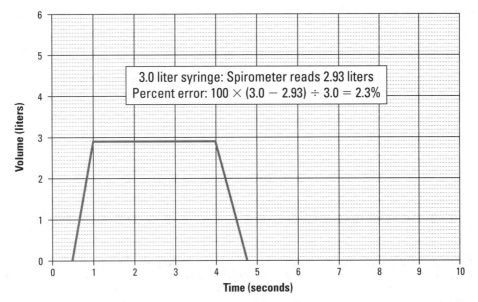

Figure 8-5 Plot of Volume Calibration of a Spirometer Showing the Percent Error Computation Falling Within the ± 3% Range of Accuracy Specified by the American Thoracic Society.

Source: National Institute for Occupational Safety and Health. (2003). NIOSH spirometry training guide—unit three. The quality assurance program. Publication No. 2004-154c. Atlanta, GA: Centers for Disease Control and Prevention.

The gold standard for spirometer flow calibration is based on a computer-controlled air pump that generates 24 standard expiratory waveforms to evaluate device response. Using this device, the ATS recommends a flow accuracy standard of ±5% of the reading or ±0.2 L/sec, whichever is greater. Since this calibration equipment is expensive and not readily available, an acceptable alternative for assessing flow linearity is to expel the full volume from the 3.0-L calibrated syringe over three different time intervals (different injection speeds) into the spirometer. The common time intervals are 0.5 seconds (equivalent to 6 L/sec, the highest flow), 6 seconds (equivalent to 0.5 L/sec, the lowest flow), and somewhere in between. Volume linearity is demonstrated if the recorded volume deviates by no more than 100 mL from the 3.0-L target volume. In addition, any deviations from the target volume should be unrelated to the expiratory flow (a rough index of flow linearity). Computerized spirometers that provide for flow calibration typically include prompted routines to guide you through this process and maintain the appropriate time interval or flow.

You should record the results of the leak test and volume and flow calibration daily on a QC log. If repeated checks indicate that the spirometer is no longer accurate, and you cannot identify any mechanical cause for the inaccuracy, you will need to recalibrate the device.

Obtaining Valid Test Results

Because forced expiratory maneuvers are technique dependent, obtaining accurate data depends on (1) proper instruction and coaching of the patient, and (2) recognition and correction of errors due to poor or incorrect patient performance. Your goal is to obtain at least three error-free maneuvers that meet basic acceptability standards. An FVC maneuver meets acceptability standards if it is free of the following common validity errors:

- A slow or a false start to the maneuver (back extrapolated volume ≥ 5% of FVC or 150 mL)
- Coughing during the maneuver
- Breathing during the maneuver
- Variable effort (e.g., prematurely ending exhalation)
- Exhalation time less than 6 seconds

Although many computerized spirometers automatically check the acceptability of each maneuver according to these criteria, the NBRC expects that you can recognize these problems by manually inspecting the FVC graph. **Table 8-6** depicts the most common validity errors that you will encounter when measuring a patient's forced vital capacity.

After obtaining the acceptable maneuvers, you need to ensure the reproducibility of the patient's efforts. *You ensure reproducibility by confirming that the two largest values for both the FVC and FEV₁ are within 0.150 L (150 mL) of each other.* If both of these criteria are not met, you must continue testing until either both criteria are met or the patient cannot continue.

Table 8-6 Common Validity Errors Occurring During Measurement of Forced Vital Capacity

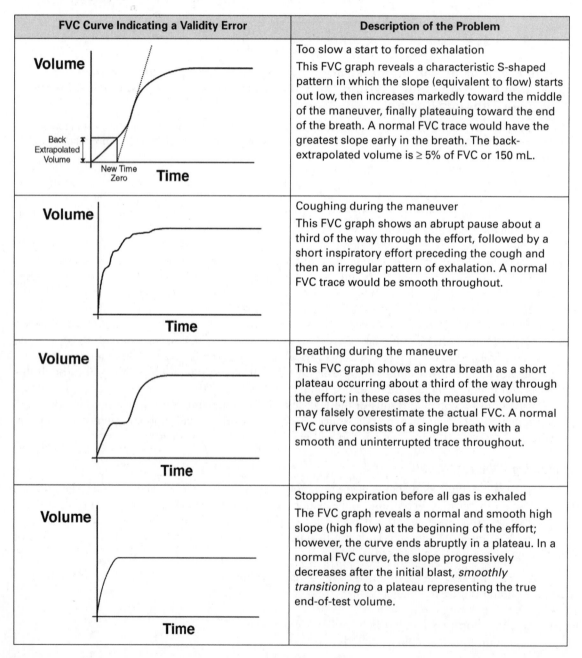

FVC Curve Indicating a Validity Error	Description of the Problem
Volume / Back Extrapolated Volume / New Time Zero / Time	**Too slow a start to forced exhalation** This FVC graph reveals a characteristic S-shaped pattern in which the slope (equivalent to flow) starts out low, then increases markedly toward the middle of the maneuver, finally plateauing toward the end of the breath. A normal FVC trace would have the greatest slope early in the breath. The back-extrapolated volume is $\geq$ 5% of FVC or 150 mL.
Volume / Time	**Coughing during the maneuver** This FVC graph shows an abrupt pause about a third of the way through the effort, followed by a short inspiratory effort preceding the cough and then an irregular pattern of exhalation. A normal FVC trace would be smooth throughout.
Volume / Time	**Breathing during the maneuver** This FVC graph shows an extra breath as a short plateau occurring about a third of the way through the effort; in these cases the measured volume may falsely overestimate the actual FVC. A normal FVC curve consists of a single breath with a smooth and uninterrupted trace throughout.
Volume / Time	**Stopping expiration before all gas is exhaled** The FVC graph reveals a normal and smooth high slope (high flow) at the beginning of the effort; however, the curve ends abruptly in a plateau. In a normal FVC curve, the slope progressively decreases after the initial blast, *smoothly transitioning* to a plateau representing the true end-of-test volume.

Mechanical Ventilators

Quality control of mechanical ventilators involves a procedure called *operational verification*. Operational verification of ventilators that lack microprocessor self-test programming is a manual procedure based on manufacturer's recommendations and incorporated into the standard operating procedures of your respiratory care department. Microprocessor-based ventilators are generally capable of semi-automated operational verification procedures.

Manual Ventilator Operational Verification

Table 8-7 outlines the basic manual operational verification procedure for ventilators that lack microprocessor self-test programming, adapted from recommendations disseminated by the Emergency Care Research Institute.

Operational Verification of Microprocessor Ventilator

Most microprocessor-controlled ventilators perform two types of operational verifications: a power-on self-test (POST) and an extended self-test (EST). Both of these QC procedures should be performed according to the manufacturer's recommendations.

A POST generally tests microprocessor function, zeros the sensors, and performs some basic checks related to patient functions, such as leak tests. You should always confirm a successful POST before applying a ventilator to a patient and whenever you change the circuit.

Typically, an EST first performs a POST, followed by a series of more comprehensive function checks. You should perform an EST between each application of a ventilator on different patients. Extended self-testing of ventilators also should be fully documented in writing, with all records maintained as a vital part of the QC program. Any ventilator that fails any portion of a self-test should be taken out of service for repair and replaced with a unit that has successfully completed operational verification.

Gas Analyzers

Oxygen Analyzers

The most commonly used oxygen analyzers today are the electrochemical analyzers (Clark electrode or polarographic analyzer) and galvanic fuel cells. Both of these analyzers measure the partial pressure of oxygen. They are accurate at any altitude as long as they are calibrated at the altitude at which the measurement is made. Polarographic analyzers require an external power source to maintain the chemical reaction in the electrode. Galvanic cells do not require an external power source for analysis. Both require external power to operate any alarms.

Most O_2 analyzers are calibrated in four steps:

1. Expose the sensor to a contained source of 100% O_2 (e.g., in a plastic bag or glove)
2. After the reading stabilizes, adjust the analyzer to 100%
3. Remove the sensor from the 100% O_2 source
4. After restabilization, confirm a reading of 21% (± 2%)

Calibration should occur under the same conditions under which measurement will occur (i.e., the same temperature, atmospheric pressure, and humidity). **Table 8-8** (see page 253) summarizes the common causes of O_2 analyzer calibration problems and measurement errors and how to correct them.

Other Gas Analyzers

In addition to O_2 analysis, you may be asked to use selected specialty gas analyzers to measure N_2, He, CO, and NO/NO_2 concentrations in the PFT lab or at the bedside. Chapter 6 provides details on the analysis method used to measure these gases, as well as the applicable performance standards and calibration methods.

Table 8-7 Manual Operational Verification of Non-Microprocessor-Based Ventilators

Component or Function	Operational Verification Procedure
Battery test/ power loss alarm	With the unit turned on, disconnect and then reconnect the power source while the ventilator is not in use on a patient. The machine's battery backup and its disconnection alarms should function appropriately.
F_{IO_2}/O_2 analyzer	See the *Gas Analyzers* section in this chapter.
Audible and visual alarms	*Gas supply:* disconnect the high pressure O_2 supply hose and, separately, the air supply hose (if used). Appropriate alarm(s) should result. Reconnect the hoses.
	Low pressure, low exhaled volume, disconnect alarms: connect the ventilator to a test lung and set a stable minute volume; momentarily disconnect the circuit to check for the appropriate activation of all alarms.
	Apnea alarm: connect the ventilator to a test lung with the SMIV rate = 2/min to a test lung and trigger the ventilator 8–12 times, then cease triggering to confirm appropriate activation of the alarm.
	High-pressure alarm: momentarily occlude the circuit to check for the appropriate activation of all audible and visual alarms.
	Inverse I:E ratio alarm: momentarily adjust the peak flow to create an inverse-ratio condition and confirm appropriate activation of the alarm.
Proximal airway pressure display	Connect the ventilator to a test lung and momentarily disconnect the pressure line or inspiratory limb of the circuit; the pressure display should read zero (± 1 cm H_2O). Set the PEEP level to 10 cm H_2O and trigger several breaths; the pressure display should rise and then return to the appropriate baseline (± 1 cm H_2O) at the end of each breath.
PEEP control	Connect the ventilator to a test lung, set a PEEP level of 5 cm H_2O, and trigger several breaths; the pressure display should rise and then return to 5 cm H_2O (± 1 cm H_2O) at the end of each breath. Repeat at PEEP = 10 and PEEP = 15 cm H_2O.
Leak tests	Perform either or both of these tests as the machine allows: *Occlusion method:* occlude the patient connection, set the pressure limit and tidal volume to their maximum levels and the peak flow and rate to their minimum levels, and initiate a breath. The pressure limit should reached the maximum set level, and the high pressure alarm should activate. *Plateau pressure method:* set the inspiratory pause to ≥ 2 seconds. When the ventilator triggers, observe the plateau pressure for stability; a drop of 10% or more during the pause indicates a leak.
Modes	Use a test lung to verify proper operation of all ventilator modes.
Ventilator rate (and rate display)	Count the number of breaths delivered during a convenient interval, timed using a clock or watch with a second hand. The measured rate should be within 1 breath per minute of the rate setting and rate display.
Delivered volume	Set the ventilator to a specific volume, connect a Wright respirometer to the ventilator outlet, and trigger the ventilator; all measurements should be within 5% of the setting.
Volume display	Connect a test lung to the circuit, cycle the machine, and compare the measured exhaled tidal volume and minute volume to their respective settings.
Sensitivity	Put the ventilator into an assist mode. Squeeze and release the test lung; an inspiration should result when the airway pressure or flow drops to the intended sensitivity level.
Filters	Ensure that a high-efficiency particulate-air (HEPA) filter is present on the main inspiratory line.

Adapted from: Emergency Care Research Institute. (1998). Minimum requirements for ventilator testing. *Health Devices,* 27(9–10): 363–364.

Table 8-8 Troubleshooting Electrochemical and Fuel Cell O₂ Analyzers

Problem	Possible Cause	Suggested Solutions
Cannot calibrate to 21% O_2	• Probe not exposed to room air • Bad probe (electrode or cell) • Water condensation on probe membrane	• Ensure probe is exposed to room air • Recharge/replace probe • Dry probe membrane
Cannot calibrate to 100% O_2	• Low battery • Probe not exposed to 100% O_2 • Bad probe (electrode or cell) • Water condensation on probe membrane	• Replace battery • Ensure probe is exposed to 100% O_2 • Recharge/replace probe • Dry probe membrane
Measured %O_2 differs from expected value	• Low battery • Analyzer not calibrated • O_2 delivery device malfunction • Bad probe (electrode or cell)	• Replace battery • Calibrate analyzer • Ensure proper function of delivery device • Recharge or replace probe
Analyzer reads 0% O_2	• Low battery • Probe not plugged into analyzer • Dead battery • Dead probe	• Replace battery • Plug probe into analyzer • Replace battery • Recharge or replace probe

Adapted from: Branson, R. D., Hess, D., & Chatburn, R. L. (1998). *Respiratory Care Equipment* (2nd ed.). Philadelphia: Lippincott.

Noninvasive Monitors

Pulse Oximeters

Pulse oximeter readings are based on measurement of *relative* light intensities, as opposed to absolute values. For this reason, they do not require "true value" calibration, as previously described for blood gas analyzers. Instead, in most clinical settings the following simple operational verification procedure is sufficient:

1. Connect the device to a normal person
2. Compare the pulse reading with the actual pulse measured manually
3. Check and confirm an SpO_2 reading of 97–100%
4. Confirm loss of signal detection by removing the device

An incorrect pulse rate, SpO_2 below 97%, or failure to detect loss of signal indicates a malfunctioning oximeter that should be taken out of service. **Table 8-9** identifies other common problems with oximeters and their solutions.

Transcutaneous PCO₂/PO₂ Monitors

The selection, use, and troubleshooting of transcutaneous PCO_2/PO_2 monitors is covered in Chapter 6. As with blood gas analyzers and capnographs, obtaining accurate data from these monitors requires proper setup and calibration (also described in Chapter 6). Careful preparation of the skin and proper placement of the electrode(s) are prerequisites to obtaining good data. The site selected should have good capillary blood flow and allow for an airtight seal.

Transcutaneous PCO_2/PO_2 technology has continuously improved over the past several decades, making these systems easier and more reliable to use. In particular, modern transcutaneous sensors are smaller, require less frequent changing/calibration (twice a day) and membrane replacement (at least every 2 weeks), operate at lower temperatures (42°C), and can achieve capillary arterialization in as little as 3 minutes.

Table 8-9 Common Operational Problems with Oximeters and their Solutions

Problem	Solution
The oximeter continues to "search" but cannot find a pulse or there is a pulse displayed but no SpO_2	• Readjust the sensor or apply it to a new site that has better perfusion. • Check and confirm that the detector "windows" are free of dirt or debris. Make sure the sensor is plugged in to the monitor. • Check the sensor for damage and replace if needed.
The heart rate and SpO_2 readings fluctuate rapidly	• Usually due to motion artifact (resolved when patient stops moving). • Use an oximeter with Masimo signal extraction technology (SET).
The oximeter reading seems to be inaccurate	• Check whether the oximeter pulse rate is the same as that determined by a cardiac monitor; if they are different, the sensor may need to be adjusted or replaced. • Check and confirm that the sensor is shielded from bright light.
The SpO_2 differs from that provided in a blood gas report	• Remember that SaO_2 value generated by a blood gas analyzer is a computed value, not a measured value • Better to compare the SpO_2 to hemoximeter measurement of SaO_2. • Use the difference between the SaO_2 and SpO_2 to "calibrate" the oximeter.

Capnometers/Capnographs

A capnometer measures exhaled CO_2 concentrations. A capnograph is a capnometer that graphically displays the expired CO_2 concentrations breath by breath. Details on the use of these devices are covered in Chapter 13. Here we focus on the procedures used to ensure the quality of monitoring information provided by capnographs.

To obtain accurate CO_2 concentrations and partial pressures with a capnograph, you must properly set up the device, calibrate it, and maintain it while in use. Setup should follow the manufacturer's recommendations. Differences in setup, calibration, and maintenance vary depending on whether the capnograph uses mainstream or sidestream technology.

Capnographs that incorporate mainstream sensors are used primarily for intubated patients, with the sensor placed at the artificial airway connection. Placement distal to the airway can result in inaccurate measurements due to rebreathing. To avoid condensation affecting the reading, most mainstream sensors are heated. For this reason, you must allow adequate warm-up time before operation, as recommended by the manufacturer. Accurate readings also require the proper-size sensor for the patient. Mainstream sensors can be applied to nonintubated patients using a mask or mouthpiece; however, accurate readings in such patients require supplemental O_2 flows of 6 L/min or higher to prevent rebreathing due to the added mechanical deadspace.

Capnographs using sidestream technology can be applied to intubated patients but are most useful for ventilatory monitoring of nonintubated patients. Newer low-flow sidestream capnographs that employ disposable nasal sampling cannulas can be used with infants, children, and adults. The primary problem with sidestream systems is occlusion of the sampling tubing with condensate. Manufacturers address this problem by using water traps, moisture-absorbing filters, and/or nafion tubing (which absorbs both water vapor and liquid water and transfers it via evaporation to the surrounding atmosphere). Sampling tube obstruction also can occur if it becomes twisted or kinked. Use of the recommended condensate prevention methods and proper tube placement can help avoid occlusion of sidestream sampling systems.

Most modern capnographs automatically zero themselves at startup and during regular use. Automatic zeroing is accomplished by aspirating air through a CO_2 scrubber. As with blood gas analyzer calibration, this one-point method adjusts only the offset (baseline drift) and does not properly correct instrument gain, which is required for accurate readings of CO_2 concentrations above zero.

To assess and adjust a capnograph's gain, you need to measure a known concentration of CO_2. Most sidestream capnographs use a precision gas mixture of 5% CO_2 in air for this "high" calibration. Based on Dalton's law, at sea level (760 mm Hg), the P_{CO_2} of a 5% CO_2 concentration equals 38 mm Hg (ATPD). The most often cited standard for capnograph calibration is ±0.3%, or a range of 4.7–5.3% (36–40 mm Hg). For sidestream capnographs, calibration must be performed using the same sampling tubing used when the analyzer is connected to the patient. This is because aspiration through the sampling tubing creates a pressure difference that can affect the P_{CO_2} measurement.

Also, as with blood-gas analyzers, to *verify* calibration you need to confirm accuracy at *three levels* of measurement. For those manufacturers recommending calibration verification, both a 5% and 10% CO_2 mixture (P_{CO_2} = 76 mm Hg) CO_2 are used. Note that all gas calibration of capnographs is conducted at ambient pressure and temperature, *dry* (ATPD). Since capnographs normally measure and report CO_2 concentrations and partial pressures at BTPS, calibration routines must account for the difference in P_{CO_2} values between BTPS and ATPD conditions.

Instead of using precision gases for calibration, some mainstream capnographs employ filters to simulate the infrared absorption of various CO_2 concentrations. Alternatively, some capnographs store initial calibration results in nonvolatile memory and use this information to automatically adjust both the offset and gain of the analyzer with each use, or with a change in the sensor.

Gas Delivery and Metering Devices

A key responsibility for all respiratory therapists is the safe and effective delivery of medical gases to patients. For this reason, you must be familiar with a wide variety of delivery devices and medical gas supply systems. Chapter 6 provides details on the selection and application of these systems and devices. Here we emphasize standards and procedures to ensure safe and accurate delivery of medical gases.

Several nongovernmental agencies, such as the Compressed Gas Association (CGA), National Fire Protection Association (NFPA), International Standards Organization (ISO), American Society of Mechanical Engineers (ASME), and the Joint Commission (TJC), have published standards for the safe use and maintenance of the various systems used to get medical gases to the patient's bedside. Based on these standards, the following general quality assurance recommendations apply:

- Medical gas distribution systems require alarms to monitor the operating supply, reserve supply, and line pressures. Monitoring must consist of two separate locations to ensure continuous surveillance. Critical care areas will have their own monitoring system with audible and visual (non-cancelable) for pressure changes greater than 20% from normal operating pressure.
- Periodic testing and inspection of piping systems should be done and recorded. This should include station outlets for insertion, locking of the gas connector, gas leakage, wear, and damage.
- Indexed safety connections to prevent inadvertent delivery of the wrong gas should never be circumvented.
- If compressed gas cylinders are used, rules and regulation for cylinder safety promulgated by the CGA's Handbook of Compressed Gases must be followed.
- If portable compressors are used for delivery of compressed air, manufacturer's recommendations for preventive maintenance must be followed.
- Medical gas regulators and flowmeters require periodic preventive/restorative maintenance to ensure proper function. Periodic checking of indicated flow should be performed using a calibrated rotameter whenever a device appears damaged or its function is questioned.

COMMON ERRORS TO AVOID

You can improve your score by avoiding these mistakes:

- Never aspirate an arterial blood gas sample or mix it if it contains air bubbles.
- Do not use any gas analyzer that is not or cannot be calibrated at two points in the range of expected results.
- Do not use any pH/blood gas analyzer for reporting results if the most recent quality control results violate any of the rules for acceptable performance.
- Never proceed with pulmonary function testing if the spirometer has an uncorrected leak.
- Never apply a ventilator to a patient if it has failed its operational verification testing.
- Never circumvent medical gas connection safety systems (e.g., PISS, DISS).

SURE BETS

In some situations you can always be sure of the right approach to a clinical problem or scenario:

- Always perform a two-point calibration prior to using any gas analyzer or monitor.
- Always use tonometry whenever the accuracy of a blood gas analyzer's PO_2 and PCO_2 measurements is in doubt.
- Always document the patient's FIO_2, oxygen delivery device, mode of ventilation, and the results of any related assessments made when obtaining a blood sample for analysis.
- Always perform leak testing on spirometers before volume calibration.
- Always perform an operational verification test prior to using a mechanical ventilator on any patient.
- Always include a statement about test quality in the final report of every pulmonary function test.
- When establishing quality assurance programs, an assessment of the competency of the technician(s) must be performed initially and periodically thereafter.

PRE-TEST ANSWERS AND EXPLANATIONS

Below are this chapter's pre-test answers and explanations. Be sure to review each answer's explanation thoroughly to help you understand why it is correct. If the explanation is still unclear to you, review the chapter contents or the references and/or refer to this chapter's supplemental resources on the CD.

8-1. **Correct Answer: D.** Using the minimum amount of heparin. To avoid pre-analytical errors associated with air contamination of a blood gas sample, you should fully remove any air bubbles, cap the syringe quickly, and mix the sample only after all air has been removed.

8-2. **Correct Answer: A.** Analyze the sample immediately. ABG errors caused by blood metabolism are time and temperature dependent. It is important to analyze all ABG samples immediately on receipt in the lab after transport with minimal delay. If this is not possible, the sample should be kept in an ice/water bath and analyzed as soon as possible.

8-3. **Correct Answer: A.** Every 2 hours. Both transcutaneous PCO_2 and PO_2 electrodes are heated to 44°C to "arterialize" the capillary blood. As a result of the increased temperature at the site the electrodes must be moved frequently, every 2 hours for neonates and every 2–4 hours for adults.

8-4. **Correct Answer: B.** ± 2%. There are two common types of electrochemical oxygen analyzers: the polarographic (Clark) electrode and the galvanic fuel cell. Under ideal conditions of temperature, pressure, and relative humidity, both types are accurate to within 2% of the actual concentration.

8-5. **Correct Answer: C.** HbO_2 levels. Levels of HbO_2 values for samples contaminated with air bubbles should be questioned. Levels of HbCO, metHb, SHb, and total Hb are unaffected by air contamination. Additionally, inadequate mixing of either a syringe or capillary sample just prior to analysis will result in erroneous total hemoglobin measurements.

8-6. **Correct Answer: D.** Precision flowmeter. To assess the output or flow accuracy of a Bourdon gauge regulator used for O_2 transport, you would use a precision (calibrated) flowmeter.

8-7. **Correct Answer: D.** Control media calibration verification. To periodically confirm the validity of a blood gas analyzer, you would perform a calibration verification using control media. Calibration verification requires analysis of at least three materials with known values (controls) spanning the entire range of results expected for clinical samples. At least one control should be analyzed every 8-hour shift. All three levels of the control media are analyzed at least once every 24 hours.

8-8. **Correct Answer: B.** 3% or 50 mL, whichever is greater, using a 3-liter syringe. American Thoracic Society (ATS) recommendations for diagnostic spirometers are that calibration checks should be within 3% or 50 mL, whichever is larger.

8-9. **Correct Answer: B.** Between patient uses. All ventilators should be tested after each use to verify performance before the unit is used on another patient. A complete operational verification procedure, based on the manufacturer's recommendations, should be performed each time. These procedures should be detailed in the health care facility's policies and procedures manual.

8-10. **Correct Answer: A.** Calibrate the sensor. If a galvanic cell oxygen analyzer reads 18% when exposed to ambient air, it should first be recalibrated to 20.9%. Replace the sensor only if an analyzer fails to calibrate at 21% and 100% oxygen.

POST-TEST

A post-test for this chapter that includes automated scoring and feedback is available on the accompanying CD. Be sure to complete this additional assessment to confirm your mastery of this chapter's objectives.

REFERENCES

American Association for Respiratory Care. (1996). Clinical practice guideline. Spirometry, 1996 Update. *Respiratory care, 41,* 629–636.

American Association for Respiratory Care. (2001). Clinical practice guideline. Blood gas analysis and hemoximetry: 2001 revision and update. *Respiratory care, 46,* 498–505.

American Association for Respiratory Care. (2004). Clinical practice guideline. Transcutaneous blood gas monitoring for neonatal and pediatric patients: 2004 revision and update. *Respiratory care, 49,* 1070–1072.

Branson, R. D., Hess, D., & Chatburn, R. L. (1998). *Respiratory care equipment* (2nd ed.). Philadelphia: Lippincott.

Emergency Care Research Institute. (1998). Minimum requirements for ventilator testing. *Health devices, 27,* 363–364.

Madama, V. C. (1998). *Pulmonary function testing and cardiopulmonary stress testing* (2nd ed.). Albany, NY: Delmar.

Miller, M. R., Hankinson, J., Brusasco, V., et al. (2005). Standardisation of spirometry. *European respiratory journal, 26,* 319–338.

National Institute for Occupational Safety and Health. (2003). NIOSH Spirometry Training Guide. NIOSH Publication No. 2004-154c. Atlanta, GA: Centers for Disease Control and Prevention.

Ruppel, G. L. (2009). *Manual of pulmonary function testing* (9th ed.). St. Louis: Mosby.

Scanlan, C. L. (1999). Analysis and monitoring of gas exchange. In Scanlan, C. L., Wilkins, R. L., & Stoller, J. K. (Eds.). *Egan's fundamentals of respiratory care* (7th ed.). St. Louis: Mosby.

White, G. C. (2005). *Equipment theory for respiratory care* (4th ed.). Albany, NY: Delmar Cengage Learning.

Initiation and Modification of Therapeutic Procedure

Maintain Records and Communicate Information

Louis M. Sinopoli

INTRODUCTION

Maintaining accurate records and properly communicating information is an essential part of your job. Without proper record keeping, the therapy you provide may not be reimbursable, the hospital may get cited for improper record keeping, and most important, it may result in harm to your patients. It is for these reasons that the NBRC defines record keeping and communication as key entry-level skills that are tested on the CRT exam.

This section of the CRT exam can be difficult because it requires knowledge of many facts, standards, and requirements for maintaining records and communication with other health care workers, patients, and family members. In addition, the sections on *Accept and Verify Patient Care Orders* and *Apply Computer Technology to Patient Safety Initiatives* are new to the NBRC CRT exam in 2009. These skill areas require that you apply the rules and standards for record keeping and communication while paying great attention to detail. A small mistake, especially in real life, can result in large consequences for your patient, your hospital, and your career.

If you are not familiar with all the new rules and standards for record keeping and communication, you may need to spend a larger portion of your exam preparation time on this topic. Areas you will need to emphasize include charting rules and standards, communication and coordination of patient care, and patient education, including smoking cessation education.

OBJECTIVES

After completion of this chapter, you should demonstrate the knowledge needed to:

1. Accept and verify patient care orders
2. Record therapy and results using conventional terminology
3. Communicate information regarding a patient's status to appropriate members of the health care team
4. Apply computer technology to patient safety initiatives and to document patient management
5. Communicate results of therapy and modify therapy according to protocol(s)
6. Explain planned therapy and goals to the patient in understandable terms
7. Educate the patient and family concerning smoking cessation and disease management

WHAT TO EXPECT ON THIS CATEGORY OF THE CRT EXAM

Number of questions: 5
Level of questions: 40% recall, 60% application

WHAT'S NEW FOR 2009

As of July 2009, this section of the NBRC CRT examination includes the following *new content areas*:

- Accept and verify patient care orders
- Apply computer technology to patient safety initiatives, e.g., drug dispensing, order entry

PRE-TEST

Carefully respond to each of the following questions. After completing the pre-test, compare your answers to those provided at the end of this chapter. Then thoroughly review each answer's explanation to help understand why it is correct.

9-1. On checking a ventilator patient's progress notes, you see that the attending physician's treatment plan includes starting spontaneous breathing trials. Your most appropriate action is to do which of the following?
  A. Begin a spontaneous breathing trial immediately
  B. Wait until after the patient's sedation is discontinued
  C. Check to verify that a valid physician's order is present
  D. Review the plan changes with the patient's nurse

9-2. After completing a ventilator check, you note that you incorrectly computed the patient's compliance in a prior entry. Which of the following is the most appropriate course of action?
  A. Inform the medical director of the error
  B. Erase the error and write over it with the correction
  C. Copy the entire ventilator sheet over to correct the error
  D. Line out the error, write the word "error," and correct and initial it

9-3. When *must* you contact the ordering physician when implementing a respiratory care treatment protocol?
  A. After your initial assessment of the patient
  B. Whenever a change in therapy is needed
  C. Prior to providing the initial therapy
  D. Whenever a limit or boundary rule takes effect

9-4. A prescription for an aerosolized drug for a patient under your care is complete except for the actual drug dosage. Which of the following is the appropriate action to take in this case?
  A. Use the standard dosage listed in the package insert
  B. Ask your medical director to rewrite the prescription
  C. Contact the ordering physician for clarification
  D. Postpone the therapy until the following day

9-5. The best way to routinely communicate a patient's clinical status to the appropriate members of the health care team is by reporting information:
  A. To the respiratory therapy supervisor
  B. To the next shift of respiratory therapy staff
  C. In the respiratory therapy department records
  D. In the patient's chart

9-6. If you are giving routine therapy and note adverse changes in the patient's condition, you should do which of the following?
  I. Notify the nurse who is responsible for the patient
  II. Contact the physician if a change in therapy seems warranted
  III. Record the patient's reactions in the chart
  A. II only
  B. I and III only
  C. II and III only
  D. I, II, and III

9-7. Midway through an aerosol drug treatment via intermittent positive pressure breathing (IPPB), a patient complains of dizziness and tingling in her fingers. After stopping the therapy and adjusting the equipment to correct the problem and completing the treatment, you should record which of the following in the chart?

    I. Medication used during the treatment

    II. The patient's pulse and blood pressure before and after the treatment

    III. The nature of the problem and the way in which it was corrected

    A. I and II only
    B. I and III only
    C. II and III only
    D. I, II, and III

9-8. When assessing a patient after a treatment, you note a significant deterioration in vital signs. The most appropriate action in this case is to:

    A. Call for the institution's rapid response team
    B. Report the findings to the next shift of respiratory therapy staff
    C. Chart the findings as an unexpected response to therapy
    D. Orally communicate the findings to the patient's physician

9-9. When a patient refuses to take a treatment, you should do which of the following?

    A. Notify the nurse in charge and chart the patient's refusal
    B. Give the treatment anyway and record that it was done
    C. Ask the head nurse to convince the patient to take the treatment
    D. Leave the patient's room and discontinue the therapy

9-10. Which of the following represents a charting entry that would be placed in the "S" portion of a problem-oriented (SOAP) record entry?

    A. Color of patient's sputum
    B. The patient is not tolerating weaning
    C. Patient states, "I'm short of breath"
    D. Perform another ABG after next attempt

WHAT YOU NEED TO KNOW: ESSENTIAL CONTENT

Accept and Verify Patient Care Orders

All respiratory care is normally provided by order of the patient's personal doctor or attending physician. In some settings, respiratory care orders also may originate from other licensed health care providers, such as nurse practitioners (NPs) or physician assistants (PAs).

Accepting Orders

Your state licensure regulations and institutional policies will dictate if you can accept orders from other health care professionals and may vary according to whether the order is written or verbal. If you can accept orders, they must come from an authorized health care provider with prescribing privileges. You cannot accept orders transmitted to you via unauthorized third parties, such as registered nurses. If an order is transmitted to you via a third party, you must verify the order in the patient's chart before proceeding. In most institutions, orders written by medical students must be countersigned by a physician before you are allowed to carry them out. You also should not accept blanket orders. Examples of blanket orders include "continue previous medications" or "resume preoperative orders."

Regarding verbal or telephone orders, if the "doctor is in the house" and the situation is not an emergency, it's best to secure a regular written order. If a verbal order is required and you are authorized to take it, you must avoid transcription errors. The Joint Commission recommends the following procedure for taking verbal orders properly:

1. While speaking with the prescribing physician or health care provider, write or type the complete order into the applicable section of the patient's record.
2. Read the order back to the originator exactly as written (and clarify as needed).
3. Have the originator confirm the accuracy of the order as read back.
4. Write the time and date of the order with the name and credentials of originator, specify "read back and confirmed," and provide your signature and credentials.

Verifying Orders

Regardless of their source or route of transmission, it is your duty to assure that all respiratory care orders are accurate and complete. Although the components vary according to what is being prescribed, a complete written order generally includes the following elements:

- Date and time of order
- Name of therapy or diagnostic test being prescribed
- Requisite details for therapy (e.g., ventilator settings) or conditions for diagnostic testing
- Frequency of therapy or testing (if intermittent)
- Name, signature, and credentials of the ordering health care provider

If the order is for a drug (including oxygen), it must contain the following additional information:

- Drug name
- Route of administration
- Dose/concentration (for O_2 the liter flow or FIO_2)

If the order is for mechanical ventilation, the AARC recommends that it include at least one and ideally both of the following:

- Desired range for $PaCO_2$ and/or desired range for PaO_2 or oxygen saturation
- ventilator variables to initiate or manipulate in order to achieve desired blood gas results (e.g., mode, tidal volume, airway pressure, ventilatory frequency, or FIO_2)

Should any of these elements be missing, the order is incomplete and you should contact the prescriber for clarification before implementing the request. The same procedure applies if the order falls outside established institutional standards. For example, if the order specifies a drug dosage higher than that recommended for the patient's size or age or includes a ventilator mode or setting not normally applied in similar cases, you should contact the physician and request an explanation before proceeding further.

Recording Therapy and Results

As both clinician and NBRC candidate, you must be up to date on all the rules, standards, and regulations governing record keeping and communicating in the health care setting. Many of these rules are legal or regulatory, and breaking them can have grave consequences. Not only might a hospital's accreditation or licensure be jeopardized, but your legal right to practice respiratory care could be revoked by your state licensure board. In order to prepare for this area of the NBRC CRT exam, you must become familiar with the basic information needed to properly record therapy using conventional terminology as required in the health care setting and/or by regulatory agencies.

As is frequently the case on the NBRC exam, memorization of these facts is important, but it is only a small part of the thinking skills tested in this section. Of the five questions included in this part of the exam, only two are at the recall level. This means you also must be able to apply information about record keeping and communication to patient care situations.

Basic Rule for Medical Record Keeping

Good record keeping begins with careful attention to detail, requires proper use of terminology and abbreviations, and involves knowledge of how to make needed corrections or deletions to a patient's record. Basic rules for medical record keeping include all of the following:

1. For paper records, print or write your entries legibly in the applicable section of the chart (see Chapter 3 for details on the structure of medical records). Sign each entry with one initial, your last name, and your credential/title (CRT, Resp Care Student, etc.), such as S. Smith, CRT. Agency policy may require supervisors to countersign student entries.
2. Never use ditto marks.
3. Never try to erase an entry. Erasures provide reason to question the information if the chart is used later for QA purposes or in court. If a mistake is made, draw a single line through the mistake and print the word "error" above it. Then continue your charting in a normal manner.

4. Make entries after completing each patient task, and sign your name correctly after each entry.
5. Be exact in noting the time, effect, and results of all treatments and procedures.
6. Record patient complaints and general behavior. Describe the severity, type, location, onset, and duration of pain. Describe clearly and concisely the character and amount of secretions (see Chapter 4 for details).
7. Do not leave blank lines in the chart. Draw a line through the center of an empty line or part of a line. This prevents charting by someone else in an area signed by you.
8. Use institutionally accepted standard abbreviations and avoid banned abbreviations.
9. Never use future tense, as in "patient will receive treatment after lunch."
10. Spell correctly. If you are not sure about the spelling of a word, use a dictionary.

Each institution establishes its own list of accepted abbreviations, which you are obliged to follow. Due to variations among institutions, the NBRC avoids using all but the most common general abbreviations on its exams, such as ECG or STAT.

However, *the NBRC does expect that you know all standard respiratory care abbreviations and symbols*, which are used on the agency's exams. A complete list of the abbreviations and symbols applicable to respiratory care (adapted from recommendation of the ACCP-ATS Committee on Pulmonary Nomenclature) is published in *Respiratory Care*, the official journal of the American Association for Respiratory Care. This list is available online at http://www.rcjournal.com/guidelines_for_authors/symbols.pdf and is reproduced on the CD accompanying this book.

Based on growing safety concerns due to serious errors associated with written miscommunications, the Joint Commission has established a list of banned abbreviations and symbols. **Table 9-1** specifies the Joint Commission's official "do not use" abbreviations and symbols, and includes an additional set of those being considered for exclusion in the future. This list applies to all orders and all medication-related documentation that is handwritten (including free-text computer entry) or appears on pre-printed forms. A comprehensive list of error-prone abbreviations, symbols, and dose designations specifically associated with medication errors is provided by the Institute for Safe Medication Practices (ISMP); see this chapter's reference list.

Normally, if an order contains a prohibited notation, you must confirm the intent of the order before proceeding. The exception is when order confirmation might delay essential or emergency patient treatment. In these cases, if in your judgment the order is clear and complete and any delays to obtain confirmation would place the patient at greater risk, then you should carry out the order and obtain confirmation as soon as possible thereafter.

Specifying Therapy Administered

There is a common saying in health care that "if it wasn't charted, it wasn't done!" This saying has care-related, financial, and legal implications. First, if you fail to chart a therapy or medication you have provided, your patient may receive additional treatment that is unnecessary and may be harmful. Second, if a procedure is not charted, the hospital may not be able to get reimbursed for the services provided. Last, should any legal questions ever arise, the medical record becomes the primary evidence about the care you or the hospital provided.

For all these reasons, *whenever you provide therapy to or obtain diagnostic information from a patient, you must record the relevant details and, as necessary, communicate this key information to other members of the patient's health care team*. This is how everyone involved in the patient's care will know exactly what was done when, and how the patient responded. To that end, whenever you provide therapy to or obtain diagnostic information from a patient you must record at least the following information:

1. Specific therapy or diagnostic test administered
2. Date and time of therapy or test administration
3. Medication name, dose, and concentration if applicable
4. Patient response to therapy or test results (covered in subsequent section)

Table 9-1 The Joint Commission's Recommended List of Banned Abbreviations

Do Not Use	Potential Problem	Preferred Term
Official Do Not Use Abbreviations and Symbols		
U,u (for unit)	Mistaken as zero, four, or cc	Write "unit"
IU (for international unit)	Mistaken as IV (intravenous) or 10 (ten)	Write "international unit"
Q.D. (QD, q.d., qd) Q.O.D. (QOD, q.o.d., qod) (Latin abbreviations for once daily and every other day)	Mistaken for each other. The period after the Q can be mistaken for an "I" and the "O" can be mistaken for "I."	Write "daily" or "every other day"
Trailing zero (X.0 mg) Note: Prohibited only for medication-related notations	Decimal point is missed	Never write a zero by itself after a decimal point (X mg)
Lack of leading zero (.X mg)	Decimal point is missed	*Always* use a zero before a decimal point (0.X mg)
MS MSO$_4$ MgSO$_4$	Confused for one another; can mean morphine sulfate or magnesium sulfate	Write "morphine sulfate" or "magnesium sulfate"
Additional Abbreviations and Symbols for Possible Exclusion		
μg (for microgram)	Mistaken for mg (milligrams) resulting in 1000-fold dosing overdose	Write "mcg"
c.c. (for cubic centimeter)	Mistaken for U (units) when poorly written	Write "mL" or "milliliters"
> (greater than) < (less than)	Misinterpreted as the number "7" (seven) or the letter "L"	Write "greater than" Write "less than"
Abbreviations for drug names	Misinterpreted due to similar abbreviations for multiple drugs	Write drug names in full
Apothecary units	Unfamiliar to many practitioners; confused with metric units	Use metric units
@	Mistaken for the number "2" (two)	Write "at"

A patient's refusal of therapy must also be charted, along with any rationale the patient might provide, such as pain or discomfort. You must also notify the patient's nurse orally whenever a treatment is refused.

Ventilator management represents a special case of record keeping, because it normally involves using a flow sheet. A typical ventilator flow sheet provides sequential row or column data entry that concisely combines the "therapy" (ventilator settings) information with the patient response information (monitoring data).

As with lists of accepted abbreviations, each institution usually develops its own ventilator flow sheet. Obviously, all such flow sheets must include the appropriate patient identifying information. Typically, each entry must specify the date and time at which the information was logged and by whom (signature or initials, depending on institutional policy). In terms of additional information, most institutions follow the recommendations established by the AARC in their clinical practice guideline on patient-ventilator system checks, as summarized in **Table 9-2**.

Table 9-2 Key Information Elements for Recording Patient-Ventilator System Checks (Flow Sheets)

Ventilator Settings (should include but not be limited to the following)	Patient Observation/Response (should include but not be limited to the following)
• F_{IO_2} • Humidifier temperature setting (when applicable) • Mode of ventilation • Set frequency • Peak, mean, and baseline airway pressures and presence of auto-PEEP (if applicable) • Set peak inspiratory pressure limit and pressure support level, if applicable • Set tidal volume (if applicable) • Delivered tidal volume (measured or calculated) • Set high variables (if applicable) • Set minute ventilation (if applicable) • Set minimum mandatory minute ventilation (if applicable) • Set inspiratory-flow rate and waveform (if applicable) • Set continuous-flow rate (for IMV mode, if applicable) • Set I:E ratio, percent inspiration, or inspiratory and expiratory times • Set sensitivity threshold (if applicable) • Documentation of alarm settings and activation of appropriate alarms	• Breath sounds • Spontaneous respiratory rate, volume, and pattern • Chest motion • Pallor, skin color • Patient's level of consciousness or remarks • Endotracheal tube cuff pressure • Stability and position of the tube • Volume and consistency of secretions • Results of bedside pulmonary function evaluations • Any untoward effects of disconnection from ventilator during bedside procedures • Documentation of oxygenation and ventilation status (e.g., ABGs, pulse oximetry, capnometry) • Documentation of patient-ventilator synchrony during assisted or supported breaths • Documentation of time of last HME and/or circuit change • Condition of ancillary equipment (e.g., chest tube apparatus and manual resuscitator)

Noting and Interpreting the Patient's Response to Therapy

All documentation of patient encounters must include assessment of the results of your intervention and the patient's response to it. At a minimum this means charting the outcomes of therapy and recording any adverse reactions encountered during or after the intervention. In addition, for most bedside encounters you also should assess and record the patient's vital signs, breath sounds, and the volume and quality of secretions (see Chapters 4 and 13 for pertinent details). If available, objective data derived from pulse oximetry, ECG monitoring, and capnography should also be documented. Last, your charting responsibilities also require that you verify all computations and note any erroneous data.

Effects of Therapy, Adverse Reactions, and Patient's Subjective and Objective Response

In terms of documenting the effects of therapy, what you need to chart depends on (1) the expected outcomes of the prescribed procedure; (2) what parameters you should be monitoring prior to, during, and after the procedure; and (3) what measures are available to evaluate the expected outcomes. In addition, the NBRC expects that you will properly chart any adverse reactions the patient may exhibit during or after the procedure.

For most respiratory care procedures, essentially all this key information is provided in the clinical practice guidelines published by the AARC and linked to from the CD accompanying this text. Each guideline provides pertinent information on the expected outcomes (*Indications and Assessment of Outcomes*), what to monitor (*Monitoring*), and what adverse reactions to look for (*Hazards/Complications*). For example, were you to suction a patient receiving ventilatory support, the applicable AARC guideline would direct you to document whether one or more of the following outcomes was achieved:

- Improved breath sounds
- Decreased peak pressure (or increased tidal volume if pressure-limited ventilation)
- Improved ABGs or SpO_2
- Removal of secretions

In order to monitor for adverse effects, you also would need to assess the patient's:

- Skin color
- Respiratory rate and pattern
- Hemodynamic parameters
- EKG, if available
- Sputum characteristics
- Cough effort
- Intracranial pressure (if indicated and available)

Based on the information provided by these additional monitoring parameters, you would include in your chart entry the occurrence of any of the following adverse effects:

- Hypoxemia
- Cardiac dysrhythmias
- Changes in blood pressure
- Cardiac or respiratory arrest
- Atelectasis
- Bronchospasm
- Bleeding
- Elevated intracranial pressure

An alternative record-keeping format that goes beyond simply charting outcomes and adverse reactions is the problem-oriented method, also called the SOAP format. SOAP stands for:

S: Subjective data
O: Objective data
A: Assessment
P: Plan

Table 9-3 describes the components of the problem-oriented method based on the SOAP acronym, with examples of how such information typically would be recorded in the patient's chart for a specific problem—in this example, an asthma patient's breathing effort.

When using this method it is best to phrase the plan element of your chart entry as a recommendation. For example, if your plan involves changing the therapy, it is best to put it in the form of a recommendation so that if the physician disagrees, the record reflects a tone of discussion as opposed to disagreement.

Whether or not your institution uses the problem-oriented approach, you should still incorporate the basic SOAP actions both into your daily clinical care and whenever responding to NBRC exam questions. **Figure 9-1** outlines this process. First, identify the patient's problem or the objective of the prescribed therapy. Then collect the information needed to assess the patient (subjective and objective). Next, analyze this information by comparing your findings to the patient's problem or the therapy objective. Finally, develop your care plan, communicate it to others, and implement it after physician approval. As indicated in Figure 9-1, you should repeat the data collection and analysis as needed and modify or update your plan accordingly until the patient's problem is resolved or the objectives are achieved.

Verifying Computations and Noting Erroneous Data

Many procedures within your scope of practice require that you use or derive information based on computations. As with any data recorded in the patient record, all computations must be precise and accurate. If you are the one making the measurements, you must use the proper tools and techniques for precision, and check your results in order to ensure accuracy. Never report data about which you are unsure. And if you mistakenly record inaccurate data, you must follow the applicable rules for correcting charting errors, as previously described.

Several examples of NBRC-type questions designed to assess your skill in verifying computations and noting erroneous data are provided in Chapter 2 (Test-Taking Tips and Techniques). In the section on *Specific Tips for Common NBRC-Type Items* you will find good examples of questions that

Table 9-3 Components of the Problem-Oriented Method for Medical Record-Keeping

Element	Description	Charting Example
S: Subjective data	Qualitative information collected from the patient in response to questions or based on the judgment of the clinician	S = "Patient states his breathing is better today and he has not had to use his Proventil MDI."
O: Objective data	Objective data collected by the therapist via physical exam or instrumentation	O = "The patient's FEV_1 has increased from a low of 700 mL on admission to 2500 mL (70% predicted) after the 10/5 3 PM treatment; minimal wheezing on auscultation."
A: Assessment	Conclusions based on the goal of therapy and the subjective and objective information gathered	A = "Patient's asthma appears under control and need for PRN MDI reliever medication has diminished."
P: Plan	Recommendations for how to proceed with the patient's respiratory care	P = "Recommend continuing therapy and discussing discharge planning and patient education with the patient's attending physician."

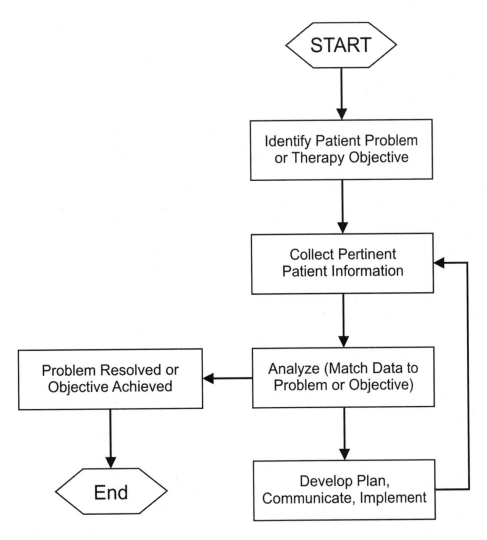

Figure 9-1 The Basic Problem-Oriented Approach to Patient Care.

test your ability to (1) recognize and/or deal with conflicting data (*Data Just Don't Jive*); (2) recognize plainly incorrect data (*Errors, Errors Everywhere!*) and (3) identifying and deriving essential but missing information (*Don't Know What You're Missing!*).

To do well on these questions, you must first know how to apply the common formulas and equations likely to appear on the CRT exam, as reviewed in Chapter 20 of this text. In addition, whenever a question involves any numeric data you should follow three key steps:

1. Inspect the data for obvious errors (i.e., values that simply could not exist). An example would be a PaO_2 of 200 torr on a patient breathing room air.
2. Inspect the data for discrepancies (i.e., two or more values in conflict). An example would be a patient with a reported PaO_2 of 50 torr and an SaO_2 of 95%.
3. Review the numbers to see what, if anything, is missing—missing data may be the key to solving the problem. An example would be assessing the mechanics of a patient on a ventilator with a peak pressure = 50 cm H_2O, PEEP = 10 cm H_2O, and V_T = 400 mL. Missing is the patient's compliance = 400 mL/(50–10) cm H_2O = 10 mL/cm H_2O. Compared with a normal of about 100 mL/cm H_2O, this is a *very low* value.

Communicating Information

The Joint Commission defines effective communication as being timely, accurate, complete, unambiguous, and understood by the recipient. Effective communication among health professionals can reduce errors, improve patient safety, and help assure the quality of care. The NBRC assesses your communication skills in the following three areas:

1. Reporting the patient's clinical status
2. Coordinating the patient's care
3. Planning for patient discharge

If your written plan includes any recommendations for a change in therapy, you should communicate this directly to the prescribing physician as soon as possible. Likewise, any unexpected response to therapy or adverse effects noted when charting a patient encounter should also be communicated orally to the patient's attending physician and nurse. In general, the more serious the problem, the sooner these key people should be informed. In particular, *if it is clear that the patient's vital signs are deteriorating, you should call for your institution's rapid response team.*

As a key member of the health care team, you should also participate in coordinating the patient's care. Your responsibility is to work with the patient's nurse and/or attending physician to schedule the therapy you provide at times (1) least likely to conflict with other treatments, tests, or meals and (2) most likely to coincide with either the administration or holding of medications. For example, you would avoid performing postural drainage and directed coughing on a post-op patient immediately after a meal, but you would normally want to schedule this therapy to coincide with prior administration of pain medication. However, you would want to wait until after sedatives have been held back from a patient on a ventilator (a "sedation vacation") before implementing a spontaneous breathing trial.

Another key aspect related to coordinating patient care is the patient "handoff." Common patient handoffs that you participate in include shift change reporting, taking temporary responsibility for a fellow therapist's patients for a short time, receiving a patient in or from a specialized care unit, and having other health care professionals take over during emergency procedures such as resuscitation. If you are handing-off a patient to another health care professional, you must provide accurate information about the patient and his or her current condition and treatment, as well as any recent or anticipated changes. To assure that effective communication occurs, the recipient of the handoff needs to verify the received information via either repeat-back (for oral handoffs) or read-back (for written handoffs).

Applying Computer Technology to Medical Record Keeping

The electronic medical record (EMR) is a reality in many hospitals across the county. If you don't have an EMR system in your facility, you will soon. EMR systems are used to document patient care, monitor workload assignments, and assure patient safety (e.g., for drug dispensing and order entry). Security and privacy are two important elements of using and maintaining the EMR. Security issues that directly affect you include unauthorized access, lost passwords, and compliance with regulations such as the Health Insurance Portability and Accountability Act, or HIPAA (see the accompanying box for a summary of the HIPAA provisions). Maintenance of data security and patient privacy is taken very seriously, with many health care providers employing zero-tolerance policies, implementing fines or even job termination for violations.

The Health Insurance Portability and Accountability Act (HIPAA): Key Provisions

Information Security and Use

- The integrity of patient information must be assured via proper access control, data encryption, and backup procedures.
- Security programs for protected health information must be monitored by a security officer.
- Strict security measures must be in place for access to and transmission of patient information over the Internet.
- The use of patient information is limited to reasons of treatment, payment, and routine health care operations.
- Health care providers must give notice of policies regarding information disclosure to their patients.

Patient Privacy Rights

- Patients have the right to access their health information.
- Patients may review and request amendments to their health information.
- Patients must be informed by health care providers about their information disclosure policies.
- Patients may limit the scope of data disclosed to other health care providers.
- Patient authorization is required to use or disclose information for a purpose other than treatment, payment, or operations.

Most EMR systems also provide automated alerts to prescribing health care professionals. Some alerts warn of potentially dangerous medication conflicts. Other alerts track order dates. For example, if an order for respiratory care is about to expire, the EMR system will alert the physician to evaluate the order for renewal. When such alerts occur, you should communicate with the patient's physician regarding continuation or modification of the current therapy and document this interaction in the medical record. Depending on institutional policy, EMR systems may also allow you to record a physician's verbal order and verify it with your electronic signature. Normally, this is followed by an electronic alert to the prescribing physician to cosign the verbal order.

When giving medications to a patient, you should know that some EMR systems require two separate entries. In these systems you must first record the drug information in the medication administration record, where all drugs that the patient receives are recorded. Second, you will need to chart the treatment separately in the either the respiratory care notes or the general patient care notes, whichever are used for recording therapy in your institution. In these cases, both entries must be made correctly in order for the procedure to be considered properly documented.

Explaining Planned Therapy and Goals to Patients

The effectiveness of most respiratory care modalities depends on patient cooperation. Good patient cooperation requires that the patient understand both the procedure itself and the goals of therapy. Thus, to provide effective respiratory care you must properly explain to your patients both what needs to be done and why.

The Joint Commission considers good communication with patients and their families an essential safety strategy. The better patients and their family members understand the care provided, the more likely it is that they will recognize adverse events, hazardous conditions, or potential treatment errors. You should always encourage patients and their family members to report any concerns they might have about their condition, their treatment, or any related safety issues.

A particularly important safety issue for patients receiving respiratory care is infection control. The Joint Commission specifically recommends that you explain to your patients and their families all infection control measures they need to implement, including good hand hygiene practices, respiratory hygiene/cough etiquette, and any transmission-based precautions applicable to the patient's condition (see Chapter 7).

Questions in this section are likely to focus on your ability to "translate" therapeutic goals and/or procedural terminology into terms a layperson can understand. To do so, you'll need to (1) know the methods and expected outcomes of the applicable procedures and (2) be able to use appropriate language to express this information to patients and their families. *The key is always to avoid using medical terminology.* **Table 9-4** provides examples of proper and improper patient explanations of planned therapy and its goals.

Communicating Results of Therapy and Alter Therapy According to Protocol(s)

Special considerations apply to medical record keeping when implementing a respiratory care protocol. As recommended by the AARC, the main requirements for documenting protocols are:

1. Date and time of protocol initiation
2. Pertinent medical history and physical examination
3. Pertinent diagnostic results
4. Management plan details
5. Physician notification criteria (i.e., guidelines for physician notification of patient status change)
6. Adverse reaction, if any, and remedial steps taken
7. Notification of physician, nurse, and other appropriate health care professionals
8. Required departmental documentation
9. Signature with credential

When implementing a protocol, make sure you are familiar with the limits (also called boundaries) within which you are permitted to make independent adjustments, as well as what conditions require physician notification. For example, in a mechanical ventilation protocol, you may find a boundary rule like this:

If more than 50% O_2 is needed to maintain an $SpO_2 \geq 88\%$, inform the ordering MD.

Table 9-4 Proper and Improper Patient Explanation for Incentive Spirometry

Improper Explanation	Proper Explanation
Ms. Smith, your doctor has ordered incentive spirometry treatments for you. These treatments will help prevent you from getting atelectasis. The treatment requires that you perform a sustained maximum inspiratory maneuver, or SMI. This device will measure your inspiratory capacity as you perform the SMI.	Ms. Smith, your doctor has ordered deep breathing exercises for you. These exercises will help prevent your lungs from collapsing, which can lead to pneumonia. All you need to do is take a few slow, deep breaths in. I'll also encourage you to briefly hold your breath after you take in all the air you can, then slowly exhale. This little device will show us how well you are doing.

If you were to implement a protocol containing this rule, as long as you could maintain a satisfactory SpO_2 on an FIO_2 of 0.50 or less, you would be permitted to independently modify the O_2 setting on the ventilator. In contrast, if your assessment indicated that the patient needed more than 50% O_2 to ensure adequate arterial saturation, you would need to notify the ordering physician and determine an alternative approach that might be outside the protocol boundary, such as adding PEEP.

Educating the Patient and Family

You can expect that questions on this part of the CRT exam will address providing education on smoking cessation and disease management. Disease management is covered in Chapter 13, as related to participation in pulmonary rehabilitation. Here we focus primarily on smoking cessation.

A prerequisite to any well-planned education effort is assessing the patient's learning needs, as discussed in Chapter 4. In regard to smoking cessation, your assessment of the patient's learning needs should ideally reveal a desire to quit. Family members can be very helpful in motivating patients to stop smoking, and their assistance should be sought whenever needed.

For patients hesitant to quit smoking, you'll need to motivate them by explaining the health consequences of not doing so, as well as the significant benefits that come from giving up the habit. For these patients the U.S. Department of Health and Human Services recommends an educational strategy based upon the five R's: *relevance*, *risks*, *rewards*, *roadblocks*, and *repetition*. **Table 9-5** describes the components of this five-pronged strategy.

Table 9-5 Using the Five R's to Motivate Patients to Quit Smoking

Component	Description
Relevance	Encourage the patient to indicate why quitting is personally **relevant**. Motivational information has the greatest impact if it is relevant to a patient's disease status or risk, family or social situation (e.g., having children in the home), health concerns, age, sex, and other important patient characteristics (e.g., prior quitting experience, personal barriers to quitting).
Risks	Ask the patient to identify the **negative consequences** of tobacco use. Suggest and highlight those consequences that seem most relevant to the patient. Acute risks include shortness of breath, exacerbation of asthma, harm to pregnancy, impotence, and increased serum CO levels. Long-term risks include heart attacks and strokes, lung and other cancers, COPD, etc. Environmental risks include lung cancer and heart disease in spouses; higher rates of smoking by children; increased risk for low birth weight, sudden infant death syndrome, asthma, middle ear disease, and respiratory infections in the children of smokers. Be sure to emphasize that smoking low-tar/low-nicotine cigarettes or use of smokeless tobacco, cigars, or pipes will not eliminate these risks.
Rewards	Ask the patient to identify potential **benefits** of stopping tobacco use. Suggest and highlight those that seem most relevant to the patient (e.g., quitting will improve health, improve sense of smell, cause food to taste better, and improve self-esteem; home, car, clothing, and breath will smell better; the patient will no longer have to worry about quitting, set a good example for kids, have healthier babies and children, avoid exposing others to smoke, feel better physically, perform better in physical activities, and have reduced wrinkling/aging of skin).
Roadblocks	Ask the patient to identify **barriers** or impediments to quitting and note elements of treatment (problem solving, pharmacotherapy) that could address these barriers. Typical barriers might include withdrawal symptoms, fear of failure, weight gain, lack of support, depression, and enjoyment of tobacco.
Repetition	**Repeat** the above motivational interventions as needed.

Once the patient has expressed a desire to quit smoking, you should recommend to the patient's physician implementation of a comprehensive treatment program that includes both counseling and pharmacologic support. Pharmacologic treatment of nicotine dependence is covered in Chapter 19.

According to the U.S. Department of Health and Human Services, counseling and behavioral therapies that can significantly motivate patients to stop smoking include:

- Provision of practical counseling (problem-solving/skills training)
- Provision of "intra-treatment" social support
- Helping the patient obtain "extra-treatment" social support

Table 9-6 outlines and defines the major components involved in each of these strategies and provides practical examples of discussion points or suggestions to share with the patient.

COMMON ERRORS TO AVOID

You can improve your score by avoiding these mistakes:

- Never accept an incomplete order, a blanket order, or an order transmitted to you via an unauthorized third party.
- Never use medical or technical terms with patients or their families when explaining procedures or providing patient education.
- Never erase entries in a medical record; instead, always line it out and write "error" above the line-out (your institution may also require that you initial this entry).
- Avoid using any banned abbreviations and request clarification if an order contains them.
- Never allow unauthorized individuals access to any patient's health care information.

SURE BETS

In some situations you can always be sure of the right approach to a clinical problem or scenario:

- Always read back and confirm a telephone order, and note the phone order in the chart.
- Always contact the physician and request an explanation before proceeding with any order that falls outside established standards, such as the normal drug dosage.
- Always document each patient encounter with an assessment of the intervention and the patient's response to it.
- Always chart a patient's refusal of therapy and the reason, if provided.
- Always communicate any recommendations for a change in therapy directly to the prescribing physician as soon as possible.
- Always verify that the appropriate information has been received by those to whom you "hand off" a patient.
- Always notify the physician if any significant change occurs when managing a patient via a respiratory care protocol.
- Always respect patients' privacy rights and their right of access to their own health information.
- Always recommend both counseling and pharmacologic support for patients who desire to quit smoking.

PRE-TEST ANSWERS AND EXPLANATIONS

Below are this chapter's pre-test answers and explanations. Be sure to review each answer's explanation thoroughly to help you understand why it is correct. If the explanation is still unclear to you, review the chapter contents or the references and/or refer to this chapter's supplemental resources on the CD.

9-1. **Correct answer: C.** Check to verify that a valid physician's order is present. All respiratory care is normally provided by order of the patient's personal doctor or attending physician. A progress note or plan is not the same as an order. Before initiating any therapeutic or diagnostic procedure, you need to check to see that a valid physician order is present.

Table 9-6 Counseling and Behavioral Therapies for Smoking Cessation

Component	Discussion Points or Suggestions
Practical Counseling (Problem-Solving/Skills Training) Treatment	
Identify events, internal states, or activities that increase the risk of smoking or relapse.	• Negative effect • Being around other smokers • Drinking alcohol • Experiencing urges • Being under time pressure
Identify and practice coping or problem-solving skills. Typically, these skills are intended to cope with danger situations.	• Learning to anticipate and avoid temptation • Learning cognitive strategies that will reduce negative moods • Accomplishing lifestyle changes that reduce stress, improve quality of life, or produce pleasure • Learning cognitive and behavioral activities to cope with smoking urges (e.g., distracting attention)
Provide basic information about smoking and successful quitting.	• The fact that any smoking (even a single puff) increases the likelihood of full relapse • Withdrawal symptoms typically peak within 1–3 weeks after quitting • Withdrawal symptoms include negative mood, urges to smoke, and difficulty concentrating • The addictive nature of smoking
Intra-Treatment Supportive Interventions	
Encourage the patient in the quit attempt.	• Note that effective tobacco dependence treatments are now available • Note that half of all people who have ever smoked have now quit • Communicate belief in patient's ability to quit
Communicate caring and concern.	• Ask how patient feels about quitting • Directly express concern and willingness to help • Be open to the patient's expression of fears of quitting, difficulties experienced, and ambivalent feelings

Encourage the patient to talk about the quitting process.	• Ask about:
	  • Reasons the patient wants to quit
	  • Concerns or worries about quitting
	  • Success the patient has achieved
	  • Difficulties encountered while quitting

Extra-Treatment Supportive Interventions	
Train patient in support solicitation skills.	• Show videotapes that model support skills • Practice requesting social support from family, friends, and coworkers • Aid patient in establishing a smoke-free home
Prompt support seeking.	• Help patient identify supportive others • Call the patient to remind him/her to seek support • Inform patient of community resources such as hotlines/helplines
Physician arranges outside support.	• Mail letters to supportive others • Call supportive others • Invite others to cessation sessions • Assign patients to be "buddies" for one another

9-2. **Correct answer: D.** Line out the error, write the word "error," and correct and initial it. The ventilator flow sheet is part of the patient record and represents a legal document. Consequently, whenever errors are detected, the error should be lined out, the word "error" should be noted, the corrected information should be given, and the therapist correcting the error should write his or her initials.

9-3. **Correct answer: D.** Whenever a limit or boundary rule takes effect. When implementing a protocol, you must know the limits (also called boundaries) within which you are permitted to make independent adjustments, as well as know what conditions require physician notification. In general, if your assessment indicates that the patient's response strays outside any of the protocol's defined boundaries, you cannot proceed until you notify the ordering physician and determine a new course of action.

9-4. **Correct answer: C.** Contact the ordering physician for clarification. The minimum requirements for a proper prescription for respiratory care-related drugs include the following: (1) the drug name, (2) the drug dosage/concentration, (3) the frequency of administration, (4) the route of administration, and (5) the signature of the prescribing physician. Always seek clarification from the patient's physician if the order does not specify this necessary information.

9-5. **Correct answer: D.** Recording information in the patient's chart. The patient's chart is an official record of their ongoing progress and course of treatment. Consequently, the best way to routinely communicate a patient's clinical status is by accurately recording all essential information in the patient's medical record.

9-6. **Correct answer: D.** I, II, and III. When noting an adverse change in a patient's condition, the therapist should notify the nurse, contact the physician (if a therapy change is warranted), and record the reaction in the patient's chart. If the patient becomes unstable due to the adverse change, the therapist should also stay with the patient until he or she is stable or help arrives. Recording this information in the medical record is a very important part of making sure that vital patient information is communicated among all health care professionals providing care to the patient.

9-7. **Correct answer: D.** I, II, and III. If any adverse reaction is noted to a patient receiving therapy, the treatment should initially be stopped, the patient assessed, the problem corrected. Once the patient is stable, the therapy can be completed. All of these points should be recorded in the patient's medical record.

9-8. **Correct answer: A.** Call for the institution's rapid response team. Any unexpected response to therapy or adverse effects noted when charting a patient encounter should also be communicated orally to the patient's physician and nurse. In general, the more serious the problem, the sooner these key people should be informed. However, if it is clear that the patient's vital signs are deteriorating, do not wait to inform the doctor. Instead, call for your institution's rapid response team.

9-9. **Correct answer: A.** Notify the nurse in charge and chart the patient's refusal. When a patient is intent on refusing treatment, the nurse should be notified immediately and the refusal must be noted in the patient's medical record.

9-10. **Correct answer: C.** Patient states, "I'm short of breath." Color of sputum can be verified by others and should appear in the Objective portion of the SOAP. "Not tolerating weaning" is a qualitative judgment and therefore belongs in the Analysis portion of a SOAP. "Perform another ABG after next attempt" is a statement that fits best in the Plan portion of the SOAP.

POST-TEST

A post-test for this chapter that includes automated scoring and feedback is available on the accompanying CD. Be sure to complete this additional assessment to confirm your mastery of this chapter's objectives.

REFERENCES

American Association for Respiratory Care. (n.d.). Guidelines for preparing a respiratory care protocol (RC protocol). Retrieved October 10, 2008, from http://www.aarc.org/members_area/resources/protocol_guidelines.html

American Association for Respiratory Care. (1992). Clinical practice guideline. Patient-ventilator system checks. *Respiratory care, 37*, 882–886.

American Association for Respiratory Care. (1997). Respiratory care standard abbreviations and symbols. *Respiratory care, 42*, 637-642.

Fiore, M. C., Baker, T. B., Jaén, C. R., et al. (2008). *Treating tobacco use and dependence: 2008 update*. Rockville, MD: U.S. Department of Health and Human Services, Public Health Service.

Institute for Safe Medication Practices. (2008). List of error-prone abbreviations, symbols and dose designations. Retrieved October 1, 2008, from http://www.ismp.org/tools/errorproneabbreviations.pdf

Institute of Medicine. (1991). *The computer-based patient record: An essential technology for health care*. Washington, DC: National Academy Press.

Joint Commission. (2007). *2008 National patient safety goals*. Chicago: Joint Commission.

Mallin, R. (2002). Smoking cessation: Integration of behavioral and drug therapies. *American family physician, 65*, 1108–1114, 2002.

Piper, M. E., Fox, B. J., Fiore, M. C. (2001). Strategies for smoking cessation. *Pulmonary and Critical Care Update, Lesson 13, Volume 15*.

University of California San Diego, Respiratory Services. (2008). *Respiratory care patient-driven protocols* (3rd ed.). Dallas, TX: Daedalus Enterprises.

Weed, L. L. (1970). *Medical records, medical education, and patient care: The problem-oriented record as a basic tool*. Chicago: Year Book Medical Publishers.

Wilkins, R. L., Stoller, J. K., & Kacmarek, R. M. (Eds.). (2009). *Egan's fundamentals of respiratory care* (9th ed.). St. Louis: Mosby.

Wood, L. A., & Rambo, B. J. (1977). *Nursing skills for allied health services*. (2nd ed.). Philadelphia: W. B. Saunders.

CHAPTER

10

Maintain Patent Airway/ Care of Artificial Airways

Salomay R. Corbaley
Craig L. Scanlan

INTRODUCTION

As indicated in the ABC's of resuscitation, maintaining a patent airway and caring for artificial airways are critical components of good respiratory care. It is for this reason that the NBRC devotes a specific section of the CRT exam to this topic. If you have not had much experience in this area, then you need to concentrate on this chapter. You must be familiar with the many types of artificial airways available and how to properly place, maintain, and remove these devices. In addition, since maintenance of normal airway function depends on proper humidification, you also need to be proficient in this area.

OBJECTIVES

After completion of this chapter, you should demonstrate the knowledge needed to:

1. Properly position a patient
2. Insert oro- and nasopharyngeal airways
3. Perform endotracheal intubation
4. Assess tube placement
5. Maintain position in the airway and appropriate cuff inflation of:
   a. Endotracheal tube
   b. Tracheostomy tube
   c. Laryngeal mask airway (LMA)
   d. Esophageal-tracheal Combitube®
6. Perform tracheostomy care
7. Change tracheostomy tubes
8. Maintain adequate humidification
9. Perform extubation

WHAT TO EXPECT ON THIS CATEGORY OF THE CRT EXAM

Number of questions: 7
Level of questions: about 30% recall, 30% application, 40% analysis

WHAT'S NEW FOR 2009

As of July 2009, this section of the NBRC CRT examination includes the following *new content areas*:

- Performing endotracheal intubation
- Laryngeal mask airway (LMA)
- Esophageal-tracheal Combitube®
- Performing tracheostomy care

PRE-TEST

Carefully respond to each of the following questions. After completing the pre-test, compare your answers with those provided at the end of this chapter. Then thoroughly review each answer's explanation to help understand why it is correct.

10-1. A patient suddenly loses consciousness. Which of the following is the first procedure you should perform to maintain an open airway in this patient?
A. Inserting a laryngeal mask airway
B. Applying the "jaw thrust" maneuver
C. Inserting an oropharyngeal airway
D. Applying the "head-tilt/chin-lift" maneuver

10-2. A patient in the intensive care unit exhibits signs of acute upper airway obstruction and is concurrently having severe seizures that make it impossible to open the mouth. In this case, what is the adjunct airway of choice?
A. Oral endotracheal tube
B. Nasopharyngeal airway
C. Tracheostomy tube
D. Oropharyngeal airway

10-3. An oropharyngeal airway is *least* appropriate for a patient who:
A. Is having seizures
B. Requires manual ventilation
C. Is conscious and alert
D. Is heavily sedated

10-4. When ventilating a patient with a bag-valve resuscitator through a laryngeal mask airway (LMA), you note significant air leakage. Which of the following should be your first approach to eliminating this leakage?
A. Bag slowly to reduce peak pressure
B. Add more air to LMA the cuff
C. Pull the tube out 2–3 cm
D. Lower the cuff pressure

10-5. Which of the following should be prescribed in order to provide adequate humidification to an intubated patient?
A. Inspired gas with 100% relative humidity
B. Inspired gas with an absolute humidity greater than 30 mg/L
C. Inspired gas through a cold bubble humidifier
D. Tracheobronchial suctioning

10-6. When checking for proper placement of an endotracheal tube in an adult patient on chest X-ray, it is noted that the distal tip of the tube is 3 cm above the carina. Which of the following actions is appropriate?
A. None, since the tube is properly positioned in the trachea
B. Withdraw the tube by 4–5 cm (using tube markings as a guide)
C. Withdraw the tube by 1–2 cm (using tube markings as a guide)
D. Advance the tube by 1–2 cm (using tube markings as a guide)

10-7. After insertion of a esophageal-tracheal Combitube®, you begin ventilation through the #1 pharyngeal airway connection. Your partner reports an absence of breath sounds and the presence of gurgling over the epigastrium. In order to provide effective ventilation, you should:
A. Deflate the large (#1) cuff
B. Withdraw the Combitube® 3–4 cm
C. Ventilate through the other (#2) tube
D. Deflate the small (#2) cuff

10-8. Significant overinflation of an endotracheal tube cuff may cause which of the following?
   A. Laryngospasm
   B. Tissue damage
   C. Tachycardia
   D. Stridor

10-9. Which of the following devices are contraindicated for a patient whose upper airway has been bypassed?
   A. A hygroscopic condenser humidifier
   B. A heated large-volume jet nebulizer
   C. A simple bubble humidifier
   D. A heated cascade humidifier

10-10. The methylene blue test is used to confirm:
   A. "Leakage" type aspiration
   B. Tracheal granuloma
   C. Infection
   D. Artificial airway obstruction

WHAT YOU NEED TO KNOW: ESSENTIAL CONTENT

Position Patients Properly

Proper patient positioning is an essential component of emergency airway management. Proper patient positioning is also important in preventing ventilator-associated pneumonia (VAP) and managing conditions that cause hypoxemia or abnormally increase the production of respiratory tract secretions. **Table 10-1** summarizes the various conditions in which special patient positioning may be required and the rationale for each.

Insert Oro- and Nasopharyngeal Airways

During resuscitation efforts, if you cannot establish a patent airway by proper positioning, then you will need to consider inserting an artificial airway. In this situation, the two most common artificial airways used are the oropharyngeal and nasopharyngeal airways.

Oropharyngeal Airways

Oropharyngeal airways are used during resuscitation to prevent upper airway obstruction when providing bag-valve-mask ventilation. These devices also may be used as a "bite block" in intubated patients who are heavily sedated or unconscious. In addition, oropharyngeal airways may be indicated in patients who are having a seizure or when a comatose patient develops upper airway occlusion.

Selecting an Appropriate-Sized Oropharyngeal Airway
- Preliminary selection should be based on patient's age or size (refer to **Table 10-2** on page 282).
- Tailor the size to the patient by measuring from the corner of the mouth to the angle of the jaw.
- An airway that is too large or too small can worsen airway obstruction.

Inserting and Securing Oropharyngeal Airways
- Insert either with the distal tip pointing up or from the side.
- Advance the device to the base of the tongue.
- Rotate the airway into place so that it holds the tongue away from the back of the pharynx.
- The airway should always be placed midline into the patient's mouth.
- Do not tape over the center opening of the airway (the opening can be used to pass a suction catheter).

Troubleshooting Oropharyngeal Airways
- If airway obstruction due to the tongue is not relieved:
  ○ Remove the airway and reinsert, making sure it extends past the base of the tongue and is not pressing the tongue into the airway.

Table 10-1 Conditions Necessitating Special Patient Positions

Condition or Situation	Position	Rationale
Resuscitation	Head-tilt/chin-lift maneuver (all rescuers)	Helps displace the tongue away from the posterior pharyngeal wall
	Jaw thrust without head extension (health care provider)	Minimizes neck movement in patients with suspected cervical spine injury
	Recovery position (lateral recumbent) with victim placed on side and with the lower arm in front of the body	Helps maintain a patent airway and reduces the risk of airway obstruction and aspiration in unresponsive adults with normal breathing and effective circulation
Endotracheal intubation	"Sniffing" position (i.e., neck hyperextended with pillow or towel under the head)	Aligns upper airway structures with larynx and trachea, facilitating tube insertion; *not* to be used with suspected cervical spine injury
Prevent VAP	Elevating the head of the bed 30° or more (unless contraindicated)	Helps prevent gastric reflux aspiration and improves the distribution of ventilation and the efficiency of diaphragmatic action
ARDS	Prone position (consider only if ARDS ventilator protocol cannot provide satisfactory oxygenation)	Recruits collapsed lung units and shifts blood flow away from shunt regions, thus improving V/Q balance and oxygenation
Unilateral lung disease	Left or right lateral decubitus position with the good lung down[a]	Improves oxygenation by diverting most blood flow and ventilation to the dependent (good) lung
Postural drainage	Varies according to lobe or segment being drained (see Chapter 11 for details)	Vertical alignment of the lobar or segmental bronchus facilitates drainage into the mainstem bronchi for removal by coughing or suctioning
Directed coughing	Sitting or semi-Fowler's position, with knees slightly flexed, forearms relaxed, feet supported	Aids exhalation and facilitates thoracic compression during coughing

a. Exceptions to the "keep the good lung down" rule include lung abscess or bleeding, in which the good lung normally is kept in the up position to prevent blood or pus from entering the good lung. Likewise, in infants with unilateral pulmonary interstitial emphysema (PIE), the good lung normally is kept in the up position.

- ○ Recheck the size of the airway:
  - • If the airway is too long, it will block the airway itself.
  - • If it is too short, it can force the tongue back against the posterior pharynx.
- • If the patient gags or otherwise does not tolerate the airway, remove the airway immediately to avoid vomiting.
  - ○ Maintain the airway by repositioning the head.
  - ○ Make sure the airway is not too small, as it can slip into the throat and cause obstruction.

Table 10-2 Recommended Sizes for Oro- and Nasopharyngeal Airways Based on Patient's Age or Size

Patient Age or Size	Oropharyngeal Airway	Nasopharyngeal Airway
Premature infant	40 mm/00	n/a
Newborn–1 year	50 mm/0	n/a
1–3 years	60 mm/1	n/a
3–6 years	60 mm/1	n/a
8 years	70 mm/2	n/a
12 years	70 mm/2	5 (20 Fr)
16 years	80 mm/3	6 (24 Fr)
Adult female	80 mm/3	6 (24 Fr)
Adult male	90 mm/4	7 (28 Fr)
Large adult	100 mm/5	8–9 (32–36 Fr)

Nasopharyngeal Airways

A nasopharyngeal airway also is used during resuscitation to prevent upper airway obstruction, most often when an oropharyngeal airway is contraindicated. These situations include mouth or jaw trauma, or when the patient is conscious. Nasopharyngeal airways are also indicated when a patient exhibits acute upper airway obstruction and is having severe seizures that prevent opening the mouth. Last, a nasopharyngeal airway is a good option to prevent trauma in patients requiring frequent nasotracheal suctioning.

Selecting an Appropriate-Sized Nasopharyngeal Airway
- Preliminary selection should be based on patient's age or size (refer to Table 10-2).
- Tailor the size to the patient by measuring from the nares to the earlobe.
- Select the largest diameter will fit into the inferior meatus without being forced.

Inserting and Securing Nasopharyngeal Airways
- Prior to inserting a nasopharyngeal airway, you may want to advance a suction catheter through the nose to determine which side is more patent.
- You need to lubricate the device with water-soluble gel before inserting.
- The patient's head should be tilted slightly backward.
- Follow the *floor* of the nasal passage and insert with the bevel facing medially.
- Do not force the airway past nasal obstructions; you may find that a slight rotating action will facilitate advancement through a tight opening.
- Once inserted, a safety pin attached to the flange can prevent slippage into the nose.
- When suctioning through a nasopharyngeal airway:
  - Secure the end of the airway to prevent it from moving back and forth.
  - Always lubricate the suction catheter.
- Never lavage through a nasopharyngeal airway.

Troubleshooting Nasopharyngeal Airways
- If the airway will not pass through the selected nostril/naris:
  - Make sure the airway is well lubricated.
  - Try the patient's other nostril/naris.
  - Try a smaller-diameter airway.
  - The patient may have a deviated septum.

- If a suction catheter will not pass through the airway:
  - Lubricate the catheter with water-soluble gel.
  - Remove and reinsert the airway in the other nostril/naris.
  - Replace the airway with a larger one.
- If swelling of the nasal mucosa narrows the airway passage, do not try to replace the airway; notify the physician.

Hazards and Complications

- Nasopharyngeal airways normally are *not* used in children under 12 years of age.
- You should not insert a nasopharyngeal airway if the patient has nasal trauma, or if the nasal passages are blocked or damaged (e.g., for a patient with a deviated septum).
- If the patient experiences excessive bleeding or tissue trauma, notify the physician.

Endotracheal Intubation

In the NBRC hospital, respiratory therapists must be skilled in endotracheal intubation. For this reason, you can expect to see several questions on this procedure on the CRT exam, either in this section or in Chapter 18 (Act as an Assistant to the Physician Performing Special Procedures). The difference is that in this section of the exam the focus is on you performing the procedure independently, whereas Chapter 18 questions concentrate on assisting with the procedure.

Intubation Equipment

The first step in performing endotracheal intubation is gathering and confirming the function of necessary equipment. Chapter 6 summarizes the general indications for, selection, use, and troubleshooting of endotracheal tubes. The accompanying box lists the key equipment involved.

Equipment Needed for Routine Endotracheal Intubation

CDC barrier precautions (e.g., gloves, gowns, masks, eyewear)

towels (for positioning)

stethoscope

oxygen flowmeter and connecting tubing

bag-valve-mask (BVM) manual resuscitator

vacuum source/suction apparatus (e.g., regulator, portable pump)

suction catheters (e.g., flexible suction catheters, Yankauer tip)

local anesthetic spray*

water-soluble lubricating jelly*

laryngoscopes (2) with assorted blades, batteries, and bulbs*

endotracheal tubes (at least 3 different sizes)*

stylet(s)*

Magill forceps*

syringe*

devices used to confirm placement (e.g., EDD, CO_2 detector, light wand)

tape and/or ET tube holders(s)*

oropharyngeal airways and/or bite blocks*

*Typically included on an intubation tray.

The size of tubes available on the intubation tray depends on the patient's age and/or size.

Table 10-3 specifies the recommended endotracheal (ET) tube sizes for the full range of patients you will encounter, as well as their normal insertion lengths. You should select an appropriate-size tube, but have available at least one size larger and one size smaller. Note that you normally select a cuffed

Table 10-3 Recommended Endotracheal Tube Sizes and Insertion Lengths Based on Patient's Age or Size

Patient Age of Size	ET Tube (mm ID[a])	ET Tube length cm[b]
Premature infant	2.5–3.0 uncuffed	9–11
Newborn–1 year	3.0–4.0 uncuffed	11–12
1–3 years	4.0 uncuffed	11–13
3 yrs	4.5 uncuffed	12–14
5 yrs	5.0 uncuffed	13–15
6 yrs	5.5 uncuffed	14–16
8 yrs	6.0 cuffed	15–17
12 yrs	6.5 cuffed	17–19
16 yrs	7.0 cuffed	18–20
Adult female	7.0–8.0 cuffed	19–21
Adult male	8.0–9.0 cuffed	21–23
Large adult	8.5+ cuffed	23+

a. ID = internal or inside diameter.
b. From incisors to tube tip in trachea; for the nasotracheal route (adults), add 2 cm to insertion length.

tube (6.0 mm and larger) for intubating adults and children down to about 8 years old. *Use uncuffed tubes (< 6.0 mm) for smaller children, toddlers, and infants.*

Table 10-4 provides more detail on the accessory equipment needed for endotracheal intubation, including its selection, use, and troubleshooting.

Intubation Procedure

The accompanying box outlines the basic steps in orotracheal intubation. The nasotracheal route is discouraged because (1) the incidence of VAP and other infections (sinusitis and otitis media) is higher; (2) smaller/longer ET tubes are required, which increases airway resistance; and (3) necrosis of the nasal septum and external meatus may occur.

Table 10-4 Accessory Equipment Needed for Endotracheal Intubation

Description	Selection and Use	Troubleshooting
Laryngoscope		

• Used to visualize the glottis
• Consists of a handle with batteries and a blade with a light source
	• Curved/MacIntosh blade inserted into vallecula at base of tongue; lifts epiglottis indirectly
	• Straight/Miller blade positioned directly under the epiglottis, which is directly lifted
	• Blade selection based on personal preference (most clinician use a straight blade for infants)
	• Size based on age: premi: 0; infant: 1; 3–12 mo: 1–1½; child: 2; adult: 3; large adult: 4
		• To prevent aspiration, always confirm that the light bulb is tightly screwed in (not necessary with fiberoptic scopes)
		• If the bulb does not light:
		  • Recheck the handle/blade connection, then
		  • Replace the blade, then
		  • Replace the batteries, then
		  • Check/replace the bulbs

(continues)

Table 10-4 Accessory Equipment Needed for Endotracheal Intubation (continued)

Description	Selection and Use	Troubleshooting
Stylet		
• Adds rigidity and maintain the shape of an ET tube during insertion	• Used only for oral intubation	• To prevent trauma, make sure stylet tip does not extend beyond ET tube tip; either: • Use stylet flange OR • Bend stylet at right angle at the ET tube adaptor
McGill Forceps		
• Used to manipulate the ET tube during nasal intubation by direct visualization	• Once the tip of the ET tube is in the oropharynx, insert the laryngoscope, and visualize the glottis • Use the forceps to grasp the tube just above the cuff and direct it between the cords	• To prevent trauma, never use forceps without direct visualization and avoid forceful movements
Squeeze-Bulb EDD		
• Self-inflating rubber bulb with 15-mm ID connector used to detect esophageal intubation • Not recommended for children < 1 year old	• Connect squeezed bulb to ET tube • If bulb quickly re-expands the tube is in an airway • If the bulb does not re-expand, tube is in esophagus	• Re-expansion does not confirm tracheal placement; always check breath sounds and confirm with X-ray
Colorimetric CO_2 Detector		
• Disposable CO_2 indicator used to confirm ET tube placement in airway	• Select correct type based on patient size/weight • Place between the ET tube and BVM • Correct tube position indicated when indicator changes color from purple to tan/yellow as patient is ventilated	• Failure to change color can occur even with proper tube position during cardiac arrest (false negative) • Color change can occur with improper tube placement in mainstem bronchus (false positive)
Light Wand		
• A flexible stylet with a lighted bulb at the tip passed with ET tube to confirm placement in trachea	• Characteristic glow (the "jack-o'-lantern" effect) under the skin confirms placement in trachea • No glow is observed if the tube is in the esophagus	• Does not confirm tracheal placement; always check breath sounds and confirm with X-ray
Bite Block/Tube Holder		
• Stabilizes oral ET tube, prevents biting on tube, minimizes tube movement/ accidental extubation	• Options include: • Oropharyngeal airway taped to ET tube • Flanged plastic tub holder with straps	• Gagging response may require sedation • Can make provision of oral care difficult

---

Basic Procedure for Orotracheal Intubation

Equipment and Patient Preparation

1. Verify, interpret, and evaluate doctor's order or protocol
2. Select, gather, assemble, and check the required equipment
3. Decontaminate hands and apply standard/transmission-based precautions as appropriate
4. Identify patient, introduce self and department
5. Provide for sedation/topical anesthetic or vasocontrictor, if indicated
6. Test laryngoscope and endotracheal tube cuff
7. Lubricate endotracheal tube/stylet

Assessment and Implementation

8. Assess patient
9. Position patient in sniffing position
10. Clear airway
11. Anesthetize airway
12. Hyperoxygenate patient
13. Insert laryngoscope into the oropharynx
14. Expose and lift epiglottis; visualize cords
15. Insert ET tube between the vocal cords until cuff disappears (2–3 cm beyond cords)
16. Inflate the cuff using minimal leak or minimal occluding volume method
17. Provide ventilation and 100% O_2
18. Observe, auscultate chest for symmetrical ventilation; auscultate epigastrium
19. Verify tube placement (breath sounds, chest wall movement, EDD, CO_2 detector, light wand)

Follow-up

20. Hyperoxygenate between attempts if necessary
21. Mark proximal end of tube
22. Secure and stabilize tube
23. Aspirate trachea
24. Provide postintubation care
25. Place patient on appropriate oxygen/humidification/ventilation device
26. Provide for postintubation chest X-ray
27. Reposition tube, if needed
28. Maintain/process equipment
29. Dispose of infectious waste and decontaminate hands
30. Record pertinent data in chart and departmental records
31. Notify appropriate personnel and make any needed recommendations or modifications to patient care plan

---

Key considerations related to ET tube placement include the following:

- To test the ET tube cuff, either observe for deflation over several minutes or immerse the tube in sterile saline and observe for air leakage.
- During oral intubation of an adult, the ET tube should be advanced into the trachea until the cuff has passed the vocal cords by 2–3 cm.

- The tip of an ET tube should be positioned in the trachea about 4–6 cm above the carina (use of light wand can help verify position).
- The average length from the teeth (incisors) to the tip of a properly positioned oral ET tube in adult males is between 21 and 23 cm, and 19 and 21 cm in adult females.
- After tube passage and cuff inflation, listen for equal and bilateral breath sounds and look for chest wall motion while the patient is being manually ventilated by bag.
- Air movement or gurgling sounds over the epigastrium indicate possible esophageal intubation.
- Decreased breath sounds and chest movement on the left side indicate that right mainstem bronchial intubation may have occurred.
- To correct right mainstem intubation, withdraw the tube slowly and listen for the return of left-side breath sounds.
- Consider using a squeeze-bulb esophageal detection device, colorimetric CO_2 detector, or light wand to assess tube placement.
- If the suction catheter will not pass when aspirating the trachea after tube placement, the tube may be kinked or have become displaced from the trachea.
- There are only two ways to confirm proper tube placement: chest X-ray or fiberoptic laryngoscopy; on the X-ray, the tube tip should be positioned about 4–6 cm above the carina, usually between thoracic vertebrae T2 and T4.
- Because the ET tube tip moves up and down as the patient's head and neck moves, you should also check the position of the head and neck when reviewing an X-ray for tube placement.
- If the ET tube is malpositioned, remove the tape and reposition the tube, using the cm markings as a guide, and confirm the new position via either a chest X-ray or fiberoptic laryngoscopy.

Tracheotomy

Tracheotomy is a surgical procedure that creates an opening, or *stoma*, through the neck tissues and into the trachea, normally below the cricoid cartilage. The stoma is created either by surgical incision or percutaneous dilation. The most common indications for tracheotomy are the need for long-term positive pressure ventilation or the need for a permanent artificial airway.

Standard Tracheostomy Tubes

Tracheostomy tubes are placed through a stoma into the trachea and secured around the neck. Tracheostomy tubes (also called trach tubes) are sized by *internal diameter* (ID) in millimeters (mm) using the International Standards Organization (ISO) diameter-based system. **Table 10-5** provides general guidelines for trach tube selection based on the ISO sizing system. Note that most trach tubes designed for infants and small children (ISO size 5 or smaller) have too narrow an ID to hold an inner cannula.

When a doctor selects a trach tube for a patient, primary consideration is given to the outside diameter, especially for cuffed tubes. In general, *a trach tube's OD needs to be no more than two-thirds to three-quarters of the internal diameter of the trachea*. A bigger tube will impede airflow through the upper airway when the cuff is deflated, while a smaller tube may require unacceptably high cuff pressures to achieve an adequate seal.

Key points in the placement and management of standard tracheostomy tubes include the following:

- To ease insertion and to guard against cuff perforation from sharp edges of cartilage, the trach cuff should be tapered back by using the fingers to gently "milk" it away from the distal tip of the outer cannula as it its deflated.
- When a trach tube is inserted, a blunt obturator is placed in the tube.
  - The rounded end of the obturator extends beyond the tube tip, thus preventing tissue trauma ("snowplowing") during insertion.
  - The obturator is removed immediately after tube insertion.
  - The obturator should be kept at the bedside in case the tube comes out and needs to be reinserted.

Table 10-5 Common Tracheostomy Tube Sizes

Patient Age or Size	ISO Size[a]	ID without inner cannula (mm)	Approximate ID with inner cannula (mm)[b]	Approximate OD (mm)[b]
Premature infant	2.5	2.5	n/a	4.5
Newborn infant	3.0	3.0	n/a	5.0
	3.5	3.5	n/a	5.5
Toddler/small child	4.0	4.0	n/a	6.0
School-age child	4.5	4.5	n/a	7.0
	5	5	n/a	7.5
Adolescent/small adult	6	6	4–5	8.5
	7	7	5–6	9–10
Adult	8	8	6–7	10–11
	9	9	7–8	11–12
Large adult	10	10	8–9	13–14

a. ISO standards require that both ID without inner cannula and its OD in mm be display on neck plate.

b. Dimensions vary somewhat by manufacturer.

- The flange at the proximal end of some trach tubes can be adjusted to customize the fit of the tube and assure proper placement of the distal end in the trachea (generally needed for severely obese patients or those with abnormally thick necks).
  - Tape or use hook-and-loop ties attached to the flange and around the patient's neck to secure the tube in place.
  - Ties should be changed as needed, for comfort and cleanliness.
- As with ET tubes, placement of tracheal tubes should be verified by X-ray (a radiopaque material is embedded in the tube).
- If the trach tube has an inner cannula, slide it into the outer cannula and lock it into place to complete the airway.
  - The inner cannula has a standard 15-mm OD connector for respiratory equipment.
  - To prevent disconnection of the inner cannula, accidental extubation, or tracheal damage, always avoid pulling on or rocking the inner-cannula connection to respiratory equipment.
  - The inner cannula periodically should be removed and cleaned to prevent obstruction by secretions.
  - A correctly sized spare inner cannula (and spare tubes in the same size and one size smaller) should *always* be kept at the bedside.

Providing Tracheotomy Care

Optimum care of patients with artificial tracheal airways involves provision of adequate humidification, suctioning as needed, and regular cuff management, all discussed subsequently. For patients with trach tubes, the NBRC also expects that you be skilled in basic tracheostomy care. In general, you should provide tracheostomy care whenever the stoma dressing becomes soiled. Key considerations involved when providing tracheotomy care include the following:

A. Equipment and supplies needed (most items provided in trach care kits):
1. Replacement inner cannula (properly sized)
2. Clean tracheostomy ties or a replacement hook-and-loop tube holder
3. Pre-cut sterile tracheostomy dressing (do NOT cut a plain gauze pad, as the fibers may be aspirated into the airway)
4. Sterile trach brush or sterile pipe cleaners

5. Sterile cotton-tipped applicators
6. Sterile gauze pads
7. ½-strength hydrogen peroxide
8. Sterile basin
B. Basic procedure:
1. Remove old dressing, being careful to keep tracheostomy tube in place
2. Clean around tube at stoma site with the hydrogen peroxide solution
3. Remove the inner cannula and insert its replacement
    a. Clean the inner cannula in hydrogen peroxide with the trach brush or pipe cleaners
    b. Rinse the inner cannula thoroughly with sterile water
    c. Dry the inner cannula using a sterile gauze sponge
4. Replace the inner cannula
5. Place a clean tracheostomy dressing under the flange (insert from below)
6. Change the tube ties/holder as necessary
    a. While changing the tube ties or holders, *always have a second person hold the tube in place*
    b. *Never* tie tracheostomy ties with a bow; instead, *always use a square knot*
7. Ensure that the tube is secured in the proper position

Changing Tracheostomy Tubes

In addition to providing trach care, in the NBRC hospital you are expected to be skilled in changing these tubes in patients with established stomas. A tube change is indicated if the cuff is damaged and cannot be inflated or if the physician wants to switch to a different-size or different-type tube, e.g., a fenestrated or "talking" tube. Key points to remember when changing a trach tube are outlined in the accompanying box.

Key Steps in Changing a Tracheostomy Tube

1. Perform a surgical hand scrub

2. Follow appropriate barrier precautions, including use of sterile gloves

3. Suction the patient before deflating the cuff

    a. First remove accumulated secretions above the cuff

    b. Then perform tracheal aspiration

4. Open the new trach tube box, removing the tube and placing it on a sterile field

5. Check the tube for cuff leaks; deflate the cuff completely while "tapering" it back toward the flange

6. Attach new, clean tracheostomy ties

7. Remove the inner cannula, insert the obturator, and lubricate the tube/obturator tip

8. Position the patient in semi-Fowler's position with the neck slightly extended

9. Loosen or untie the old ties and deflate the cuff fully

10. Remove the oxygen or humidity therapy device

11. Remove the old trach tube

12. Visually inspect the stoma for bleeding or infection

13. Insert the new tube with a slightly downward motion

14. Remove the obturator and insert the inner cannula

15. Inflate the cuff if ordered, ensure proper placement, and secure the tube in place

16. Restore the patient to the previous oxygen or humidity therapy device

---

Specialized Tracheostomy Airways

This section of the CRT exam may also assess your knowledge of two specialized tracheostomy airways: the fenestrated tracheostomy tube and the tracheostomy button.

Fenestrated Tracheostomy Tubes

Fenestrated tracheostomy tubes are indicated to (1) facilitate weaning from a trach tube or (2) to support patients needing intermittent (e.g., nocturnal) ventilatory support. As illustrated in **Figure 10-1**, a fenestrated tracheotomy tube has an opening in the posterior wall of the outer cannula above the cuff. Removal of the inner cannula opens the fenestration. When the cuff is deflated and a cap is used to plug the tube's exterior opening, air can move freely between the trachea and upper airway through the fenestration and around the cuff. Removal of the plug allows access for suctioning, while reinsertion of the inner cannula closes the fenestration and allows for positive pressure ventilation.

Troubleshooting of fenestrated tracheostomy tubes is similar to that described for regular tracheostomy tubes. The most common problem with fenestrated tracheostomy tubes is malpositioning of the fenestration, such as between the skin and the stoma, or against the posterior wall of the trachea. This can result in respiratory distress when the tube is plugged and the cuff deflated. Repositioning the tube, as confirmed by fiberoptic bronchoscopy, solves this problem in most cases. Alternatively, if the tube has an adjustable flange, modifying its position can help align the fenestration in the middle of the trachea.

Respiratory distress also can occur if the tube cuff is not completely deflated prior to plugging its outer cannula. To avoid this problem:

- Always make sure that the cuff is fully deflated before plugging the tube
- Attach a warning tag to the tube cap/plug

With most fenestrated tubes, you should insert the inner cannula when suctioning the patient. This prevents the catheter from getting caught in the fenestration(s). Newer fenestrated tubes overcome this problem by providing multiple smaller openings as opposed to one large hole.

When soft tissues are obstructing the fenestration, you may feel resistance when inserting the inner cannula. To avoid tissue damage, never force the inner cannula during insertion. If you feel abnormal resistance when placing the inner cannula, withdraw it and notify the patient's physician immediately.

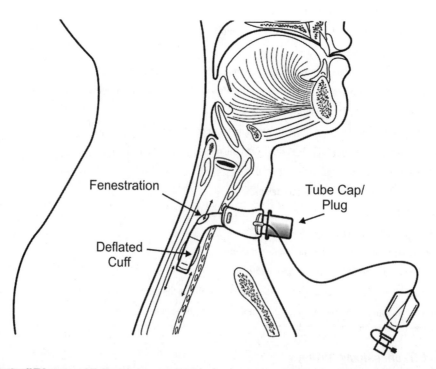

Fenestration

Tube Cap/ Plug

Deflated Cuff

Figure 10-1 "Plugged" Fenestrated Tracheostomy Tube in Place with Cuff Deflated.

Tracheostomy Buttons

Tracheostomy buttons are small tubes used to maintain an open stoma after the tracheostomy tube is removed. The patient can eat, breathe, and cough normally, but the stoma is available in case the airway needs to be reestablished quickly (i.e., to bypass laryngeal or upper airway obstruction, or for suctioning or ventilatory support). Regarding placement:

- The cannula is slightly flared at the outer end to prevent it slipping into the trachea.
- The inner end is flanged to keep it in place against the tracheal wall.
- Spacers of various widths are used to make sure the cannula is at the appropriate depth and does not obstruct the airway.
- A plug that fits into the cannula can be used to seal the button, forcing patient to breathe and cough normally via the upper airway.
- A standard 15-mm connection can be used to deliver positive pressure ventilation if needed; however, leakage through the nose and mouth must be overcome for ventilation to be effective.
- A one-way valve can be used to allow inspiration through the button but block expiration; when used properly, this valve allows the patient to talk, eat, and cough normally.

To avoid obstruction and assure patency of a trach button, one should regularly pass a suction catheter through the tube. If respiratory distress occurs when the plug is open, the tube is probably protruding too far into the trachea and will need to be repositioned by changing the number of spacers. As with fenestrated trach tubes, proper placement is confirmed using fiberoptic bronchoscopy.

Tracheal Airway Cuff Management

As previously indicated, optimum care of patients with artificial tracheal airways involves good cuff management. When cuff pressures exceeds 20–25 mm Hg, capillary blood flow is obstructed (ischemia), causing tissue ulceration and necrosis. When cuff pressures are too low, leakage-type aspiration can occur, which can cause pneumonia or pulmonary abscess. The goal is to achieve an adequate seal at the lowest possible pressure, ideally no higher than 20–25 mm Hg. The cuff management procedures most often used are the (1) minimal leak technique (MLT) and the (2) minimal occluding volume (MOV) method.

Equipment Needed

The following equipment is needed to adjust cuff pressures via either the MLT or MOV method:

- A three-way stopcock
- A 10- or 20-mL syringe
- A pressure manometer
- A stethoscope

Note that a commercially available bulb device that combines the functions of the stopcock, syringe, and pressure manometer is used in many institutions.

Key Elements in the Procedure

The following are the key elements involved in managing tracheal airway cuff pressures:

1. To avoid aspiration of supraglottic secretions when the cuff pressure is lowered, always suction the patient's pharynx before measuring the cuff pressure.
2. Attach the syringe and pressure manometer to the stopcock; the stopcock valve indicator should be positioned so that all three ports are open.
3. Attach the tapered stopcock port to the cuff's pilot tube valve, being sure that the valve opens and the connection is leak free.
4. With the stopcock open to the syringe, manometer, and cuff, you can add or remove air while observing the pressure changes on the manometer.
5. Place your stethoscope over the lateral surface of the upper trachea.
   a. If you hear gurgling or airflow at peak inspiratory pressure, slowly inflate the cuff until these sounds stop (indicating a leak-free seal).

- If a minimal leak is the goal (MLT):
  - Add just enough air to stop the sounds at peak inspiration.
  - Remove air while observing the pressure on the manometer until the sounds return at peak inspiration.
  - If the cuff pressure is less than 25 cm H_2O, you have achieved the desired minimal link.
- If the minimal occluding volume is the goal (MOV):
  - Add just enough air to stop the sounds at peak inspiration.
  - Observe/record the pressure on the manometer.

  b. If you hear no gurgling sounds during positive pressure breaths:
  - If a minimal leak is the goal (MLT):
    - Remove air while observing the pressure on the manometer until the sounds return at peak inspiration.
    - If the cuff pressure is less than 25 cm H_2O, you have achieved the desired minimal link.
  - If the minimal occluding volume is the goal (MOV):
    - Remove air until the sounds return at peak inspiration.
    - Add just enough air to stop the sounds at peak inspiration.
    - Observe/record the pressure on the manometer.

6. Enter/record on the patient record/flow sheet: the method used (MLT or MOV) and cuff pressure.

Note that some cuff management protocols require that you measure the volume leak. The volume leak is the difference between the patient's expired volume at MOV and that at the cuff inflation pressure corresponding to minimal leak. *Most of these protocols define a minimal leak as being less than 10% of the delivered volume.*

Additional fine points in the procedure that may appear on the CRT exam include the following:

- Simply attaching the measurement system to the pilot tube evacuates some volume from the cuff and lowers its pressure; for this reason, *you should always adjust the pressure to the desired level, never just measure it.*
- Most manometers used for cuff pressure management are calibrated in cm H_2O, not mm Hg.
  - 20–25 mm Hg (ischemia pressure) equals about 27–34 cm H_2O (factor = 1.36)
  - Most hospitals and the NBRC set 25 cm H_2O as the "high-end" pressure
- Any change in ventilator settings that alters peak inspiratory pressure will require a readjustment of the cuff pressure.
- Cuff pressures exceeding 20–25 mm Hg may occur when:
  - using high peak pressures
  - the tracheal tube is too small for the patient's airway
- Ideally, if you know in advance that higher pressures will be required to ventilate a patient, you should recommend a tracheal tube that provides a suction lumen above the cuff (a CASS tube).
- If the tracheal tube is too small, you can recommend replacing it with a larger one; otherwise you will have to keep pressures at or below 25 cm H_2O and tolerate any air leakage.

Recent research indicates that leakage aspiration around tracheal tube cuffs is a contributing factor to VAP. Based on this knowledge, many authors now recommend abandoning the MLT and instead using the MOV method. Others are recommending always maintaining cuff pressures at 20–25 cm H_2O. However, even at these pressures, folds that normally occur in low-pressure cuffs may still allow some leakage. For these reasons, the best approach is probably to use tracheal tubes that provide a suction lumen above the cuff (CASS tubes). When attached to a low-level vacuum (typically −20 mm Hg), these devices continuously aspirate subglottic secretions and may help prevent VAP.

Some clinicians also recommend recording and tracking the cuff inflation *volume* needed to achieve MOV or MLT. *Increases in inflation volume over time likely indicate tracheal dilation,* which can lead to permanent damage like tracheomalacia. Unfortunately, this technique requires completely emptying the cuff each time the measurement is made, which significantly increases the danger of aspiration. Since this hazard outweighs the potential benefits of this procedure, it is not recommended.

Some spontaneously breathing patients will have cuffed tracheal airways in place, usually tracheostomy tubes. Generally, these airways are used to protect the lower airway from aspiration and/or to allow for frequent tracheal suctioning. For these patients, cuff inflation pressures should be adjusted to the lowest pressure needed to prevent aspiration. To confirm that the cuff is inflated enough to prevent aspiration, perform the methylene blue test, normally done by order of the physician. To perform this test:

1. Inflate the cuff to the desired pressure
2. Have the patient swallows a small amount of methylene blue dye that has been added to water
3. Suction the patient's trachea through the artificial airway

You will know that aspiration is occurring if you obtain blue-tinged secretions during the suctioning. If you confirm aspiration, you must try to minimize it. The following approaches can be used:

- Perform oropharyngeal suctioning (above the tube cuff) as needed.
- During/after oral feeding, elevated the head of the bed and increase cuff pressure
- Switch the patient to a tracheal airway that continually aspirates subglottic secretions
- Insert a feeding tube into the duodenum (confirm its position by X-ray)

Alternative Cuff Designs

Several different cuff designs can help avoid pressure trauma to the tracheal mucosa. These include the Lanz and Kamen-Wilkinson tubes. The Lanz tube incorporates an external pressure-regulating valve and control reservoir designed to automatically maintain cuff pressure at approximately 30 cm H_2O. The Kamen-Wilkinson tube has a foam cuff that seals the trachea at atmospheric pressure. With the Kamen-Wilkinson tube:

- Prior to insertion, you *deflate* the cuff with a syringe and close off the pilot tube
- Once the tube is positioned properly in the trachea, you open the pilot tube to the atmosphere and allow the foam to expand against the tracheal wall

Troubleshooting Tracheal Airways

Basic troubleshooting of artificial airways is covered in Chapter 6. Here we cover three of the most critical problems in depth: (1) cuff leaks, (2) accidental extubation, and (3) an obstructed airway.

Cuff Leaks

Cuff leaks are among the most common serious problems with tracheal airways. On ventilator patients, a leak in the cuff itself, the pilot tube, or the one-way valve will result in a potentially large loss of delivered volume and/or inability to maintain the preset pressure limit. With both ventilator- and spontaneously breathing patients, cuff leaks also can lead to aspiration. Key points you need to address when dealing with leaks include the following:

- Small/slow leaks are evident when cuff pressure decrease between readings.
- Your first step is to try to reinflate the cuff, while checking the pilot tube and valve for leaks.
  - If the leak is at the one-way valve, attach a stopcock to its outlet.
  - If the leak is in the pilot tube, place a needle (with stopcock) in the pilot tube distal to the leak.
- Usually, one of these methods will allow you to reinflate the cuff and thus avoid reintubation.
- A large cuff leak ("blown cuff") makes it impossible to pressurize the cuff.
- A ventilator patient with a blown cuff will exhibit a large volume loss and/or drop in delivered inspiratory pressure and have decreased breath sounds as well as significant leakage/gurgling around the tube.
- A patient with a blown cuff normally requires reintubation. Using a tube exchanger will make oral reintubation easier for the patient.

Because the clinical signs of partial extubation are essentially the same as those observed with a blown cuff, do not recommend reintubation until you confirm that a cuff leak is the real problem.

- Before presuming a cuff leak, attempt to advance the tube slightly and reassess the leak and equality of breath sounds in both lung fields.
- Next, rule out or correct any pilot tube or valve leakage.
- Finally, try to measure the cuff pressure.
- If you cannot maintain cuff pressure (confirming a large leak), the patient must be reintubated.

Accidental Extubation

Accidental extubation (including self-extubation) can be minimized by attention to the following:

- The integrity of the securing tube tape or ties
- The avoidance of traction on the tube connector
- The adequacy of sedation
- The appropriate use of restraints

Accidental extubation can occur even with proper attention to these preventive measures. It can be partial or complete. As indicated previously, the clinical signs of partial extubation are essentially the same as those observed with a blown cuff. For this reason, the first step in dealing with this problem is to rule out a large cuff leak by quickly measuring the cuff pressure.

If partial extubation of an ET tube is confirmed, you should deflate the cuff, remove the securing tape, and try to reposition the tube back into the trachea. If this does not reestablish the airway, you'll need to extubate the patient, provide bag-and-mask ventilation with oxygen, then consider reintubation.

If accidental extubation occurs in a patient with a tracheostomy whose tract is fresh:

- Call the attending surgeon to replace the tube
- Occlude the stoma with a sterile petroleum jelly gauze pad
- Provide bag-and-mask ventilation with oxygen as needed

On the NBRC exam, if the stoma is well established, you are expected to obtain a sterile tube of the same size or one size smaller and follow the procedure for changing tracheostomy tubes.

Dealing with an Obstructed Airway

Tracheal tube obstruction can be caused by:

- Kinking of the tube
- Patient biting down on the tube (*ET tubes only*)
- Malpositioning of the tube tip against the tracheal wall (mainly trach tubes)
- Herniation of the cuff causing occlusion of the tube tip
- Compression of the tube due to cuff overinflation (mainly silicone ET tubes)
- Inspissated secretions, mucous, or blood clots plugging the tube lumen

Figure 10-2 provides a general algorithm for dealing with potential obstruction of ET or tracheostomy tubes in patients receiving ventilatory support. Typically, such patients will exhibit signs of severe respiratory distress. However, since many problems can cause respiratory distress—including a malfunctioning ventilator—*the first step is always to remove the patient from the ventilator, bag them manually with 100% O$_2$, and reassess the situation.* If no improvement is noted, you then progress through the algorithm, reassessing the adequacy of ventilation at each step.

Ultimately, you may reach the point at which the only viable solution is to remove the tube. Once you remove an obstructed tube, you should first try to reestablish ventilation and oxygenation, normally using a resuscitation bag and face mask. For trach patients, you may need to close off the stoma with a petroleum jelly gauze pad. Once the patient is stabilized, a new tube can be reinserted.

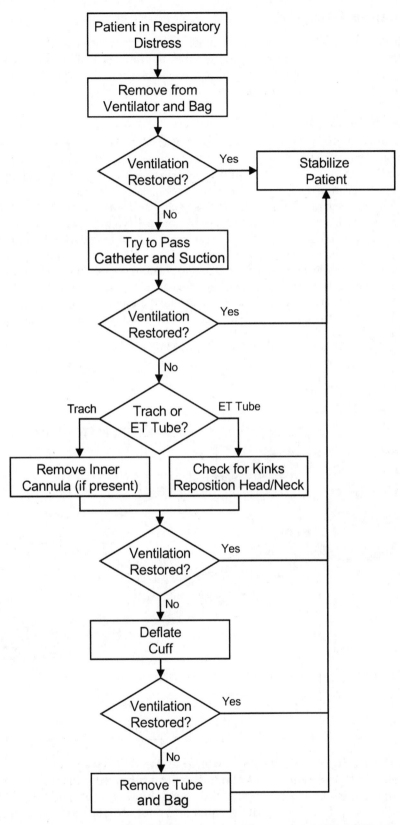

Figure 10-2 General Algorithm for Dealing with an Obstructed Artificial Tracheal Airway.

Alternative Emergency Airways

Oral endotracheal intubation is the procedure of choice in emergency situations requiring airway protection and artificial ventilation. However, effective with the July 2009 CRT exam administration, the NBRC expects you to be proficient with two alternative emergency airways: (1) the laryngeal mask airway and (2) the esophageal-tracheal Combitube®.

Laryngeal Mask Airway (LMA)

As depicted in **Figure 10-3**, a laryngeal mask airway (LMA) consists of a tube and mask with an inflatable cuff that is blindly inserted into the pharynx. When properly positioned and with the cuff inflated, the mask seals off the laryngeal inlet. This effectively bypasses the esophagus and provides a direct route for bag-valve ventilation via the standard 15-mm connector.

The LMA is used primarily by anesthesiologists as an alternative to endotracheal intubation during surgery. Because it allows rapid airway access without a laryngoscope, the LMA also is used for emergency airway management of unconscious patients in whom tracheal intubation cannot be performed or fails ("can't ventilate, can't intubate"). Because the LMA does not prevent aspiration, its use in emergency airway management must always take into account the potential risk of regurgitation. Unfortunately, the presence of a gastric tube does not eliminate and may even increase the risk of aspiration in patients with LMAs. For these reasons, when tracheal intubation cannot be performed and the risk of aspiration is known to be high, the esophageal-tracheal Combitube® may be a better choice.

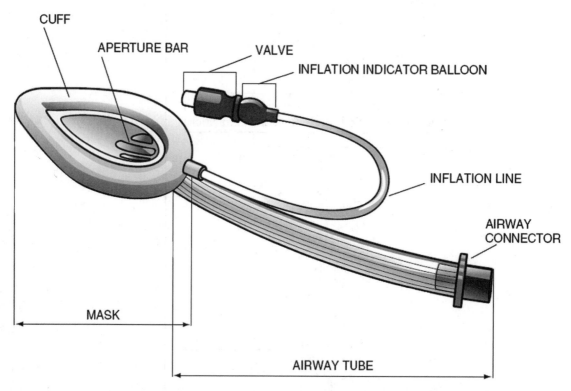

Figure 10-3 The Components of the Laryngeal Mask Airway (LMA). This device consists of a tube and mask with an inflatable cuff. The tube provides a standard 15 OD mm airway connector for attaching an anesthesia machine or ventilation equipment. The mask is inflated via an inflation line with a valve and pilot indicator balloon, much like those used on ET tubes. The mask portion fits into the pyriform sinus, over the opening into the larynx. The aperture bars, used mainly in the reusable versions, help prevent the epiglottis from obstructing the inlet to the mask.

Source: Courtesy of the Laryngeal Mask Company Limited, San Diego, CA.

You should avoid using the LMA to establish an emergency airway in patients who are conscious, who have intact gag reflexes, or who resist insertion. You also should avoid using an LMA in patients who will need tracheobronchial suctioning. The LMA should not be inserted in patients with trauma to or obstructive lesions of the mouth or pharynx. Last, the LMA is a poor choice in patients with decreased pulmonary or thoracic compliance who need positive pressure ventilation, since the high peak pressures required to ventilate these patients will breach the mask seal around the larynx.

Proper size selection is critical to effective use of the LMA. **Table 10-6** specifies the appropriate-size LMA based on patient size and weight as well as the maximum cuff inflation volume for each size.

Key points related to the use of the LMA are summarized as follows:

Preparation

- Choose an LMA appropriate for the patient's size and weight (see Table 10-6).
- Always have a spare LMA ready for use; ideally, have one size larger and one smaller.
- Fully deflate the cuff by pulling back firmly on the deflating syringe until it forms a smooth wedge shape without any wrinkles; insertion of an LMA with a partially deflated cuff can obstruct the airway by pushing down on the epiglottis.
- Lubricate the posterior tip of the cuff using a water-soluble gel—*posterior surface only.*
- Preoxygenate the patient and implement standard monitoring procedures.

Insertion

- Use the "sniffing position" for insertion (i.e., extension of the head with flexion of the neck).
- During insertion, use your fingers to keep the mask and tube pressed against the palato-pharyngeal curve (i.e., upward [cranially] and posteriorly).
- Avoid excessive force during insertion.

Inflation

- After insertion, inflate the cuff with just enough air to achieve a cuff pressure of 60 cm H_2O.
- During cuff inflation, avoid holding the tube, as this may prevent the mask from settling into the correct position.
- The cuff volume needed to obtain a seal varies according to the size of the patient and LMA: volumes in Table 10-6 are maximum values *not to be exceeded;* lesser volumes are often sufficient to obtain a seal and/or achieve 60 cm H_2O cuff pressure.
- During cuff inflation of a properly positioned LMA, you should observe a slight outward movement of the tube.

Table 10-6 Laryngeal Mask Airway Sizes and Maximum Cuff Inflation Volumes[a]

Patient Size	LMA Airway Size	Max Cuff Volume
Neonate/infant up to 5 kg	1	4 mL
Infants 5–10 kg	1 1/2	7 mL
Infants/Children 10–20 kg	2	10 mL
Children 20–30 kg	2 1/2	14 mL
Children 30–50 kg	3	20 mL
Adults 50–70 kg	4	30 mL
Adults 70–100 kg	5	40 mL
	6	50 mL

a. These are maximum clinical volumes that should never be exceeded. It is recommended the cuff be inflated to 60 cm H_2O intracuff pressures.

- Avoid LMA cuff pressures greater than 60 cm H_2O; excessive pressures can cause malpositioning and/or damage to the pharynx or larynx

Assessing and Ensuring Correct Placement

- Correct placement is indicated if you observe chest expansion during inspiration and can auscultate breath sounds; additional indicators of proper positioning include:
  - Not being able to see any portion of the cuff in the oral cavity
  - Observing a smooth oval swelling in the neck area around the thyroid cartilage
- Malpositioning causing leakage is indicated by either decreased tidal volumes or expired CO_2 levels.
- Malpositioning causing obstruction typically results in a prolonged expiratory phase and/or increased peak pressures during positive pressure ventilation.
- If an incorrectly placed LMA cannot be properly positioned, you should remove and reinsert it.

Fixation

- After ensuring correct placement, insert a bite block before taping the LMA in place; do not use an oropharyngeal airway as a bite block since it can cause malpositioning of the airway.
- You can make a temporary bite block by rolling together three or four 4×4 gauze pads.
- Secure the LMA in place using adhesive tape while applying gentle pressure to the airway tube as it is fixed (to assure that the tip of the mask is pressed against the esophageal sphincter).
- Keep the bite block in place until the LMA airway is removed.

Providing Positive Pressure Ventilation (PPV)

- To avoids leaks during PPV, use slow inflation, keep peak inspiratory pressures less than 20–30 cm H_2O, and limit delivered tidal volume to no more than 8 mL/kg.
- Leaks during PPV are most likely due to upward displacement of the mask.
- If a leak occurs during PPV:
  - Assure that the airway is securely taped in place.
  - Readjust the position of the airway by pressing the tube downward.
  - Resecure the airway in its new position.
  - *Do not simply add more air to the cuff* (this can worsen the leak by pushing the cuff away from the larynx).

Troubleshooting

- If airway problems persist or ventilation is inadequate, the LMA should be removed and an airway established by some other means.
- The presence of a gastric tube does not eliminate and may even increase the risk of aspiration.
- If regurgitation occurs:
  - Do not remove the LMA.
  - Place the patient in a head-down or side-lying position and temporarily disconnect the all ventilation equipment so that gastric contents are not forced into the lungs.
  - Reposition the device to assure that the distal end is lying against the upper esophageal sphincter and secure it in place.
  - Suction through the airway tube.
  - Prepare for immediate tracheal intubation.

Removal

- Consider removing the LMA only after the patient's upper airway reflexes have returned.
- Prior to removing an LMA, gather the equipment needed for suctioning and tracheal intubation.
- Avoid suctioning the airway tube with the LMA airway in place (this may provoke laryngospasm).
- Deflate the cuff and simultaneously remove the device.

- Verify airway patency and unobstructed ventilation.
- Perform oropharyngeal suctioning as needed.

Esophageal-Tracheal Combitube® (ETC)

Like the LMA, the esophageal-tracheal Combitube® (ETC) is an alternative to endotracheal intubation for emergency ventilatory support and airway control, designed to be inserted blindly. The ETC is the standard alternative to endotracheal intubation in the pre-hospital/emergency medicine setting. In the hospital, it is a good choice for patients who are difficult to intubate due to trauma, bleeding, vomiting, or other factors that make visualization of the vocal cords impossible. As with the LMA, the ETC should not be inserted in conscious patients or those with intact gag reflexes. It is contraindicated for infants and small children and for patients with esophageal trauma or disease.

As depicted in **Figure 10-4**, the ETC is a double-tube, double-cuff airway. This design assures effective ventilation regardless of whether the airway ends up in the esophagus or trachea. In either case, the pharyngeal balloon fills the space between the tongue and soft palate, thus eliminating the need for a mask. If the airway is inserted into the esophagus, the distal cuff seals off this passageway and ventilation is provided via the holes in the mid-portion of the pharyngeal tube, below the pharyngeal balloon. If the ETC is inserted into the trachea, it functions as an endotracheal tube, with the distal cuff sealing the lower airway and preventing aspiration.

The ETC comes in two sizes: 37 and 41 French. The manufacturer recommends using the 37 French version (Combitube SA®) on patients 4–5 feet tall, with the 41-French version for taller patients. Recent studies indicate that the 37-French version suffices for patients from 4 to 6 feet tall and thus is the preferred size for all but the largest patients.

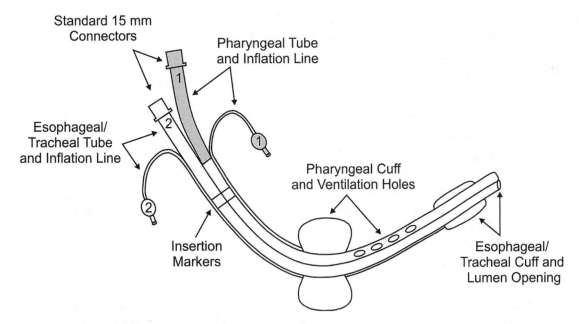

Figure 10-4 Esophageal-Tracheal Combitube®. The Combitube® is a double-tube, double-cuff airway. The #1 pharyngeal tube (longer blue connector) has a large volume cuff, includes a set of ventilation holes toward its mid-portion, and terminates in a dead-end. The shorter, clear #2 tracheal/esophageal tube has a regular volume cuff and beveled opening at its distal tip. Both cuffs have inflation lines and pilot balloons, ringed insertion markers, and standard 15 mm OD connectors for attaching respiratory equipment at their proximal ends. Accessory equipment provided with the airway includes 2 inflation syringes (large and small), a suction catheter, and an aspiration deflection elbow.

The basic procedure for inserting the ETC is the same for both sizes, except for the cuff inflation volume. The key steps in this procedure are outlined in the accompanying box.

Procedure for Insertion of an Esophageal-Tracheal Combitube®

1. Open the airway and suction mouth and oropharynx

1. Have the patient ventilated with 100% oxygen for at least 2–3 minutes

3. Select and assemble the correct-size airway, attaching the large syringe to the blue pharyngeal cuff (#1) and the small syringe to the white tracheal/esophageal cuff (#2)

4. Test the device by inflating both cuffs and removing syringes from check valves

5. Fully withdraw the air from both cuffs and leave assembled to speed insertion

6. Attach the aspiration deflection elbow to the shorter (#2) white tube

7. Lubricate the tube tip and pharyngeal balloon with water-soluble jelly

8. Place the head in a neutral position and pull the patient's mandible and tongue forward between the thumb and fingers

9. Place the tip of the airway into the mouth and align it along the midline

10. Gently guide the tube inward and downward along the palate and posterior surface of the oropharynx, using a curving motion

11. Advance the tube until the upper teeth or gums are aligned between the two black-ringed insertion markers

12. Do not force the tube; if resistance is met, withdraw the tube, reposition the head and retry

13. If unable to place the tube within 30 seconds, ventilate patient with O_2 for 1–2 minutes and retry

14. Limit insertion attempts to two unless directed to make further attempts

15. Inflate the cuffs:

    a. 41 Fr: large balloon (#1 cuff)—100 mL; small balloon (#2 cuff)—15 mL

    b. 37 Fr: large balloon (#1 cuff)—85 mL; small balloon (#2 cuff)—12 mL

16. Begin ventilating through the longer blue pharyngeal tube (#1)

17. Assess placement by:

    a. Observing the chest rising and falling

    b. Listening for bilateral lung sounds

    c. Listening over epigastrum for air gurgling in stomach

    d. Using a colorimetric CO_2 detector

18. If there are bilateral lung sounds, no stomach sounds, and good chest rise (indicating esophageal placement), continue ventilating with 100% O_2 through the #1 tube

19. If chest movement and lung sounds are absent, and/or if there are gurgling sounds over the stomach (indicating tracheal placement):

    a. Remove the aspiration deflection elbow

    b. Ventilate through the shorter tube (#2)

    c. Reconfirm adequacy of ventilation

20. Once adequate ventilation is confirmed, secure tube with tape or tube holder and continue providing essential life support

---

Note that the majority of blind intubation attempts with the ETC end up in the esophagus. *It is for this reason that the initial attempt at ventilation should always be via the longer (blue) #1 pharyngeal tube.* As an added benefit, if you confirm that the airway is in the esophagus, you can use the #2 tracheal/esophageal tube to relieve any gastric distention that may have occurred during bag-valve-mask ventilation. To do so, remove the aspiration deflection elbow and insert the suction catheter that comes with the airway into the #2 tube to between the two insertion markers. Then connect the catheter to a vacuum regulator set to low for several minutes. Once the gastric distention is relieved, you should remove the catheter. Do not use continuous suction.

If you cannot ventilate through either connector, the tube is likely inserted too far, causing the large proximal cuff to obstruct the glottis. To correct this problem, withdraw the tube 2–3 cm at a time while ventilating through connector #1 until breath sounds are heard over the lungs. If this procedure does not solve the problem or if ventilation becomes more difficult after insertion, you should remove the ETC and reestablish the airway by any alternative means available.

To switch a patient from an ETC to an oral endotracheal tube, the airway normally must be in the esophagus. In this case, gather and prepare all equipment needed for endotracheal intubation, and aspirate any stomach contents through the #2 tracheal/esophageal tube. To intubate while the ETC is in place, you must first deflate the large #1 pharyngeal cuff. This will allow for laryngoscopy while the #2 ETC cuff keeps the esophagus occluded. Alternatively, as long as stomach contents have been aspirated, you can consider removing the ETC before proceeding with endotracheal intubation.

The ETC should be removed when the patient regains consciousness, begins biting or gagging on the tube, or requires endotracheal intubation. Since regurgitation can occur with ETC removal, you must have suction equipment set up for immediate use. Normally, before removal, the patient is log rolled to the side. You then fully deflate both cuffs until the pilot balloons are completely collapsed and gently remove the ETC while suctioning the airway.

Maintaining Adequate Humidification

According to the AARC, humidity therapy is indicated either to humidify dry medical gases or to overcome the humidity deficit when bypassing the upper airway. In addition, ensuring adequate humidification can facilitate the mobilization of secretions. Heated humidification also can be used to treat hypothermia and bronchospasm associated with inhaling cold air.

Humidification Needs

Table 10-7 specifies the temperature and relative and absolute humidity levels recommended by site of delivery. As evident, when you deliver medical gases via the patient's upper airway, heat and humidity needs are less, due to the effectiveness of the nose in providing the necessary heat and moisture. Indeed, a humidifier normally is *not* needed when delivering O_2 to the upper airways:

- At low-flow O_2 (£ 4 L/min)
- Via air-entrainment devices providing less than 50% O_2
- Via O_2 masks in emergency situations or for short time periods (hours)

In contrast, if the patient's upper airway has been bypassed via tracheal intubation, you must compensate for the humidity deficit by providing more heat and humidity. *For this reason, the use of unheated active humidifiers is contraindicated in patients with bypassed upper airways.*

Selecting a Humidification Strategy

Figure 10-5 provides a decision algorithm to assist you in selecting the appropriate humidification strategy. The key information needed to make your decision includes (1) whether or not the patient has an artificial tracheal airway, (2) the thickness of secretions, (3) the gas flow, (4) the need for and duration of mechanical ventilation, and (5) the presence of contraindications against using an HME. To use the algorithm, answer each question posed with a "yes" or "no" and follow the prescribed branch.

Table 10-7 Recommended Levels of Heat and Humidity Needed for Adequate Humidification

Delivery Site	Temperature Range	Relative Humidity	Minimum H2O Content
Nose/mouth	20–22°C	50%	10 mg/L
Trachea	32–35°C	100%	30 mg/L

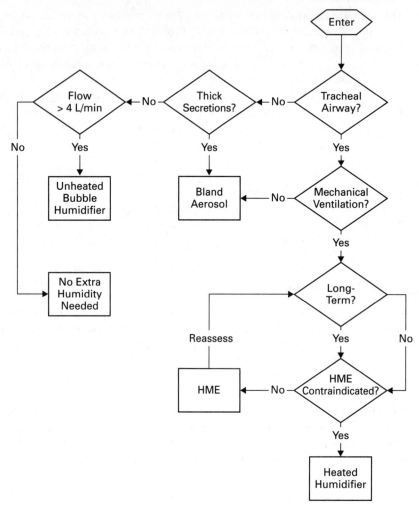

Figure 10-5 Selection of Humidification Devices.

Spontaneously Breathing Patients

For patients with intact upper airways with normal secretions receiving O_2 at flows greater than 4 L/min, a simple unheated bubble humidifier is all that is needed. In spontaneously breathing patients with either thick secretions or those with a tracheal airway, bland aerosol therapy is the most common option for humidifying medical gases. Airway appliances used to deliver bland aerosol therapy include the aerosol mask, face tent, T-tube, and tracheostomy mask (**Table 10-8**). As with humidifiers, heat can be added using an appropriate heating element.

Patients Requiring Ventilatory Support

All patients needing ventilatory support via a tracheal airway require a humidifier system in the ventilator circuit. For these patients, you can provide humidification using either a heated passover humidifier or an HME. **Figure 10-6** provides a simple algorithm for determining which of these systems to use. In general, you can begin with an HME unless it is contraindicated. Since HME performance varies, *be sure that the HME you select meets or exceeds the 30 mg/L standard for humidification of gases delivered to the trachea.*

If an HME is contraindicated, you should start the patient on a heated humidifier. Contraindications to HME use include thick or bloody secretions, hypothermia (< 32°C), large tidal volumes (> 1000 mL), and large system leaks. Should one or more of these contraindications occur at any time during patient management, or if the HME needs to be changed frequently (> 4 times per day), you should switch to a heated humidifier.

Table 10-8 Selection of Airway Appliances for Bland Aerosol Therapy

Airway Appliances	Best Use
Aerosol mask	Short-term application to most patients with intact upper airways
Face tent	Patients with intact upper airways who do not tolerate an aerosol mask
T-tube	Patients who are orally or nasally intubated or have a tracheostomy and need moderate to high F_{IO_2}
Tracheostomy mask	Patients with a tracheostomy for whom precise or high F_{IO_2} are not needed; also ideal when you need to avoid traction on the airway

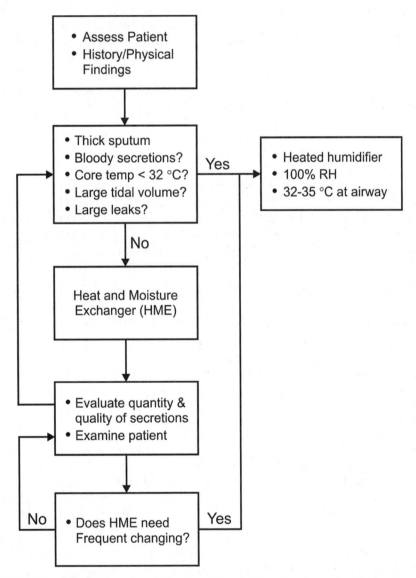

Figure 10-6 Decision Algorithm for Selecting Humidifier Systems for Patients with Artificial Tracheal Airways.

Adapted from: Branson R. D., Davis K., Campbell R. S., Johnson D. J., & Porembka D. T. (1993). Humidification in the intensive care unit: prospective study of a new protocol utilizing heated humidification and a hygroscopic condenser humidifier. *Chest, 104*, 1800–1805.

HMEs require minimal troubleshooting. HMEs increase deadspace by 30–70 mL, but this is a problem mainly with infants and small children. With these patients, you need to select the correct-size HME and adjust the inspired tidal volume to compensate for the added deadspace. HME deadspace also can impact adults receiving small tidal volumes, as occurs when applying ARDS protocols. Increasing the V_T or pressure to adjust for the added deadspace is contraindicated in these patients. For this reason, when using a low-V_T protocol, you should use a heated humidifier.

HMEs also increase flow resistance through the breathing circuit by about 1–3 cm H_2O/L/sec, which is not a problem for most adults. However, if mucous accumulates in the HME, resistance can increase over time, increasing airway pressures during volume-controlled ventilation and potentially decreasing delivered volume during pressure-controlled ventilation. You can verify this problem by visually inspecting the HME and correct it by replacing the device with a new one.

Heated passover humidifiers can be used by themselves or in conjunction with heated-wire circuits. In the absence of heated wires, use of a heated humidifier will always cause condensation in the circuit (refer to Figure 6-1). Heated-wire circuits provide more accurate control over inspired gas temperatures and prevent water condensation in the tubing. In addition, heated-wire circuits reduce water usage and decrease long-term cost. However, there are reports of heated wires actually melting the delivery tubing and causing dangerous circuit leaks. To avoid this potentially serious problem:

1. Never use reusable wires with disposable breathing circuits
2. Ensure that heating wires are threaded evenly along the tubing and not bunched up
3. Never cover the heated-wire circuit with towels, drapes, or linens

Some patients receiving long-term noninvasive ventilation may also require extra humidification, especially those using oral interfaces or those residing in dry climates. *HMEs are generally contraindicated for these patients*, due to both the flow leakage that occurs in NPPV circuits as well as the added deadspace and flow resistance that these devices create. For these patients you should use a simple passover humidifier. Since the upper airway is not being bypassed, an unheated system generally provides adequate humidification and avoids the problems associated with condensation. However, if dry supplemental O_2 is being provided or the patient has a problem with secretion retention, you may want to consider a heated humidifier. To prevent condensation problems with these systems, be sure to place the humidifier *below* both the ventilator and the patient.

Perform Extubation

Removal of a tracheal tube should be considered only in patients who:

- Can maintain adequate oxygenation and ventilation without ventilatory support
- Are at minimal risk for upper airway obstruction
- Have adequate airway protection and are at minimal risk for aspiration
- Can adequately clear pulmonary secretions on their own

In regard to the patient's ability to maintain adequate oxygenation and ventilation, this should be demonstrated via spontaneous breathing trials. To assess the risk for upper airway obstruction, you can perform a cuff-leak test. To do so, fully deflate the tube cuff and completely occlude the ET tube at its outlet. If air leakage occurs (a "positive" cuff-leak test), then the airway most likely is patent. A positive gag reflex and the ability of the patient to raise the head off the bed indicate adequate airway protection. Last, the ability to clear secretions is evident if the patient is alert, coughs deeply on suctioning, and can generate a maximum expiratory pressure (MEP) greater than 60 cm H_2O.

Key considerations in performing extubation include the following:

- Needed equipment:
  - Suctioning apparatus and suction kits
  - Oxygen and aerosol therapy equipment
  - Bag-valve-mask
  - Small-volume nebulizer with racemic epinephrine
  - An intubation tray (in case reintubation is required)

- Patient preparation:
  - Suction the ET tube and pharynx to above the cuff
  - Provide 100% O_2 for 1–2 minutes after suctioning
- Extubation procedure:
  - Fully deflate the cuff
  - Remove securing tape or device
  - Simultaneously have the patient cough while you quickly pull the tube
- Follow-up:
  - Provide cool, humidified O_2 via aerosol mask at a higher F_{IO_2} than prior to extubation
  - Assess breath sounds and vital signs
  - Encourage the patient to cough
  - Analyze arterial blood gases as needed
  - If stridor develops, recommend treatment with aerosolized racemic epinephrine
  - Recommend that the patient be NPO (except for sips of water) for 24 hours

The most serious complication that can occur with extubation is laryngospasm. Should laryngospasm occur, you should initially provide positive pressure ventilation with a BVM with 100% O_2. If laryngospasm persists, the doctor may need to paralyze the patient with a neuromuscular blocking agent and reintubate.

COMMON ERRORS TO AVOID

You can improve your score by avoiding these mistakes:

- Never place or keep an oropharyngeal airway in a conscious patient.
- Never use McGill forceps during intubation without direct visualization.
- Never tie tracheostomy ties with a bow; instead, always use a square knot.
- Never force the inner cannula of a tracheostomy tube during insertion, nor pull on or rock it when attaching equipment.
- Never just measure cuff pressure; always adjust the pressure if it is not correct.
- Never use more than 60 cm H_2O to inflate an LMA cuff.
- Never cover a heated-wire breathing circuit with towels, drapes, or linens.
- Never extubate a patient without being prepared to reintubate.

SURE BETS

In some situations you can always be sure of the right approach to a clinical problem or scenario:

- Always be sure a nasopharyngeal airway is well lubricated before insertion.
- Always keep an obturator and unopened tubes in the same size and one size smaller at the bedside of patients with tracheostomies.
- Always use the lowest cuff inflation pressures needed to protect the airway and provide for adequate ventilation.
- Always suction the patient's oropharynx before you measure cuff pressure or extubate.
- Always provide 100% O_2 to patients prior to suctioning and before/after extubation.
- Always pass a suction catheter through artificial tracheal airways regularly to ensure patency.
- Always make sure that the cuff of a fenestrated trach tube is fully deflated before plugging it.
- Always provide all patients receiving ventilatory support via an artificial tracheal airway at least 30 mg/L water vapor (equivalent to 100% relative humidity at 32–35°C).

PRE-TEST ANSWERS AND EXPLANATIONS

Below are this chapter's pre-test answers and explanations. Be sure to review each answer's explanation thoroughly to help you understand why it is correct. If the explanation is still unclear to you, review the chapter contents or the references and/or refer to this chapter's supplemental resources on the CD.

10-1. **Correct Answer: D.** Applying the "head-tilt/chin-lift" maneuver. The initial procedure used to maintain an open airway in an unconscious patient is the "head-tilt/chin-lift" maneuver. This maneuver helps displace the tongue away from the posterior pharyngeal wall.

10-2. **Correct Answer: B.** Nasopharyngeal airway. When the mouth is unavailable as a route for airway access, you should try the nose. In this case, a nasopharyngeal airway would help overcome upper airway obstruction and can be easily inserted.

10-3. **Correct Answer: C.** Is conscious and alert. Oropharyngeal airways can provoke a gag reflex and possible vomiting and should therefore generally not be used in conscious patients.

10-4. **Correct Answer: A.** Bag slowly to reduce peak pressure. To avoid leaks during positive pressure ventilation through an LMA, you should use slow inflation, keep peak inspiratory pressures less than 20–30 cm H_2O, and limit delivered tidal volume to no more than 8 mL/kg. If a leak persists in spite of these efforts to limit pressure/volume, you should readjust the tube's position by pressing it downward and resecuring it. Do *not* add more air to the LMA cuff, since this can worsen the leak by pushing the cuff away from the larynx.

10-5. **Correct Answer: B.** Inspired gas with an absolute humidity greater than 30 mg/L. To provide adequate humidity to an intubated patient, strive to provide a gas with an absolute humidity of at least 30 mg/L. Inspired gas with 50% relative humidity or that provided through a cold bubble humidifier provides an absolute humidity of about 15–20 mg/L. If administered to a patient with a bypassed upper airway, this level of humidity can cause damage to the tracheal mucosa and impair mucociliary clearance.

10-6. **Correct Answer: C.** Withdraw the tube by 1–2 cm (using tube markings as a guide). The tip of an endotracheal or tracheostomy tube should be positioned 4–6 cm above the carina. If the tube is malpositioned, the therapist should gain physician permission to remove the old tape and reposition the tube using the markings on the tube as a guide. This often requires two people to prevent extubation. The new position should again be confirmed by X-ray or laryngoscopy.

10-7. **Correct Answer: C.** Ventilate through the other (#2) tube. After insertion of a esophageal-tracheal Combitube®, you normally begin ventilation through the #1 pharyngeal airway connection. If you detect no chest motion or breath sounds via this route, or if there are stomach sounds present, the tube is in the trachea and you should switch to ventilating the patient via the shorter esophageal/tracheal tube (labeled as #2).

10-8. **Correct Answer: B.** Tissue damage. Tracheal wall tissue damage can occur as a result of overinflating the cuff of an endotracheal tube, because pressures significantly above 20–25 cm H_2O can decrease or occlude capillary blood flow.

10-9. **Correct Answer: C.** A simple bubble humidifier. When the upper airway has been bypassed, the only way to prevent a large humidity deficit is to provide inspired gases at or near BTPS conditions. This is not possible with a simple (unheated) bubble humidifier. Instead, either a heated humidifier (cascade or wick), hygroscopic condenser humidifier, or heated large-volume jet nebulizer must be used. These systems are capable of controlling temperature and humidity levels and providing saturated gases at or near the normal body temperature.

10-10. **Correct Answer: A.** "Leakage" type aspiration. The methylene blue test can help determine if "leakage" aspiration is occurring. Methylene blue may be added to the patient's feedings or swallowed by the patient in a small amount of water. Once the dye is introduced, the patient's trachea is suctioned through the artificial airway. If blue-tinged secretions are retrieved while suctioning, aspiration is occurring.

POST-TEST

A post-test for this chapter that includes automated scoring and feedback is available on the accompanying CD. Be sure to complete this additional assessment to confirm your mastery of this chapter's objectives.

REFERENCES

American Association for Respiratory Care. (2007). Clinical practice guideline. Removal of the endotracheal tube: 2007 revision and update. *Respiratory care, 52*, 81–93.

American Association for Respiratory Care. (1995). Clinical practice guideline. Management of airway emergencies. *Respiratory care, 40*, 749–760.

American Association for Respiratory Care. (1992). Clinical practice guideline. Humidification during mechanical ventilation. *Respiratory care, 37*, 887–890.

American Heart Association. (2005). Guidelines for cardiopulmonary resuscitation and emergency cardiovascular care: Part 7.1: Adjuncts for airway control and ventilation. *Circulation, 112* [Suppl. 1], IV-51-IV-57.

Blazer, C. *Quick reference to respiratory therapy equipment assembly and troubleshooting.* St. Louis: Mosby, 1994.

Brain, A., Denman, W. T., Goudsouzian, N. G. *Laryngeal mask airway instruction manual.* San Diego, CA: LMA North America, 1999.

Branson, R. D. (1999). Humidification for patients with artificial airways. *Respiratory care, 44*, 630–642.

Brimacombe, J. R., Brain, A. I. J., & Berry, A. (1997). Nonanesthetic uses. In J. R. Brimacombe (Ed.), *The laryngeal mask airway: A review and practice guide.* Philadelphia: Saunders.

Burton, G. G., & Hudogkin, J. E. (Eds. (1984). *Respiratory care: A guide to clinical practice* (2nd ed.) Philadelphia: Lippincott.

Butler, T. J., Close, J. R., Close, R. J. (1998). *Laboratory exercises for competency in respiratory care,* Philadelphia: FA Davis.

Centers for Disease and Prevention. (2003). Guidelines for environmental infection control in healthcare facilities: Recommendations of CDC and the healthcare infection control practices advisory committee (HICPAC). *Morbidity and mortality weekly report,* 52 (No. RR-10), 1–48.

Chatburn, R. L., & Primiano, F. P. (1987). A rational basis for humidity therapy. *Respiratory care,* 32, 249–253.

Divatia, J. V., & Bhowmick, K. (2005). Complications of endotracheal intubation and other airway management procedures. *Indian journal of anaesthesia, 49*, 316–317.

McPherson, S. P. (1995). *Respiratory care equipment* (5th ed.). St. Louis: Mosby.

Scanlan, C. L., West, G. A., von der Heydt, P. A., & Dolan, G. K. (1984). *Respiratory therapy competency evaluation manual.* Boston: Blackwell Scientific.

Wilkins, R. L., Stoller, J. K., & Kacmarek, R. M. (Eds.). (2009). *Egan's fundamentals of respiratory care,* (9th ed.). St. Louis: Mosby.

Remove Bronchopulmonary Secretions

Brian X. Weaver
Albert J. Heuer

INTRODUCTION

Many of your patients will require your assistance in removing bronchopulmonary secretions in order to maintain a patent airway. In this section of the NBRC exam, you will be tested on your knowledge of this type of therapy, including postural drainage, percussion, and vibration, as well as directed coughing and the use of adjunct mechanical devices to aid secretion clearance. Also included in this section are questions on the use of drugs or bland water aerosols to facilitate secretion clearance. All of these techniques are ultimately intended to improve ventilation and gas exchange. As such, they represent a small but important component of the CRT exam that is deserving of your careful attention.

OBJECTIVES

After completion of this chapter, you should demonstrate the knowledge needed to:

1. Perform postural drainage, percussion, and vibration
2. Instruct and encourage bronchopulmonary hygiene techniques
3. Perform airway clearance using mechanical devices
4. Clear secretions via suctioning:
   a. Oropharyngeal
   b. Nasotracheal
   c. Artificial airways
5. Administer aerosol therapy with prescribed medications

WHAT TO EXPECT ON THIS CATEGORY OF THE CRT EXAM

Number of questions: About 4 questions; typically 1 recall and 3 application

WHAT'S NEW FOR 2009

As of July 2009, this section of the NBRC CRT examination includes the following *new content area*:

- Airway clearance using mechanical devices

PRE-TEST

Carefully respond to each of the following questions. After completing the pre-test, compare your answers to those provided at the end of this chapter. Then thoroughly review each answer's explanation to help understand why it is correct.

11-1. An adult male requires postural drainage of the posterior basal segments bilaterally. The doctor's order is complete and you have performed all pre-treatment assessments and taken all needed precautions. To properly position this patient, you should:
    I. Elevate the foot of the bed 30 degrees
    II. Keep the bed flat but put a pillow under the patient's hips
    III. Have the patient lie supine with a pillow under the hips
    IV. Have the patient lie prone with a pillow under the hips
A. I and II only
B. III and IV only
C. I and IV only
D. II and III only

11-2. By placing a patient in the prone position with a pillow under the abdomen and keeping the bed level, you would be targeting what segment in postural drainage?
A. Lateral basal segment of lower lobes
B. Superior segment of lower lobes
C. Apical segment of upper lobes
D. Posterior segment of upper lobes

11-3. All of the following are needed for an effective cough *except*:
A. A closed glottis
B. Compression phase
C. Explosive exhalation
D. Low inspiratory volumes

11-4. Which of the following should you do in order to properly perform nasotracheal suctioning on an adult patient?
    I. Lubricate the catheter
    II. Apply suction for less than 15 seconds
    III. Preoxygenate and postoxygenate the patient
    IV. Instruct patient to exhale and hold breath
A. I and IV only
B. I, II, and III
C. III and IV only
D. I, III, and IV

11-5. The administration of what aerosolized drug is most appropriate to thin secretions and help in the removal of a mucous plug?
A. Albuterol
B. Ipratropium bromide
C. Acetylcysteine (Mucomyst)
D. Racemic epinephrine

11-6. A morning X-ray confirms bilateral infiltrates in the posterior segments of the upper lobes of a 30-year-old female patient. What postural drainage position should you use to drain these segments?
A. Prone with a pillow under her hips
B. Sitting position leaning forward on a pillow
C. The foot of the bed raised 18 inches and the patient on her left side
D. Supine with a pillow under her legs

11-7. Which of the following bronchial hygiene techniques is most suitable for small infants?
A. Postural drainage, percussion, and vibration
B. Positive expiratory pressure
C. Aggressive suctioning with a 14-Fr catheter
D. High-frequency oscillation

11-8. During your morning patient assessments you suction a 7-month-old nasally intubated patient. After assembling the needed equipment and following all precautions you begin the procedure. For this patient, what are the appropriate pressure and time limits for this procedure?
A. Suction at a pressure range of −40 to −60 mm Hg, limiting the time to 30 seconds
B. Suction at a pressure range of −80 to −100 mm Hg, limiting the time to less than 10–15 seconds
C. Suction at a pressure range of −100 to −120 mm Hg and continuing until you observe secretions in the suction catheter
D. Suction at a pressure range of −60 to −80 mm Hg, limiting the time to less than 10–15 seconds

11-9. Which of the following is a possible complication of postural drainage, percussion, and vibration?
  - **I.** Pulmonary barotrauma
  - **II.** Acute hypotension during procedure
  - **III.** Dysrhythmias
  - **IV.** Fractured ribs
  - **A.** I and III only
  - **B.** I, II, and III
  - **C.** I, II, III, and IV
  - **D.** II, III, and IV

11-10. To remove accumulations of subglottic secretions from above the cuff of intubated patients, you should recommend which of the following?
  - **A.** Intrapulmonary percussive ventilation (IPV)
  - **B.** Use of a tracheal tube with a suction port above the cuff
  - **C.** Aggressive tracheal suctioning with saline lavage
  - **D.** Frequent oropharyngeal suctioning with a Yankauer tip

WHAT YOU NEED TO KNOW: ESSENTIAL CONTENT

Selecting the Best Approach

There are a variety of specific techniques that constitute bronchial hygiene therapy. Some of the most important factors in determining which technique to use are the patient's age, preexisting conditions, and personal preference. **Table 11-1** indicates the recommended bronchial hygiene techniques for the most common disorders that often require secretion clearance. In some cases, you may combine these methods to achieve optimum results.

Bronchial hygiene is often ordered by protocol, given your discretion as to the selection and implementation of therapy, and its evaluation. **Figure 11-1** provides a sample algorithm for a bronchial hygiene protocol that directs your decision making based on the patient's diagnosis, volume of sputum produced, and ability to cough effectively.

Postural Drainage, Percussion, Vibration, and Turning

Postural drainage, percussion, and vibration (PDPV) techniques help you loosen and clear secretions from a patient's respiratory tract. Doing so can help reduce infection, enhance ventilation, and improve both pulmonary function and gas exchange.

Table 11-1 Bronchial Hygiene Techniques

Condition	Recommended Technique
Cystic fibrosis, bronchiectasis	
Infants	PDPV
3–12 year olds	PEP, PDPV, HFO
> 12 years old	AD, PEP, PDPV, HFO
Adult, living alone	PEP, HFO (flutter valve)
Atelectasis	PEP, PDPV, T&R
Asthma (with mucous plugging)	PEP, PDPV, HFO
Neurologic abnormalities (spasticity, bulbar palsy, aspiration-prone)	PDPV, suction, MI-E, T&R
Musculoskeletal weakness (muscular dystrophy, myasthenia, poliomyelitis)	PEP, MI-E, T&R

Abbreviations: PDPV, postural drainage, percussion, and vibration; PEP, positive expiratory pressure; AD, autogenic drainage; MI-E, mechanical insufflation-exsufflation; HFO, high-frequency oscillation (flutter valve, interpulmonary percussive ventilation); T&R, turning and rotation.

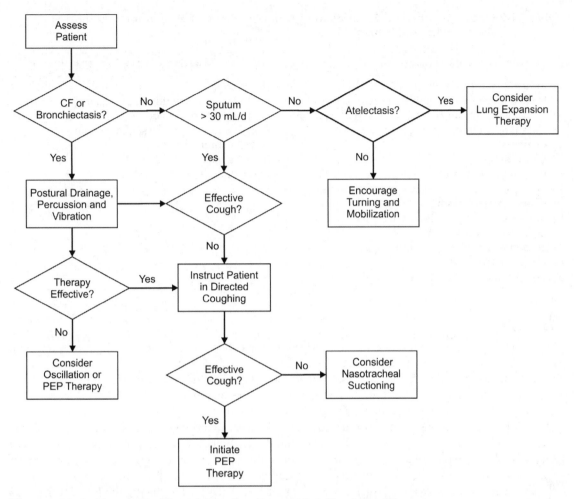

Figure 11-1 Example Algorithm for Bronchial Hygiene Therapy.

CF = cystic fibrosis; PEP = positive expiratory pressure.

Adapted from: Burton, G. G., Hodgkin, J. E., & Ward, J. (1997). *Respiratory care: a guide to clinical practice.* (4th ed.). Philadelphia: J. B. Lippincott.

Indications

PDPV is indicated in conditions that increase the likelihood of mucous plugging and atelectasis. These may include:

- Retention of secretion and difficulty clearing the airways
- An inability to turn or change position
- Artificial airways
- Atelectasis caused by a mucous plug or obstruction
- Patients with conditions that increase the amount and thickness of secretions

Contraindications, Hazards, and Complications

Before proceeding with PDPV, you need to consider both the contraindications and hazards and complications of this therapy. **Table 11-2** provides a summary of these considerations, as defined by the AARC.

Table 11-2 Contraindications, Hazards, and Complications of Postural Drainage, Percussion, and Vibration

Contraindications	Hazards and Complications
• Intracranial pressure (ICP) > 20 mm Hg • Head and neck injury until stabilized • Active hemorrhage with hemodynamic instability • Recent or acute spinal surgery or active hemoptysis • Empyema • Bronchopleural fistula • Pulmonary edema or large pleural effusions • Pulmonary embolism • Rib fracture, with or without flail chest • Osteomyelitis of the ribs • Osteoporosis • Coagulopathy • Complaint of chest wall pain	• Hypoxemia • Acute hypotension during procedure • Pulmonary hemorrhage • Pain or injury to muscles, ribs, or spine • Vomiting and aspiration • Bronchospasm • Dysrhythmias

Procedure

The accompanying box outlines the basic procedure for PDPV. As indicated in this procedure, you should monitor the patient's clinical status before, during, and after the therapy. Your monitoring of patients should include their overall appearance, vital signs, breathing pattern, and pulse oximetry. If the patient shows any signs of distress, you should stop the treatment, remain with and monitor the patient, and promptly notify the nurse and physician.

Most of the positions used in postural drainage are logical and involve aligning the affected segment and/or side in the "up" position. This way gravity can help move secretions toward the trachea and airway opening to facilitate removal. For example, the position for draining the posterior segment of the lower lobes includes placing the foot of the bed 18 inches above the head, thus raising the affected lung regions above the larger airways and trachea. Each position is usually held for up to 15 minutes depending on patient tolerance. **Figure 11-2** depicts the most commonly recommended positions for draining various lobes and segments of the lung.

Many forms of bronchial hygiene therapy need to be scheduled to account for meals ands/or pain medications. Generally, PDPV should be done either before or 60–90 minutes after meals. Also, patients receiving pain management will tend to tolerate percussion and vibration better if you perform it 30–60 minutes after administration of pain medication.

During drainage, additional assistance may be needed to help mobilize the secretions being retained in the lung. Percussion can mechanically dislodge secretions and enable them to drain more easily. With this technique, you use your cupped hands to deliver rapid, repetitive impacts on the chest wall over the targeted segment. As described in Chapter 6, in place of your cupped hands, you may select mechanical devices such as pneumatic or electrical percussors or—for infants or children—small rubber cups. However, there is little evidence supporting the superiority of any of these devices over manual percussion. For this reason, your selection and use of these devices should be guided by patient preference, convenience, and availability.

Vibration involves rapid shaking motion performed against the chest wall over the affected area *during expiration*. It may be performed manually or with a mechanical device. In combination with percussion and other secretion-clearance aids, vibration can help you loosen the patient's secretions, particularly if they are copious and thick.

Instead of intermittent application of postural drainage, some critical care units implement turning and rotation protocols to help prevent retained secretions and atelectasis in patients prone to these complications. This procedure involves rotating the patient's body around its longitudinal axis. Turning can be done manually (with pillows or a foam wedge) or with the assistance of a specially equipped

---

Postural Drainage, Percussion, and Vibration

Equipment and Patient Preparation

1. Verify, interpret, and evaluate doctor's order or protocol; determine lobes/segments to be drained by reviewing chest X-ray results, progress notes, and diagnosis; scan chart for any possible contraindications

2. Coordinate therapy:

    • Either before meals and tube feedings or 1 to 1½ hours after meals

    • With pain medication, as needed

3. Select, gather, assemble, and check the required equipment: blood pressure manometer, percussor (if needed), and pulse oximeter (see Chapter 6)

4. Decontaminate hands and apply standard/transmission-based precautions as appropriate

5. Identify patient, introduce self and department

6. Explain/demonstrate procedure and confirm patient understanding

Assessment and Implementation

7. Assess patient pulse, respirations, blood pressure, breath sounds, SpO₂, color, level of dyspnea, and ability to cooperate

8. Instruct patient in diaphragmatic breathing and coughing (by demonstration)

9. Position patient for segmental/lobar drainage, beginning with most dependent portions first

10. Reassess patient response and tolerance

11. Modify position to accommodate patient's response, if needed

12. Encourage maintenance of proper breathing pattern

13. Perform percussion over properly identified areas as indicated

14. Perform vibration over correct area during expiration, if needed

15. Maintain position for appropriate time interval (minimum 5–10 min) as tolerated

16. Encourage and assist patient with coughing

17. Examine (collect) sputum

18. Reposition patient and repeat procedure as indicated and tolerated

19. Return patient to comfortable position

20. Reassess patient

Follow-up

21. Maintain/process equipment

22. Dispose of infectious waste and decontaminate hands

23. Record pertinent data in chart and departmental records

24. Notify appropriate personnel and make any recommendations or modifications to patient care plan as indicated

Adapted from: Scanlan, C. L., West, G. A., von der Heydt, P. A., & Dolan, G. K. (1984). *Respiratory therapy competency evaluation manual.* Boston: Blackwell Scientific.

---

bed. As an added but significant benefit, proper turning and rotation helps prevent bed sores in immobile patients.

Assessment

To assess the effectiveness and outcome of PDPV, you should monitor several indicators. Changes in the chest X-ray and vital signs, including SpO₂, can all be monitored noninvasively and provide an

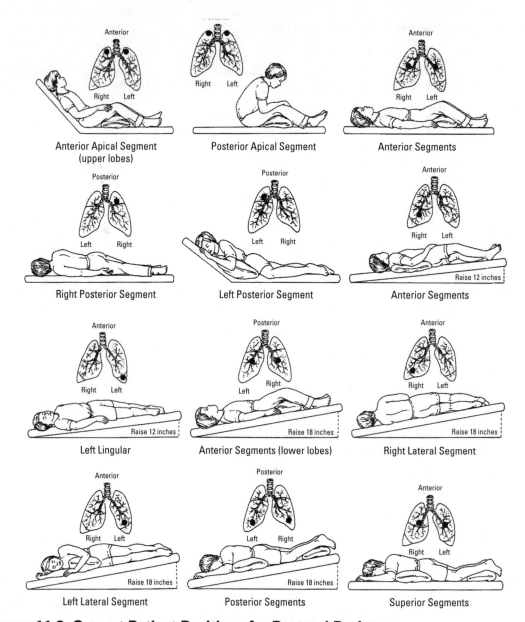

Figure 11-2 Correct Patient Positions for Postural Drainage.

Source: Potter, P. A,. & Perry, A. G. (1997). Patient positions for postural drainage. In B. J. Kozier, G. Erb, A. J. Berman, & S. Snyder. *Fundamentals of nursing: concepts, process and practice.* (4th ed.). St. Louis: Mosby. Courtesy of Elsevier Ltd.

excellent source of information about the progress of the patient. Sputum production and auscultation provide a very good gauge to determine if the therapy is progressing successfully. In general, when the sputum production drops below 30 mL/day and the patient can generate an effective spontaneous cough, you should recommend that PDPV be discontinued.

Instruct and Encourage Bronchopulmonary Hygiene Techniques

PDPV only moves secretions into the patient's large airways. From there, the secretions are normally cleared by spontaneous coughing. Since not all patients know how to cough effectively, it is your job to instruct and encourage them to use this important secretion clearance mechanism. If patients cannot cough effectively, manual removal of secretions via suctioning may be required, as described later in this chapter.

Cough-related training techniques that the NBRC expects you to be familiar with include directed coughing, the forced expiratory technique, the abdominal thrust maneuver, and autogenic drainage.

Directed Cough

A normal cough has the following three phases:

1. Deep inspiration
2. Compression against a closed glottis
3. Explosive exhalation

In patients with a normal cough, the explosive exhalation helps loosens the secretions in the smaller airway, moving them into the trachea and pharynx for expectoration or swallowing. However, some patients have trouble with one or more of the phases of coughing. Patients with recent thoracic or abdominal surgery may have trouble with the inspiratory and expiratory phases of coughing. For them, splinting the incision site with a pillow often permits them to generate a more effective cough. Patients with neuromuscular disorders may also have an ineffective cough. For them, the coughing technique may need to be modified by supplementing the explosive phase with an abdominal thrust or by adding mechanical assistance, as discussed later in this chapter.

Forced Expiratory Technique (FET)

The AARC describes the forced expiratory technique or FET as "huff coughing" in order to distinguish it from a normal cough in which high flows are generated by gas compression against a closed glottis. The FET consists of 2–3 forced exhalations, or huffs, *with the glottis open*, followed by a rest period. This process is repeated until the secretions have moved up into the pharynx, where they can be cleared by the patient via expectoration. The FET is best suited for post-op patients for whom explosive exhalation is very painful, and COPD patients prone to airway closure on forced exhalation.

Abdominal Thrust

The abdominal thrust maneuver uses the diaphragm to help compress the air in the lungs and airways to augment expiratory flow. To perform this maneuver, you push on the upper abdomen in synchrony with the explosive phase of the patient's own cough effort. You should not push down on the belly; instead, the motion should be upward toward the epigastrium. This technique is contraindicated in patients with abdominal trauma, surgical incisions, or certain gastrointestinal conditions.

The accompanying box outlines the basic procedure for directed coughing, including incorporation of the FET technique and abdominal thrust maneuver, as needed.

Directed Cough

Equipment and Patient Preparation

1. Verify, interpret, and evaluate doctor's order or protocol
2. Scan chart for diagnosis and any other pertinent data and notes
3. Select, gather, assemble, and check the required equipment: pillows, tissues, and waste receptacle
4. Decontaminate hands and apply standard/transmission-based precautions as appropriate
5. Identify patient, introduce self and department
6. Explain/demonstrate procedure and confirm patient understanding

Assessment and Implementation

7. Assess patient
8. Position patient in Fowler's position (or side-lying position with knees bent)

(continues)

9. Instruct patient in effective use of diaphragm

10. Demonstrate cough phases

11. Instruct the patient regarding incisional support (postoperative splinting)

12. Encourage deep inspiration, inspiratory hold

13. Assure forceful contraction of abdominal muscles

14. Observe and correct common errors

15. Modify technique as appropriate to patient:

   • Instruct the patient in the forced expiratory technique (huffing)

   • Provide manually assisted cough, using epigastric pressure (abdominal thrust) or external lateral compression of the thoracic cage

   • With tracheostomy, provide manually assisted deep inspiration using a manual resuscitator bag in conjunction with manually assisted cough techniques

16. Reassess patient and reinstruct as needed

17. Repeat procedure as indicated and tolerated

18. Examine (collect) sputum

Follow-up

19. Return patient to comfortable position

20. Maintain/process equipment

21. Dispose of infectious waste and decontaminate hands

22. Record pertinent data in chart and departmental records

23. Notify appropriate personnel and make any necessary recommendations or modifications to the patient care plan

Autogenic Drainage

Autogenic drainage is usually combined with directed coughing. This procedure consists of three phases. In phase one, the goal is to loosen mucous by the patient taking a full inspiratory capacity breath. During phase two, the patient breathes at a low volume to allow mucous to build in the airways. During the final phase of autogenic drainage the patient "stacks" three breaths on top of each other, followed by a cough, which may require your assistance. Some studies suggest that this procedure can be as effective as postural drainage, percussion, and vibration, but is more difficult to apply because it requires patient cooperation.

The rationale for this technique is that the appropriately rapid air flow may mobilize secretions by shearing them from the bronchial walls and transporting them from the peripheral airways to the mouth. The specific style of breathing described is performed at different lung volumes, usually starting within the expiratory reserve volume (ERV) and progressing into the inspiratory reserve volume (IRV). This technique is summarized below.

   • Inspire a deeper than normal breath; about 1.5–2 times tidal volume
   • Exhale in a gentle but active way to:
      ○ Achieve the highest possible expiratory air flow simultaneously in different generations of the bronchi
      ○ Keep bronchial resistance low
      ○ Avoid bronchospasm and dynamic airway collapse

Mechanical Devices to Facilitate Secretion Clearance

Equipment designed to aid in secretion clearance includes high-frequency chest wall oscillation (HFCWO) systems, simple and vibratory PEP devices, the intrapulmonary percussive ventilation (IPV) device, and the mechanical insufflator-exsufflator (MI-E). Details on the selection, setup, application, and troubleshooting of HFCWO systems, PEP devices, and IPV devices are provided in Chapter 6.

Table 11-3 lists the contraindications and hazards/complications associated with airway-clearance devices that apply positive pressure during breathing (PEP, IPV, and mechanical insufflation). Here we focus on application of the mechanical insufflator-exsufflator.

Mechanical insufflation-exsufflation, also known as MI-E or cough assist (**Figure 11-3**), involves the application of alternating positive and negative pressure to the airway to help increase expiratory flows and remove secretions. This noninvasive therapy can be applied with a variety of patient interfaces, including a mask or mouthpiece for spontaneously breathing patients or a standard 15-mm adaptor for artificial airways. The inspiratory and expiratory time and pressure can be manually adjusted or pre-set for models with auto mode. Because it is noninvasive, cough assist has a low infection risk and therefore should be considered for patients who frequently need help with secretion removal, such as those with advanced neuromuscular disorders. The major features of MI-E therapy are as follows:

Indications

- Weak cough effort as suggested by maximum expiratory pressure less than 60 cm H_2O or peak cough flow (similar to peak flow) approximately less than 270 L/min

Contraindications

- History of bullous emphysema
- Susceptibility to pneumothorax or pneumomediastinum
- Recent barotrauma

Key Elements of Procedure

- Test equipment by turning it on, occluding the circuit and toggling between inhalation and exhalation.
- Adjust initial inhalation/exhalation pressures to between 10 and 15 cm H_2O.
- If auto mode, set inhale time and exhale time to 2–3 seconds.
- Connect circuit interface to patient's airway.
- Adjust airway inhalation pressures between 15 and 40 cm H_2O and exhalation pressures between 35–45 cm H_2O (in general, the lowest pressures needed to effectively remove secretions should be used).
- Administer 4–6 cycles of insufflation/exsufflation.
- Remove visible secretions from airway or tubing.
- Return patient to prescribed mode of ventilation and oxygen.
- Assess patient and repeat as appropriate.

Table 11-3 Contraindications and Hazards/Complications Associated with Airway Clearance Devices Using Positive Pressure

Contraindications	Hazards and Complications
• Patients unable to tolerate the increased work of breathing (e.g., acute asthma, COPD) • Intracranial pressure (ICP) > 20 mm Hg • Hemodynamic instability • Recent facial, oral, or skull surgery or trauma • Acute sinusitis • Epistaxis • Esophageal surgery • Active hemoptysis • Nausea • Known or suspected tympanic membrane rupture or other middle ear pathology • Untreated pneumothorax	• Increased work of breathing • Increased intracranial pressure • Cardiovascular compromise • Myocardial ischemia • Decreased venous return • Air swallowing • Claustrophobia • Skin breakdown and discomfort from mask • Pulmonary barotrauma

Recommended Modifications

- As an alternative to a 15-mm adaptor, treatment can be applied to patients with ET or trach tubes by adapting to inline/suction catheter for easy removal of secretions.
- Higher exhalation pressures may be required to overcome the increased resistance of ET or trach tubes.
- When administering therapy to patients with a trach, you should include a means for collecting secretions such as a sputum trap.

Clearance of Secretions via Suctioning

If directed coughing techniques and the use of adjunct devices designed to facilitate secretion removal are ineffective, you may need to consider suctioning. Suctioning is used as needed on all patients with artificial tracheal airways. In addition, patients with certain neuromuscular disorders or those with conditions causing an increase in the volume or thickness of secretions may also require suctioning.

Chapter 6 provides details on the selection, use, and troubleshooting of the equipment used for suctioning, including both vacuum systems and suction apparatus. Here we focus on the procedures that you employ to prevent or remove retained secretions.

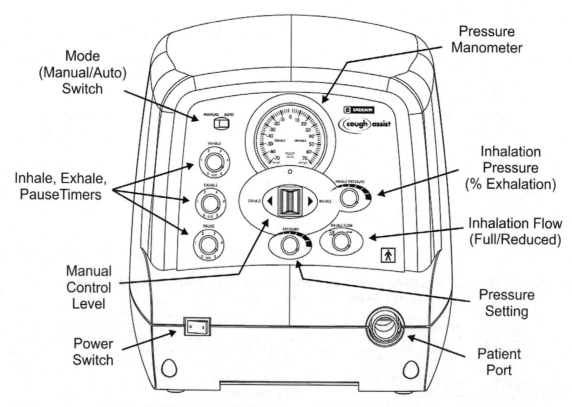

Figure 11-3 Cough-Assist or Mechanical Insufflation-Exsufflation (M-IE) Device.
Mask and large-bore tubing attach to the patient port. Power switch turns unit on/off. The mode switch toggles between automatic and manual modes. The pressure setting varies the inhalation and exhalation pressures together, while the inhalation pressure knob adjusts this value to a percent of the exhalation pressure. Inhalation flow can be switched between full or reduced. Three timers allow adjustment of the inhalation, exhalation, and pause time. A pressure manometer calibrated in cm H_2O displays the pressure changes.

Adapted from: Cough Assist™. User's Guide. Cambridge, MA: J.H. Emerson Co.

Indications and Hazards

Several clinical clues indicate the need for suctioning:

- Presence of a weak, loose cough
- Auscultation revealing rhonchi
- Direct observation of secretions in the mouth or oropharynx
- Fremitus (vibrations) felt on the chest wall
- Patient feedback suggesting retained secretions

For patients receiving mechanical ventilation, an increase in peak pressure (volume-limited ventilation) or a decrease in delivered volume (pressure-limited ventilation) may indicate the presence of secretions. Additionally, less-specific indications for excessive secretions may be deterioration in pulse oximetry readings or arterial blood gases and a chest X-ray indicating atelectasis.

Suctioning is among the most dangerous procedures that you perform. Potential hazards and complications associated with the various suctioning methods include the following:

- Oxygen desaturation
- Trauma to the oral, tracheal, or bronchial mucosa
- Cardiac arrest
- Respiratory arrest
- Cardiac dysrhythmias
- Bronchospasm or bronchoconstriction
- Airway infection
- Bleeding or hemorrhage from the airway
- Hypertension
- Hypotension
- Infection
- Elevated ICP
- Pulmonary atelectasis

Careful implementation of patient safety measures before, during, and after the procedure, as well as careful monitoring throughout, can prevent or minimize most of these potential risks. In most cases, the danger associated with *not* clearing retained secretions far outweighs these potential hazards. It is for this reason that there are few or any absolute contraindications to clearing retained secretions by suctioning.

Routes for Suctioning

You can suction secretions from a patient's mouth and pharynx or trachea and bronchi. Tracheobronchial suctioning is normally performed through an artificial airway, but it can be accomplished via the nasal route.

Oropharyngeal Suctioning

Oropharyngeal suctioning involves the removal of excessive secretions, vomit, and/or food particles from the oral cavity and pharynx. For this reason, you normally need to use a rigid catheter with a larger diameter lumen, such as a Yankauer suction tip (**Figure 11-4**). With a Yankauer tip, you can reach the back of the oropharyngeal cavity and remove both liquid secretions and moderately large particulate matter. An alternative for removing liquid secretions from the posterior pharynx is to thread

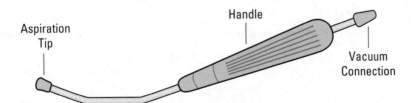

Figure 11-4 Yankauer Suction Tip.

a large flexible suction catheter through an oro- or nasopharyngeal airway into this region. If there is vomitus in the oral cavity that is too thick to pass through a Yankauer tip, some clinicians suggest using the large-bore semi-rigid tubing that connects to a vacuum collection bottle for aspirating this material.

Suctioning Through a Tracheal Airway

Equipment and Patient Preparation

1. Select, gather, assemble, and check the required equipment (see Chapter 6)
   - Suction source (portable suction pump, wall regulator/collector)
   - Suction equipment (e.g., catheters, collection traps)
2. Decontaminate hands and apply standard/transmission-based precautions as appropriate
3. Identify patient, introduce self and department
4. Explain/demonstrate procedure and confirm patient understanding

Assessment and Implementation

5. Assess patient for adequate oxygenation, cardiac rhythm, need for suction
6. Adjust suction to appropriate level
7. Position patient
8. Hyperoxygenate and hyperinflate patient for at least 1 minute
9. Put on sterile gloves
10. Maintain sterile technique throughout procedure
11. Pour sterile water into sterile container
12. Attach sputum trap to suction source (if required)
13. Attach catheter to suction source
14. Reassure patient; disconnect oxygen or ventilator source
15. Insert catheter with suction port open into airway and advance until resistance is met
16. Withdraw catheter 1–2 cm
17. Apply suction continuously while withdrawing the catheter for less than 10–15 seconds
18. Reassess patient
19. Lavage with sterile saline, if indicated
20. Hyperoxygenate and hyperinflate patient for at least 1 minute
21. Rinse catheter with sterile solution and repeat if necessary
22. Reassess patient airway and patient periodically; reinstruct if necessary
23. Reassure patient, resume oxygen or ventilator source

Follow-up

24. Restore patient to prior status
25. Return F_{IO_2} to prior settings
26. Maintain/process equipment and supplies
27. Dispose of infectious waste and decontaminate hands
28. Record pertinent data in chart and departmental records
29. Notify appropriate personnel and make any necessary recommendations or modifications to the patient care plan

Adapted from: Scanlan, C. L., West, G. A., von der Heydt, P. A., & Dolan, G. K. (1984). *Respiratory therapy competency evaluation manual.* Boston: Blackwell Scientific.

Suctioning Through a Tracheal Airway

Suctioning of patients through endotracheal or tracheostomy tubes is the most common procedure used to help prevent retained secretions. The accompanying box outlines the essential steps in this procedure.

Essentially all suction systems have an adjustable suction setting. You should set the vacuum pressure to the lowest level needed to effectively remove the secretions. For centrally piped vacuum systems, the recommended negative pressure range for adults is between −100 and −120 mm Hg and −80 and −100 mm Hg for children. Negative pressure applied to the infant airway generally should be limited to −60 to −80 mm Hg. To assure that there is adequate space for gas to flow around the catheter and prevent atelectasis, always select a suction catheter with an outside diameter (OD) no larger than ½ the inner diameter of the patient's artificial airway. **Table 11-4** lists the recommended suction catheter diameters to be used with tracheal tubes in the 2.5- to 9.5-mm ID range. Alternatively, you can quickly estimate the correct catheter size in French units (Fr): simply double the internal diameter (ID) of the tracheal tube and select the next smallest catheter size. For example, to suction a patient with a 6.0-mm tracheal tube:

$$2 \times 6 = 12$$
Next smallest catheter size = 10 Fr

In regard to suctioning patients receiving mechanical ventilation with 5 or more cm H_2O PEEP, the AARC recommends that you assure that adequate PEEP levels are maintained during the procedure. The best way to do so is to use a closed suction system. These systems also may offer the advantage of less chance of cross-contamination and may help lower the incidence of ventilator-associated pneumonia.

Figure 11-5 depicts the key components of a closed suction system for use on ventilator patients (a separate model is available for spontaneous breathing patients with trach tubes). Key points to help assure effectiveness and safety when using this device include the following:

- Select the correct version of the system (versions for trach patients have shorter catheters).
- Always set the pressure on the suction regulator with the thumb valve fully depressed.

Table 11-4 Recommended Suction Catheter Diameters

Tracheal Tube (ID mm)	Suction Catheter (OD French)
2.5–3.0	5
3.0–4.0	6
4.0	6
4.5	8
5.0	8
5.5	10
6.0	10
6.5	12
7.0	12
8.0	14
8.5	16
9.0	16
> 9.0	16
8.5–9.5	16

- Apply closed suction to patients receiving ventilatory support only with a mode that either (1) provides continuous flow through the circuit or (2) will trigger and provide flow during suctioning (avoid pure volume control mode).
- Always be sure to stabilize the airway when suctioning by keeping firm hold of the T-piece with your nondominant hand while inserting or withdrawing the catheter.
- To avoid bunching of the sleeve from limited insertion depth, advance the catheter from at or near the airway connection about 2 inches at a time.
- To avoid trauma and minimize dangerous vagal responses, many clinicians recommend using closed systems with cm markers for adults (required for infants) and limiting insertion depth to 2 cm beyond the tip of the ET.
- Always be sure to fully withdraw the catheter at the end of the procedure (indicated by visualizing the black marking ring); if the catheter is not fully withdrawn, increased airway pressure and work of breathing may occur.
- However, be careful not to withdraw the catheter too far; if you do so, the catheter side holes may pass the seal and allow gas from the ventilator to enter the sleeve.
- Always lock the thumb valve in the OFF position at the end of the procedure; failure to do so could result in accidental application of suction.
- To clear the catheter after withdrawal, instill at least 5 mL normal saline through the lavage port while applying continuous suction; always cap the lavage port after use.
- Change the closed suction system as per manufacturer recommendations or institutional protocol.

A common problem in intubated patients is leakage of subglottic secretions past the tracheal tube cuff. These secretions can contaminate the lower respiratory tract and are thought to be a major contributing factor in the development of ventilator-associated pneumonia (VAP). Although frequent oropharyngeal suctioning can help prevent accumulation of subglottic secretions, it cannot remove them.

For this reason, many VAP protocols call for continuous aspiration of subglottic secretions (CASS). As depicted in **Figure 11-6**, this is accomplished using specially designed tracheal tubes that incorporate a suction port just above the cuff. You connect this lumen via its separate suction line to a standard wall suction unit and set it to apply continuous low suction, normally 20 mm Hg. In order to avoid any confusion over various connecting lines (cuff inflation line, feeding lines, etc.) you should label the CASS suction port clearly.

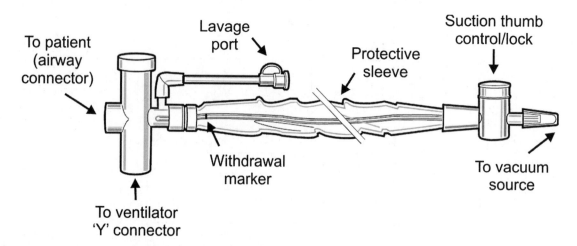

Figure 11-5 Closed Suction System.

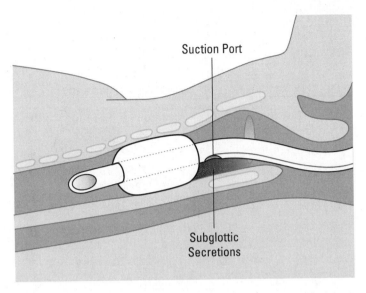

Suction Port

Subglottic
Secretions

**Figure 11-6 Endotracheal Tube Designed for Continuous Aspiration of
Subglottic Secretions (CASS).**

Nasotracheal Suctioning

Nasotracheal suctioning is the most common method used to clear secretions in patients who do not
have artificial airways, but do have an ineffective cough. Contraindications for nasotracheal suctioning include the following:

- Occluded nasal passages
- Nasal bleeding
- Epiglottitis or croup
- Acute head, facial, or neck injury
- Coagulopathy or bleeding disorder
- Laryngospasm
- Irritable airway
- Surgery
- Gastric surgery with high anastomosis

With a few exceptions, the procedure is similar to that employed to suction through a tracheal
airway. To minimize the risk of spreading nasopharyngeal bacteria into the lungs, many protocols include having patients blow their noses and rinse their mouths and throats with an antiseptic mouthwash
prior to the procedure. To avoid airway trauma, you should lubricate the catheter with a sterile, water-
soluble jelly before insertion. If frequent secretion clearance is required, you can minimize airway
trauma by keeping a nasopharyngeal airway in place and suctioning through it. In this case, you should
lubricate the catheter with sterile water, not water-soluble jelly.

To increase the likelihood of the catheter entering the trachea, you must position the patient properly. As indicated in **Figure 11-7**, a modified sniffing position should be used, with the neck slightly hy-
perextended and the tongue displaced forward. If the patient cannot displace his or her tongue, you
may need to manually put it forward (using a 4 × 4 gauze pad) during insertion. You then should advance the catheter slowly during inspiration (to assure abduction of the vocal cords). In most patients,
vigorous coughing confirms that you have passed through vocal cords and are in the trachea.

Assessment

You judge the effectiveness of suctioning by assessing the amount of secretions removed, as well as
changes in breath sounds, vital signs, and oxygenation. For a patient being mechanically ventilated in

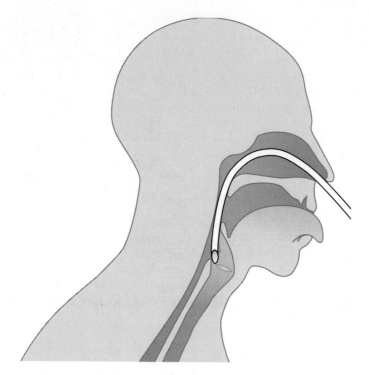

Figure 11-7 Patient Positioning for Insertion of a Nasotracheal Suction Catheter.

a volume-limited mode, removal of retained secretions usually reduces peak airway pressures, whereas patients receiving pressure-limited ventilation may experience an increase in delivered volume. Ultimately, the benefits of bronchial hygiene, including suctioning, may be seen in improved aeration on the chest X-ray and an overall improvement in clinical status.

Administer Aerosol Therapy with Prescribed Medications

Bland Aerosols

For patients with bypassed upper airways or those otherwise predisposed to retain secretions, bland aerosol therapy may be helpful. If properly administered, bland aerosol therapy may benefit the patient in one or more of the following ways:

- Ease of secretion clearance
- Decreased work of breathing
- Improved vital signs
- Decreased stridor
- Improved arterial blood gas values
- Improved oxygen saturation as indicated by pulse oximetry (SpO_2)

Due to its potential in some patients to cause bronchoconstriction, bland aerosol therapy is contraindicated in patients with a history of airway hyperresponsiveness. In addition to this potential problem, other potential hazards of bland aerosol therapy include the following:

- Infection
- Overhydration
- Patient discomfort
- Caregiver exposure to contagious microorganisms
- Airway edema/increased airway resistance

Details on the specific equipment used for aerosol therapy are discussed in Chapter 6. To provide bland aerosol therapy, you generally provide continuous therapy via a large-volume jet nebulizer filled with sterile water. If only intermittent therapy is required, you may instead apply individual treatments via a small-volume jet or ultrasonic nebulizer delivering sterile normal saline or water. Because the desired site of deposition for these bland aerosols is the larger airways, the targeted aerosol size is a mass median diameter (MMAD) of 5 microns or larger. If the goal is to induce coughing and obtain sputum for laboratory examination (sputum induction), you should use either a high-density ultrasonic water aerosol or a hypertonic saline solution (typically 5%).

Administration of Prescribed Agents

Administration of aerosolized medications delivery is covered in Chapter 12. In this section of the CRT exam, the focus is primarily on the use of aerosolized medications to aid in removal of bronchopulmonary secretions.

The agents most commonly used to mobilize and remove secretions fall into the following categories: bronchodilators, mucolytics, steroids, and diluting agents. These agents and their roles in bronchial hygiene are summarized in **Table 11-5**.

Bronchodilators such as albuterol are designed to dilate or open the airways, which when coupled with the thinning action of mucolytics may aid secretion clearance. The most common mucolytic agents are acetylcysteine (Mucomyst) or dornase alfa (Pulmozyme), which work directly on the mucous to reduce its viscosity. These agents are often used in patients with conditions like cystic fibrosis or those with abnormally thick secretions not easy managed with bland aerosol therapy. Two other types of aerosolized agents that may be helpful in secretion removal are corticosteroids and diluting agents such as hypertonic saline. By reducing airway inflammation, inhaled steroids help maintain airway patency and may reduce secretions production. Diluting agents such as aerosolized saline work by thinning secretions and thus helping with mucous removal.

Table 11-5 Selected Aerosol Agents Used to Facilitate Secretion Clearance

Agent	Classification	Example	Role in Bronchial Hygiene
Bronchodilators	Sympathomimetics	Albuterol	Dilates airways
	Parasympatholytics	Ipratropium Bromide	Dilates airways
	Xanthines	Theophylline	Dilates airways
Steroids	Corticosteroids	Fluticisone	Anti-inflammatory; dilates airways and reduces mucous production
	Nonsteroidals	Cromolyn sodium	Anti-inflammatory; reduces mucous production and prevents bronchoconstriction
Mucolytic	Mucolytics	Acetylcysteine Dornase alpha	Thins mucous (*note:* acetylcysteine can cause bronchospasm and should therefore be ordered with a bronchodilator such as albuterol)
Diluting agents	Expectorants	Hypertonic saline	Dilutes mucus by drawing fluid from airway lining

COMMON ERRORS TO AVOID

- Avoid performing postural drainage, particularly in a head-down position, in the presence of an intracranial pressure (ICP) greater than 20 mm Hg or an unstable head or neck injury, with an active hemorrhage, or in the presence of hemodynamic instability.

- Don't apply an abdominal thrust maneuver to help clear secretions on a patient with abdominal trauma or surgical incisions.
- Avoid using positive expiratory pressure (PEP) adjuncts on patients with acute exacerbations of asthma or COPD, or on any patient who cannot tolerate the short-term added work of breathing caused by these devices.
- Don't use excessive suction pressures on patients; many hazards may be avoided. In general, suction pressures should never exceed −120 mm Hg for adults, −100 mm Hg for children, and −80 mm Hg for infants.
- Avoid applying suction to the airway for more than 15 seconds for each attempt.
- Avoid performing percussion and vibration therapy immediately before or after meals.

SURE BETS

In some situations you can be sure of the right approach to a clinical problem or scenario:

- Always monitor a patient before, during, and immediately following bronchial hygiene therapy to assure that they are tolerating the therapy. Such assessment should include their overall appearance, vital signs, breath sounds, and possible other indicators, such as pulse oximetry.
- Always remember that if a patient appears to be having an adverse reaction to bronchial hygiene therapy, stop the therapy, stay with the patient and monitor him or her, help stabilize the patient, and immediately notify the nurse and physician.
- Always consider that a patient with recent thoracic or abdominal surgery may have trouble with the inspiratory and expiratory phases of coughing. For such patients, splinting the incision site with a pillow often permits them to generate a more effective cough.
- Always recognize that some patients with an ineffective cough may need help both loosening secretions through percussion and vibration as well as clearing mucous through such means as cough assist or suctioning.
- Always remember that patients with a weak cough, rhonchi, visible secretions, or fremitus (vibrations) on the chest wall may need bronchial hygiene therapy.
- Always oxygenate a patient with an F_{IO_2} of 100% for at least a minute before each suction attempt.
- Always consider recommending the addition of bland aerosol and the administration of prescribed agents such as bronchodilators and mucolytics if a patient is unable to clear secretions in spite of percussion, vibration, and turning, as well as other adjuncts such as PEP and cough assist.
- Always remember that the effectiveness of bronchial hygiene therapy can be assessed through an improvement in breath sounds, vital signs, oxygenation, and overall appearance.

PRE-TEST ANSWERS AND EXPLANATIONS

Below are this chapter's pre-test answers and explanations. Be sure to review each answer's explanation thoroughly to help you understand why it is correct. If the explanation is still unclear to you, review the chapter contents or the references and/or refer to this chapter's supplemental resources on the CD.

11-1. **Correct answer: C.** I and IV only. In order to drain the posterior basal segments, a patient should be prone for the posterior and in Trendelenburg position (30° down tilt) with a pillow under the hips for the basal segments.

11-2. **Correct answer: B.** Superior segment of lower lobes. The superior segments of the lower lobes are drained in a flat prone position with a pillow under the abdomen.

11-3. **Correct answer: D.** Low inspiratory volumes. The effectiveness of a cough requires proper integration of three phases: inspiratory component, compression phase, and finally the explosive exhalation. Energy is transferred to the mucous and it is expelled from the airway. Strong abdominal muscles to generate large volumes with glottis closure will generate high intra-alveolar pressures and a good cough.

11-4. **Correct answer: B.** I, II, and III. When applying nasotracheal suctioning, the patient should be pre- and post-oxygenated, and the suction catheter tip should be prelubricated. As with tracheal suctioning in general, the time for applying suction should not exceed 15 seconds.

11-5. **Correct answer: C.** Acetylcysteine (Mucomyst). Acetylcysteine breaks the disulfide bonds in mucous, thereby helping thin and mobilize secretions in patients with mucous plugs.

11-6. **Correct answer: B.** Sitting position leaning forward on a pillow. To drain the posterior segments of the upper lobes, the proper patient position should be sitting on a chair leaning forward on a pillow.

11-7. **Correct answer: A.** Postural drainage, percussion, and vibration. Of the choices available, the bronchial hygiene technique that is most suitable for small infants is postural drainage, percussion, and vibration. Positive expiratory pressure and high-frequency oscillation are generally not used on infants, and aggressive suctioning, especially with a large catheter, would be potentially harmful.

11-8. **Correct answer: D.** Suction at a pressure range of –60 to –80 mm Hg, limiting the time to less than 10–15 seconds. The normal pressure range for adults is –100 to –120 mm Hg, for children –80 to –100 mm Hg, and for infants –60 to –80 mm Hg. The patient should be preoxygenated with 100% oxygen for at least a minute, and the total suction time should be limited to no more than 10–15 seconds on each attempt.

11-9. **Correct answer: D.** II, III, and IV. Major hazards and complications of postural drainage, percussion, and vibration include hypoxemia; acute hypotension during the procedure; pulmonary hemorrhage; pain or injury to muscles, ribs, or spine; vomiting and aspiration; bronchospasm; dysrhythmias.

11-10. **Correct answer: B.** Use of a tracheal tube with a suction port above the cuff. A common problem in intubated patients is leakage of subglottic secretions past the tracheal tube cuff. These secretions can contaminate the lower respiratory tract and are thought to be a major contributing factor in the development of ventilator-associated pneumonia (VAP).

POST-TEST

A post-test for this chapter that includes automated scoring and feedback is available on the accompanying CD. Be sure to complete this additional assessment to confirm your mastery of this chapter's objectives.

REFERENCES

American Association for Respiratory Care. (1991). Clinical practice guideline. Postural drainage therapy. *Respiratory care, 36*, 1418–1426.

American Association for Respiratory Care. (1993). Clinical practice guidelines. Endotracheal suctioning of mechanically ventilated adults and children with artificial airways. *Respiratory care, 38*, 500–504.

American Association for Respiratory Care. (1993). Clinical practice guideline. Directed cough. *Respiratory care, 38*, 495–499.

American Association for Respiratory Care. (1993). Clinical practice guideline. Use of positive airway pressure adjuncts to bronchial hygiene therapy. *Respiratory care, 38*, 516–521.

American Association for Respiratory Care. (2003). Clinical practice guidelines. Bland aerosol administration: 2003 revision and update. *Respiratory care, 48*, 529–533.

American Association for Respiratory Care. (2004). Clinical practice guidelines. Nasotracheal suctioning: 2004 revision and update. *Respiratory care, 49*, 1080–1084.

Hardy, K. A., & Anderson, B. D. (1996). Noninvasive clearance of airway secretions. *Respiratory care clinics of north america, 2*, 323–345.

Lapin, C. (2002). Airway physiology, autogenic drainage, and active cycle of breathing. *Respiratory care, 47*, 778–779.

Murry, J. F., & Nadel, J. A. (1994). *Textbook of respiratory medicine*. Philadelphia: W. B. Saunders.

Wilkins, R. L., Stoller, J. K., & Kacmarek, R. M. (Eds.). (2009). *Egan's fundamentals of respiratory care*. (9th ed.). St. Louis: Mosby.

Wyka, K. A., Mathews, P. J., & Clark, W. F. (2002). *Foundations of respiratory care*. Albany: Delmar.

Achieve Adequate Respiratory Support

Craig Scanlan
Roy Mekaru

INTRODUCTION

Achieving adequate respiratory support is one of many critical roles that respiratory therapists provide to help assure quality care. Although this area is not one of the major areas on the CRT exam, its content is very broad in scope and emphasizes application-level questions. New additions to what is tested for in this area include high-frequency ventilation, as well as disease-specific protocols for mechanical ventilation. Also, new to some candidates will be coverage of newer modes of mechanical ventilation such as airway pressure release ventilation (APRV) and new drugs you may be expected to administer by the inhalation route. Good preparation for the CRT exam requires that you devote sufficient attention to this area to master its content.

OBJECTIVES

After completion of this chapter, you should demonstrate the knowledge needed to:

1. Instruct a patient in
   a. Deep breathing and incentive spirometry techniques
   b. Inspiratory muscle training techniques
2. Initiate and adjust
   a. IPPB therapy
   b. Continuous mechanical ventilation settings
   c. Noninvasive ventilation
   d. Elevated baseline pressure (e.g., CPAP, PEEP)
3. Select ventilator graphics (e.g., waveforms, scales)
4. Apply disease-specific ventilator protocols
5. Initiate and select appropriate settings for high-frequency ventilation
6. Initiate and modify weaning procedures
7. Administer medications:
   a. Aerosolized
   b. Dry powder preparations
   c. Via endotracheal instillation
8. Administer oxygen
9. Position patient to minimize hypoxemia
10. Prevent procedure-associated hypoxemia

WHAT TO EXPECT ON THIS CATEGORY OF THE CRT EXAM

Number of questions: 8
Level of questions: about 25% recall, 60% application, 15% analysis

WHAT'S NEW FOR 2009

As of July 2009, this section of the NBRC CRT examination includes the following *new content areas*:

* Initiate and select appropriate settings for high-frequency ventilation
* Administer medications as dry powder aerosols and via endotracheal instillation
* Apply disease-specific ventilator protocols (e.g., ARDS-Net protocol)

PRE-TEST

Carefully respond to each of the following questions. After completing the pre-test, compare your answers to those provided at the end of this chapter. Then thoroughly review each answer's explanation to help understand why it is correct.

12-1. While suctioning a patient receiving ventilatory support, you note the heart rate increases abruptly from 92 to 145 beats per minute. Which of the following actions could help prevent or minimize this problem?
  A. Recommend an IV dose of atropine before suctioning
  B. Instill lidocaine (Xylocaine) into the trachea before suctioning
  C. Increase the oxygen concentration immediately before suctioning
  D. Give the patient two MDI puffs of beclomethasone before suctioning

12-2. An ARDS patient is receiving ventilatory support with 100% oxygen and PEEP at the recommended high limit of the protocol (25 cm H_2O) but remains dangerously hypoxemic. Long plateau pressures and inverse ratio ventilation have been tried, but without success. Which of the following should you recommend to improve this patient's oxygenation?
  A. Increase the mandatory rate
  B. Put the patient in the prone position
  C. Administer a paralytic agent
  D. Increase the pressure limit

12-3. Which of the following is the appropriate load to establish for patients receiving inspiratory muscle training?
  A. At least 33% of the predicted inspiratory capacity (IC)
  B. At least 10–15 ml/kg of predicted body weight (PBW)
  C. At least 30% of the maximum inspiratory pressure (MIP/PImax)
  D. At least –25 cm H_2O, as measured by a calibrated manometer

12-4. To obtain the most effective ventilation, a patient with severe emphysema should be instructed to:
  A. Inhale slowly
  B. Exhale slowly
  C. Hold every third breath
  D. Breathe as deeply as possible

12-5. For which of the following patients would you carefully monitor cardiovascular function during application of intermittent positive pressure breathing (IPPB)?
  I. A patient suffering from low blood pressure
  II. A patient with poor vasomotor tone
  III. A patient with cardiac insufficiency
  A. I and II only
  B. II and III only
  C. I and III only
  D. I, II, and III

12-6. An adult patient in respiratory failure has the following ABGs on a simple O_2 mask at 8 L/min: pH = 7.19; $Paco_2$ = 68 torr; HCO_3 = 28 mEq/L; Pao_2 = 85 torr. The attending physician orders intubation and ventilatory support. Which of the following modes of support are appropriate for this patient?

    I. CMV at a frequency of 12/min
    II. IMV at a frequency of 12/min
    III. CPAP with 10 cm H_2O pressure

A. I or II only
B. II or III only
C. I or III only
D. I, II, or III

12-7. A doctor asks you to decrease the $Paco_2$ of a patient receiving high-frequency ventilation oscillation ventilation (HFOV). You should consider all of the following adjustments *except*:

A. Increasing the power/amplitude
B. Decreasing the frequency
C. Deflating the ET tube cuff
D. Decreasing the bias flow

12-8. A patient with congestive heart failure is coughing up large quantities of pink, frothy sputum. ABG values on simple mask O_2 at 7 L/min are as follows:

pH	7.44
$Paco_2$	29 torr
HCO_3	20 mEq/L
BE	−3 mEq/L
Pao_2	46 torr
Sao_2	76%

Which of the following treatments would you recommend?
A. Nonrebreathing mask at 12 L/min and postural drainage therapy
B. Intermittent positive pressure breathing (IPPB) with compressed air
C. Starting intrapulmonary percussive ventilation to clear secretions
D. Mask continuous positive airway pressure (CPAP) with 80% O_2

12-9. A patient during CPR can not have an intravenous line started. The physician wants to administer nalaxone because the patient is suffering from a morphine overdose. What is an alternative route of administration?

A. Nasogastric (NG) tube
B. Feeding tube
C. Aerosol
D. Endotracheal tube

12-10. Data for a patient being mechanically ventilated are below.

Ventilator Settings		Blood Gases	
Mode	CMV-AC	pH	7.55
V_T	900 ml	$Paco_2$	20 torr
Set rate	10	HCO_3	17 mEq/L
Actual rate	20	Pao_2	125 torr
FIO_2	0.35	Sao_2	99%

Based on this information, you would suggest which of the following?
A. Add 5 cm H_2O PEEP
B. Add deadspace to the breathing circuit
C. Change to the IMV mode with a set rate of 10 breaths/min
D. Set the FIO_2 to 0.25

12-11. During a patient-ventilator check in the ICU, you observe the following settings and monitored parameters on a 70-kg (154-lb.) patient receiving ventilator support:

Mode	SIMV
V_T	600 mL
Mandatory rate	10
Total rate	38
PEEP	8 cm H_2O
Minute volume	10 L/min

Which of the following actions would you recommend at this time?
A. Switch to assist/control mode
B. Decrease the mandatory rate
C. Add pressure support
D. Increase the PEEP level

12-12. Data for a 63-kg (140-lb.) patient receiving ventilatory support with 10 cm PEEP are as follows:

Ventilator Settings		Blood Gases	
Mode	SIMV	pH	7.45
V_T	600 ml	$Paco_2$	36 torr
Rate	10	HCO_3	25 mEq/L
Fio_2	0.70	Pao_2	55 torr
PEEP	5 cm H_2O	Sao_2	100%

Which of the following changes should you recommend at this time?
A. Lower the V_T
B. Increase the rate
C. Increase PEEP
D. Decrease the Fio_2

12-13. Which of the following best describes the way a patient should perform incentive spirometry?
A. The patient should exhale maximally and hold it for at least 5 seconds
B. The patient should inhale normally hold it for several seconds
C. The patient should hold a maximum inspiratory capacity (IC) breath for at least 5 seconds
D. The patient should repeat maximum inspiratory and expiratory efforts for 10–15 seconds

12-14. An ARDS patient is receiving ventilatory support with 100% oxygen and 20 cm H_2O PEEP with a plateau pressure of 30 cm H_2O, but remains dangerously hypoxemic. Which of the following should you recommend to improve this patient's oxygenation?
A. Using inverse ratio ventilation (I:E > 1:1)
B. Putting the patient in the prone position
C. Administering a paralytic agent
D. Increasing the pressure limit

12-15. You are called to the ER to help in the assessment and care of a patient admitted with severe pulmonary edema. While starting an intravenous line, the physician tells you to give the patient O_2. You should provide oxygen to this patient via a:
A. Nonrebreathing mask at 15 L/min
B. Nasal cannula at 6 L/min
C. Simple face mask at 7 L/min
D. 50% air-entrainment mask

12-16. A patient receiving bilevel positive airway pressure for acute respiratory failure has a Pao_2 of 48 torr on 65% O_2 with IPAP = 20 cm H_2O and EPAP = 5 cm H_2O. To raise this patient's Pao_2, you should recommend:
A. Increasing the Fio_2 to 0.80
B. Increasing IPAP to 25 cm H_2O
C. Increasing EPAP to 10 cm H_2O
D. Decreasing IPAP to 15 cm H_2O

12-17. A patient who is receiving 0.5 mL isoetharine (Bronkosol) in 3 mL of normal saline three times a day to relieve bronchospasm complains of nervousness and palpitations after therapy. You should consider recommending all of the following to the patient's doctor *except*:
A. Substituting levalbuterol (Xopenex) for the isoetharine
B. Decreasing the dose of isoetharine to 0.25 mL
C. Substituting budesonide (Pulmicort) for the isoetharine
D. Substituting albuterol (Proventil) for the isoetharine

12-18. A doctor institutes volume control ventilation for an 80-kg (176-lb.) ARDS patient. Which of the following is the maximum pressure you should aim to achieve in this patient?
A. 50 cm H_2O peak pressure
B. 30 cm H_2O plateau pressure
C. 40 cm H_2O peak pressure
D. 50 cm H_2O plateau pressure

12-19. A patient receiving mechanical ventilation has the following ventilator settings and arterial blood gas results:

Ventilator Settings		Blood Gases	
Mode	SIMV	pH	7.26
V_T	750 ml	$Paco_2$	56 torr
Set rate	4	HCO_3	22 mEq/L
Spontaneous rate	0	Pao_2	92 torr
Fio_2	0.55	Sao_2	96%

Which of the following should you recommend?
A. Increasing the inspiratory time
B. Increasing the tidal volume to 800 mL
C. Decreasing the Fio_2 to 0.50
D. Increasing the SIMV rate

12-20. Thirty minutes into a spontaneous breathing trial to determine if a patient can be removed from ventilatory support, you note a 15-torr rise in the $Paco_2$, an increase in the rate of breathing from 20 to 35 breaths per minute, and greater dependence on accessory muscle use. Based on these observations, you should recommend:
A. Continuing the trial and carefully monitoring the patient for an additional 30 minutes
B. Ending the trial and returning the patient to a full ventilatory support mode
C. Adding 10 cm H_2O pressure support and obtaining another ABG to assess the effect
D. Ending the trial and restoring the patient to partial support to exercise the diaphragm

WHAT YOU NEED TO KNOW: ESSENTIAL CONTENT

Instruct Patients in Deep Breathing/Muscle Training

Deep breathing, incentive spirometry, and respiratory muscle training are used in both the acute care and rehabilitation settings. In acute care, these methods can aid secretion clearance, prevent or treat post-op atelectasis, and improve aerosol drug delivery. In the rehabilitation setting, breathing and muscle training exercises can improve the efficiency of ventilation and exercise tolerance.

Deep Breathing Exercises

Breathing exercises work by imposing resistance to muscle contraction. Initially, this resistance helps the patient focus on the appropriate muscle action. Over time, inspiratory breathing exercises can increase the strength and endurance of the diaphragm and increase exercise tolerance.

There are two types of inspiratory breathing exercises: diaphragmatic (abdominal) breathing and lateral costal breathing. Both are intended to promote effective use of the diaphragm, with less emphasis on the accessory muscles of inspiration. As an added benefit, inspiratory breathing exercises can improve the efficiency of ventilation by increasing V_T and decreasing the rate of breathing.

Key steps in teaching diaphragmatic breathing include the following:

- Place the patient in a semi-Fowler's position, with forearms relaxed and knees bent.
- Position your hand on the patient's upper abdomen, below the xiphoid.
- Encourage the patient to inhale slowly through the nose and "push out" against your hand.
- Provide progressive resistance to the abdominal movement until end-inspiration.
- Repeat this exercise (with rest as needed) until satisfactory movement is achieved.

As with any teaching process, you should first demonstrate this technique on yourself, while explaining both the "why" and "how" to the patient. As the patient's performance improves, you can extend the exercise time. You should also assist ambulatory patients in diaphragmatic breathing while standing and walking. Your goal is to get patients performing these exercises on their own. In the rehabilitation setting, patients can create the resistance using a small weight (about 5 lbs.) placed over the upper abdomen and progressively increase the load as their diaphragm strengthens.

Lateral costal breathing exercises aim to enhance expansion of the costal margins, which also increases diaphragmatic excursion and strength. These exercises are a good alternative to the diaphragmatic method, especially for patients who have undergone abdominal surgery. The technique is similar to that used in teaching diaphragmatic breathing, but with the resistance applied by both hands "cupping" the lower rib edges. As you apply increasing resistance during inspiration, you instruct the patient to slowly "breathe around the waist" and push out against your hands. As with the diaphragmatic method, your goal is to teach patients to perform these exercises on their own.

Expiratory breathing technique is also important, especially for COPD patients. Exhalation through pursed lips increases "back pressure" in the airways during exhalation and can help lessen the air-trapping that tends to occur in these patients. Pursed-lip breathing also decreases expiratory flow, which prolongs the expiratory time and decreases the rate of breathing. In combination, these effects can improve ventilation and may help diminish the sensation of dyspnea. When teaching pursed-lip breathing, you should have the patient aim for an expiratory time that is at least 2–3 times longer than inspiration, while avoiding strenuous expiratory effort.

Incentive Spirometry

Incentive spirometry (IS) uses simple disposable indicator devices to help patients perform slow, deep breaths accompanied by a breath hold (a sustained maximal inspiration). IS is used primarily in the acute care setting for patients at risk for or diagnosed with atelectasis, typically those who have undergone thoracic or abdominal surgery. IS cannot be performed with patients who cannot cooperate or generate an inspiratory capacity that is at least a third of their predicted values. The primary hazard of IS is discomfort due to pain. Improperly administered IS can result in hyperventilation and fatigue.

Chapter 6 provides details on the selection, use, and troubleshooting of incentive spirometry equipment. The accompanying box outlines the basic procedure for incentive spirometry.

Incentive Spirometry Procedure

Equipment and Patient Preparation

1. Verify, interpret, and evaluate doctor's order or protocol

2. Scan chart for diagnosis and other pertinent data and notes

3. Select, gather, assemble, and check the required equipment

4. Decontaminate hands and apply standard/transmission-based precautions as appropriate

5. Identify patient, introduce self and department

6. Explain/demonstrate procedure and confirm patient understanding

Assessment and Implementation

7. Assess patient progress by the following:

   a. Pain medication schedule

   b. Chest X-ray report

   c. Patient's temperature

   d. Preoperative evaluation of volumes and capacities

   e. Patient's vital signs

   f. Auscultation of breath sounds

8. Assemble the incentive spirometer

9. Instruct the patient on the use and frequency of the incentive spirometer

   a. Include breath hold for 5–10 seconds

   b. Repeat the procedure 6–10 times per hour; allow adequate recovery time between breaths to prevent hyperventilation

---

(continues)

10. Assist patient in splinting thoracic/abdominal surgical incisions to minimize pain

11. Have the patient demonstrate the procedure

12. Measure the achieved volume

13. Instruct the patient to cough; observe for any sputum production

14. Reassess the patient

Follow-up

15. Maintain/process equipment

16. Dispose of infectious waste and decontaminate hands

17. Record pertinent data in chart and departmental records

18. Notify appropriate personnel and make any necessary recommendations or modifications to the patient care plan

Adapted from: Scanlan, C. L., West, G. A., von der Heydt, P. A., & Dolan, G. K. (1984). *Respiratory therapy competency evaluation manual.* Boston: Blackwell Scientific.

After preliminary patient instruction and confirmation of proper incentive breathing technique, you should arrange for periodic patient visits to monitor therapy compliance and provide additional instruction as needed. During such visits, you should encourage increasing the inspiratory volume goal. Other key points that can help assure effective outcomes with IS include the following:

- If ordered for a surgical patient, instruction ideally should occur pre-operatively.
- To confirm patient understanding, always require a "return demonstration" of the procedure by the patient.
- To obtain an accurate measure of the patient's inspired volume, attach a one-way breathing valve and calibrated respirometer to the incentive breathing device.
- If on initial assessment the patient cannot cooperate or cannot generate an inspiratory capacity at least 33% of predicted, recommend IPPB as an alternative.
- If the patient is also having difficulty with retained secretions, recommend combining IS (or positive expiratory pressure therapy) with bronchial hygiene measures.
- Recommend discontinuation when clinical signs indicate resolution of atelectasis, e.g.:
  ○ Resolution of fever
  ○ Improvement in breath sounds
  ○ Normal chest X-ray
  ○ Improved arterial blood oxygenation

In addition, see Chapter 14 for discussion of various modifications you can make to tailor incentive spirometry to meet individual patient needs.

Inspiratory Muscle Training Techniques

Inspiratory muscle training (IMT) has largely replaced manual breathing exercises as the method of choice to help COPD patients manage their dyspnea, increase their exercise tolerance, and enhance their health-related quality of life. IMT may also improve patients' diaphragmatic function in some neuromuscular disorders and may aid in weaning ventilator-dependent patients.

There are two types of IMT devices: flow and threshold resistors. These are similar in concept to the resistors used to deliver positive expiratory pressure therapy (PEP), as discussed in Chapter 6. The difference is that with IMT, the patient *inhales* against the flow or threshold resistance. For IMT, the spring-loaded threshold resistor is preferred since it can be adjusted to a specific negative opening pressure. This assures a relatively constant muscle load that is independent of flow. In addition, because threshold resistor IMT allows for short inspiratory times, patients find it easier to maintain a breathing pattern that includes a prolonged expiratory phase, which is critical for those with COPD.

Key points needed to assure effective outcomes with IMT include the following:

- Before implementing IMT, train the patient in proper diaphragmatic breathing.
- Measure the patient's maximum inspiratory pressure (MIP/PImax) with a calibrated manometer.

- Encourage slow breathing (< 10–12 breaths/min) through the device with minimal initial resistance.
- Once the patient becomes accustomed to the device, slowly increase the resistance load until the inspiratory pressure is at least 30% of the MIP/PImax.
- After confirming the load setting and patient's ability to independently perform the procedure, instruct the patient to perform 10- or 15-minute exercise sessions once or twice per day.
- To help motivate the patient and assist you in progress monitoring, encourage the patient to maintain a detailed treatment log (including session dates and durations).
- If the MIP does not improve, interview the patient and inspect the log to determine the reason for failure—failure is usually due to the patient's noncompliance with the exercise plan.

Table 12-1 summarizes IMT parameter recommendations from various sources. Note in particular that patients will progressively lose any health-related benefit if they cease training.

Initiate and Adjust Mechanical Ventilation

IPPB Therapy

Intermittent positive pressure breathing (IPPB) is the application of positive pressure breaths to a patient via a pressure-cycled ventilator. IPPB is indicated to:

- Improve lung expansion in patients with atelectasis who cannot use other methods, such as incentive spirometry
- Aid in delivery of aerosolized drugs (usually when other methods have failed)
- Provide short-term ventilatory support for patients with acute hypercapnic respiratory failure or chronic muscle weakness

In terms of providing short-term ventilatory support, IPPB has for the most part been replaced with noninvasive positive pressure ventilation, as discussed later in this section. **Table 12-2** specifies the major contraindications and hazards associated with IPPB. Among the contraindications listed, only an untreated tension pneumothorax is an absolute contraindication.

Table 12-1 Recommended Inspiratory Muscle Training Parameters

Parameter	Consideration	Recommendation
Mode	Type of device	Threshold or flow-resistor (calibrated threshold preferred; if using a flow resistor, you will need to attach a calibrated manometer to the device's monitoring port)
Intensity	Load against which the person is exercising	Minimum of 30% of PImax (lower initial intensity may be needed with severe COPD patients); increase PImax by 5% per week as tolerated
Frequency/duration	Number of sessions/day	1–2 training sessions per day, depending on patient exercise tolerance
	Length of sessions	Total of 30 min per day (divided over 1–2 sessions); initial sessions may need to be limited to 3–5 minutes
	Number of days/week	4–6 days of training sessions per week according to patient tolerance
	Weeks of training	Continue indefinitely to maintain training benefits; functional improvement usually requires at least 5 weeks of training, and most benefits are lost after 6 months without training

Table 12-2 Contraindications and Hazards/Complications Associated with IPPB

Contraindications	Hazards/Complications
• Tension pneumothorax (untreated) • Intracranial pressure (ICP) > 15 mm Hg • Hemodynamic instability • Recent facial, oral, or skull surgery • Tracheoesophageal fistula • Recent esophageal surgery • Active hemoptysis • Radiographic evidence of bleb	• Increased airway resistance/work of breathing • Barotrauma, pneumothorax • Nosocomial infection • Hyperventilation or hypocarbia • Hyperoxia when oxygen is the gas source • Gastric distention • Impedance of venous return • Air trapping, auto-PEEP, overdistended alveoli

Equipment used to provide IPPB includes pneumatic or electrically powered pressure-cycled devices. Pneumatic IPPB devices (Bird Mark 7/8 and Bennett PR series) are typically driven by oxygen and use air entrainment to enhance flow and lower the F_{IO_2}. Electrically powered IPPB devices like the Bennett AP-5 use a small compressor to deliver room air to the patient. All IPPB devices provide user control over the peak inspiratory (cycle) pressure and incorporate a small-volume nebulizer for delivery of aerosolized drugs. Some IPPB devices provide additional control over the sensitivity or trigger level, inspiratory flow and flow waveform, and expiratory flow (i.e., expiratory retard). Airway interfaces common to all IPPB devices include mouthpieces, flanged mouthpieces, masks, and 15-mm ET tube adaptors. Flanged mouthpiece or masks are used for patients unable to maintain a seal with a simple mouthpiece or mouthpiece with noseclips.

With the exception of F_{IO_2} control, which device you use to deliver IPPB is less important than your skill in its application. Key points in ensuring effective IPPB include the following:

- After assembly, confirm proper operation of the equipment.
- Assess the patient before therapy (vital signs and breath sounds).
- Record the relevant outcome measure at baseline:
  - Tidal volume, inspiratory capacity for treating atelectasis
  - Peak flow or $FEV_1\%$ for bronchodilator therapy
- Adjust settings initially at a low pressure (~ 10–15 cm H_2O) with moderate flow.
- Instruct patient to insert the mouthpiece and maintain a tight seal (apply noseclips, mouth flange, or mask as needed).
- Instruct patient to inhale slightly until the machine triggers on and allow the machine to augment inspiration; measure and note the inspiratory volume.
- Adjust the sensitivity as needed to facilitate triggering.
- Adjust the pressure and flow until the tidal volume is 2–3 times the baseline value without patient discomfort.
- Instruct the patient to avoid forceful exhalation and breathe slowly (to prevent hyperventilation).
- Reassess the patient's vital signs, breath sounds, inspiratory capacity/expiatory flows.
- Observe for any adverse reactions.

To check the IPPB device's function, manually trigger the machine on and confirm that it cycles off when the circuit is obstructed. If the machine does not cycle off with the circuit obstructed, check for leaks, most commonly at the tubing connections to the nebulizer or expiratory valve. If the device includes any rate controls, make sure they are turned off. If there is a nebulizer control, make sure that it is on and that aerosol is being produced. Start therapy with an initial sensitivity of about −2 cm H_2O, with the cycle pressure set between 10 and 20 cm H_2O and with a moderate flow (if adjustable).

In terms of F_{IO_2} control, you should try to match the $O_2\%$ during IPPB to the patient's O_2 therapy prescription, if any. With pneumatic units, you can deliver either 100% O_2 or an air mixture with an F_{IO_2} that varies between 0.40 and 0.60. The air-mix control also affects the amount and pattern of inspiratory flow. In the air-mix modes, flow capability is higher and the pattern of flow more normal (decelerating ramp). When air mix is off, available flow is less. In addition, Bird IPPB devices set to deliver pure source gas provide a less desirable square wave (constant flow) flow pattern.

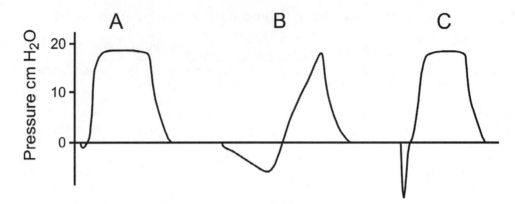

Figure 12-1 Graphic Depiction of IPPB Pressure Patterns. (A) A normal pattern with quick on-triggering, followed by a relatively rapid pressure rise and ending in a short plateau. (B) "Scalloping" of the pressure waveform after machine triggering indicating inadequate flow. (C) A large drop in airway pressure below zero before the breath starts indicating inadequate sensitivity or a malfunctioning breathing valve.

In order to provide a precise F_{IO_2} with pneumatically powered IPPB units, you must attach them to an O_2 blender and set them to deliver pure source gas (air mix off). Moderate but inexact O_2 concentrations can be achieved with electrically powered IPPB units by bleeding 100% O_2 into the delivery circuit, usually via the nebulizer.

During therapy, you should carefully observe the IPPB unit's pressure manometer for the changes occurring during breathing. As indicated in **Figure 12-1**, the goal is to achieve quick and near-effortless on-triggering, followed by a relatively rapid pressure rise and ending in a short plateau (pattern A). In pattern B, airway pressure drops below zero after the breath starts. This "scalloping" of the pressure waveform indicates that the patient's flow exceeds that provided by the machine (i.e., there is inadequate flow to meet patient's demand). Normally, if you observe this condition you should either coach the patient to relax and let the machine do the work or increase the inspiratory flow. Pattern C demonstrates a different problem needing your attention. Here the large drop in airway pressure below zero *before the breath starts* indicates improper triggering, usually corrected by increasing the sensitivity. The same situation can occur if the IPPB breathing valve malfunctions or is sticking. A malfunctioning valve usually indicates improper assembly, whereas a sticking value most often signifies accumulation of dirt or aerosolized drug residue on its surface. In either case, the device should be replaced with one that properly triggers on and cycles off. For more details on the various modifications you can make to tailor IPPB therapy to meet individual patient needs, refer to Chapter 14.

Continuous Mechanical Ventilation Settings

There is no more important area to emphasize in preparing for the CRT exam than initiating and adjusting mechanical ventilation settings. Questions assessing your ability in this area appear in this section as well as in three other content areas, as covered in Chapters 14–16. The bottom line is that candidates who cannot properly select appropriate modes and set and adjust ventilator parameters will not be able to pass the CRT exam. The accompanying box outlines the basic procedure for initiating ventilatory support.

Ventilator Initiation

Equipment and Patient Preparation

1. Verify, interpret, and evaluate doctor's order or protocol

2. Review any pertinent information (e.g., history and interview, lab data, X-rays) in the patient's chart

3. Select, gather, assemble, and check the required equipment

---

(continues)

4. Decontaminate hands and apply standard/transmission-based precautions as appropriate

5. Identify patient, introduce self and department

6. Explain/demonstrate procedure and confirm patient understanding

7. Connect the ventilator to the appropriate emergency electrical outlets

8. Connect the high-pressure lines to the appropriate 50-psi gas source outlets

9. Turn on the ventilator and verify proper ventilator function

Assessment and Implementation

10. Evaluate the patient by performing

    a. Assessment of vital signs

    b. Physical assessment of the chest

    c. Auscultation

    d. ECG, blood gases, or noninvasive monitoring of CO_2 and SpO_2

11. Select appropriate ventilator mode for patient

12. Select the initial ventilator settings appropriate for mode

13. Set initial alarm parameter

14. Analyze/confirm F_{IO_2}

15. Reassess the patient, including oxygenation, ventilation, mechanics, and hemodynamics

16. Adjust ventilator settings to assure adequate ventilation and oxygenation

Follow-Up

17. Maintain/process equipment

18. Dispose of infectious waste and decontaminate hands

19. Record pertinent data in chart and departmental records

20. Notify appropriate personnel and make any necessary recommendations or modifications to the patient care plan

Adapted from: Scanlan, C. L., West, G. A., von der Heydt, P. A., & Dolan, G. K. (1984). *Respiratory therapy competency evaluation manual.* Boston: Blackwell Scientific.

Chapter 8 covers procedures for verifying proper ventilator function prior to application. Chapters 13–15 discuss how to monitor and adjust alarm settings. Here we focus on selecting the appropriate ventilator mode, setting initial ventilator parameters, and making basic adjustments to assure adequate ventilation and oxygenation.

In terms of modes of ventilation, the NBRC hospital expects you be familiar with all common modes, including control mode, assist/control mode, SIMV, pressure support ventilation, CPAP, and bi-level positive airway pressure (BiPAP™). Given their growing usage, you also may be expected to understand dual breath modes such as pressure-regulated volume control (PRVC) as well as the newer bi-level mode called airway pressure release ventilation (APRV).

Table 12-3 describes each of these modes of ventilation, specifies their appropriate use, and defines their advantages and disadvantages. You should apply this information when confronted with CRT exam questions asking you to select or recommend the most appropriate mode for an individual patient. According to the AARC, mechanical ventilation should be individually tailored to each patient's needs. Generally this means that in the early stages of acute respiratory failure, you should select or recommend a mode that provides full ventilatory support, such as assist/control or normal-rate SIMV. As the patient improves and is able to carry more of the ventilatory load, you should begin using modes that allow or encourage spontaneous breathing (partial ventilatory support).

In addition, the mode selected should be familiar to the staff responsible for applying it. Based on these principles, you can expect the NBRC to emphasize selection of either volume- or pressure-oriented assist/control or SIMV (with or without pressure support) for most patients needing ventilatory support. You should also apply PEEP to these patients if they require more than 50% O_2 to

Table 12-3 Modes of Ventilation

Description	Recommend or Use	Advantages	Disadvantages
Control Mode			

• Patient breathes at rate and time interval set on ventilator
• No patient triggering
• All machine (mandatory) breaths
• Provides full ventilatory support
• May target either volume (VCV) or pressure (PCV)
	• When full ventilator support is needed but the rate and/or ventilatory pattern must be controlled or patient effort eliminated; i.e., in patients with:
	  • Inverse I:E ratio ventilation
	  • Permissive hypercapnia
	  • Hyperventilation in brain injury
	  • Flail chest
	  • Hyperventilation syndrome
	  • Seizure disorders
		• Rate, ventilatory pattern, and $Paco_2$ controlled
		• Eliminates work of breathing (as long as patient makes no efforts)
		• Allows for "abnormal" patterns such as inverse I:E ratio
			• Poorly tolerated by most patients
			• Patient efforts result in asynchrony ("fighting the ventilator") and increased work of breathing
			• May require heavy sedation or neuromuscular paralysis

Assist/Control Mode (A/C)			
• Ventilator provides a baseline or guaranteed rate, which the patient can exceed by triggering additional breaths • All machine (mandatory) breaths • Provides full ventilatory support if baseline rate normal • May target either volume or pressure	• When full ventilator support is needed but patient's rate results in acceptable Pco_2 (*note:* has largely been replaced by normal-rate SIMV)	• Patient controls own rate and CO_2 level • May avoid need for sedation or paralysis • Guaranteed baseline rate if patient's rate falls or apnea occurs	• Hyperventilation can occur at high triggering rates (e.g., due to anxiety, fear, pain, hypoxemia) • Asynchronous breathing (improper machine sensitivity or flow) • Asynchrony may increase work of breathing and O_2 consumption • May worsen auto-PEEP in COPD patients
Synchronous Intermittent Mandatory Ventilation (SIMV)			
• The patient breathes spontaneously between machine breaths synchronized to patient effort • Provides full ventilatory support at normal rates; partial support at lower rates • Machine breaths may target either volume or pressure • Spontaneous breaths may be pressure supported	• When full ventilator support is needed but patient's spontaneous rate would result in hyperventilation on A/C • To provide for incremental lowering of ventilatory support levels (weaning)	• Allows graded levels of ventilatory support • Spontaneous breathing allowed; patient controls rate and pattern • Decreased need for sedatives or relaxants • Less "fighting" of ventilator • Lower mean pleural pressures than with A/C	• Hypoventilation a hazard at low rates (adequate minute ventilation not guaranteed) • Some systems increase work of breathing • Asynchronous breathing can still occur during machine breaths (improper machine sensitivity or flow)

(continues)

Table 12-3 Modes of Ventilation (continued)

Description	Recommend or Use	Advantages	Disadvantages
Pressure Support Ventilation (PSV)			
• Patient-triggered, pressure limited, flow-cycled spontaneous breaths • V_T depends on pressure level and patient effort • Normally provides partial ventilatory support; full support only if pressure high enough to yield normal V_Ts (PSVmax)	• To overcome the imposed work of breathing caused by small artificial airways and/or ventilator circuits (low PSV) • To boost the spontaneous V_T of patients receiving SIMV • To provide for incremental lowering of ventilatory support levels (weaning)	• Patient controls the rate of breathing, and the inspiratory time and flow • As compared with unsupported spontaneous breaths, results in lower rate, higher V_T, less respiratory muscle activity, and lower O_2 consumption • Improves respiratory muscle conditioning, facilitates weaning.	• Without backup rate, hypoventilation can occur • Variable V_T and $\dot{V}_E$ • If rise time to pressure limit cannot be adjusted, asynchrony may occur • In COPD patients, flow cycling to end inspiration may either require active effort or be prolonged
Pressure-Regulated Volume Control (PRVC)			

• A form of pressure control (patient- or time-triggered, pressure-limited and time-cycled ventilation) in which the pressure limit is automatically adjusted breath-to-breath to maintain a target tidal volume	• For patients:
	  • requiring the lowest possible pressure and a guaranteed consistent V_T
	  • with acute lung injury/ARDS
	  • requiring high and/or variable inspiratory flow
	  • with changing C_L or Raw (*note:* may be *less* suitable for patients with asthma or COPD)
		• Lower PIP that VCV or PCV; lower incidence of barotrauma
		• Pressure automatically adjusted for changes in C_L and Raw within a set range
		• Provision of near-constant V_T
		• Patient controls rate and $\dot{V}_E$
		• Automatic decrease in ventilatory support as the patient improves
		• Decelerating flow pattern (improves gas distribution, patient-ventilator synchrony, reduces work of breathing)
		• Duration of ventilation may be less than VCV or PCV
			• Variable patient effort will result in variable V_T and possible asynchrony
			• Severe increase in Raw or decrease in C_L may result in high/unsafe PIP or (based on upper pressure limit setting) a delivered V_T < set V_T
			• When patient demand is increased, pressure level may diminish when support is most needed
			• As pressure level drops, Pmean drops, possibly causing hypoxemia
			• May cause or worsen auto-PEEP
			• May be tolerated poorly in awake, non-sedated patients

(continues)

Table 12-3 Modes of Ventilation (continued)

Description	Recommend or Use	Advantages	Disadvantages
Continuous Positive Airway Pressure (CPAP)			
• The application of positive pressure to the airway throughout the spontaneous breathing cycle • May be provided by either demand-flow or continuous-flow systems	• For patients with CHF/pulmonary edema (short-term application) • For patients with sleep apnea (nocturnal application) • To decrease hypoxemia due to shunting in patients with adequate spontaneous ventilation (e.g., ARDS, IRDS)	• Provides increased PaO_2 for a given FIO_2 • Can increase lung compliance • Can decrease work of breathing	• Increases mean pleural pressure, ICP, pulmonary vascular resistance • Decreases venous return • Increases incidence of barotrauma • Hypoventilation (adequate $\dot{V}E$ not guaranteed) • Continuous flow systems make monitoring ($\dot{V}E$, VD/VT) difficult
Bi-Level Positive Airway Pressure (BiPAP™)			
• Patient-triggered, pressure-limited breaths with positive pressure maintained throughout the expiratory phase • Equivalent to pressure-support ventilation with CPAP; IPAP = pressure limit, EPAP = CPAP level • VT depends on pressure difference (IPAP – EPAP) and patient effort • May include timed-triggered backup mode	• For noninvasive support of patients with acute ventilatory failure • To avoid intubation of COPD patients requiring ventilatory support for acute or chronic ventilatory failure • To avoid reintubation of patients who develop mild to moderate hypercapnia or hypoxemia after extubation • For patients with CHF or pulmonary edema (short-term application) • For patients with sleep apnea (nocturnal application)	• Fewer hazards than invasive ventilatory support • Patient controls the rate of breathing, and the inspiratory time and flow	• Requires cooperative patient with adequate secretion clearance • Most systems have limited FIO_2 capability ($\leq 60\%$) • Most systems have limited pressure capabilities (≤ 40 cm H_2O) • Airway interface problems can cause discomfort, tissue damage, leaks

(continues)

Table 12-3 Modes of Ventilation (continued)

Description	Recommend or Use	Advantages	Disadvantages
Airway Pressure Release Ventilation (APRV)			
• Equivalent to CPAP with regular, brief, intermittent releases in airway pressure to baseline • Technically time-triggered, pressure-limited, time-cycled with spontaneous breathing • Often referred to as "inverted IMV" (based on graphic appearance)	• For patients with: • ALI/ARDS, especially when Pplat > 30 cm H_2O • refractory hypoxemia due to collapsed alveoli • massive atelectasis	• Lower PIP/Pplat than VCV, PCV • Less impact on hemodynamics than VCV, PCV • Reduced risk of ventilator-associated lung injury • Allows for spontaneous breathing throughout the ventilatory cycle • improves V/Q matching, oxygenation • May decrease physiologic deadspace, lower $\dot{V}E$ needs • Reduces the need for sedation and paralysis • Improves patient-ventilator synchrony (compared with IR-PCV)	• VT delivery depends on CL, Raw, and patient's spontaneous effort • Does not completely support CO_2 removal; relies on spontaneous breathing • Could be harmful to patients with high Raw (as in COPD or asthma) • Caution should be used with hemodynamically unstable patients • Auto-PEEP is usually present • Asynchrony can occur if spontaneous breaths are out of sync with release time

maintain adequate arterial oxygenation. In the NBRC hospital, CPAP (with backup ventilation) is the mode of choice for critically ill patients who have *adequate ventilation* but who due to shunting need extra support for oxygenation. Bi-level positive airway pressure is normally the mode of choice when noninvasive ventilation is indicated (as discussed subsequently).

In terms of selecting volume or pressure as the target for machine breaths, your choice depends on the ordering physician's clinical goals. Specifically, if CO_2 elimination is the primary goal and patient comfort and lung distention are secondary issues, then volume-targeted ventilation is the best choice. In contrast, if patient-ventilator synchrony is important and CO_2 elimination is of lesser concern, then pressure-targeted ventilation is the most appropriate approach. Other ways to enhance patient-ventilator synchrony and minimize imposed work include proper setting of the ventilator trigger, application of PEEP to overcome auto-PEEP, matching the flow pattern to the patient's demand, and avoiding air trapping by ensuring adequate expiratory time.

To help avoid ventilator-associated lung injury due to overdistention, patients requiring high peak or plateau pressures when receiving volume-targeted ventilation should probably be switched to pressure-targeted ventilation (PCV or PRVC) at a safe pressure limit—i.e., 30 cm H_2O or less. In terms of initial adult ventilator settings, the AARC provides the following general guidelines:

1. *Volume vs. Pressure as Target:* Volume ventilation may be used for the majority of patients, but pressure-ventilation (PCV or PRVC) should be considered if peak pressures rise over 40 cm H_2O or Pplat is greater than 30 cm H_2O.
2. *Tidal Volume:* Set VT between 4 and 12 mL/kg of predicted body weight (PBW), while maintaining plateau pressure less than 30 cm H_2O and ΔP less than 20 cm H_2O.

3. *Minute Ventilation:* For males $\dot{V}_E$ (L/min) = 4.0 × BSA (body surface area via DuBois nomogram); for females $\dot{V}_E$ = 3.5 × BSA, while maintaining plateau pressure less than 30 cm H_2O and ΔP less than 20 cm H_2O.

4. *Respiratory Rate:* 8–26/min adjusted to achieve optimum total cycle time and maintain desired minute ventilation, while maintaining plateau pressure less than 30 cm H_2O and ΔP less than 20 cm H_2O.

5. *F_{IO_2}:* Initial setting of 0.60–0.90 until results from arterial blood gases (ABGs) can be obtained and the setting adjusted.
   a. Initial ABG should be obtained 15–45 minutes after initiating ventilation.
   b. After correlating pulse oximetry with initial ABG results, maintain Sp_{O_2} at or above patient's normal or less than 90% Sp_{O_2}.
   c. PEEP 5–15 cm H_2O. Set initial PEEP at 5 cm H_2O, unless otherwise indicated. Higher PEEP may be required with acute lung injury or ARDS (see ARDS protocol).

6. *Pressure Support:* 8–20 cm H_2O. Maintain Pplat less than 30 cm H_2O and ΔP less than 20 cm H_2O. Pressure support should be adjusted to reduce work of breathing and patient fatigue and support effective ventilation.

7. *I:E Ratio:* normally less than 1:1 (e.g., 1:3); the I:E ratio should be optimized along with total cycle time to provide optimum mean airway pressure, lung filling, lung emptying (minimizing air trapping/auto-PEEP), and patient/ventilator synchrony.

In regard to adjusting ventilator settings, your primary goals are to (1) achieve acceptable arterial blood gases and (2) minimize or eliminate dyspnea, accessory muscle use, and paradoxical breathing. **Table 12-4** specifies the target blood gas values recommended by the AARC for the four most common categories of adult patients requiring ventilatory support.

According to the AARC, ventilator adjustments should be made as follows:

1. Regular assessment of general appearance, vital signs, breath sounds, and hemodynamic stability should be evaluated prior to and during any ventilator adjustments.

2. For a pH of 7.30 or less and confirmed respiratory cause, increase rate to a maximum of 24 breaths per minute until pH is greater than 7.30. If further adjustment is needed, increase V_T until PIP is greater than or equal to 40 cm H_2O or Pplat is greater than or equal to 30 cm H_2O. If unable to maintain these parameters, consider permissive hypercapnia.

3. For a pH of 7.45 or greater and confirmed respiratory cause, reduce rate to a minimum of 8 breaths per minute or until pH is less than 7.45. After rate is decreased to 8 breaths per minute, if pH is still greater than or equal to 7.45, reduce volume to a minimum of 4 mL/kg (PBW).

4. Pa_{O_2} or Sp_{O_2} should be maintained based on patient's targeted values (Table 12-4). Hemoglobin should be checked to assure the absence of anemia. Hemodynamic data should be checked to assure adequate circulation.

5. If Pa_{O_2}/F_{IO_2} ratio is less than or equal to 300 or should an F_{IO_2} = 0.5 with PEEP = 12 cm H_2O be insufficient to maintain an acceptable arterial oxygenation, you should contact an intensivist or pulmonologist and consider the ARDS Protocol.

Table 12-4 Target Blood Gas Values for Adult Patients Receiving Mechanical Ventilation

Patient Category	pH	Pa_{CO_2}	Pa_{O_2}	Sp_{O_2}
Normal	7.35–7.45	35–45 torr	≥ 80 torr	92–97%
COPD	7.30–7.45	45–55 torr; adjust to pH range	55–75 torr	> 89%
Open heart	7.35–7.50	35–50 torr	≥ 65 torr	90–95%
ARDS[a]	7.30–7.45	Adjust to pH range	≥ 55 torr	≥ 88%
a. See ARDS protocol in this chapter.				

The NBRC hospital generally follows these guidelines, with the following key points helpful in answering adult ventilator initiation/adjustment questions likely to appear on the CRT exam:

- Ventilator initiation
  - Unless otherwise indicated, start all patients on *full ventilatory support* (pressure or volume-targeted assist-control or normal-rate SIMV)
  - For volume-targeted ventilation (except ARDS), set the initial V_T to 8–10 mL/kg PBW
  - For pressure-targeted ventilation, set the initial pressure limit to 20–30 cm H_2O
  - Unless otherwise indicated, start all patients on a high F_{IO_2} (≥ 0.60)
  - Unless otherwise indicated, start all patients on 5 cm H_2O PEEP ("physiologic" PEEP)
- Ventilator adjustment
  - To adjust Pa_{CO_2}/pH, change the rate; change the V_T/pressure limit only if rate changes at the limits (8–24/min) do not achieve the desired results
  - To adjust Pa_{O_2}/Sa_{O_2}:
    - If satisfactory Pa_{O_2}/Sa_{O_2} can be maintained with $\leq 50\%$ O_2, change the F_{IO_2}
    - If satisfactory Pa_{O_2}/Sa_{O_2} cannot be maintained with $\leq 50\%$ O_2, add PEEP

Table 12-5 extends these general guidelines and provides details on the typical initial settings for each major mode of mechanical ventilation, as well as the mode-specific adjustments needed to assure adequate ventilation and oxygenation.

Noninvasive Ventilation

Noninvasive ventilation is the delivery of assisted mechanical ventilation without the need for an artificial tracheal airway. **Table 12-6** (see page 351) lists the major advantages and limitations of noninvasive ventilation.

There are two primary types of noninvasive ventilation: negative and positive pressure. Noninvasive negative pressure devices include the iron lung or tank ventilator, chest curiass, and pneumosuit. Most noninvasive positive pressure ventilation (NPPV) is delivered using ventilators capable of providing and independently regulating the pressure support and CPAP levels (bi-level positive pressure ventilation, or BiPAP™). *Application of NPPV requires that the patient have control over upper airway function, be able to manage secretions, and be cooperative and motivated.*

The primary indications for NPPV are to:

- Reverse hypercapnic respiratory failure (pH < 7.35 but > 7.20)
- Reverse hypoxemic respiratory failure (P/F ratio < 200)
- Treat acute cardiogenic pulmonary edema
- Facilitate earlier weaning/extubation of COPD patients from invasive support
- Alleviate breathlessness and fatigue in terminally ill patients

NPPV may also be useful in supporting patients with chronic hypoventilation syndromes or slowly progressive respiratory failure due to neuromuscular disorders or thoracic wall deformities.

Contraindications for NPPV include the following:

- Respiratory arrest
- pH < 7.20
- Uncooperative patient
- Inability to protect airway or clear secretions
- Upper airway obstruction
- Hemodynamic instability/hypotension
- Uncontrolled arrhythmias
- Active upper gastrointestinal bleeding
- Facial burns or trauma
- Need for airway protection/at high risk for aspiration

Table 12-5 Typical Adult Setting and Basic Adjustment of Common Ventilatory Modes

Settings	Control Mode	Assist/Control Mode
Tidal volume (if VCV)	8–10 mL/kg PBW; 4–6 mL/kg in ARDS/ARF (ARDS protocol)	8–10 mL/kg PBW; 4–6 mL/kg in ARDS/ARF (ARDS protocol)
Pressure limit (if PCV)	20–30 cm H_2O	20–30 cm H_2O
Rate	8–24/min	8–24/min
Trigger/sensitivity	n/a	1–2 cm H_2O < baseline (pressure); 1–3 L/min < baseline (flow)
Flow, I-time, I:E	Set initially to achieve I:E ≤ 1:1 (e.g., 1:2, 1:3)	Set to achieve I:E ≤ 1:1 (e.g., 1:2, 1:3)
Flow waveform	Square or decelerating (VCV only)	Square or decelerating (VCV only)
F_{IO_2}	As needed to maintain Pa_{O_2} ≥ 60 torr, Sa_{O_2} ≥ 90% ARDS F_{IO_2}/PEEP combinations (ARDS protocol)	As needed to maintain Pa_{O_2} ≥ 60 torr, Sa_{O_2} ≥ 90 ARDS F_{IO_2}/PEEP combinations (ARDS protocol)
PEEP	5–10 cm H_2O, then as needed to maintain oxygenation with F_{IO_2} ≤ 50% when possible ARDS F_{IO_2}/PEEP combinations (ARDS protocol) As needed to balance auto-PEEP	5–10 cm H_2O, then as needed to maintain oxygenation with F_{IO_2} ≤ 50% when possible ARDS F_{IO_2}/PEEP combinations (ARDS protocol) As needed to balance auto-PEEP
To adjust pH/P_{CO_2}	To lower P_{CO_2} or raise pH: increase V_E (increase V_T, rate, and/or pressure limit) To raise P_{CO_2} or lower pH: decrease V_E (decrease V_T, rate, and/or pressure limit)	To lower P_{CO_2} or raise pH: increase V_E (increase V_T, rate, and/or pressure limit) To raise P_{CO_2} or lower pH: decrease V_E (decrease V_T, rate, and/or pressure limit) If P_{CO_2} remains low, consider adding mechanical deadspace If respiratory alkalosis persists, consider switching to SIMV
To adjust Pa_{O_2}/Sa_{O_2}	If simple V/Q imbalance and F_{IO_2} ≤ 0.50, raise F_{IO_2} If shunting present (Pa_{O_2} ≤50 torr, F_{IO_2} ≥ 0.50), increase PEEP When oxygenation improves, first decrease F_{IO_2} until ≤ 0.50, then lower PEEP	If simple V/Q imbalance and F_{IO_2} ≤ 0.50. raise F_{IO_2} If shunting present (Pa_{O_2} ≤ 50 torr, F_{IO_2} ≥ 0.50), increase PEEP When oxygenation improves, first decrease F_{IO_2} until ≤ 0.50, then lower PEEP

(continues)

Table 12-5 Typical Adult Setting and Basic Adjustment of Common Ventilatory Modes (continued)

Settings	Control Mode	Assist/Control Mode
Comments	Can limit inspiratory volume (VCV) or pressure (PCV) Control mode usually requires patient sedation or paralysis When switching from VCV to PCV, use Pplateau as target (if ≤ 35 cm H_2O) Use lower tidal volumes/higher rates in acute lung injury/ARDS (ARDS protocol) Manipulate flow/I-time to prevent auto-PEEP PaO_2 ≥ 50 torr, SaO_2 ≥ 85% acceptable in ARDS	Can limit inspiratory volume (VCV) or pressure (PCV) Respiratory alkalosis is a common problem; see adjusting $PaCO_2$ above COPD patients prone to auto-PEEP on A/C; consider SIMV instead Provide adequate flow (VCV) to prevent scalloping of inspiratory pressure curve (usually ≥ 60 L/min) When switching from VCV to PCV, use Pplat as target Use lower V_T/higher rates in acute lung injury/ARDS (ARDS protocol) PaO_2 ≥ 55 torr, SaO_2 ≥ 88% acceptable in ARDS (ARDS protocol)

Settings	Intermittent Mandatory Ventilation (SIMV)	Pressure Support Ventilation (PSV)
Tidal volume (if VCV)	8–10 mL/kg PBW for machine breaths; 4–6 mL/kg in ARDS/ARF	n/a
Pressure limit (if PCV)	20–30 cm H_2O for machine breaths	When used simply to augment spontaneous breaths (e.g., with IMV), increase until tachypnea and/or accessory muscle use diminished or eliminated When used as full support mode (PSVmax), set to achieve V_T of 6–10 mL/kg
Rate	8–24 breaths/min for full ventilatory support; < 8 for partial support or weaning	n/a (patient determined); however, must provide backup ventilation for critically ill patients who could become apneic
Trigger/sensitivity	1–2 cm H_2O < baseline (pressure); 1–3 L/min < baseline (flow)	1–2 cm H_2O below baseline (pressure); 1–3 L/min below baseline (flow)
Flow, I-time, I:E	Set to achieve I:E ≤ 1:1 (e.g., 1:2, 1:3) on machine breaths	n/a (flow is machine-determined; I-time depends on patient); however, if pressure slope or rise time can be set, adjust for patient comfort and to avoid scalloping or early peaking
Flow waveform	Square or decelerating (VCV only)	n/a
FIO_2	As needed to maintain PaO_2 ≥ 60 torr, SaO_2 ≥ 90% ARDS FIO_2/PEEP combinations (ARDS protocol)	As needed to maintain PaO_2 ≥ 60 torr, SaO_2 ≥ 90%

(continues)

Table 12-5 Typical Adult Setting and Basic Adjustment of Common Ventilatory Modes (continued)

Settings	Intermittent Mandatory Ventilation (SIMV)	Pressure Support Ventilation (PSV)
PEEP	5–10 cm H_2O, then as needed to maintain oxygenation with $F_{IO_2} \leq 50\%$ when possible ARDS F_{IO_2}/PEEP combinations (ARDS protocol) As needed to balance auto-PEEP	5–10 cm H_2O, then as needed to maintain oxygenation with $F_{IO_2} \leq 50\%$ when possible As needed to balance auto-PEEP
To adjust pH/P_{CO_2}	To lower P_{CO_2} or raise pH: increase V_E (increase V_T, rate, and/or pressure limit) To increase P_{CO_2} or lower pH: decrease V_E (decrease V_T, rate, and/or pressure limit) Do NOT add mechanical deadspace to IMV circuits to increase P_{CO_2} If tachypnea persists, increase machine rate or add/increase pressure support	To lower P_{CO_2} or raise pH: increase pressure limit To increase P_{CO_2} or lower pH: decrease pressure limit
To adjust P_{aO_2}/S_{aO_2}	If simple V/Q imbalance and $F_{IO_2} \leq 0.50$, raise F_{IO_2} If shunting present ($P_{aO_2} \leq 50$ torr, $F_{IO_2} \geq 0.50$), increase PEEP When oxygenation improves, first decrease F_{IO_2} until ≤ 0.50, then lower PEEP	If simple V/Q imbalance and $F_{IO_2} \leq 0.50$, raise F_{IO_2} to raise P_{aO_2} If shunting present ($P_{aO_2} \leq 50$ torr, $F_{IO_2} \geq 0.50$), increase PEEP When oxygenation improves, first decrease F_{IO_2} until ≤ 0.50, then lower PEEP
Comments	Can limit inspiratory volume or pressure for machine breaths Provide adequate flow (VCV) to prevent scalloping of inspiratory pressure curve during machine breaths (usually ≥ 60 L/min) Low levels of pressure support (5–8 cm H_2O) are usually applied to spontaneous breaths When switching from VC-IMV to PC-IMV, use Pplat as target Use lower tidal volumes/higher rates in acute lung injury/ARDS $P_{aO_2} \geq 55$ torr, $S_{aO_2} \geq 88\%$ acceptable in ARDS For weaning, first decrease IMV rate until ≤ 2 breaths/min, then lower pressure support to no less than 4–5 cm H_2O above PEEP	$P_{aO_2} \geq 55$ torr, $S_{aO_2} \geq 88\%$ acceptable in ARDS

(continues)

Table 12-5 Typical Adult Setting and Basic Adjustment of Common Ventilatory Modes (continued)

Settings	Pressure-Regulated Volume Control (PRVC)	Continuous Positive Airway Pressure (CPAP)
Tidal volume (if VCV)	Set *targeted* V_T to 8–10 mL/kg PBW; 4–6 mL/kg in ARDS/ARF (ARDS protocol)	n/a (patient determined)
Pressure limit (if PCV)	20–30 cm H_2O (in PRVC mode, ventilator delivers pressure of up to 5 cm H_2O below upper pressure alarm limit)	For obstructive sleep apnea: titrate to eliminate apneas, desaturations, arousals (usually in the 8–12 cm H_2O range) For hypoxemic respiratory failure/ARDS: as needed to maintain oxygenation with $FIO_2 \leq 50\%$ when possible
Rate	8–24 breaths/min	n/a (patient determined)
Trigger/sensitivity	1–2 cm H_2O < baseline (pressure); 1–3 L/min < baseline (flow)	For demand flow systems: 1–2 cm H_2O < baseline (pressure); 1–3 L/min < baseline (flow)
Flow, I-time, I:E	1:2 (I-time = 33%); consider longer I-time no intrinsic PEEP, no bronchospasm, and poor oxygenation	n/a (flow is machine-determined; I-time depends on patient); however, if pressure drops by ≥ 2 cm H_2O during inspiration, increase sensitivity (demand flow systems) or system flow (continuous-flow systems)
Flow waveform	Pattern not settable (decelerating); if adjustable, increase time set to 5% initially	n/a
FIO_2	As needed to maintain $PaO_2 \geq 60$ torr, $SaO_2 \geq 90$ ARDS FIO_2/PEEP combinations (ARDS protocol)	As needed to maintain $PaO_2 \geq 60$ torr, $SaO_2 \geq 90\%$ Usually room air for obstructive sleep apnea Use $FIO_2 = 1.0$ for CHF/pulmonary edema applications (short-term)
PEEP	5–10 cm H_2O, then as needed to maintain oxygenation with $FIO_2 \leq 50\%$ when possible If ARDS FIO_2/PEEP combinations (ARDS protocol) As needed to balance auto-PEEP	Patient-dependent; cannot be adjusted by clinician If PCO_2 rises and respiratory acidosis persists, provide ventilatory support (BiPAP™, SIMV, A/C)
To adjust pH/PCO_2	To lower PCO_2 or increase pH: increase V_E (increase targeted V_T, rate, and/or pressure limit) To raise PCO_2 or lower pH: decrease V_E (decrease targeted V_T, rate, and/or pressure limit) If Pplat exceeds 30–35 cm H_2O, consider APRV If respiratory alkalosis persists, consider switching to SIMV-PC	n/a (ventilation provided by patient)

(continues)

Table 12-5 Typical Adult Setting and Basic Adjustment of Common Ventilatory Modes (continued)

Settings	Pressure-Regulated Volume Control (PRVC)	Continuous Positive Airway Pressure (CPAP)
To adjust Pao_2/Sao_2	If simple V/Q imbalance and $Fio_2 \leq$ 0.50, raise Fio_2 If shunting present ($Pao_2 \leq 50$ torr, $Fio_2 \geq 0.50$), increase PEEP When oxygenation improves, first decrease Fio_2 until ≤ 0.50, then lower PEEP	If simple V/Q imbalance and $Fio_2 \leq$ 0.50, raise Fio_2 If shunting present ($Pao_2 \leq 50$ torr, $Fio_2 \geq 0.50$), increase CPAP When oxygenation improves, first decrease Fio_2 until ≤ 0.50, then lower CPAP $Pao_2 \geq 55$ torr, $Sao_2 \geq 88\%$ acceptable in ARDS
Comments	Can be used in control, A/C, or SIMV modes When switching from VCV to PCV, use Pplat as target Use lower targeted V_T/higher rates in ARDS (ARDS protocol) $Pao_2 \geq 55$ torr, $Sao_2 \geq 88\%$ acceptable in ARDS	Must provide apnea alarm and backup ventilation for critically ill patients

Settings	Bi-Level Positive Airway Pressure (BiPAP™)	Airway Pressure Release Ventilation (APRV)
Tidal volume	(if VCV) Function of patient effort and ΔP (IPAP – EPAP); aim for 6–8 mL/kg	n/a
Pressure limit (if PCV)	Initial IPAP = 10 cm H_2O; adjust to normalize pH/Pco_2 (below)	P-high = 25–35 cm H_2O
Rate	Guarantee minimum of 8 breaths/min (A/C or S/T mode)	Depends on T-high and T-low
Trigger/sensitivity	n/a (machine determined)	1–2 cm H_2O < baseline (pressure); 1–3 L/min < baseline (flow)
Flow, I-time, I:E	n/a for spontaneous breaths; in timed mode (T), start with %I-time in the 20–30% range	T-high = 4.0 sec (use lower T-high for infants/children—e.g., 2 sec) T-low (release time) = 0.5–0.8 (0.2–0.6 sec for infants/children) T-low should limit expiratory flow to about 50–75% of peak value as indicated on the flow × time graphic display
Flow waveform	n/a (machine determined; some other manufacturers provide a rise-time adjustment—e.g., Healthdyne Quantum PSV)	n/a
Fio_2	As needed to maintain $Pao_2 \geq 60$ torr, $Sao_2 \geq 90\%$	
PEEP	Initial EPAP = 5 cm H_2O; adjust to maintain $Pao_2 \geq 60$ torr, $Sao_2 \geq 90\%$; keep ΔP (IPAP – EPAP) ≥ 5 cm H_2O	P-low = 0 H_2O

(continues)

Table 12-5 Typical Adult Setting and Basic Adjustment of Common Ventilatory Modes (continued)

Settings	Bi-Level Positive Airway Pressure (BiPAP™)	Airway Pressure Release Ventilation (APRV)
To adjust pH/P_{CO_2}	To lower P_{CO_2} or raise pH: increase IPAP To raise P_{CO_2} or lower pH: decrease IPAP	To lower P_{CO_2} or increase pH: decrease T-high (no shorter than 3 sec in adults) or increase P-high in 2–3 cm H_2O increments; also check T-low and, if possible, increase to allow more time for exhalation To raise P_{CO_2} or lower pH: increase T-high in increments of 0.5–2.0 sec or decrease P-high in 2–3 cm H_2O increments (*note:* in ALI/ARDS it may be better to accept hypercapnia than to reduce P-high so much that oxygenation becomes impaired)
To adjust Pa_{O_2}/Sa_{O_2}	If simple V/Q imbalance and F_{IO_2} < 0.50, raise F_{IO_2} If shunting present (Pa_{O_2} ≤ 50 torr, F_{IO_2} ≥ 0.50), increase EPAP (keep ΔP ≥ 5 cm H_2O) When oxygenation improves, first decrease F_{IO_2} until ≤ 0.50, then lower EPAP	To increase Pa_{O_2}: • increase F_{IO_2} • increase P-high in 2-cm H_2O increments • increase T-high slowly (in 0.5-sec increments) • decrease T-low (increases auto-PEEP) in 0.1-sec increments (*note:* this may reduce V_T and raise Pa_{CO_2})
Comments	For acute hypercapnic respiratory failure, gradually increase IPAP until spontaneous rate is below 25 breaths/min or until the estimated V_T exceeds spontaneous by 30–50% After initial stabilization, an ABG is obtained to assess the effect of ventilation on Pa_{CO_2}, with a target reduction of 5–10 torr	When switching from VCV, use Pplat as P-high (≤ 35 cm H_2O) As patient improves, increase reduce support as tolerated by: • Lowering F_{IO_2} to < 50% • Increasing T-high in 0.5- to 2.0-sec increments (target 12–15 sec) • Lowering P-high in 2-cm H_2O increments (target: 6–12 cm H_2O)

PBW, predicted body weight males = 50 + 2.3 [height (in) – 60]; PBW, females = 45.5 + 2.3 [height (in) – 60]); A/C, assist/control ventilation; ARF, acute respiratory failure; I-time, interval time; VCV, volume control ventilation; PCV, pressure control ventilation; Pplat, plateau pressure; P-high, APRV high pressure; P-low, APRV low/release pressure; T-high, APRV release interval (time between releases); T-low, APRV release time

Table 12-6 Advantages and Limitations of Noninvasive Ventilation

Advantages	Limitations
• Avoidance of intubation-related trauma • Preservation of airway defenses • Lower incidence of nosocomial pneumonia • Permits normal speech and eating • Reduces the need for sedation • Facilitates the weaning process • Shorter duration of ventilation/LOS • Reduces costs	• Can be used only in cooperative patients • Does not provide direct airway access • Increases the risk of secretion retention • Requires more caregiver time (initially)

Chapter 6 provides details on both the common circuitry and interfaces used with NPPV. Because the airway interface defines NPPV, technically any ventilator or mode can be applied noninvasively. However, pressure-support ventilation (PSV) has become the norm for providing NPPV. When combined with an elevated baseline pressure (PSV + CPAP), this approach is commonly called bi-level positive airway pressure (BiPAP™). BiPAP™ can be delivered by most ICU ventilators, but more commonly is provided by electrically powered pressure generators. These dedicated NPPV systems are less expensive, simpler to use, and more portable than general-purpose critical care ventilators.

Table 12-5 outlines the typical initial settings and basic ways to adjust NPPV/BiPAP™. Additional key pointers related to application of NPPV include the following:

- Confirm that the patient is alert and has intact upper airway function/secretion control.
- Position the patient in a high semi-Fowler's (sitting) position if possible.
- Choose the best interface (generally an oronasal/"full" face mask for acute respiratory failure).
- Hold the NPPV interface in place (without strapping) until the patient gets accustomed to it.
- Keep IPAP levels less than 20–25 cm H_2O (esophageal opening pressure).
- Improvement in blood gases is important; however, resolution of dyspnea, tachypnea, and/or accessory muscle use also indicate success.
- Adjust ventilation (Pa_{CO_2}, pH) via IPAP and ΔP.
- Adjust oxygenation (Pa_{O_2}/Sa_{O_2}) via F_{IO_2} and EPAP.
- If any factor that contraindicates NPPV develops during administration (e.g., unconsciousness or vomiting), consider intubation and conventional mechanical ventilation.
- If despite proper application of NPPV hypercapnia progresses, oxygenation worsens, hemodynamic instability develops, or the patient becomes severely agitated, recommend intubation and conventional mechanical ventilation.

Elevated Baseline Pressure (CPAP, PEEP)

Whereas CPAP is a mode of ventilation, PEEP is an "add-on" that can be applied to any mode. Both methods maintain the baseline airway pressure above atmospheric pressure. Strictly speaking, CPAP involves *spontaneous breathing at an elevated baseline pressure*. CPAP is indicated to treat sleep apnea and acute cardiogenic pulmonary edema, as well as manage refractory hypoxemia in patients with adequate ventilation, such as infants with hyaline membrane disease. PEEP also is used on patients with refractory hypoxemia (e.g., $Pa_{O_2} \leq 50$ torr or $F_{IO_2} \geq 0.50$) but for whom additional "machine" breaths are needed to assure adequate ventilation. PEEP also helps lower F_{IO_2} needs (and avoid oxygen toxicity), as well as improve patient-ventilator synchrony (by decreasing auto-PEEP).

CPAP and PEEP can have detrimental effects. Both increase mean pleural pressure. Higher mean pleural pressures can increase intracranial pressure (ICP) and pulmonary vascular resistance, and decrease venous return and cardiac output. Last, CPAP and PEEP can increase the risk of barotrauma.

In the management of sleep apnea, you titrate the CPAP pressure until obstructive events are abolished or controlled, up to a maximum of 20 cm H_2O (see Chapter 4 for details of CPAP titration). When using CPAP to treat cardiogenic pulmonary edema, you apply 5–15 cm H_2O and adjust as needed to help maintain an adequate Pa_{O_2}/Sp_{O_2} and eliminate the signs of pulmonary edema, such as frothy sputum and end-inspiratory crackles. When used to manage infants with hyaline membrane disease, you typically start CPAP at 5 cm H_2O and gradually increase it as needed to:

- Stabilize F_{IO_2} requirements ($F_{IO_2} \leq 0.60$ with $Pa_{O_2} > 50$ torr)
- Reduce the work of breathing as indicated by:
  - A decrease in respiratory rate
  - A decrease in the severity of retractions, grunting, and nasal flaring
- Improve lung aeration (as indicated by chest X-ray)

Application of low levels of PEEP (typically 5 cm H_2O) to all adult patients receiving ventilatory support has become a standard of care in most hospitals, including the NBRC hospital. This level of PEEP helps maintain the FRC and prevents airway closure/auto-PEEP, while presenting minimal hazards for most patients. Higher PEEP levels are indicated when satisfactory arterial oxygenation cannot be achieved at O_2 concentrations less than 50% (indicating hypoxemia due to shunting).

Deciding when to apply PEEP is easy; determining how much PEEP to use is difficult. The problem is that too little PEEP may not overcome shunting, while too much can cause overdistention, worsen preexisting lung injury, and decrease O_2 delivery to the tissues. "Optimum" PEEP represents the end-expiratory pressure level that maximizes patient benefits while minimizing risk.

Currently, there are four ways to determine optimum PEEP, any of which can appear on the NBRC CRT exam. These four different methods define optimum PEEP as the pressure level that:

1. Maximizes O_2 delivery to the tissues
2. Yields the highest static total compliance
3. Provides the maximum volume change for a given ΔP
4. Exceeds the lower inflection point (LIP) on the pressure-volume curve

Method #1 is based on the fact that oxygen delivery to the tissues is a function of the patient's cardiac output (CO) and arterial O_2 content (CaO_2), i.e.,

$$O_2 \text{ delivery} = CO \times CaO_2$$

In general, as PEEP levels rise, so too does the patient's arterial O_2 content (good!). However, the higher the PEEP level, the greater the potential negative effect on cardiac output (bad!). Based on these relationships, PEEP is optimized when the desired increase in CaO_2 is not offset by decreases in CO. To make this determination, the patient must have a pulmonary artery catheter in place so that you can measure both cardiac output and the mixed venous O_2 content. You then apply incremental levels of PEEP while simultaneously measuring these parameters and the arterial O_2 content via an A-line. Compute O_2 delivery at each PEEP increment, with optimum PEEP defined as that level with the highest O_2 delivery. Fortunately, if the NBRC tests you on this approach, it will not have you perform computation but rather query you on what to do if either cardiac output or blood pressure should fall when raising PEEP levels. Since a fall in cardiac output or blood pressure likely means a decrease in O_2 delivery, should this occur, the correct action is to decrease PEEP back to its prior setting.

Methods 2–4 all use measures of respiratory mechanics to determine optimum PEEP. The conventional technique involves raising PEEP while simultaneously measuring the patient's static compliance [$VT/(Pplat - PEEP)$] during volume-targeted ventilation. An example of this type of PEEP study as it might appear on the NBRC CRT exam is depicted below:

PEEP (cm H_2O)	VT (mL)	PIP (cm H_2O)	Pplat (cm H_2O)
0	600	30	20
5	600	36	24
10	600	41	27
15	600	45	33
20	600	49	41

First, you can disregard the peak pressure (PIP)—it's there to confuse you. What you are interested in is the numerator in the formula for static compliance (i.e., Pplat – PEEP). *Since the tidal volume is constant, the smaller this difference, the greater the compliance*, as indicated below:

Pplat (cm H_2O)	PEEP (cm H_2O)	Pplat – PEEP (cm H_2O)	C_{L+T} (mL/cm H_2O)
20	0	20	30
24	5	19	32
27	10	17	35
33	15	18	33
41	20	21	29

Based on this method, the optimum PEEP for this patient would be 10 cm H_2O, the PEEP level yielding the highest compliance.

What if the patient is receiving pressure-target ventilation? In this case you can use method #3, which applies the same basic concept as just discussed. With this method, however, *rather than maintain a constant volume, you maintain a constant ΔP* (pressure limit − PEEP), typically 15 or 20 cm H_2O. You then assess the exhaled V_T, with the largest change representing the optimum PEEP.

For obvious reasons, this approach is called the equal pressure method. An example of the equal pressure method for determining optimum PEEP as it might appear on the NBRC CRT exam is depicted below:

PEEP (cm H_2O)	PIP (cm H_2O)	V_T (mL)
0	15	350
5	20	390
10	25	410
15	30	430
20	35	380

Using this approach, the optimum PEEP for this patient is 15 cm H_2O, corresponding to the maximum volume change for a given ΔP (in this case 15 cm H_2O).

The last method for determining optimum PEEP (method #4) requires plotting of a static pressure-volume curve for the patient's respiratory system, as depicted in **Figure 12-2**. Note first that the slope of any line on this graph equals compliance ($\Delta V/\Delta P$). Second, the curve exhibits the typical "S" shape, with a low slope (low compliance) at low pressures/volumes, changing over to a steep slope (high compliance) at moderate volumes/pressures, then changing back to a low slope (low compliance) at high pressures/volumes. In theory, the low compliance at low lung volumes is due to the high opening pressures required to expand collapsed alveoli. As more and more alveoli open (alveolar recruitment), the curve steepens and enters the "sweet spot" for efficient mechanics of breathing, where compliance is at a maximum. However, like any elastic structure, the lungs eventually reach their limit of expansion, signaled by a rapid leveling off of the pressure-volume curve at high volumes—i.e., overdistention. Here any small increase in volume results in a large change in pressure.

The lower inflection point (LIP or *Pflex*) of the curve corresponds to the changeover from low to high compliance at low lung volume, representing maximum alveolar recruitment. Based on these concepts, optimum PEEP is the *lowest pressure* needed to exceed LIP or Pflex. Clinically, we maintain PEEP 2–3 cm H_2O above the LIP or Pflex in order to keep alveoli open, while avoiding overdistention.

Unfortunately, this procedure is very complicated, requiring sedation or paralysis of the patient and either incremental or gradual inflation with a calibrated super syringe. Moreover, the curve you obtain often is not as "clean" as that depicted in Figure 12-2 and thus subject to variable interpretation. It is for this reason that methods 1–3 for determining optimum PEEP are more likely to appear on the CRT exam and be tested at the application level, as discussed here. If they appear at all, questions on using the static pressure-volume curve to determine optimum PEEP will likely be at the recall level.

Select Ventilator Graphics

The ventilator graphics display incorporated into most critical care ventilators provides the following essential monitoring capabilities:

- Checking/confirming and fine tuning ventilator function
- Assessing patients' respiratory mechanics
- Evaluating patients' responses to therapy
- Troubleshooting patient-ventilator interaction

The interpretation and use of ventilator graphics is covered in detail in Chapters 13 and 14. Here we address only how to select graphic displays according to the information you need.

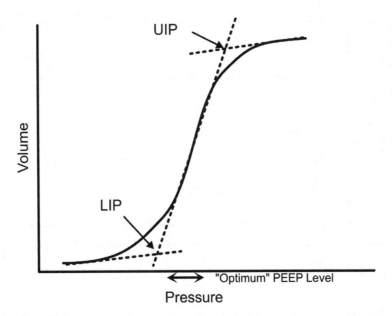

Figure 12-2 Idealized Static Pressure-Volume Curve of the Respiratory System. The points at which the slope of the curve changes are called inflection points. (Note that these points are not on the curve itself, but extrapolated from tangents of the curve.) Optimum PEEP is the lowest pressure needed to exceed LIP.

LIP = lower inflection point representing the changeover from low to high compliance at low lung volume; UIP = upper inflection point representing the changeover from high compliance to low compliance at high lung volume.

There are two major types of ventilator graphics: scalar (time-based) and X-Y (loops). As depicted in **Figure 12-3**, scalar graphics plot pressure, volume, and/or flow on the Y-axis against time on the X-axis. On most ventilators, you can set the graphics screen to display one or more of these three parameters. Note that most ventilators allow you to change the time scale (sweep speed) for displaying scalar graphics. Changing the time scale by selecting a faster speed gives you a closer look at individual breath waveforms, whereas selecting a slow sweep speed can help you identify trends.

X-Y or loop graphics simultaneously display two variables plotted on the X- and Y-axes. The two most common loop graphics are pressure (X-axis) vs. volume (Y-axis) and volume (X-axis) vs. flow (Y-axis). **Figure 12-4** (see page 357) depicts a representative X-Y plot of volume vs. pressure (for the same patient and same conditions as in Figure 12-3). **Table 12-7** (see page 357) provides guidance on which graphic display to select, based on your monitoring needs.

Apply Disease-Specific Ventilator Protocols

The NBRC exam expects you to be familiar with selected disease-specific protocols, the most important of which is the National Heart, Lung, and Blood Institute (NHLBI) ARDS protocol. This protocol helps increase survival of ARDS patients by maintaining adequate oxygenation while preventing ventilator-associated lung injury. You should consider implementing this protocol for any patient who exhibits an acute onset of respiratory distress not associated with heart failure and has:

- A Pa_{O_2}/F_{IO_2} less than 300 (signifying acute lung injury)
- Bilateral diffuse infiltrates on X-ray consistent with pulmonary edema

Basic ventilator setup and adjustment is as follows:

1. Calculate predicted body weight (PBW).

Males = 50 + 2.3 [height (inches) – 60]
Females = 45.5 + 2.3 [height (inches) – 60]

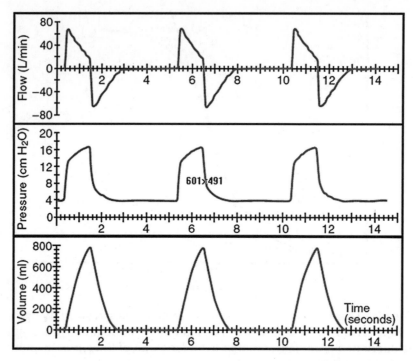

Figure 12-3 Scalar Graphic Display of Flow, Pressure and Volume Versus Time. The flow and pressure waveform indicate pressure-limited ventilation with 4 cm H₂O PEEP.

From: White, G. C. (2003). *Basic clinical lab competencies for respiratory care* (4th ed.). © 2003 Delmar Learning, a part of Cengage Learning, Inc. Reproduced with permission. www.cengage.com/permissions.

2. Select assist/control (volume-targeted) mode.
3. Set initial VT to 8 ml/kg PBW.
4. Reduce VT by 1 mL/kg at intervals of no more than 2 hours until VT = 6mL/kg PBW.
5. Set initial rate to approximate baseline V̇E (no greater than 35/min).
6. Adjust VT and rate to achieve pH and plateau pressure goals below.
7. Set inspiratory flow rate above patient demand (usually > 80 L/min).

To assure adequate oxygenation, the goal is to maintain a Pao_2 between 55 and 80 torr or an Spo_2 between 88% and 95%. To achieve these targets, you raise or lower Fio_2 and PEEP according to the combinations specified in Table 12-8. The higher PEEP options (lower row) should be considered in patients with high Fio_2 needs who are hemodynamically stable and have no underlying barotrauma.

To help prevent lung injury, you should keep the plateau pressure less than or equal to 30 cm H₂O and measure it every 4 hours and after each change in PEEP or VT. The following guidelines apply to adjusting Pplat:

- If Pplat is greater than 30 cm H₂O: decrease VT in 1 mL/kg steps to a minimum of 4 ml/kg
- If Pplat is less than 25 cm H₂O: if VT is less than 6 mL/kg, increase VT by 1 mL/kg until Pplat is greater than 25 cm H₂O or VT equals 6 mL/kg
- If Pplat is less than 30 cm H₂O and breath stacking occurs: consider increasing VT in 1-mL/kg increments (maximum = 8 mL/kg)

In terms of acid-base balance, the goal is to keep the pH between 7.30 and 7.45. If the pH rises above 7.45 (rare), you should decrease the ventilator rate. Otherwise:

- If the pH between 7.15 and 7.30: increase rate until pH > 7.30 or $Paco_2$ < 25 (max rate = 35)
- If rate equals 35 and $Paco_2$ is less than 25: consider giving $NaHCO_3$

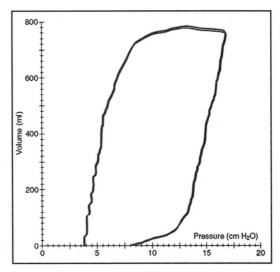

Figure 12-4 X–Y Graphic Display of Pressure-Volume Loop During Mechanical Ventilation. The right side upswing is the inspiratory portion with the downswing to the left being the expiratory return to baseline pressure of about +4 cm H_2O (PEEP).

From: White, G. C. (2003). *Basic clinical lab competencies for respiratory care* (4th ed.). © 2003 Delmar Learning, a part of Cengage Learning, Inc. Reproduced with permission. www.cengage.com/permissions.

- If pH is less than 7.15: increase rate to 35
- If pH remains less than 7.15 and $NaHCO_3$ is being given: increase VT in 1-ml/kg steps until pH is greater than 7.15 (Pplat target may be exceeded)

You should adjust the ventilator flow (VCV) or I-time (interval time) so that the I:E ratio is between 1:1 and 1:3. If the patient is at maximum FIO_2 (1.0) and PEEP (24 cm H_2O), adjust the I:E ratio to 1:1. Weaning patients off the NHLBI ARDS protocol is described in a subsequent section of this chapter.

Table 12-7 Common Usage for Scalar and X-Y Loop Graphic Displays

Display	Select When Need To
Scalar Graphics	
Flow vs. time	• Identify presence of auto-PEEP (expiratory) • Identify flow starvation (VCV) • Assess/adjust rise time (PCV, PSV) • Identify asynchrony
Pressure vs. time	• Confirm PIP and PEEP level • Visually assess mechanics using PIP-Pplat (~ Raw) and Pplat – PEEP (~ C_{L+T}) • Assess sensitivity/trigger response • Identify asynchrony
Volume vs. time	• Identify leaks • Identify asynchrony
X-Y Loop Graphics	
Pressure (X-axis) vs. volume (Y-axis)	• Assess overall work of breathing • Identify overdistension • Assess trigger work • Adjust PSV levels
Volume (X-axis) vs. flow (Y-axis)	• Assess bronchodilator response • Identify presence of auto-PEEP • Identify leaks

Table 12-8 NHLBI ARDS Protocol FIO₂/PEEP Combinations

F_{IO_2}	0.3	0.4	0.4	0.5	0.5	0.6	0.7	0.7
PEEP	5	5	8	8	10	10	10	12
	12–14	*14*	*16*	*16*	*18–20*	*20*	*20*	*20*
F_{IO_2}	0.7	0.8	0.9	0.9	0.9	1.0	1.0	1.0
PEEP	14	14	14	16	18	20	22	24
	20	*20–22*	*22*	*22*	*22*	*22*	*22*	*24*

Initiate and Select Appropriate Settings for High-Frequency Ventilation

The primary mode of high-frequency ventilation in current use is high-frequency oscillation ventilation (HFOV). HFOV was initially used only for infants and children but is now being applied to adults. For this reason, you need to be familiar with both applications.

HFOV is designed to promote gas exchange by maintaining alveolar recruitment while minimizing the cyclical lung expansion/contraction characterizing conventional positive pressure ventilation. Instead of providing 6–10 mL/kg tidal volumes, HFOV provides CO_2 elimination by the application of rapid "push-pull" pressure oscillations to the airway. In theory, this approach can help prevent ventilator-associated lung injury, especially that associated with the repetitive stress of conventional tidal volume exchange at low lung volumes.

In general, HFOV is indicated for infants, children, and adults with hypoxemic respiratory failure who have not responded to more conventional methods of improving oxygenation. This includes patients receiving VCV or PCV who:

- Need high concentrations of O_2 (F_{IO_2} > 0.60; P/F ratio < 200)
- Require high airway pressures/reverse I:E (Pmean > 25 cm H_2O)
- Remain hypoxemic on high PEEP (20–25 cm H_2O)

In terms of specific diagnoses, HFOV should be considered for adults and children with severe ARDS or air-leak syndromes causing hypoxemia. Among infants, HFOV has been successfully applied to patients with severe IRDS, meconium aspiration syndrome, pulmonary interstitial edema, congenital diaphragmatic hernia, and pulmonary hypoplasia. Relative contraindications for HFOV include obstructive lung disease and an abnormally elevated ICP.

The main determinant of oxygenation during HFOV is the mean airway pressure (Pmean). The settings that affect ventilation/CO_2 elimination in this mode are the amplitude and frequency of the pressure oscillations. Increasing the amplitude and decreasing the oscillation frequency lowers the $PaCO_2$, whereas decreasing the amplitude and increasing frequency raises the $PaCO_2$.

Table 12-9 Guidelines for Initial HFOV Settings

Setting	Patient Category			
	Preterm	*Term*	*Child*	*Adult*
FIO_2[a]	1.0	1.0	1.0	1.0
Frequency (Hz)	15	10	6–8	5–6
% I-time	33% (1:2)	33% (1:2)	33% (1:2)	33% (1:2)
Power/amplitude[b]	2–3	3–4	4–5	5–6
Pmean (cm H_2O)[c]	8–10	8–10	10–15	15–20
Bias flow (L/min)	8–15	10–20	15–25	> 25

a. Set FIO_2 to 1.0 or match to patient's current level.
b. Adjust to get chest "wiggle."
c. Set 1–5 cm H_2O higher than Pmean on VCV or PCV.

Based on different amplitude and pressure needs, there are different versions of HFOV ventilators available for infants/children and adults. **Table 12-9** provides general guidelines for initial HFOV for infants, children, and adults. In most cases, you set the initial FIO_2 to 1.0 or match the patient's current O_2%, then immediately titrate it down by adjusting the Pmean.

You set the frequency in Hz (cycles/sec). For example, you often start preterm infants on HFOV at a rate of 15 Hz, which equals 15 cycles/sec × 60 sec/min = 900 cycles/min. Recommended HFOV frequencies vary inversely with patient size and weight.

Under current guidelines, you keep the percentage of I-time constant at 33% (I:E = 1:2) across all patient categories. Increasing the I-time to 50% (I:E = 1:1) has been used to improve oxygenation but may increase air trapping and increase the incidence of pulmonary barotrauma.

The HFOV power setting varies the displacement of the diaphragm/piston used to generate airway oscillations (i.e., the "push-pull" amplitude). You adjust this power setting from 1 to 10, using higher levels for larger patients. Changes in the power setting are monitored by a digital display of amplitude, as measured by ΔP in cm H_2O. You determine the proper power level by observing its effect on the chest wall. Specifically, HFOV power should be high enough to create visible chest vibrations. In infants, this "wiggle" should extend from the shoulders to the umbilicus, and in adults to the mid-thigh region. Alternatively, some clinicians suggest adjusting *adult* HFOV power levels to achieve a ΔP equal to the patient's $PaCO_2$ + 20 (e.g., if the patient has a $PaCO_2$ of 60 torr, you would set the power to achieve an amplitude of 80 cm H_2O).

The initial Pmean setting depends on patient size and varies between 8 and 20 cm H_2O. If you are switching from conventional ventilatory support, you initially should set the Pmean 2–4 cm H_2O *higher* than that occurring during VCV or PCV and adjust it as needed to keep the SaO_2 at 88% or higher.

As with conventional mechanical ventilation, once you start a patient on HFOV, you adjust the parameters to normalize blood gases. **Table 12-10** specifies the adjustments needed to raise or lower the $PaCO_2$ and PaO_2/SaO_2. Note first that frequency changes during HFOV affect CO_2 elimination in a manner opposite to that observed during conventional mechanical ventilation—i.e., *decreasing the HFOV frequency tends to lower the $PaCO_2$, while increasing the HFOV frequency tends to raise the $PaCO_2$*. Note also the unique use of a cuff leak for lowering the $PaCO_2$ during HFOV. Generally this approach is used only if the patient remains severely hypercapnic (pH < 7.2) despite use of the maximum power/amplitude and lowest frequency settings. Because a cuff leak during HFOV tends to lower Pmean, this parameter may need to be readjusted to maintain adequate oxygenation.

To apply these guidelines to adults who deteriorate while receiving HFOV:

- If oxygenation worsens, increase Pmean in 3–5 cm H_2O increments every 30 minutes until maximum is reached (45–55 cm H_2O).
- Accept hypercapnia if pH can be kept above 7.25 (permissive hypercapnia).

Table 12-10 Adjusting Blood Gas Parameters on HFOV

Parameter	To Raise	To Lower
Paco$_2$ (ventilation)	↓ power/amplitude (ΔP) ↑ frequency	↑ power/amplitude (ΔP) ↓ frequency deflate cuff
Pao$_2$/Sao$_2$ (oxygenation)	↑ Pmean ↑ Fio$_2$ ↑ I-time[a]	↓ Fio$_2$ ↓ Pmean
a. Consider only as last resort; may increase air trapping and lead to barotraumas.		

- If hypercapnia worsens (but pH > 7.2), increase power/ΔP in 10 cm H$_2$O increments every 30 minutes up to maximum power setting; if hypercapnia persists after reaching maximum ΔP, consider decreasing frequency to 3 Hz.
- If severe hypercapnia (pH < 7.2) persists, bag patient, set power to maximum, set frequency to 3 Hz, and allow a cuff leak around the ET tube.
- Any abrupt rise in Paco$_2$ may indicate obstruction of the ET tube.

Initiate and Modify Weaning Procedures

According to the AARC, patients receiving mechanical ventilation for respiratory failure should undergo a weaning assessment whenever the following criteria are met:

1. Evidence for some reversal of the underlying cause of respiratory failure
2. Adequate oxygenation, e.g.:
    a. Pao$_2$/Fio$_2$ > 150–200
    b. PEEP ≤ 5–8 cm H$_2$O
    c. Fio$_2$ ≤ 0.4–0.5
3. pH ≥ 7.25
4. Hemodynamic stability (no myocardial ischemia or significant hypotension)
5. The capability to initiate an inspiratory effort

In terms of the method for weaning acutely ill patients who meet these criteria, daily *spontaneous breathing trials* (SBTs) provide the quickest route for discontinuing mechanical ventilation. Tracking measures such as vital capacity and MIP/NIF while the patient is receiving ventilatory support can provide useful insight about weaning potential. However, a carefully monitored SBT provides the most valid information for deciding whether or not a patient can stay off the ventilator. And because SBTs are most successful when implemented by nonphysicians using defined protocols, you can expect the NBRC to assess your ability to perform independently in this area.

Spontaneous breathing modes used in SBT weaning protocols include (1) straight T-tube breathing, (2) CPAP, (3) pressure support, or (4) pressure support + CPAP (i.e., BiPAP™). Based on current evidence, no one approach is better than another. However, provision of an elevated baseline pressure may improve breath triggering in patients who experience auto-PEEP.

SBT protocols vary somewhat by institution and unit—e.g., surgical vs. medical ICU. **Figure 12-5** provides a decision-making algorithm for a typical spontaneous breathing trial protocol. All such protocols involve initial assessment of the patient to assure that he or she is ready to wean, using criteria like those recommended by the AARC. The next step normally is application of a brief (2–5 minute) supervised period of carefully monitored spontaneous breathing. During this "screening" phase, you assess the patient's breathing pattern, vital signs, and comfort level.

If the patient tolerates the screening phase, you continue the SBT for at least 30 minutes, but no more than 120 minutes. During this period you provide encouragement to the patient, obtain an ABG,

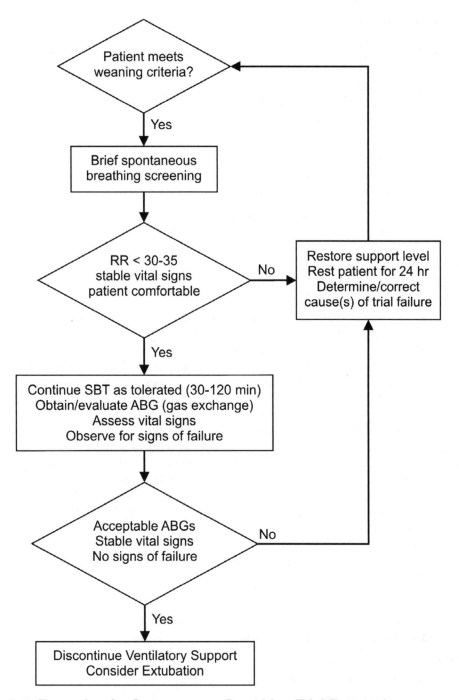

Figure 12-5 Example of a Spontaneous Breathing Trial Protocol.

and intermittently monitor heart rate, blood pressure, and respiratory rate. Objective physiologic measures indicating a successful SBT include the following:

- Acceptable gas exchange
  - $SpO_2 \geq 85–90\%$ or $PaO_2 \geq 50–60$ torr
  - $pH \geq 7.32$
  - Increase in $PaCO_2 \leq 10$ torr

- Stable hemodynamics
  ○ Heart rate < 120–140 beats/min; change < 20%
  ○ Systolic blood pressure < 180–200 mm Hg and > 90 mm Hg; change < 20%
  ○ No vasopressors required
- Stable ventilatory pattern
  ○ Respiratory rate ≤ 30–35 breaths/min
  ○ Change in respiratory rate < 50%

If these objective indicators are not met, you should return the patient to a sufficient level of ventilatory support to maintain adequate oxygenation and ventilation and prevent muscle fatigue. Even when the patient meets these physiologic measures, you may need to discontinue the SBT if you note one or more of the following subjective indicators of intolerance/failure:

- Change in mental status (e.g., somnolence, coma, agitation, anxiety)
- Onset or worsening of discomfort
- Diaphoresis
- Signs of increased work of breathing:
  ○ Use of accessory respiratory muscles
  ○ Thoracoabdominal paradox

If a patient fails an SBT, you should work with the physician to determine the cause(s). Once these factors are identified and corrected, you should resume performing an SBT every 24 hours.

However, if the patient can maintain acceptable physiologic parameters and is able to tolerate the SBT for its full duration, you can remove ventilatory support and consider extubation. The decision whether to proceed with extubation should be a separate consideration, based on assessment of the patient's airway patency and protective reflexes, including the ability to clear secretions by coughing. Chapter 10 provides details on when and how to extubate a patient.

Procedures for ventilator-dependent patients differ somewhat from this approach. For these patients, you gradually reduce the level of ventilator support using a mode such as SIMV. Once such patients progress to the point where they can provide at least half the needed minute volume via spontaneous breathing, you can consider implementing an SBT protocol like that described above. However, rather than discontinue ventilatory support after a successful trial, you instead should implement periods of spontaneous breathing of increasing duration (e.g., 30–60–120–240 minutes), until the patient is fully liberated from the ventilator.

The NHLBI ARDS protocol follows these basic principles but uses a progressive transitioning from CPAP to pressure support to true unassisted spontaneous breathing. Details on this portion of the ARDS protocol are provided in the accompanying box.

NHLBI ARDS Protocol: Weaning Component

Criteria Indicating Readiness to Wean

1. $F_{IO_2} \leq 0.40$ and PEEP ≤ 8 cm H_2O

2. PEEP and $F_{IO_2} \leq$ previous day settings

3. Patient has acceptable spontaneous breathing efforts

4. Systolic BP ≥ 90 mm Hg without vasopressors

Procedure

I. CPAP Phase

  1. Set CPAP = 5 cm H_2O, $F_{IO_2} = 0.50$

    a. If respiratory rate < 35 for 5 min, advance to pressure support phase

---

(continues)

    b. If respiratory rate > 35 in less than 5 min, repeat trial after appropriate intervention (e.g., suctioning, analgesia, anxiolysis)

  2. If CPAP trial not tolerated, return to previous support settings

II. Pressure Support (PS) Phase

  1. Set PEEP = 5, FIO_2 = 0.50

  2. Set initial PS based on respiratory rate during CPAP trial:

    a. If CPAP respiratory rate < 25, set PS = 5 cm H_2O and go to step 3d

    b. If CPAP respiratory rate = 25-35, set PS = 20 cm H_2O, then reduce by 5 cm H_2O at ≤ 5 minute intervals until respiratory rate = 26–35, then go to step 3a

    c. If initial PS not tolerated: return to previous support settings

  3. Reduce PS (no reductions made after 1700 hours)

    a. Reduce PS by 5 cm H_2O every 1–3 hours

    b. If PS ≥ 10 cm H_2O not tolerated, return to previous support settings (reinitiate last tolerated PS level next morning and go to step 3a)

    c. If PS = 5 cm H_2O not tolerated, return to PS = 10 cm H_2O. If tolerated, 5 or 10 cm H_2O may be used overnight with further attempts at weaning the next morning

    d. If PS = 5 cm H_2O tolerated for 2 hours or more, advance to unassisted breathing trial phase

III. Unassisted Breathing Trial Phase

  1. Place on T-piece, trach collar, or CPAP ≤ 5 cm H_2O

  2. Assess for tolerance as below for 2 hours

    a. SpO_2 ≥ 90 and/or PaO_2 ≥ 60 mmHg

    b. Spontaneous VT ≥ 4 ml/kg PBW

    c. Respiratory rate ≤ 35/min

    d. pH ≥ 7.3

    e. No distress; distress = 2 or more of the following:

      • Heart rate > 120% of baseline

      • Marked accessory muscle use

      • Abdominal paradox

      • Diaphoresis

      • Marked dyspnea

  3. If tolerated, consider extubation

  4. If not tolerated, resume PS = 5 cm H_2O

Source: National Heart, Lung, and Blood Institute. ARDS Clinical Network. (2005). Mechanical ventilation protocol summary. Retrieved October 26, 2008, from http://www.ardsnet.org

Weaning from HFOV focuses mainly on oxygenation needs. As oxygenation improves in the adult HFOV patient, you should first lower the FIO_2 to 0.40, then slowly reduce Pmean by 2–3 cm H_2O every 4–6 hours until it is 20 cm H_2O or less. At this point you should consider switching the patient to PCV at a pressure limit less than or equal to 30 cm H_2O and PEEP 10–12 cm H_2O. Thereafter, weaning should follow a standard SBT protocol, as previously described.

Administer Medications

One of your most frequent tasks is administration of bronchodilators, anti-inflammatory agents, mucolytics, or anti-infective agents to patients via the inhalation route. Depending on the preparation of these drugs, they may be delivered as either liquid or dry powder aerosols. In certain circumstances, you may also administer specific drugs directly into the lungs via endotracheal instillation.

Aerosolized Drugs

Chapter 6 provides details on the selection, use, and troubleshooting of aerosol drug delivery systems, including small-volume nebulizers, metered-dose inhalers, dry powder inhalers, and accessory equipment. Chapter 11 provides guidelines on the appropriate selection of bronchodilators, mucolytics, steroids, and diluting agents and their role in bronchial hygiene. Here we focus on the specific drugs available to you and provide general pointers regarding their administration.

Table 12-11 provides details on the most common drugs you may administer by aerosol, including their generic and brand names; available preparations; recommended adult doses; onset, peak, and duration of action; and recommended frequency of administration.

Regarding use of the beta-adrenergic bronchodilators, keep in mind the following key points:

- All beta-adrenergics have some cardiovascular and CNS effects; in general, you should select those with the least beta$_1$ and most beta$_2$ effect (e.g., albuterol or its isomer levalbuterol).
- Beta-adrenergics are best used as relievers of bronchospasm; corticosteroids should be used to control reactive airway disease.
- You should tailor dosages according to individual patient response; if change in levels of FEV$_1$ are less than 12–15%, recommend increasing the dose; if cardiovascular/CNS effects are pronounced (e.g., tachycardia, palpitations, nervousness), recommend decreasing the dose.
- If also administering steroids, mucokinetics, or anti-infective agents by inhalation, always give the bronchodilator first.
- In acute exacerbations of asthma, repeat the standard dose every 20 minutes (up to 3 times) or provide continuous nebulization until symptoms are relieved.
- Long-acting beta-adrenergics such as salmeterol (Serevent) should be used for asthma only if inhaled steroids do not provide control of symptoms; provide urgent treatment if symptoms worsen while using a long-acting beta-adrenergic.
- For maintenance therapy of bronchospasm in COPD, consider an anticholinergic such as ipratropium bromide or tiotropium bromide.

In terms of administration of inhaled corticosteroids, you need to remember the following essentials:

- Inhaled corticosteroids control inflammation and are the first-line drugs for mild persistent asthma.
- Cromolyn, nedocromil, leukotriene modifiers, and sustained-release theophylline are the major alternatives to steroids for asthma patients.
- Oral medication (tablets or syrup) may be needed to supplement inhaled steroids if asthma is severe.
- With the exception of budesonide (Pulmicort), common inhaled steroids preparations are all MDI or DPI; therefore, proper technique is critical.
- Rinsing the mouth after therapy is essential in order to prevent pharyngitis and/or oral candidiasis.
- Use of spacers or valved holding chambers with MDI steroids minimizes pharyngeal deposition and the incidence of pharyngitis and candidiasis.

In administering mucokinetics, you need to be aware that:

- All mucokinetics are irritating to the airway; to prevent bronchospasm, always precede treatment with a bronchodilator.
- Acetylcysteine and sodium bicarbonate can be instilled directly into the airway via ET tube.
- Mucokinetics must always be administered in combination with bronchial hygiene measures to facilitate secretion removal.

Regarding use of inhaled anti-infective agents, keep in mind the following key points:

- Aerosolized antibiotics (Coly-Mycin, Tobramycin) are generally indicated only in cystic fibrosis patients with suspected or confirmed *Pseudomonas aeruginosa* pulmonary infections.
- If the patient is receiving several inhaled medications, the recommended order is bronchodilator first, followed by mucolytic, then bronchial hygiene therapy, then steroids, and then the aerosolized antibiotics.

Table 12-11 Medications Commonly Administered by Inhalation Route

Generic Name	Brand Name(s)	Delivery and Preparation	Adult Dose/ Frequency	Action	Comments
Beta-Adrenergic Bronchodilators					
Albuterol	Proventil Ventolin	SVN 0.5% MDI (90 mcg/puff) DPI (200 mcg/cap)	0.5 mL q 4–6 hr 2 puffs q 4–6 hr 1 puff q 4–6 hr	Onset: 5 min Peak: 30–60 min Duration: 3–8 hrs (medium)	Mild CV/CNS side effects; can be mixed with cromolyn or ipratropium
Bitolterol	Tornalate	SVN 0.2% MDI (37 mcg/puff)	1.25 mL T/QID 2 puffs q 6 hr	Onset: 3–4 min Peak: 30–60 min Duration: 5–8 hrs (Medium)	Mild CV/CNS side effects; do not mix with other drugs
Epinephrine	Adrenalin	SVN 1% (1:100)	0.25–0.5 mL PRN	Onset: 3–5 min Peak: 5–20 min Duration: 1–3 hrs (short)	Strong CV/CNS side effects
Formoterol	Foradil	DPI 25 mcg/puff	1 puff BID	Onset: 1–3 min Peak: 30–60 min Duration: 12 hrs (long)	Use only if inhaled steroids do not control the asthma; patients should seek treatment if symptoms worsen
Isoetharine	Bronkosol	SVN 1% MDI (340 mcg/ puff)	0.25–0.5 mL 1–2 puffs T/QID	Onset: 1–5 min Peak: 5–60 min Duration: 1–4 hrs (short)	Moderate CV/ CNS side effects
Levalbuterol	Xopenex	SVN 0.31, 0.63, 1.25 mg in 3 mL diluent MDI 45 mcg/puff	3.0 mL (unit dose) TID 2 puffs q 4–6 hr	Onset: 15 min Peak: 1–1/2 hrs Duration: 5–8 hrs (medium)	Mild CV/CNS side effects
Metaproterenol	Alupent Metaprel	SVN 5% MDI (650 mcg/ puff)	0.2–0.3 mL 2–3 puffs q 4–6 hr	Onset: 5–30 min Peak: 1/2–1 hr Duration: 1–6 hrs (medium)	Mild CV/CNS side effects
Pirbuterol	Maxair	MDI (200 mcg/ puff)	2 puffs q 4–6 hr	Onset: 5 min Peak: 1/2–1 hr Duration: 3–5 hrs (medium)	Mild CV/CNS side effects
Racemic epinephrine	Vaponefrin Micronephrin	SVN 2.25%	0.25–0.5 mL PRN	Onset: 3–5 min Peak: 5–20 min Duration: 0.5–2 hrs (Short)	Used for upper airway inflammation (croup, post-extubation); can cause "rebound" edema

(continues)

Table 12-11 Medications Commonly Administered by Inhalation Route (continued)

Generic Name	Brand Name(s)	Delivery and Preparation	Adult Dose/ Frequency	Action	Comments
Salmeterol	Serevent	MDI (25 mcg/puff) DPI (50 mcg/puff)	2 puffs BID 1 puff BID	Onset: 10–20 min Peak: 3 hrs Duration: 12 hrs (long)	Use only if inhaled steroids do not control the asthma; patients should seek treatment if symptoms worsen
Terbutaline Sulfate	Bricanyl	DPI (500 mcg/ puff)	2 puffs q 4–6 hrs	Onset: 5–30 min Peak:1/2–1 hr Duration: 3–6 hrs (medium)	Mild CV/CNS side effects
Anticholinergic Bronchodilators					
Ipratropium bromide	Atrovent	SVN 0.2% MDI 18 mcg/puff	2.5 mL (unit dose) T/QID 2–3 puffs T/QID	Onset: 15 min Peak: 15–90 min Duration: 4–6 hrs (medium)	For maintenance therapy of bronchospasm in COPD; can cause dryness
Tiotropium Bromide	Spiriva	DPI 18 mcg/puff	1 puff per day	Onset: 30 min Peak: 3 hrs Duration: 24 hrs (long)	Can cause dryness and paradoxical bronchospasm
Adrenergic + Anticholinergic Combinations					
Ipratropium bromide + albuterol	Combivent DuoNeb	SVN 2.5 mg albuterol + 0.5 mg ipratropium MDI 90 mcg albuterol + 18 mcg ipratropium	3 mL (unit dose) T/QID 2 puffs T/QID	As per component (see above)	As per component (see above)
Corticosteroids					
Beclomethasone	Vanceril Beclovent	MDI (40 mcg/puff) MDI (80 mcg/puff)	2 puffs BID	Varies	Have patient rinse mouth with water post Rx to prevent pharyngitis, oral candidiasis
Budesonide	Pulmicort	DPI 200 cg/puff SVN 0.25/0.5 mg/2 mL	1–3 puffs BID 2 mL (unit dose) BID	Onset: within 24 hrs Duration: varies	Have patient rinse mouth with water to prevent pharyngitis, oral candidiasis

(continues)

Table 12-11 Medications Commonly Administered by Inhalation Route (continued)

Generic Name	Brand Name(s)	Delivery and Preparation	Adult Dose/ Frequency	Action	Comments
Flunisolide	AeroBid	MDI (250 mcg/puff)	2 puffs BID	Varies	Have patient rinse mouth with water post Rx to prevent pharyngitis, oral candidiasis
Fluticasone propronate	Flovent Flovent Rotadisk	MDI 44/110/220 mcg/puff DPI 50/100/250 mcg	2 puffs QID 100 mcg inhalation BID	Onset: within 24 hrs Duration: 2–3 days	Have patient rinse mouth with water to prevent pharyngitis, oral candidiasis
Triamcinolone acetonide	Azmacort	MDI (100 mcg/ puff)	2 puffs T/QID	Varies	Have patient rinse mouth with water post Rx to prevent pharyngitis, oral candidiasis
Corticosteroids + Adrenergic Combinations					
Fluticasone + Salmeterol	Advair Diskus	100, 250, or 500 mcg fluticasone + 50 mcg salmeterol	1 puff BID	As per component	As per component
Mast Cell Stabilizers					
Cromolyn sodium	Intal	MDI 800 mcg/puff SVN 20 mg/2 mL ampule	2–4 puffs T/QID 1 ampule T/QID	Onset: 20–30 min Duration: 2–6 hr	Not for acute bronchospasm; can be mixed with albuterol
Nedocromil	Tilade	MDI 1.75 mg/puff	2–4 puffs QID	Onset: 20–30 min Duration: 3-1/4 hrs	Not for acute bronchospasm; can be mixed with albuterol
Mucokinetics					
Acetylcysteine	Mucomyst	10/20% (4-, 10-, 30-mL vials)	6–10 mL 10% T/QID—dilute 20% for equivalency	Decreases sputum viscosity on contact	Can cause bronchospasm; give bronchodilator first
Sodium bicarbonate	n/a	2% solution	2–5 mL PRN	Decreases sputum viscosity on contact	Can cause bronchospasm; give bronchodilator first

(continues)

Table 12-11 Medications Commonly Administered by Inhalation Route (continued)

Generic Name	Brand Name(s)	Delivery and Preparation	Adult Dose/ Frequency	Action	Comments
Dornase alpha	Pulmozyme	2.5 mL single-use ampule (1.0 mg/mL)	1 ampule/day or BID	Decreases sputum viscosity on contact	Can cause bronchospasm; give bronchodilator first; do not mix with other drugs
Anti-Infectives					
Colisimethate	Colistin Coly-Mycin	150 mg vials (powder); add 2 mL sterile H_2O	37.5–150 mg q 8–12 hr	Anti-pseudomonal agent	Requires valved nebulizer (Pari® Plus)
Tobramycin	Tobi	300 mg in 5 mL saline ampule	300 mg q 12 hr for 28 days, followed by 28 days off	Anti-pseudomonal agent	Many side effects; do mix with other drugs; give bronchodilator first; requires valved nebulizer (Pari® Plus)
Zanamivir	Relenza	DPI 5 mg/blister	10 mg (2 blisters) BID for 5 days	Stops viral replication (influenza A and B)	Not for use in asthma or COPD patients; if bronchospasm develops, stop therapy and treat immediately

Endotracheal Instillation

Selected drugs can be administered as liquids or "instilled" directly into the lungs via a tracheal airway. You may be asked to instill lidocaine, epinephrine, atropine, or naloxone ("LEAN") in emergency situations when IV access is not available. Guidelines for endotracheal instillation of these agents include the following:

- Make sure the dose administered is 2–2.5 times greater than the IV dose.
- Dilute the drug dose with 10 mL of sterile water or nonsterile saline for injection.
- Put the patient in a supine position (not Trendelenberg).
- Halt chest compressions.
- Instill the drug through a catheter that passes the ET tube tip.
- Immediately after instillation, provide 5–10 rapid inflations via a manual resuscitator.

Other than mucokinetics, the only other respiratory agent you may be asked to administer by endotracheal instillation is surfactant. Surfactant preparations are administered prophylactically to infants at high risk of developing respiratory distress syndrome (RDS), or as rescue therapy for those with clinical evidence of RDS. When administering instillation of surfactant to these patients, be sure to do the following:

- Take a chest X-ray before instillation to confirm ET tube position.
- Suction the infant prior to administration if necessary.

- Monitor SpO_2, ECG continuously.
- Use a 5-Fr feeding tube or suction catheter to instill the solution.
- Insert the instillation catheter up to but not past the tip of the ET tube.
- Split dose in half and instill half a dose into each dependent bronchus (turning infant from side to side).
- Administer dose as rapidly as tolerated.
- After administration, bag the infant for 1–2 minutes.
- Carefully monitor blood gases and chest wall movement during the first 3 hours after dosing.
- Adjust ventilator/FIO_2 as appropriate (patient may transiently require higher levels of ventilatory support).
- If possible, avoid suctioning for 6 hours following instillation.

Treating and Preventing Hypoxemia

You normally treat suspected or documented hypoxemia by administering oxygen. You should suspect hypoxemia whenever a patient exhibits one or more of the following signs or symptoms:

- Tachypnea
- Tachycardia
- Dyspnea
- Cyanosis
- Paleness
- Hypertension; peripheral vasoconstriction
- Restlessness
- Disorientation/confusion
- Headache
- Somnolence

You should also suspect hypoxemia in cases in which poor oxygenation is common, such as in postoperative patients and those suffering from carbon monoxide poisoning, cyanide poisoning, shock, trauma, or acute myocardial infarction. Documented hypoxemia exists regardless of condition when a patient's PaO_2 is less than 60 torr or the arterial saturation is less than 90% on room air.

In the presence of hypoxemia caused by shunting, oxygen therapy alone is of little value. You know that hypoxemia is due to shunting when the ratio of PaO_2 to FIO_2 (P/F ratio) drops below 300, equivalent to a PaO_2 of less than 300 torr on 100% O_2 (an indicator of acute lung injury). Shunting and hypoxemia are *severe* either when the P/F ratio falls below 200 (an indicator of ARDS) or you cannot maintain satisfactory arterial oxygenation on 50% or more oxygen (i.e., a $PaO_2 \leq 50$ torr or $FIO_2 \geq 0.50$). In these cases, the recommended treatment is normally CPAP or PEEP, as previously discussed. An additional method that can help raise the PaO_2 in patients suffering from refractory hypoxemia is to use patient positioning to decrease shunting.

As a respiratory therapist, many of the procedures you perform can cause or worsen hypoxemia. For this reason you are also responsible for preventing or minimizing hypoxemia associated with these procedures.

Administer Oxygen

The accompanying box outlines the basic procedure for administering oxygen.

Oxygen Therapy Procedure

Equipment and Patient Preparation

1. Verify, interpret, and evaluate doctor's order or protocol

2. Scan chart for diagnosis and any other pertinent data and notes

3. Select, gather, assemble, and check the required equipment, including the appropriate oxygen administration device

---

(continues)

4. Decontaminate hands and applies standard/transmission-based precautions as appropriate

5. Identify patient, introduce self and department

6. Explain/demonstrate procedure and confirm patient understanding, including the safety considerations regarding smoking/electrical devices

Assessment and Implementation

7. Assess the patient before beginning therapy (vital signs, color; presence of dyspnea, SpO_2)

8. Assemble the equipment as required

9. Initiate flow and apply the device to the patient

10. Confirm fit and verify patient comfort

11. Titrate flow/FIO_2 to assure adequate oxygenation/patient comfort

12. Reassess the patient after 5–10 min

13. Readjust flow/FIO_2 as needed

Follow-Up

14. Dispose of infectious waste, process contaminated equipment, and decontaminate hands

15. Record pertinent data in chart and departmental records

16. Notify appropriate personnel and make needed recommendations or modifications to the patient care plan

Adapted from: Scanlan, C. L., West, G. A., von der Heydt, P. A., & Dolan, G. K. (1984). *Respiratory therapy competency evaluation manual.* Boston: Blackwell Scientific.

When scanning the patient chart, you should look for any information that cautions against administering too much oxygen. Specifically, look for adult patients with chronic hypercapnia or newborn infants with birth weights of less than 1500 g or gestational ages less than 32 weeks. In patients with chronic hypercapnia, PaO_2s greater than 60 torr can cause ventilatory depression. In low birth weight or preterm infants, PaO_2s greater than 80 torr are associated with retinopathy of prematurity (ROP) and may contribute to development of bronchopulmonary dysplasia. In neither case, however, should you withhold supplemental oxygen if the patent needs it.

Chapter 6 provides details on the selection and troubleshooting of oxygen therapy equipment. In terms of titrating O_2 therapy, the following guidelines apply:

- In otherwise normal patients, adjust the flow/FIO_2 to the lowest level needed to maintain normal oxygenation (i.e., a PaO_2 of 80–100 torr with a saturation $\geq$ 95%).
- If you cannot maintain normal oxygenation on less than 50% oxygen, accept a PaO_2 greater than or equal to 55–60 torr with a SaO_2/SpO_2 greater than or equal to 88%.
- When treating patients with carbon monoxide poisoning, cyanide poisoning, acute pulmonary edema, shock, trauma, or acute myocardial infarction in emergency settings, provide the highest possible FIO_2.
- For patients with chronic hypercapnia, aim to keep the $PaCO_2$ in the 55–60 torr range to prevent depression of ventilation.
- In low birth weight or preterm infants at risk for ROP, your goal should be a PaO_2 in the 50–70 torr range.

Position Patient to Minimize Hypoxemia

Patient positioning can be used to alter the distribution of ventilation and perfusion and thereby improve oxygenation without raising the FIO_2. Patient positioning may also decrease the incidence of pneumonia in certain patients. Positioning techniques you need to be familiar with and their appropriate use are described in **Table 12-12**.

Table 12-12   Patient Positioning Techniques to Minimize Hypoxemia

Position	Use/Recommend	Comments
Semi-Fowler's position (head of the bed elevated ≥ 30°)	To minimize ventilator-associated pneumonia in patients receiving mechanical ventilation	• Use on all ventilator patients unless contraindicated • Helps prevent aspiration • Improves the distribution of ventilation • Enhances diaphragmatic action
Lateral rotation therapy	To prevent or minimize respiratory complications associated with immobility in bedridden patients	• Employs a bed or air mattress system that automatically turns the patient from side to side • Improve drainage of secretions within the lung and lower airways • Increases the FRC (by increasing the critical opening pressure to the independent lung) • Reduces risk of venous thrombosis and pulmonary embolism
"Keeping the good lung down"	To improve oxygenation in patients with unilateral lung disease	• Patient positioned in the left or right lateral decubitus position with the good lung down • Improves oxygenation by diverting most blood flow and ventilation to the dependent (good) lung • Exceptions in which the good lung is kept up include (1) lung abscess or bleeding and (2) unilateral pulmonary interstitial emphysema in infants
Prone positioning	To improve oxygenation in patients with ARDS and refractory hypoxemia	• Improves oxygenation by shifting blood flow to regions of the lung that are better aerated; may also improve diaphragmatic action • Facilitated by devices that support the chest and pelvis, leaving the abdomen freely suspended • Trial of "proning" recommended in ARDS patients if oxygenation inadequate on $F_{IO_2} \geq 0.6$ and PEEP $\geq$ 10 cm H_2O • Not all patients benefit; a significant increase in Pa_{O_2} (> 10 torr) in first 30 min is a good indicator of success (if tolerated) • Not recommended for patients whose heads cannot be supported in a face-down position or for those who have circulatory problems, a fractured pelvis, or are morbidly obese • Major risks include extubation, dislodgement of intravascular catheters, and impaired access to the airway for nursing and respiratory care

Prevent Procedure-Associated Hypoxemia

Hypoxemia is a complication associated with many procedures you perform, including postural drainage, suctioning, and exercise testing. In addition, in patients being treated for acute lung injury or ARDS, hypoxemia can occur whenever the patient is removed from CPAP/PEEP.

The first rule in preventing this type of hypoxemia is to assure that the patient is adequately oxygenated before implementing the procedure. For this reason, you should always monitor the patient's SpO$_2$ with a pulse oximeter prior to, during, and after any procedure that can cause hypoxemia. If the SpO$_2$ is less than 90% at the start of a procedure likely to cause hypoxemia, it's usually best to postpone implementation until the matter is discussed with the patient's physician. If a patient develops mild hypoxemia during a procedure, you should increase the FIO$_2$. If, however, a patient develops moderate to severe hypoxemia during a procedure, you should immediately stop what you are doing and provide the patient with as high an FIO$_2$ as possible.

Suctioning is a special case, because it involves both removal of oxygen and reduction of lung volume. For this reason, you should hyperoxygenate and hyperinflate the patient for at least 1 minute before suctioning and limit suction time to no more than 10–15 seconds (shorter in infants and children). Upon completion of suctioning, many clinicians recommend a recruitment maneuver to restore the patient's lung volume (discussed subsequently).

Patients receiving ventilatory support, especially with CPAP/PEEP, require additional consideration when being suctioned. First, if available, always use the "one-button" hyperoxygenation maneuver provided on most ICU ventilators. This method typically provides 100% O$_2$ for 1–2 minutes without loss of CPAP/PEEP and is always preferable to taking the patient off the ventilator. Second, you also should consider using a closed catheter suction system, especially in patients with preexisting hypoxemia. This allows you to suction patients while they are still receiving ventilatory support, including CPAP/PEEP. An alternative is to use a special swivel adapter that provides a self-sealing port through which you can pass a standard suction catheter (or bronchoscope) while the patient is still on the ventilator.

Of special concern are patients receiving low tidal volumes to protect against ventilator-associated lung injury—i.e., those being managed via the ARDS protocol previously discussed. These patients are particularly prone to loss of lung volume, due to either suctioning or being taken off the ventilator for even a short period. In these cases, you need to restore the patient's lung volume to a level consistent with efficient mechanics—i.e., on the steeper portion of the pressure-volume curve.

The method by which you restore lung volume is called a recruitment maneuver. The most widely used recruitment maneuver involves applying a high level of PEEP for a set period of time. To implement this maneuver, you:

1. Ensure hemodynamic stability
2. Set the FIO$_2$ to 1.0
3. Wait 10 minutes
4. Apply 30 cm H$_2$O PEEP (or 10 cm H$_2$O above the plateau pressure)
5. Maintain the SAA pressure for 30–45 seconds
6. Return the ventilation settings to previous levels

You will know that the recruitment is successful if the patient's oxygenation is restored or improved and the compliance increased.

COMMON ERRORS TO AVOID

You can improve your score by avoiding these mistakes:

- Never use or recommend incentive spirometry for patients who cannot cooperate.
- Never administer IPPB to a patient with an untreated tension pneumothorax.
- Never use or recommend noninvasive positive pressure ventilation (NPPV) for patients who do not have control over upper airway function or cannot manage their secretions.
- Whenever possible, avoid plateau pressures above 30 cm H$_2$O during mechanical ventilation.

- Do not use or recommend high-frequency oscillation ventilation for patients with obstructive lung disease.
- Never administer a mucokinetic agent without also providing appropriate bronchial hygiene measures to facilitate secretion removal.
- Do not use or recommend mast cell stabilizers (cromolyn sodium, nedocromil) for acute bronchospasm.
- Never mix Tobramycin (Tobi) with other drugs for inhalation.
- Avoid suctioning (if possible) for 6 hours following surfactant instillation.
- Never withhold supplemental oxygen from a patient who needs it.

SURE BETS

In some situations you can be sure of the right approach to a clinical problem or scenario:

- To confirm patient understanding of muscle training, incentive spirometry, or IPPB, always require a "return demonstration" of the procedure by the patient.
- To prevent hyperventilation during IPPB, always instruct the patient to avoid forceful exhalation and to breathe slowly.
- When initiating mechanical ventilation, always use a high FIO_2 (0.60–0.90) until an ABG can be obtained.
- Except with ARDS patients, when initiating mechanical ventilation, set the initial VT to 8–10 mL/kg PBW when targeting volume or set the pressure limit to 20–30 cm H_2O when targeting pressure.
- To adjust a patient's $PaCO_2$/pH during mechanical ventilation, always change the rate first; change the VT/pressure limit only if rate changes exceed the recommended adult limits (8–24 breaths/min) or if you do not achieve the desired results.
- Unless contraindicated, always use an oronasal/"full" face mask when initiating NPPV on patients with acute respiratory failure.
- To avoid esophageal opening/gastric distention, always keep IPAP levels during NPPV below 20–25 cm H_2O.
- Whenever a patient's cardiac output or blood pressure falls when raising the PEEP level, decrease PEEP back to its prior setting.
- Always give the bronchodilator first when ordered in combination with a mucokinetic or anti-infective agent.
- To prevent pharyngitis and oral candidiasis with inhaled steroids, always have patients rinse their mouth out after administration.
- When treating patients with carbon monoxide poisoning, cyanide poisoning, acute pulmonary edema, shock, trauma, or acute myocardial infarction in emergency settings, always provide the highest possible FIO_2.

PRE-TEST ANSWERS AND EXPLANATIONS

Below are this chapter's pre-test answers and explanations. Be sure to review each answer's explanation thoroughly to help you understand why it is correct. If the explanation is still unclear to you, review the chapter contents or the references and/or refer to this chapter's supplemental resources on the CD.

12-1. **Correct answer: C.** Increase the oxygen concentration immediately before suctioning. Most cardiac arrhythmias during suctioning are due to arterial hypoxemia. The best way to prevent or minimize arterial hypoxemia during suctioning is to preoxygenate the patient for 1–2 minutes prior to beginning the procedure. You should also keep suction time below 10–15 seconds.

12-2. **Correct answer: B.** Put the patient in the prone position. In patients with a generalized decrease in lung volume (as in ARDS), use of the prone position can improve oxygenation. The prone position probably shifts blood flow to regions of the lung that are less severely injured and thus better aerated.

With the proper equipment, "proning" may also allow the abdomen to expand more and facilitates better movement of the diaphragm. The prone position also may decrease the likelihood of further lung injury associated with positive pressure ventilation of patients with ARDS.

12-3. **Correct answer: C.** At least 30% of the maximum inspiratory pressure (MIP/PImax). For inspiratory training to be effective, the load against which the patient breathes must be sufficient to increase muscle strength. The minimal resistance load to achieve this end is an inspiratory pressure that is at least 30% of the MIP/PImax.

12-4. **Correct answer: B.** Exhale slowly. Patients with severe emphysema tend to have highly compliant (floppy) airways. As a result, to help prevent airway collapsing and air trapping, they should be instructed to exhale slowly, perhaps through pursed lips.

12-5. **Correct answer: D.** I, II, and III. IPPB can impede venous return to the heart by increasing intrathoracic pressures. Patients with poor venomotor tone or those who are already hypotensive due to conditions such as shock or cardiac insufficiency are particularly prone to this effect. For this reason, you should assess the patient's cardiovascular status before administering IPPB and monitor high-risk patients during treatment.

12-6. **Correct answer: A.** I or II only. The mode of ventilatory support initially chosen depends mainly upon the patient's underlying pathophysiologic problem. When a patient's respiratory failure is associated with hypercapnea due to inadequate alveolar ventilation—as in this case—either the CMV or IMV modes (with equivalent rate settings) may be employed.

12-7. **Correct answer: D.** Decreasing the bias flow. Increasing the HFOV power/amplitude is usually the first step to increase CO_2 elimination/lower the $Paco_2$. *Decreasing* the frequency can also lower the $Paco_2$ (note that frequency changes during HFOV affect CO_2 elimination in a manner opposite to that observed during conventional mechanical ventilation). If hypercapnia is severe despite use of the maximum power/amplitude and lowest frequency settings, you can also consider creating a cuff leak to enhance CO_2 removal. Decreasing the bias flow tends to lower the Pmean and negatively affect oxygenation.

12-8. **Correct answer: D.** Mask continuous positive airway pressure (CPAP) with 80% O_2. A patient with congestive heart failure who is coughing up pink, frothy sputum is likely suffering from acute cardiogenic pulmonary edema. The blood gas indicates a fully compensated respiratory alkalosis secondary to severe hypoxemia (due to the pulmonary edema). The goal is to restore adequate oxygenation and maintain alveolar inflation. High concentrations of oxygen combined with noninvasive positive pressure (mask CPAP or BiPAP™) are generally indicated in such instances. The positive pressure (1) helps keep alveoli open, (2) reduces venous return to the right heart, and (3) lowers pulmonary vascular pressures. This, in turn, decreases fluid movement into the interstitial space and alveoli and improves oxygenation.

12-9. **Correct answer: D.** Endotracheal tube. Some medications can be delivered via endotracheal tube. Cardiovascular medications, lidocaine, epinephrine, atropine, and nalaxone can be delivered via endotracheal tube safely.

12-10. **Correct answer: C.** Change to the IMV mode with a set rate of 10 breaths/min. The blood gas indicates a partially compensated respiratory alkalosis, most likely the result of the patient initiating 10 machine breaths above the set rate. By changing to a mode of IMV, the spontaneously initiated breaths will not be delivered at the set tidal volume, but rather the patient will receive only what he or she can draw from the circuit on such breaths. As a result, the patient's minute ventilation will be reduced.

12-11. **Correct answer: C.** Add pressure support. The key problem is the patient's rapid spontaneous rate and low spontaneous tidal volume. The spontaneous tidal volume = [total minute vol − set min vol]/[total rate − set rate] = [10,000 − 6,000]/[38 − 10] = 4,000/28 = 142 mL. To increase the spontaneous

VT, you should add pressure support. This will increase the efficiency of spontaneous ventilation and allow for a lower spontaneous rate of breathing. In fact, you can judge the effect of pressure support by the resulting decrease in rate. A good rule of thumb is to provide sufficient pressure support to assure a spontaneous rate.

12-12. **Correct answer: C.** Increase PEEP. The goal of PEEP is to achieve adequate oxygenation with a safe F_{IO_2}. In this case, the F_{IO_2} is dangerously high, but shunting persists. Given the Pa_{O_2} of 55 torr, following the 60/60 rule, the PEEP should be increased.

12-13. **Correct answer: C.** The patients should hold a maximum inspiratory capacity (IC) breath for at least 5 seconds. The "sustained maximum inspiration" underlying incentive spirometry is essentially an inspiratory capacity maneuver (IC), followed by a breath hold (10 seconds is ideal).

12-14. **Correct answer: B.** Putting the patient in the prone position. In patients with a generalized decrease in lung volume (as in ARDS), use of the prone position can improve oxygenation. The prone position probably shifts blood flow to regions of the lung that are less severely injured and thus better aerated. With the proper equipment, "proning" may also allow the abdomen to expand more and facilitates better movement of the diaphragm. The prone position may also decrease the likelihood of further lung injury associated with positive pressure ventilation of patients with ARDS.

12-15. **Correct answer: A.** Nonrebreathing mask at 15 L/min. When treating patients with carbon monoxide poisoning, cyanide poisoning, acute pulmonary edema, shock, trauma, or acute myocardial infarction in emergency settings, always provide the highest possible F_{IO_2}. Of the devices listed, only the nonrebreathing mask can deliver high F_{IO_2}s. You might also recommend CPAP with 100% O_2 for this patient, since the elevated airway pressure can help reduce venous return and alleviate pulmonary congestion.

12-16. **Correct answer: C.** Increasing EPAP to 10 cm H_2O. This patient's hypoxemia is due to shunting ($Pa_{O_2} \leq 50$ torr, $F_{IO_2} \geq 0.50$). If shunting is present when administering NPPV for acute respiratory failure, you should increase the EPAP level, while being sure to keep ΔP (IPAP − EPAP) ≥ 5 cm H_2O.

12-17. **Correct answer: C.** Substituting budesonide (Pulmicort) for the isoetharine. This patient is exhibiting undesired cardiovascular and CNS effects associated with isoetharine's moderate $beta_2$ adrenergic action. To help avoid these effects, you should generally select or recommend those agents with the least $beta_1$ and most $beta_2$ effect—e.g., albuterol or its isomer, levalbuterol. Alternatively, if cardiovascular/CNS effects are pronounced, you can recommend decreasing the dose of the drug. Substituting budesonide for the isoetharine makes no sense since budesonide is a steroid controller, not reliever.

12-18. **Correct answer: B.** 30 cm H_2O plateau pressure. According to the NHLBI protocol, the target volume for ARDS patients is 4–6 mL/kg, with a maximum plateau (alveolar) pressure of 30 cm H_2O. The ventilator rate should initially be set to match the prior $\dot{V}_E$ but can be increased as needed up to a maximum of 35 breaths/min.

12-19. **Correct answer: D.** Increasing the SIMV rate. The blood gas indicates uncompensated respiratory acidosis. As a result, the patient's minute ventilation should be increased by increasing the SIMV rate.

12-20. **Correct answer: B.** Ending the trial and returning the patient to a full ventilatory support mode. Objective physiologic measures indicating a successful SBT include acceptable gas exchange, and stable hemodynamics and ventilatory pattern. In addition, the patient should *not* exhibit any subjective indicators of intolerance or failure. In this case the rise in Pa_{CO_2} exceeds the limit (10 torr) for acceptable gas exchange, the increased rate of breathing indicates an unstable ventilatory pattern, and the greater accessory muscle use suggests intolerance of the procedure. For these reasons, you should return the patient to a level of ventilatory support that maintains adequate oxygenation and ventilation while also preventing muscle fatigue—i.e., usually a full ventilatory support mode.

POST-TEST

A post-test for this chapter that includes automated scoring and feedback is available on the accompanying CD. Be sure to complete this additional assessment to confirm your mastery of this chapter's objectives.

REFERENCES

American Association for Respiratory Care. (1991). Clinical practice guideline. Incentive spirometry. *Respiratory care, 36,* 1402–1405.

American Association for Respiratory Care. (1996). Clinical practice guideline. Selection of a device for delivery of aerosol to the lung parenchyma. *Respiratory care, 41,* 647–653.

American Association for Respiratory Care. (2002). Clinical practice guideline. Evidence-based guidelines for weaning and discontinuing ventilatory support. *Respiratory care, 47,* 69–90.

American Association for Respiratory Care. (2002). Clinical practice guideline. Oxygen therapy for adults in the acute care facility. 2002 revision and update. *Respiratory care, 47,* 717–720.

American Association for Respiratory Care, Protocol Committee; Subcommittee Adult Critical Care. (2003). *Adult respiratory ventilator protocol* (Version 1.0a).

American Association for Respiratory Care. (2003). Clinical practice guideline. Intermittent positive pressure breathing: 2003 revision and update. *Respiratory care, 48,* 540–546.

American Association for Respiratory Care. (2004). Clinical practice guideline. Application of continuous positive airway pressure to neonates via nasal prongs, nasopharyngeal tube, or nasal mask: 2004 revision and update. *Respiratory care, 49,* 1100–1108.

Butler, T. J., Close, J. R., & Close, R. J. (1998). *Laboratory exercises for competency in respiratory care.* Philadelphia: FA Davis.

Gardenhire, D. S. (2008). *Rau's respiratory care pharmacology.* St. Louis: Mosby Elsevier.

Garner, J. S., & the Hospital Infection Control Practices Advisory Committee. (1996). Guideline for isolation precautions in hospitals. *Infectious control and hospital epidemiology, 17,* 53–80.

Hodgkin, J. E., Celli, B. R., & Connors, G. (2000). *Pulmonary rehabilitation* (3rd ed.). Baltimore: Lippincott Williams and Wilkins.

National Heart, Lung and Blood Institute & ARDS Clinical Network. (2005). Mechanical ventilation protocol summary.

Pilbeam, S. P. (1998). *Mechanical ventilation.* St. Louis: Mosby.

Scanlan, C. L., West, G. A., von der Heydt, P. A., & Dolan, G. K. (1984). *Respiratory therapy competency evaluation manual.* Boston: Blackwell Scientific.

Weiner, P., & McConnell, A. (2005). Respiratory muscle training in chronic obstructive pulmonary disease: Inspiratory, expiratory, or both? *Current opinions in pulmonary medicine, 11,* 140–144.

Evaluate and Monitor Patient's Objective and Subjective Responses to Respiratory Care

CHAPTER

13

Narciso E. Rodriguez

INTRODUCTION

This chapter covers basic noninvasive and invasive procedures, as well as assessment techniques the NBRC expects you to apply when evaluating a patient's response to therapy. These techniques also provide the foundation for you to independently modify therapeutic procedures (Chapter 14), recommend modifications in the care plan (Chapter 15), and determine the appropriateness of therapy (Chapter 16). Heavy emphasis in this section should be given to high-level mastery of this content, since 80% of the CRT exam questions will involve either application or analysis.

OBJECTIVES

After completion of this chapter, you should demonstrate the knowledge needed to:

1. Recommend and review chest radiographs
2. Evaluate and monitor patient's response to therapy based on:
   a. Sputum assessment
   b. Chest radiograph
   c. Breath sounds
   d. Vital signs
   e. Cardiac rhythm
   f. Fluid balance
   g. Pulmonary function testing
   h. Laboratory blood tests results
3. Assess proper gas exchange by any of the following procedures:
   a. Blood gas puncture and analysis
   b. Pulse oximetry
   c. CO-oximetry
   d. Capnography
   e. Transcutaneous monitoring
   f. Capillary blood gas puncture
   g. Hemodynamics
4. Assess and monitor patient-ventilator interface, including integrity of artificial airways
5. Measure pulmonary compliance, measure airway resistance, and interpret normal airway graphics
6. Measure F_{IO_2} and/or liter flow

WHAT TO EXPECT ON THIS CATEGORY OF THE CRT EXAM

Number of questions: 15
Level of questions: about 20% recall, 50% application, 30% analysis

WHAT'S NEW FOR 2009

As of July 2009, this section of the NBRC CRT examination includes the following *new content areas*:

- Obtain a blood gas sample from arterialized capillary blood
- Perform:
  - Transcutaneous monitoring
  - Hemodynamic assessment
- Interpret results of:
  - Hemodynamics
  - Pulse oximetry
- Measure and record vital signs, monitor cardiac rhythm, and evaluate fluid balance (intake and output)
- Perform and interpret results of pulmonary function testing:
  - Compliance and airways resistance
  - D_{LCO}
  - Exercise
  - Bronchoprovocation studies
- Recommend blood tests (e.g., hemoglobin, potassium)

PRE-TEST

Carefully respond to each of the following questions. After completing the pre-test, compare your answers to those provided at the end of this chapter. Then thoroughly review each answer's explanation to help understand why it is correct.

13-1. The ER physician asks you to review a chest radiograph from a patient with history of severe emphysema. Which of the following findings would you expect to observe on this film?
 I. A wide mediastinum
 II. An increase in peripheral vascular markings
 III. Lowered, flattened diaphragm
 IV. An increased radiolucency in the lung fields
 V. Presence of bullae and blebs
 A. II and III only
 B. III, IV, and V
 C. II, III, and V
 D. I, II, III, IV, and V

13-2. When using a pulse oximetry device, the most common source of error and false alarms is:
 A. Patient motion artifact
 B. Presence of HbCO
 C. Presence of vascular dyes
 D. Ambient light detection

13-3. A patient receiving mechanical ventilation in the CMV control mode is making asynchronous breathing efforts against the ventilator's controlled breaths. This will result in:
 A. Decreased ventilatory drive
 B. Increased physiologic deadspace
 C. Increased work of breathing
 D. Acute metabolic acidosis

13-4. A patient on a 30% aerosol oxygen mask has the following arterial blood gas results:

pH	7.54
$Paco_2$	27 torr
Pao_2	80 torr
HCO_3	23 mEq/L
BE	−2 mEq/L

Which of the following is the correct interpretation of the arterial blood gas?
 A. Acute alveolar hyperventilation without hypoxemia

B. Partially compensated respiratory alkalosis

C. Respiratory acidemia with hypoxemia

D. Hypochloremic metabolic alkalosis

13-5. You find a patient receiving SIMV with a preset rate of 6 breaths/min, a V_T of 1000 mL, and a PEEP of 10 cm H_2O. You note a peak inspiratory pressure of 50 cm H_2O for each SIMV mechanical breath. Which of the following alarm settings are appropriate for this patient?

    I. Low exhaled minute ventilation at 8 L/min

    II. Inspiratory:expiratory (I:E) ratio alarm at 1:1

    III. High inspiratory pressure limit at 65 cm H_2O

    IV. Low PEEP/CPAP pressure alarm at 5 cm H_2O

A. I, II, and III only

B. II and III only

C. II, III, and IV only

D. III and IV only

13-6. Arterial hemoglobin saturation (%HbO$_2$) should be kept above what level in order to guarantee adequate oxygen delivery to the tissues?

A. 65%

B. 70%

C. 75%

D. 90%

13-7. A new medical resident asks for your help in calculating the static lung compliance for an ICU patient receiving volume-cycled ventilation. The patient has the following settings and monitoring data:

V_T	700 mL
Rate	12/min
Peak pressure	50 cm H_2O
Plateau pressure	30 cm H_2O
PEEP	10 cm H_2O
Mechanical deadspace	100 mL

The patient's static lung compliance is:

A. 18 mL/cm H_2O

B. 35 mL/cm H_2O

C. 22 mL/cm H_2O

D. 26 mL/cm H_2O

13-8. A doctor wants your recommendation on how to monitor the cardiopulmonary status of a patient undergoing a bronchoscopy procedure during moderate sedation. You should recommend the following:

A. Pulmonary function testing

B. Noninvasive pulse oximetry

C. Frequent ABGs via radial puncture

D. Transcutaneous Pao_2 monitoring

13-9. A patient is receiving continuous mandatory ventilation (CMV) in the control mode at a rate of 12 breaths/min. The percent inspiratory time (%I-time) is set at 20%. What is the patient's inspiratory time?

A. 0.75 sec

B. 1.00 sec

C. 1.25 sec

D. 1.50 sec

13-10. A mechanically ventilated patient is being monitored by a capnograph in the ICU. The nurse calls you STAT to the room and you note that the P_{ETCO_2} dropped suddenly from 36 to 0 torr. All of the following are possible causes of this finding *except*:

A. Ventilator disconnection

B. Increased cardiac output

C. Obstructed artificial airway

D. Cardiac arrest

13-11. During a patient-ventilator system check you notice the following airway pressures on an adult mechanically ventilated patient receiving 5 cm H_2O of PEEP:

	Time		
Measure	**0400**	**0500**	**0600**
Peak pressure (cm H_2O)	42	47	53
Plateau pressure (cm H_2O)	32	36	42

Knowing that no ventilator setting changes have been made, what is the most likely cause of these changes?

A. The patient is developing bronchospasm

B. The patient's lungs are becoming more compliant

C. The patient is performing a Valsalva maneuver

D. The patient is developing atelectasis

13-12. Common arterial sites used for percutaneous arterial blood sampling include all of the following *except*:
A. Carotid
B. Radial
C. Brachial
D. Femoral

13-13. On reviewing the blood gas report on a patient, you note a $Paco_2$ of 25 torr, a base excess (BE) of –10 mEq/L, and a pH of 7.35. You would characterize this acid-based abnormality as:
A. Compensated metabolic acidosis
B. Acute (uncompensated) metabolic acidosis
C. Compensated respiratory alkalosis
D. Acute (uncompensated) respiratory alkalosis

13-14. A first-year resident has just inserted an indwelling arterial catheter in an ICU patient. A good indication that the catheter has been successfully inserted in an artery is:
A. A positive Allen test
B. A good blood return
C. Ability to flush the line
D. Proper blood pressure and waveform

13-15. A sample obtained from the distal port of a pulmonary artery catheter has a Po_2 of 95 torr and an Hb oxygen saturation of 97%. Which of the following statements could explain these results?
I. The catheter balloon remained inflated during sampling
II. The catheter is misplaced in the right ventricle
III. The blood sample was withdrawn too quickly
IV. The patient has an abnormally low cardiac output
A. I, II, and IV
B. II, III, and IV
C. I and III only
D. I, II, and III

13-16. You need to provide continuous monitoring of the Fio_2 for a ventilator that uses a heated humidifier delivery system. The only analyzer available is a galvanic cell analyzer. Where should you place the analyzer's sensor?
A. Distal to the heated humidifier
B. On the expiratory side of the circuit
C. Proximal to the heated humidifier
D. As close to the patient as possible

13-17. All of the following statements regarding a capillary blood gas sample are true, *except*:
A. It should not be performed to assess oxygenation status
B. It should not be performed in infants less than 72 hrs old
C. It should not be performed in swollen or edematous tissue
D. It should not be performed in the posterior curvature of the heel

13-18. After performing a modified Allen test on the left hand of a patient, you note that his palm and fingers do not become pink for more than 15 seconds after releasing pressure on the ulnar artery. At this point you should:
A. Use the left brachial site for sampling
B. Repeat the test on the right hand
C. Use the femoral site for sampling
D. Go ahead and draw the sample from that site

13-19. A 20-year-old 65-kg (143-lb.) patient is receiving volume-oriented SIMV with a set rate of 14 breaths/min, a total rate of 14 breaths/min, a V_T of 500 mL, and an Fio_2 of 0.50. Blood gas results are as follows:

pH	7.52
$Paco_2$	26 torr
HCO_3	23 mEq/L
Pao_2	94 torr

What are the appropriate recommendations for you to make?
A. Decrease the SIMV rate
B. Add mechanical deadspace
C. Decrease the Fio_2
D. Add pressure support

13-20. You observe a sudden drop in the peak inspiratory pressure when monitoring a patient on volume-targeted ventilation. Which of the following may explain this change?
  I. A defective exhalation valve
  II. A burst endotracheal tube cuff
  III. A high V_T setting
  IV. Patient disconnection
  A. II and IV only
  B. III only
  C. I, II, and IV
  D. II, III, and IV

13-21. The ER physician asks you to evaluate a trauma patient who was the victim of a house fire. In order to properly evaluate the cardiopulmonary status of this patient you should perform all of the following procedures *except*:
  A. Auscultation of breath sounds
  B. Pulse oximetry
  C. Assessment of sensorium
  D. Rate, depth, and pattern of breathing

13-22. During the assessment of a mechanically ventilated patient in the ICU you notice the following vital signs:

Heart rate	118/min
BP	135/90
Set resp rate	8/min
Total resp rate	35/min
Temp	99.3°F

A surgical resident has just inserted a right pleural chest tube to drain a significant pleural effusion. At this point you should recommend that the resident:
  A. Paralyze the patient
  B. Reposition the chest tube
  C. Ask the patient to relax
  D. Assess for pain

13-23. A patient with a size 8 tracheostomy tube is being suctioned by the nurse. While suctioning the patient you observe several PVCs on the patient's monitor. You should recommend that the nurse:
  A. Use a larger suction catheter
  B. Preoxygenate the patient with 100% O_2
  C. Sedate the patient prior to suction
  D. Suction less often

13-24. A pulmonologist asks you to assess airway responsiveness during a pulmonary function exam. He wants to rule out asthma from chronic bronchitis in a patient complaining of nocturnal wheezing. You should consider all of the following tests *except*:
  A. Thoracic gas volume
  B. Graded exercise test
  C. Histamine challenge test
  D. Methacholine bronchoprovocation test

13-25. Which of the following tests should you recommend for a patient with suspected hepatitis and history of alcohol and drug abuse?
  A. Cardiac enzymes
  B. Complete blood count
  C. Liver enzymes
  D. Partial prothrombin time

WHAT YOU NEED TO KNOW: ESSENTIAL CONTENT

Recommend and Review Chest Radiographs

Chest X-rays are used to evaluate the lungs and thoracic structures. You should recommend a chest X-ray to locate lines, catheters, and tube positions; assess disease progression; and identify any pathologic lung or chest abnormalities. On the NBRC exam, X-ray findings generally will be described to you in words, not pictures. For this reason, you must familiarize yourself with the narrative descriptions of the most common normal and abnormal X-ray findings, as delineated in **Table 13-1**.

Table 13-1 Common Chest X-Ray Findings in Adults

Condition	Radiograph Findings
Abnormalities of the chest wall	• Broken ribs: consider flail chest • Kyphoscoliosis: causes lung restriction and decreases lung volumes
Acute respiratory distress syndrome (ARDS)	• Nonhomogeneous bilateral lung opacities (white-out) and infiltrates with normal heart size consistent with pulmonary edema
Airway complications	• Right or left mainstem intubation: causes the opposite lung to collapse and white out • Tracheal narrowing (tracheal stenosis) and tracheal dilation (tracheomalacia) • Tracheal edema and inflammation: croup ("steeple sign") and epiglottis ("thumb sign" on lateral neck X-ray) • Mucous plugs: cause the affected lung or lobe to collapse
Atelectasis: the collapse or loss of lung volume	• Increased radiopacity (whiteness) in the film • Air bronchograms due to tissue collapse • Elevated hemi-diaphragm on the affected side • Shift of trachea and mediastinum toward the affected side • Ribs closer together • Hyperaeration of the adjacent lung
Consolidation or infiltration: replacement of alveolar air by fluid, cells, or tissue	• Air bronchograms: airways silhouette surrounded by collapsed tissue • Increased radiopacity (whiteness) of the affected area
Congestive heart failure (CHF)	• Increased vascular markings • Cardiomegaly: increased heart size (cardio-thoracic ratio > 50%) • Kerley's B lines: engorged lymphatic vessels originating at the pleura extending into the lung parenchyma 1–2 cm • Presence of pleura effusions
Emphysema (COPD)	• Lowered, flattened diaphragms • Decreased lung markings (hyperaeration) • Increased retrosternal air space (lateral chest film) • Presence of bullae/blebs: pockets of air in the lung parenchyma • Narrow mediastinum
Pleura effusions: abnormal collection of fluid in the potential space between the parietal and visceral pleura	• Homogeneous areas of increased density that are position dependent, confirmed by a lateral decubitus chest X-ray film • Loss of sharp costo-phrenic angles • Location varies with patient position • Presence of a meniscus at the fluid surface
Pneumothorax: the presence of air in the thoracic cavity, usually in the pleural space	• Better identified in an expiratory film • Loss of peripheral lung markings • Air between the lung margin and chest wall (radiolucent space) • Mediastinal shift to the opposite side • The diaphragm may be depressed on the affected side
Pulmonary edema: abnormal accumulation of fluid in the interstitial space of the lung	• Fluffy or patchy densities in the perihilar areas and in the gravity-dependent lower lung fields • It may be accompanied by cardiomegaly, pleural effusions, and bronchograms

The chest X-ray is also the most common way to confirm proper placement of an ET or tracheostomy tube in the airway. However, you always should do your best to verify tube placement before a chest X-ray is taken. To do so, verify the presence of bilateral breath sounds and obtain a positive result using a CO_2 colorimetry device (if available). You should subsequently confirm proper ET tube position on the X-ray by locating the tube tip about 4–6 cm above the carina or between T2 and T4. This position minimizes the chances of the tube moving down into the mainstem bronchi (endobronchial intubation) or up into the larynx (extubation).

You also should be able to recommend proper X-ray positions. **Table 13-2** outlines the most common chest radiograph positions with their indications and uses.

Obtain a Blood Gas Sample

By Puncture

You obtain an arterial blood gas sample in order to measure arterial blood gas (ABG) parameters. Measured parameters include pH, $Paco_2$, and Pao_2. Calculated parameters include bicarbonate (HCO_3), base excess (BE), and hemoglobin saturation (Sao_2).

Arterial blood gases are obtained to:

- Evaluate ventilation ($Paco_2$), acid-base (pH and $Paco_2$), and oxygenation (Pao_2 and Sao_2) status, including O_2-carrying capacity (Pao_2, HbO_2, total Hb, and abnormal hemoglobins).
- Monitor and assess the patient's response to therapy and/or diagnostic tests and procedures.
- Monitor severity and progression of a documented disease process.

The radial artery is the preferred site for arterial blood sampling because (1) it is near the skin surface, (2) the ulnar artery provides for collateral circulation, and (3) the artery is not near any large veins. Other sites include the brachial, femoral, and dorsalis pedis arteries. These sites carry greater risk and should be used only by those with the proper training.

Key points in performing arterial puncture for ABG analysis include the following:

- Choose the nondominant hand first.
- Assess collateral circulation on both sides by performing the modified Allen test (**Figure 13-1**). To perform an Allen test:
  - Both the radial and ulnar arteries should be compressed at the same time while the patient clenches the fist for about 5 seconds; repeat 3 times.
  - Release compression on the ulnar artery only. The palmar surface should flush within 5–10 seconds. Prolonged delay before flushing indicates decreased ulnar artery flow.
  - If the radial artery is unsuitable as a puncture site, the other wrist should be assessed.
  - If both radial arteries lack collateral circulation, the brachial artery is the second choice, followed by the femoral artery.

Table 13-2 Common Radiograph Positions

Position	Indications/Uses
Posteroanterior (PA)	• Most commonly used position • Recommended for ambulatory patients • Taken with the patient standing upright during maximum inspiration
Anteroposterior (AP)	• Most commonly used for ICU portable films (nonambulatory patients) • The heart shadow is magnified • Film quality is inferior to PA technique
Lateral	• Indicated for visualization and assessment of the lung bases and lung tissue behind the heart in the posterior mediastinum
Lateral decubitus	• To assess for the presence of "free-fluid" or pleural effusions in the pleura space • To visualize air-fluid interfaces inside the lung

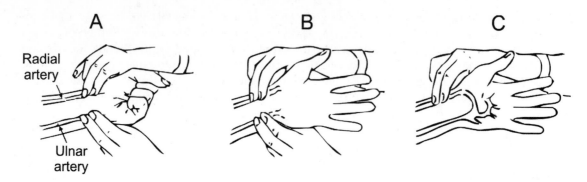

Figure 13-1 Modified Allen's Test. (A) Patient's hand clenched while you obstruct flow to both the radial and ulnar arteries. (B) The patient opens his/her hand while you maintain pressure; the hand should appear blanched. (C) Upon release of pressure on the ulnar artery, color should be restored.

Adapted from: Shapiro, B. A., Harrison, R. A., & Walton, J. R. (1977). *Clinical application of blood gases.* (2nd ed.). Chicago: Year Book Medical.

- After the puncture, the site should be compressed until the bleeding stops. Patients on anticoagulant therapy with a prolonged PT, PTT, or International Normalized Ratio (INR) may require longer compression times.
- After hemostasis is ensured, a sterile bandage should be placed over the puncture site; recheck the site after 20 minutes and document the procedure.
- The specimen should be collected with a glass or plastic syringe (3–10 mL) and should be adequately heparinized with sodium or lithium heparin.
- Air bubbles should be expelled; the needle should be capped via a capping device or using the "scoop method," and the sample should be mixed by rolling syringe for 20 seconds immediately prior to analysis.
- The sample should be stored in ice slush and analyzed within 30–45 minutes unless point-of-care analysis is being used (see Chapter 6).

Large air bubbles in the sample will invalidate the results. For this reason, if a sample contains visible air bubbles, you should discard it and obtain a new, anaerobic sample (see Chapter 8 for common related preanalytical errors). Most common complications of arterial puncture include arteriospasm, air or clotted-blood emboli, patient or sampler contamination, hematoma, hemorrhage, trauma to the vessel, arterial occlusion, infection, vasovagal response, and pain.

From Vascular Lines

Obtaining a Sample from an Arterial Line

If you need to obtain repeated arterial samples over several days, you should recommend placement of an indwelling arterial catheter, or "A-line." In the NBRC hospital you may be responsible for the insertion and care of A-lines. **Figure 13-2** depicts a typical A-line system.

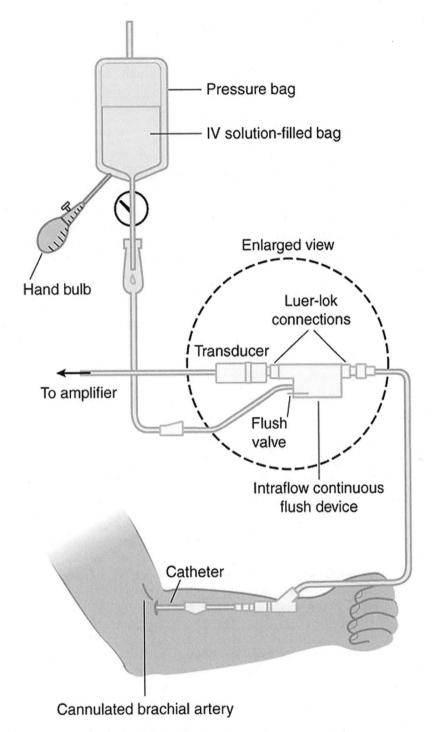

Figure 13-2 Indwelling Arterial Catheter System.

Source: Wilkins, R. L., Stoller, J. K., & Scanlan, C. L. (eds.). (2003). *Egan's fundamentals of respiratory care* (8th ed.). St. Louis: Mosby. Courtesy of Elsevier Ltd.

Insertion of an arterial line is technically difficult. Percutaneous insertion of an arterial catheter requires proper training and equipment preparation. The most common insertion sites are the radial, brachial, and femoral arteries, with the radial artery being the preferred site due to collateral circulation. The accompanying box lists the key steps involved in inserting a percutaneous arterial line.

Percutaneous Arterial Line Insertion Procedure

1. Explain procedure to the patient

2. Set up and prepare monitoring equipment (pressure bag, transducer, pressure line)

3. If using the radial artery, assess for collateral circulation (perform Allen test)

4. Palpate artery to ensure exact location

5. Using aseptic technique, prepare the insertion site by creating a sterile field

6. Use proper personal protection equipment

7. Select a small catheter (22G–23G) for the radial artery and a larger catheter (20G–21G) for large vessels like the femoral and brachial arteries

8. Insert needle and catheter into artery; if using a guide wire technique, advance the wire into the artery and observe for a flash back of blood into the catheter

9. Withdraw needle or guide wire and immediately connect the pressure line to the catheter and flush with a normal saline solution (the use of heparin solutions are *no longer* recommended)

10. Secure catheter in place and tighten all connections

11. Clean site and apply sterile dressing

12. Confirm arterial placement by monitoring pressures and waveform

13. Check for adequacy of distal blood flow

14. Observe for complications

15. Document

Prior to obtaining a sample from an arterial indwelling catheter, the following must be considered:

- The equipment and supplies needed are the same as those needed for an arterial puncture.
- Depending on the line design, a second syringe for disposing deadspace ("waste") blood may be needed.
- To draw the sample, attach the waste syringe to the stopcock port or draw the deadspace blood according to manufacturer's recommendations and line design.
- Position the stopcock so that blood flows into the syringe and the IV bag port is closed (**Figure 13-3**).
- After withdrawing the deadspace blood, attach a new heparinized syringe to the sampling port and allow 2–4 mL of arterial blood to fill the syringe.
- Reposition the stopcock handle to close off the sampling port and open the IV bag port with the flush solution.
- Disconnect the syringe, expel air bubbles from the sample, and cap or plug the syringe.
- Flush the line and stopcock with the IV solution.
- Confirm that the stopcock is open to the IV bag solution and the catheter by confirming an undampened pulse pressure waveform on the monitor graphic display.
- Place the sample in ice unless point-of-care analysis is being used, and properly dispose of waste materials.

Obtaining a Sample from a Pulmonary Artery Catheter

When obtaining a sample from a pulmonary artery (PA) or Swan-Ganz catheter, the following must be considered:

- The sample should be drawn from the catheter's distal port with the catheter's balloon deflated (refer to Chapter 4).

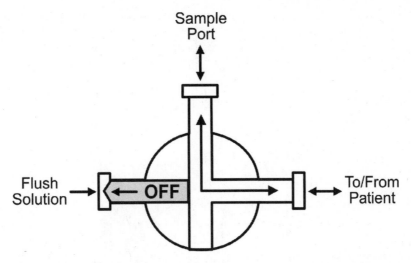

Figure 13-3 Three-Way Stopcock Positioned to Draw a Blood Sample (Off to Flush Solution).

- The sample must be drawn slowly to avoid contamination from the pulmonary capillaries; contamination will result in a falsely high oxygen level!
- Attention must be paid to the IV infusion rate through the catheter to prevent sample dilution.
- When obtaining an admixture of arterial and mixed venous blood for blood gas testing to calculate cardiac output (using the Fick equation), both samples must be drawn at the same time.

Via Capillary Puncture

Capillary blood gas sampling is a very common procedure in infants and toddlers. It is indicated when a blood sample is needed to assess ventilation and acid-base status but arterial access is not available. Capillary blood gas sampling is less invasive, quicker, and easier to perform than arterial puncture. Capillary sampling should NOT be performed:

- When accurate analysis of oxygenation is needed
- In neonates less than 24 hrs old
- Should not be performed through the following sites:
  - Along the posterior curvature of the heel (to avoid bone trauma)
  - On an infant that has just begun walking
  - On the fingers of an infant
  - In an inflamed, swollen, or edematous area
  - In a cyanotic or poorly perfused area

When obtaining a capillary blood gas sample:

- Gather the needed equipment: an appropriate-size lancet, alcohol pad, sterile gauze, adhesive bandage, and pre-heparinized capillary tube with tube caps and a metal "flea" if a delay in analysis is expected.
- Select the site (e.g., heel, great toe, earlobe). When selecting the heel, puncture the lateral sides of the heel only, avoiding the posterior curvature (see **Figure 13-4**).
- Warm the selected site for 5–10 minutes using a warm cloth or disposable warming pack to a temperature not higher than 42–45°C.
- Before performing the procedure, immobilize and secure the puncture area.
- Puncture the skin with the lancet and wipe away the first drop of blood.
- Do not squeeze the site. Always allow for free flow of blood and collect sample from the middle area of the blood drop.
- Fill the tube, place the flea inside if indicated, and cap ends.
- Unless point-of-care analysis is being performed, place the sample in an ice slush.
- Properly dispose of waste materials.

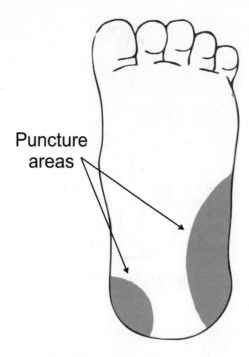

Figure 13-4 Capillary Blood Gas Sampling Sites.

Perform Blood Gas and CO-Oximetry Analysis

Blood gas and CO-oximetry analysis are complex procedures involving sample analysis, sample and equipment troubleshooting, equipment maintenance and calibration, and quality control measures. You need to be familiar with these procedures in order to ensure accurate and reliable results. The use of blood gas and CO-oximetry equipment is covered in Chapter 8.

Blood Gas Analysis

The following are key considerations in properly analyzing a blood gas sample:

- Always apply standard precautions and wear personal protection equipment.
- Confirm proper equipment functioning (Chapter 8).
- Identify the specimen and confirm all relevant information: patient's name and medical record number, FIO_2 or ventilator settings, and patient's temperature.
- Note the time at which the sample was obtained. Discard the sample if more than 60 minutes have passed.
- Inspect the sample for obvious signs of preanalytical error (refer to Chapter 8 for the most common preanalytical errors).
- Mix the sample thoroughly. This is a critical step for hemoglobin and hematocrit measurements.
- Discard a drop or two of blood from the syringe before introducing the sample.
- Analyze sample, confirm readings, and document results.
- Properly dispose of waste materials.

CO-Oximetry Analysis

CO-oximetry analysis should be performed:

- To measure actual blood oxygen content (as opposed to that computed with a simple blood gas analyzer)
- To measure levels of abnormal hemoglobins (e.g.,carboxyhemoglobin, methemoglobin, sulfhemoglobin)
- To validate pulse oximetry results (SpO_2)

CO-oximetry analysis involves the same basic steps as blood gas analysis. Unlike pulse oximeters, which use a single wavelength of light, CO-oximeters use multiple wavelengths. Doing so allows these devices to identify not only hemoglobin saturation with oxygen but also other (abnormal) chemical combinations with hemoglobin, including carboxyhemoglobin and methemoglobin. For this reason, CO-oximetry is the standard test for detecting abnormal hemoglobin saturations, as in cases of carbon monoxide (CO) poisoning. In CO poisoning, pulse oximeters tend to provide falsely high SpO_2 levels.

Typically, the blood sample undergoes analysis for total hemoglobin (total Hb, g/dL) and percentages of oxyhemoglobin saturation (SaO_2), carboxyhemoglobin saturation, methemoglobin saturation, and sulfhemoglobin saturation. In addition, total O_2 content (CaO_2 in mL/dL) of the sample is calculated (total Hb $\times$ 1.36 $\times$ SaO_2).

Interpret Blood Gas and CO-Oximetry Results

Blood Gas Analysis Interpretation

To properly assess and monitor a patient's response to therapy, you must be able to properly interpret arterial blood gas results. When assessing blood gas results, we recommend that you first assess acid-base status and then separately evaluate oxygenation.

Acid-Base Interpretation

Follow these steps to properly assess the acid-base components of an arterial blood gas:

1. Categorize the pH (high, low, or normal)
2. Determine the respiratory involvement ($PaCO_2$ high, low, or normal)
3. Determine the metabolic involvement (HCO_3 high, low, or normal)
4. Assess for compensation

Chapter 3 reviews normal arterial blood gas parameters and describes how to identify the four primary acid–base disturbances using just the pH and $PaCO_2$. Here we focus on assessing compensation for these primary disturbances and identifying combined acid–base problems.

To understand compensation, you need to know that the blood pH is controlled by a balance between the buffering and excretion of fixed acids by the kidneys and the elimination of CO_2 by the lungs. Specifically, pH is determined by the ratio of the blood buffer/base bicarbonate (HCO_3) to the dissolved CO_2 in the blood (directly proportional to the $PaCO_2$):

$$pH \approx \frac{HCO_3}{PaCO_2}$$

Compensation occurs when the system not affected by the primary disturbance attempts to restore the pH back to normal. **Table 13-3** demonstrates this concept for each of the four primary acid-base disturbances. Using respiratory acidosis as an example, if the lungs retain CO_2 (e.g., in COPD) the $PaCO_2$ rises (the primary event). Based on the balance between base (HCO_3) and acid (dissolved CO_2), a rise in the $PaCO_2$ will lower the blood pH (respiratory acidosis). To compensate, the system *not affected* (the kidneys) tries to restore the pH by increasing blood levels of HCO_3 (the compensatory response). As HCO_3 levels rise, the pH is restored back toward normal.

Table 13-3 also includes base excess (BE) measure, which is reported by most blood gas labs and normally provided by the NBRC in questions that report ABG data. The normal range for BE is $\pm$ 2 mEq/L. By combining assessment of the $PaCO_2$ and BE, you can quickly identify if compensation is occurring. *Compensation is occurring if both the $PaCO_2$ and BE are abnormally high or low.* As indicated in **Table 13-4**, if both the $PaCO_2$ and BE are high, the patient has either a compensated metabolic alkalosis or compensated respiratory acidosis. Conversely, if both the $PaCO_2$ and BE are low, the patient has either a compensated metabolic acidosis or compensated respiratory alkalosis. To determine which is the primary disturbance, simply look at the pH. If the pH is less than 7.40, the primary problem is the one that would cause acidosis. If the pH is greater than 7.40, the primary problem is the one that would cause alkalosis. You also use the pH to determine whether compensation is full or partial. Compensation is "full" if the pH is in the normal range (7.35–7.45); otherwise compensation is termed

Table 13-3 Primary Acid-Base Disorders and Compensatory Response

Acid–Base Disorder	Primary Event	Compensatory Response	Base Excess
Respiratory acidosis	$\downarrow pH = \dfrac{HCO_3^-}{\uparrow Paco_2}$	$\downarrow pH = \dfrac{\Uparrow HCO_3^-}{\uparrow Paco_2}$	$> +2$ mEq/L
Respiratory alkalosis	$\uparrow pH = \dfrac{HCO_3^-}{\downarrow Paco_2}$	$\uparrow pH = \dfrac{\Downarrow HCO_3^-}{\downarrow Paco_2}$	< -2 mEq/L
Metabolic acidosis	$\downarrow pH = \dfrac{\downarrow HCO_3^-}{Paco_2}$	$\downarrow pH = \dfrac{\downarrow HCO_3^-}{\Downarrow Paco_2}$	< -2 mEq/L
Metabolic alkalosis	$\uparrow pH = \dfrac{\uparrow HCO_3^-}{Paco_2}$	$\uparrow pH = \dfrac{\uparrow HCO_3^-}{\Uparrow Paco_2}$	$> +2$ mEq/L

$\uparrow$ = primary increase; $\downarrow$ = primary decrease; $\Uparrow$ = compensatory increase; $\Downarrow$ = compensatory decrease

"partial." In general, renal/metabolic compensation for primary respiratory disorders is slow (hours to days), whereas respiratory compensation for primary renal/metabolic disorders is fast (minutes). Indeed, a failure of the lungs to quickly compensate for a primary renal/metabolic acid–base disturbance indicates impaired pulmonary function.

If upon inspection of the ABG report you note that the $Paco_2$ and BE diverge in *opposite* directions (one abnormally high, the other abnormally low), a *combined* acid-base disturbance exists. A high $Paco_2$ and low BE define combined respiratory and metabolic acidosis, while a low $Paco_2$ and high BE define combined respiratory and metabolic alkalosis. Combined respiratory and metabolic acidosis is the most common of these disturbances, since it occurs during respiratory and cardiac arrest (cardiac arrest causes tissue hypoxia, which causes lactic acidosis).

Assessing Arterial Oxygenation

For monitoring and assessment of the patient's response to oxygen therapy, the Pao_2 and Sao_2 results always need to be compared against the Fio_2 the patient is receiving (when the ABG sample was taken). Two common formulas are used to perform this assessment: (1) the alveolar-arterial O_2 tension gradient [$P(A-a)o_2$], and (2) the ratio of Pao_2 to Fio_2 (Pao_2/Fio_2, or P/F ratio). An alternative rule of thumb (the 60-60 rule) can also be used to assess oxygenation.

To calculate a patient's alveolar-arterial O_2 tension gradient, you must first compute the alveolar oxygen tension (Pao_2). To do so, apply the alveolar air equation:

$$Pao_2 = Fio_2 (P_B - P_{H_2O}) - 1.25 \times Paco_2$$

At sea level (the most likely conditions on the CRT exam), this equation simplifies to:

$$Pao_2 = Fio_2 (713) - 1.25 \times Paco_2$$

Table 13-4 Using Base Excess to Assess for Compensation

Paco₂	BE	pH	Acid–Base Disturbance
> 45 torr	> +2 mEq/L	> 7.40	Compensated metabolic alkalosis
		< 7.40	Compensated respiratory acidosis
< 45 torr	< –2 mEq/L	> 7.40	Compensated respiratory alkalosis
		< 7.40	Compensated metabolic acidosis

As an example, if a patient breathing 100% O_2 at sea level has a P_{aO_2} of 250 torr and a P_{aCO_2} of 60 torr, the P_{AO_2} would be computed as:

$$P_{AO_2} = 1.0\ (713) - 1.25 \times 60$$
$$P_{AO_2} = 713 - 75$$
$$P_{AO_2} = 638\ torr$$

To compute the $P(A\text{-}a)O_2$, simply subtract the P_{aO_2} from the calculated P_{AO_2}. Continuing our example:

$$P(A\text{-}a)O_2 = 638 - 250$$
$$P(A\text{-}a)O_2 = 388\ torr$$

The following key points pertain to interpreting the $P(A\text{-}a)O_2$:

- A normal $P(A\text{-}a)O_2$ difference on room air is about 5–10 torr.
- A normal $P(A\text{-}a)O_2$ on 100% is about 25–65 torr.
- When the $F_{IO_2} = 1.0$, every 100 torr of $P(A\text{-}a)O_2$ corresponds to about a 5% shunt.

In our example, the $P(A\text{-}a)O_2$ of 388 torr is clearly abnormal, indicating the presence of almost a 20% shunt (388/100 = 3.8 × 5 = 19%).

Because interpretation of the $P(A\text{-}a)O_2$ depends heavily on the F_{IO_2} and is time consuming to compute, most clinicians prefer using the P/F ratio to assess oxygenation. Continuing the example, our patient's P/F ration would be computed as follows:

$$P_{aO_2}/F_{IO_2} = 250/1 = 250$$

The following key points pertain to interpreting the P/F ratio:

- A normal P/F ratio exceeds 350–450.
- A P/F ratio less than 300 indicates a moderate disturbance of oxygenation (acute lung injury).
- A P/F ratio less than 200 indicates a severe disturbance of oxygenation (consistent with ARDS).

Consistent with the prior assessment of this patient's oxygenation using the $P(A\text{-}a)O_2$, we can conclude that this patient has a moderate to severe disturbance of oxygenation.

The simplest approach (and one that will serve you well on the CRT exam) is the 60-60 rule. This rule states that if the P_{aO_2} is less than 60 torr on an F_{IO_2} greater than 0.6, then there is a severe disturbance in oxygenation, due mainly to shunting. Note that these conditions correspond to a P/F ratio less than or equal to 100.

Table 13-5 describes the three major causes of hypoxemia, the basis for their classification, and their treatment. The most common physiologic cause for a reduced P_{aO_2} is ventilation-perfusion (V/Q) imbalances. V/Q imbalances are the primary mechanism causing hypoxemia in virtually all parenchymal lung diseases, such as asthma, atelectasis, bronchitis, emphysema, pneumonia, and pulmonary embolism. V/Q imbalances generally respond well to supplemental oxygen. In contrast, when hypoxemia is due to shunting, PEEP or CPAP are needed to improve oxygenation.

Capillary Blood Gas Interpretation

When interpreting a capillary blood gas, you normally assess only the pH and P_{aCO_2}. Capillary P_{aO_2} values are questionable due to the mixed venous nature of capillary blood. Thickness of the skin and crying caused by pain will also alter the results and must be taken into consideration when interpreting capillary blood gas parameters.

CO-Oximetry Results Interpretation

Normal values for CO-oximetry are shown in **Table 13-6**. It is very important to remember the following points regarding CO-oximetry analysis:

Table 13-5 Hypoxemia Classification

Cause of Hypoxemia	Basis for Conclusion	Recommended Treatment
Hypoventilation	• Hypercapnia • Normal P(A-a)O_2 difference	Increase ventilation
V/Q imbalance	• $Paco_2$ is normal • Pao_2 is > 60 torr with an Fio_2 < 0.6 (60-60 rule)	Increase Fio_2
Shunt	• $Paco_2$ may be normal or abnormal • P(A-a) difference > 300 torr (100% O_2) • P/F ratio < 300 • Pao_2 is < 60 torr with a Fio_2 > 0.6	Add PEEP or CPAP

- Elevated blood HbCO levels can be caused by exposure to tobacco smoke, faulty gas furnaces, automobile exhaust, or smoky fires. *In this situation pulse oximetry will read falsely high* and should not be used to assess hypoxia.
- Elevated methemoglobin may be hereditary or acquired through exposure to certain chemicals (nitrites, nitrates, chlorates, quinones, aminobenzenes, nitrobenzenes, or nitrotoluenes) or drugs (benzocaine, nitroglycerin, nitroprusside).

Be sure to remember that an Sao_2 less than 85% indicates significant hypoxemia. Likewise, if the sum of the abnormal hemoglobins (HbCO + MetHb) exceeds 15%, the oxygen-carrying capacity of the blood is severely diminished. The presence of vascular dyes and high lipid intake (e.g., parenteral nutrition) can lead to falsely low total Hb and Sao_2. Last, elevated bilirubin levels (common in infants) will lead to falsely high total Hb, HbO_2, and metHb levels.

Perform Pulse Oximetry

Pulse oximetry is the assessment of arterial hemoglobin saturation using noninvasive plethysmographic and spectrophotometric methods. Whenever possible, pulse oximetry initially should be accompanied by CO-oximetry analysis of a baseline arterial blood sample. You can then "calibrate" the pulse oximeter by determining the discrepancy between the actual Sao_2 and the measured Spo_2. For example, if the pulse oximeter displays an Spo_2 of 91% and CO-oximetry on an arterial sample simultaneously yields an Sao_2 of 88%, you should subtract 3% from subsequent Spo_2 readings. Of course, any major change in patient status will require new calibration of the Spo_2 against a measured Sao_2.

Table 13-6 Normal CO-Oximetry Values

Component	Whole Blood	Normal Values
Total Hb	Newborn	14.0–24.0 g/dL
	Adult male	13.5–16.5 g/dL
	Adult female	12.0–15.0 g/dL
Sao_2 (%HbO_2)	Arterial	92%–99% (air)
O_2 content (Cao_2)	Arterial	15–23 mL/dL
%HbCO (carboxyHb)	Nonsmokers	< 1.5% of total Hb
	Smokers	1.5%–5.0% of total Hb
	Heavy smokers	5.0%–9.0% of total Hb
%MetHb		< 3% of total Hb
%SHb		0%

Pulse oximetry is indicated whenever the need exists:

- To monitor the adequacy of arterial oxyhemoglobin saturation
- To quantify the response of arterial oxyhemoglobin saturation to therapeutic intervention or to a diagnostic procedure (e.g., oxygen therapy, bronchoscopy)
- To comply with mandated regulations or recommendations by authoritative groups (e.g., moderate sedation monitoring)

When assessing and monitoring a patient with a pulse oximeter, the following steps are important to remember:

- Assess patient by measuring the patient's pulse rate manually or verifying the heart rate displayed on the ECG monitor (if applicable) to correlate with pulse oximetry readings. This helps to ensure accuracy.
- Confirm the F_{IO_2} being delivered to the patient. This must be documented upon completion of the procedure.
- Turn on the oximeter and allows for appropriate warm-up time.
- Select a site for probe application, checking for adequate perfusion. Remove patient's nail polish if necessary and clean site with alcohol prep pad.
- Attach probe to the selected site and allow for proper stabilization. Observe the pulse rate on the oximeter; correlate it with the manually measured heart rate or ECG rate.
- Record and interpret pulse rate, SpO_2, and F_{IO_2} being delivered (and turn trend monitoring on for overnight oximetry, if ordered).

Remember that the most common source of error and false alarms with pulse oximetry is motion artifacts. To overcome this problem, consider relocating the sensor to an alternative site.

Pulse oximeters provide relatively accurate (± 2–4%) estimates of oxyhemoglobin saturation, as long as there are no abnormal hemoglobins present and the perfusion is good (**Table 13-7**). To relate the SpO_2 to the approximate PaO_2, use the "40-50-60/70-80-90" rule. When applying this rule, Hb saturations of 70%, 80%, and 90% are about equal to PaO_2s of 40, 50, and 60 torr, respectively.

Normal oxyhemoglobin saturation is greater than 95% breathing room air. Levels below 90% indicate the need for supplemental oxygen therapy. Drops in oxyhemoglobin are usually the result of cardiac, pulmonary, or combined cardiopulmonary disease. Significant declines (> 5%) during exercise or sleep are abnormal. Hemoglobin saturation data must always be interpreted with knowledge of Hb/Hct levels. For example, a patient with an SpO_2 of 97% and severe anemia (Hb < 7 g/dL) is predisposed to tissue hypoxia due to reduced blood O_2 content.

Table 13-7 Most Common SpO$_2$ Reading Errors

Factor	Potential Error
Presence of HbCO (e.g., smoke inhalation injury)	Falsely high %HbO$_2$
Presence of high levels of metHb	Falsely low %HbO$_2$ if Sao$_2$ > 85% Falsely high %HbO$_2$ if Sao$_2$ < 85%
Anemia (low hematocrit)	Falsely low %HbO$_2$
Vascular dyes (e.g., methylene blue)	Falsely low %HbO$_2$
Dark skin pigmentation and nail polish	Falsely high %HbO$_2$ (3–5%)
Ambient light	Varies (e.g., falsely high %HbO$_2$ in sunlight); may also cause falsely high pulse reading
Poor perfusion and vasoconstriction	Inadequate signal; unpredictable results
Motion artifact (most common)	Unpredictable spurious readings

Source: Scanlan, C. L. Analysis and monitoring of gas exchange. In Wilkins, R. L., Stoller, J. K., & Scanlan, C. L. (Eds.). (2003). *Egan's fundamentals of respiratory care* (8th ed.). St. Louis: Mosby.

When using pulse oximetry to assess and monitor a patient's response to therapy, the greatest hazard is the device's limitations. Device limitations can result in both false negatives (normal readings in the presence of hypoxemia) and false positives (low readings when oxygenation is satisfactory). In addition, pulse oximeters provide little useful data when the PaO_2 rises above 100 torr (hyperoxia). Table 13-7 outlines the common factors causing erroneous SpO_2 readings and the expected direction of error.

Perform Capnography

Capnography involves the measurement and display of CO_2 concentrations in real time during breathing. Their primary clinical use is for patient monitoring and assessment during general anesthesia or during mechanical ventilation. Chapter 8 provides details on the design and calibration of capnographs.

Remember the following while performing a capnometry procedure:

- Calibrate the monitor according to the manufacturer's instructions.
- Connect the monitor to the patient's airway and observe the CO_2 waveform.
- Compare the monitor reading with current ABG values.
  - It is unlikely the values will match exactly. In healthy individuals $PETCO_2$ averages 1–5 torr less than arterial CO_2.
  - Consistent, close correlation of results is needed if the monitor is to provide useful information regarding changes in ventilation.

The first step in assessing end-tidal CO_2 is to determine its actual value and whether it has changed over time. **Table 13-8** differentiates between the causes of sudden and gradual changes in $PETCO_2$ readings.

Most capnographs provide continuous breath-by-breath display of inspired and exhaled CO_2 concentrations. **Figure 13-5** depicts the components of the normal CO_2 waveform for one full breathing cycle. Note that in patients with COPD, CHF, auto-PEEP, V/Q mismatch, and pulmonary emboli, a clear alveolar plateau phase may never occur. **Table 13-9** (on page 396) describes the most common scenarios found during monitoring and assessment of exhaled CO_2 levels by capnography.

There are several common problems that occur when using capnographs. **Table 13-10** (on page 397) describes these common problems, their likely causes and the appropriate actions to resolve them.

Table 13-8 Conditions Associated with Changes in $PETCO_2$

	High $PETCO_2$	Low $PETCO_2$[a]
Sudden change	• Sudden increase in cardiac output • Sudden release of a tourniquet • Injection of sodium bicarbonate	• Sudden hyperventilation • Sudden drop in cardiac output • Cardiac arrest[a] • Massive pulmonary/air embolism • Circuit leak/disconnection[a] • Esophageal intubation[a] • ET/trach tube obstruction[a]
Gradual change	• Hypoventilation • Increased metabolism/CO_2 production • Rapid rise in temperature (malignant hyperthermia)	• Hyperventilation • Decreased metabolism/CO_2 production • Decreased pulmonary perfusion • Decrease in body temperature

a. Can result in a $PETCO_2$ of 0 torr.

Source: Scanlan, C. L. Analysis and monitoring of gas exchange. In Wilkins, R. L, Stoller, J. K., & Scanlan, C. L. (Eds.). (2003). *Egan's fundamentals of respiratory care* (8th ed.). St. Louis: Mosby.

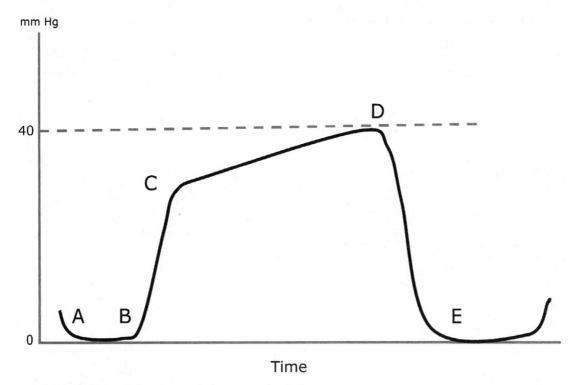

mm Hg

40

0

Time

Figure 13-5 Normal End-Tidal CO$_2$ Waveform. A to B: Exhalation of pure dead space gas. No exhaled CO$_2$ present. B to C: Combination of dead space and alveolar gas. Exhaled CO$_2$ begins to rise. C to D: Alveolar plateau. Exhalation of alveolar CO$_2$. PETCO$_2$ normally is measured at the end of the alveolar plateau. D to E: Inhalation of fresh gas (%CO$_2$ drops to zero).

Perform Transcutaneous Monitoring

Chapter 6 provides details on the indications for transcutaneous monitoring of arterial PO$_2$ and PCO$_2$, as well as the setup and assembly, use, and troubleshooting of transcutaneous monitors.

Hemodynamic Assessment

Hemodynamic assessment, including equipment needs and interpretation of vascular pressures, flows, and blood gas parameters, is covered in detail in Chapter 4.

Measure and Record Vital Signs and Cardiac Rhythm and Evaluate Fluid Balance

Vital Signs

Regular measurement of vital signs is essential in evaluating and monitoring a patient's response to therapy. Changes in patient status usually are accompanied by changes in the patient's vital signs. For example, a 20% increase in heart rate (tachycardia) above baseline when giving a bronchodilator treatment usually indicates an adverse reaction to the medication. Decreasing the dosage or changing to another bronchodilator may avoid this problem.

Normal values for vital signs are provided in Chapter 3. **Table 13-11** (on page 398) lists common causes of abnormal vital signs and their recommended solutions.

Table 13-9 Common PETCO₂ Waveform Descriptions

Event	Figures	Possible Causes
Sudden decrease of exhaled CO_2 to zero baseline		• Esophageal intubation • Disconnection from ventilator • Ventilator malfunction/failure • Obstructed/kinked ET tube
Gradual decrease of exhaled CO_2 waveform		• Hyperventilation • Hypothermia • Sedation • Hypovolemia • Decreasing CO_2
Gradual increase of exhaled CO_2 waveform		• Hypoventilation • Rising body temperature • Partial airway obstruction • Rewarming after surgery • Seizure, shivering, pain • Bicarbonate administration • COPD exacerbation • Increased cardiac output
Rise in waveform baseline		• Addition of mechanical deadspace to ventilator circuit

Monitor Cardiac Rhythm

Heart function can be affected by many respiratory therapies and interventions. For this reason, in order to properly evaluate and monitor a patient's response to therapy, you must be able to recognize major abnormal cardiac rhythms. Cardiac dysrhythmias can be classified according to their severity as lethal (causing death) and nonlethal. Using this classification, the most common dysrhythmias you can expect to see on the NBRC CRT exam include the following:

- Lethal rhythms
  - Asystole (cardiac standstill, flatline)
  - Ventricular tachycardia
  - Ventricular fibrillation
- Non-lethal dysrhythmias
  - Atrial fibrillation
  - Atrial flutter
  - Bradycardia
  - Tachycardia
  - Premature ventricular contractions (PVCs)

Lethal cardiac rhythms and their treatment are covered in Chapter 17. Chapter 4 reviews the procedure for obtaining a 12-lead ECG, as well as pointers on indentifying the major ECG abnormalities. Here we provide a brief discussion of the nonlethal dysrhythmias, along with example ECG rhythm strips.

Table 13-10 Resolving Problems When Using Capnographs

Problem	Cause	Action
Unit does not turn on	Power cable improperly attached or disconnected, or cable has faulty electrical connection	Check power cable connection and check that on/off switch is on
	Battery pack may be discharged	Replace or recharge the battery pack, or connect to AC power
	Battery pack may not be inserted properly or missing	Be sure the battery pack is inserted properly
Unit switches on but then switches off	Electrical connection is faulty, or the AC wall outlet has no power	Check connections
	Battery pack is almost discharged	Replace or recharge battery pack, or connect to AC power
	Hardware or software error	Have device serviced
CO_2 values are erratic	Mechanically ventilated patient breathing spontaneously	No action needed
	Airway/circuit leak	Check for/correct cuff or ventilator circuit leaks
	Sampling line leak (sidestream units only)	Check for/correct sampling line connections
	Water or sputum blocking the sensor window (mainstream units only)	Clean or replace sensor; recalibrate device
CO_2 values higher or lower than expected	Physiological cause	Check patient
	Ventilator malfunction	Check ventilator and patient
	Improper calibration	Recalibrate unit
	Sampling line kinked/clogged (side-stream units only–gives "0" reading)	Unkink/unclog or replace sampling line
	Moisture trap full	Replace moisture trap
	BTPS setting OFF (CO_2 values will be falsely high)	Turn BTPS correction ON

Tachycardia

- Identified in the ECG rhythm strip (**Figure 13-6** on page 399) as:
  - Rate: 100–180 beats/min
  - PR interval: usually < 0.2 sec
  - A P wave for every QRS complex
  - Shortened R-R interval (< 0.60 sec) with normal QRS complexes
- For common causes and treatment recommendations, review previous section on vital signs

Bradycardia

- Identified in the ECG rhythm strip (**Figure 13-7** on page 399) as:
  - Rate < 60 beats/min
  - Regular rhythm with a normal PR interval
  - Normal P waves followed by regular QRS complexes
  - A prolonged (> 1 sec) R-R interval
- For common causes and treatment recommendations, review previous section on vital signs

Table 13-11 Troubleshooting Changes in Vital Signs

Abnormal Vital Sign	Possible Cause	Recommendations
Increased heart rate (tachycardia)	• Anxiety • Pain • Decreased Pao_2, decreased or increased $Paco_2$ • Medications • Trauma • Fever • Failure to wean from mechanical ventilation • Ventilator asynchrony	• Relieve anxiety • Treat pain • Stabilize blood gases • Treat the fever and the cause of the fever • If failure to wean, return to previous settings • Check patient-ventilator system; obtain/evaluate ABGs
Decreased heart rate (bradycardia)	• Hypothermia • Medications • Cardiac disease • Cardiopulmonary arrest	• Provide warm blanket and fluid • Evaluate cardiac status (ECG, cardiac enzymes) • Perform CPR if needed
Increased blood pressure (hypertension)	• Anxiety • Response to decrease Pao_2, decrease $Paco_2$ • Pain • Medications • Cardiovascular disease • Trauma (sympathetic response)	• Reassure; alleviate fear • Obtain and evaluate ABG • Relieve, treat pain • Assess for cardiovascular events • Evaluate patient for cardiovascular risk factors • Recommend anti-hypertensive medications
Decreased blood pressure (hypotension)	• Hypovolemia • Trauma (bleeding) • Medications • Cardiovascular collapse	• Fluid resuscitation • Surgical intervention to stop hemorrhage • Provide CPR if necessary • Recommend vasoactive drugs to increase BP (dopamine)
Fever	• Infection • Atelectasis • Increased metabolic rate caused by increased work of breathing • Overheated humidifier	• Treat infection/review precautions • Check for mucous plugs, ET position • Check sensitivity and patient ventilator settings • Check temperature of humidifier heater
Increased respiratory rate (tachypnea)	• Anxiety or pain • Altered ventilator settings • Decreased Pao_2 or increased $Paco_2$ • Failure to wean during mechanical ventilation • Ventilator asynchrony • Change in metabolic needs	• Reassure, alleviate fear; relieve, treat pain • Check patient-ventilator settings • Obtain and evaluate ABG • If failure to wean, return to previous settings • Evaluate patient's metabolic rate
Decreased respiratory rate (bradypnea)	• Sleep • Oversedation • Decreased $Paco_2$ • Respiratory failure/arrest	• Normal observation • Reverse sedation or provide support • Restore normal ventilatory status • Provide airway support and CPR if necessary

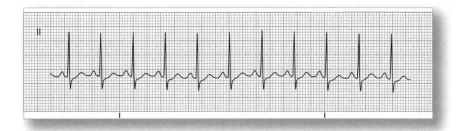

Figure 13-6 Example of Sinus Tachycardia (Rate ≈ 130/min).

Source: Garcia, T., & Miller, G. T. (2004). *Arrhythmia recognition: the art of interpretation.* Sudbury, MA: Jones and Bartlett.

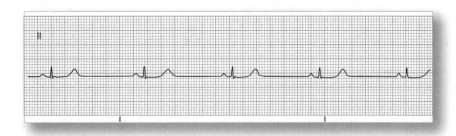

Figure 13-7 Example of Sinus Bradycardia (Rate ≈ 45/min).

Source: Garcia, T., & Miller, G. T. (2004). *Arrhythmia recognition: the art of interpretation.* Sudbury, MA: Jones and Bartlett.

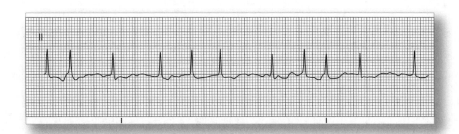

Figure 13-8 Example of Atrial Fibrillation.

Source: Garcia, T., & Miller, G. T. (2004). *Arrhythmia recognition: the art of interpretation.* Sudbury, MA: Jones and Bartlett.

Atrial Fibrillation

- Identified in the ECG rhythm strip (**Figure 13-8**) as:
  - Irregular rhythm
  - Variation in interval and amplitude in the R-R interval (> 10% variation)
  - Absent P wave with "fibrillatory" base line
- Can be a side effect of beta-adrenergic drugs. If occurs during the treatment, stop the treatment, stabilize the patient, and notify the physician.
- If already present before the therapy, assess heart rate, patient history, and consult with patient's nurse and physician before administering treatment.
- If it occurs during any other respiratory therapy procedure, stop the procedure, stabilize the patient, and notify the physician.

Atrial Flutter

- Identified in the ECG rhythm strip (**Figure 13-9**) as:
  - The classic " sawtooth" pattern seen in between the QRS complexes
  - The absence of a PR interval
- Causes and treatment recommendations are the same as with atrial fibrillation.

Premature Ventricular Contraction (PVC)

- Identified in the ECG rhythm strip (**Figure 13-10**) as:
  - Abnormal QRS complexes (> 0.12 sec in width).
  - Underlying rhythm is usually regular but becomes irregular with a PVC.
  - No P wave present before the PVC.
  - T waves are deflected in an opposite direction following the PVC.
- PVCs can be caused by anxiety, caffeine, tobacco, alcohol, and certain medications such as beta-agonist bronchodilators and theophylline.
- PVCs can also be caused by myocardial ischemia, acidosis, electrolyte imbalance, hypoxia, and direct stimulation of the myocardium.
- Many respiratory procedures can cause hypoxemia (e.g., suctioning) or myocardial stimulation (e.g., postural drainage, percussion on patients with CVP or PA catheters).
- If PVCs occur while performing any respiratory procedure, stop, stabilize the patient, and notify the physician immediately.
- If the PVCs are due to myocardial stimulation from a central vascular line, assess line position and recommend repositioning the line if necessary.

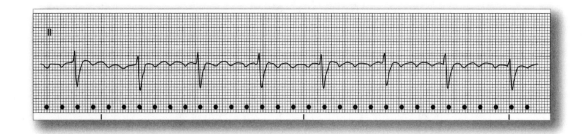

Figure 13-9 Example of Atrial Flutter with 4:1 Conduction Ratio.

Source: Garcia, T., & Miller, G. T. (2004). *Arrhythmia recognition: the art of interpretation.* Sudbury, MA: Jones and Bartlett.

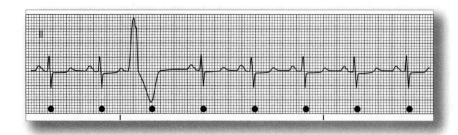

Figure 13-10 Example of a Sinus Rhythm with a Premature Ventricular Contraction (PVC).

Source: Garcia, T., & Miller, G. T. (2004). *Arrhythmia recognition: the art of interpretation.* Sudbury, MA: Jones and Bartlett.

Evaluate Fluid Balance

Chapters 3 and 15 cover normal and abnormal fluid balance and its evaluation.

Perform and Interpret Results of Pulmonary Function Testing

Indications, procedures, and interpretation of spirometry, static lung volumes, D_{LCO}, and exercise testing are covered in detail in Chapter 4. In addition, the NBRC also expects you to be familiar with bronchoprovocation studies. Bronchoprovocation studies are used to identify and assess airway responsiveness. You may want to recommend a bronchial challenge test to:

- Differentiate asthma from chronic bronchitis
- Quantify the severity of airway responsiveness
- Screen individuals who may be at risk from environmental or occupational exposure to allergens
- Identify exercise-induced bronchospasm

Table 13-12 describes some of the most common techniques that can be used to assess airway hyperreactivity.

Recommend Blood Tests

Blood test results can add significant information when making decisions about objective and subjective responses to respiratory care. Normal values for laboratory blood tests are discussed in Chapter 3. **Table 13-13** lists some of the most common lab tests you may want to recommend according to the scenario and patient assessment.

Observe Changes in Sputum Characteristics

As discussed in Chapter 4, assessing the volume, color, consistency, and odor of expectorated sputum is a key component in the overall evaluation of the patient and should be conducted whenever secretion clearance takes place. In addition, the NBRC expects that you can relate the characteristics of the patient's sputum to the need for specific diagnostic tests or treatments. Typically, if you determine that a patient has mucopurulent or purulent sputum (indicating a potential pulmonary infection), you should recommend a chest X-ray, Gram stain, and culture and sensitivity testing. Depending on the lab results, you might also recommend antibiotic therapy. If, in contrast, you observe a patient with pink, watery, frothy sputum and signs or symptoms of heart failure (indicating acute pulmonary edema), you should recommend high concentrations of oxygen, ideally with CPAP or BiPAP™.

Table 13-12 Common Bronchial Challenge Tests

Test	Description
Methacholine challenge	• Assesses changes in airway caliber with increasing concentrations of methacholine • Patients with hyperreactive airways will show early changes at low dosages • A 20% decrease in FEV_1 is considered a positive result • The methacholine concentration at which a 20% decrease in FEV_1 occurs is called the "provocative concentration," or PC20
Histamine challenge	• Uses histamine sulfate instead of methacholine • Flushing and headaches are two common side effects from histamine inhalation • Performed in a similar fashion as the methacholine test • A 20% decrease in FEV_1 is considered a positive result
Exercise challenge	• Indicated to assess exercise-induced bronchospasm (EIB) • A resting ECG should be done prior to the test to rule out possible contraindications • A treadmill or a cycle ergometer can be used • The test should not last more than 8 minutes • Bronchospasm usually occurs 5 to 10 minutes after cessation of the exercise • A drop in FEV_1 of 10–15% is consistent with increased airway sensitivity

Table 13-13 Blood Tests Recommendations

Patient Scenario	Recommended Blood Test
Post-op patient with low-grade fever	• White blood cell count with differential to rule out possible bacterial pneumonia • Blood cultures
Fluid balance disturbances	• Electrolytes to assess possible causes of fluid imbalance • Hematocrit to assess level of hemodilution or hemoconcentration
Decreased or absent urine output over time	• BUN and creatinine to assess for possible renal failure or renal disease
Chest pain due to suspected myocardial infarction or ischemia	• Cardiac enzymes to assess for cardiac muscle damage • Electrolytes
Suspected hepatitis, history of alcohol or drug abuse	• Liver enzymes (AST) to assess liver function
Patients with acid-based disturbances	• ABG • Electrolytes
Occurrence of PVCs or cardiac dysrhythmias without previous history of cardiac disease	• Electrolytes to assess for potassium
Patients on anticoagulation therapy or uncontrolled bleeding	• Prothrombin time (PT) • Partial prothrombin time (PTT) • International normalize ratio (INR)

Auscultate Chest and Interpret Changes in Breath Sounds

You perform chest auscultation to identify normal or abnormal lung and heart sounds. The NBRC CRT exam typically incorporates breath sounds within patient monitoring and assessment scenarios to guide your decision making and to provide insights as to the underlying pathologic process. To score high in this area, you need to pay close attention to these "clues" during patient assessment and always evaluate the breath sounds in the clinical context in which they are given.

Technique

While you are assessing breath sounds:

- When possible, the patient should be sitting upright in a relaxed position.
- The patient should breathe deeply than normal through an opened mouth. Inhalation should be active, with exhalation passive.
- The diaphragm (breath sounds) or bell (heart sounds) must be placed directly against the chest wall. The tubing should not rub against any objects, since this may produce extraneous sounds.
- Auscultation should include all lobes on the anterior, lateral, and posterior chest.
- Auscultation should begin at the base (because certain sounds here can be altered by subsequent deep breaths), comparing side with side, and working toward the top.
- At least one full inspiratory-expiratory cycle should be evaluated at each position.

The following must be assessed and noted:

- The pitch (frequency)
- The intensity (loudness)
- Any other distinctive characteristics
- Comparison of the duration of the sound's inspiratory and expiration components

Classification of Breath Sounds

Normal breath sounds are described in Chapter 4. Here we focus on abnormal or *adventitious* breath sounds. Most adventitious breath sounds are classified as being either continuous or discontinuous.

Continuous breath sounds are characterized by their pitch. High-pitched continuous sounds are called *wheezes*, while low-pitched continuous sounds are called *rhonchi*. Another abnormal continuous loud, high-pitched sound heard primarily over the larynx and trachea during inhalation is *stridor*.

Discontinuous sounds are intermittent, crackling, or bubbling sounds of short duration. The term *crackles* (rales) is used for discontinuous breath sounds. **Table 13-14** summarizes the likely mechanisms, characteristics, and causes of these adventitious breath sounds.

Observe for Signs of Patient-Ventilator Asynchrony

Patient-ventilator asynchrony occurs when a patient's spontaneous respiratory efforts are no longer in synchrony with that of the ventilator. Because patient-ventilator asynchrony is a frequent event in critical care, you must be able to recognize and effectively manage this problem. Here we focus on recognizing asynchrony and differentiating among its various causes. More detail on solving patient-ventilator asynchrony problems is provided in Chapter 14.

The most common manifestations of patient-ventilator asynchrony include agitation and respiratory distress. In its most severe form, patients experiencing asynchrony may appear to be fighting or "bucking" the ventilator. Agitation can be recognized by irregular patient movements and/or facial signs of pain, discomfort, or distress. Additional physical signs of respiratory distress include tachypnea, diaphoresis, nasal flaring, accessory muscles use, intercostal retractions, rib cage-abdominal paradox, tachycardia, and blood pressure changes. Asynchrony also is often evident when viewing the ventilator's graphic display monitor (see Chapter 14).

Table 13-14 Adventitious Breath Sounds

Lung Sounds	Likely Mechanism	Characteristics	Causes
Wheezes	Rapid airflow through obstructed airways	High-pitched; usually expiratory	Asthma, congestive heart failure, bronchitis
Stridor	Rapid airflow through obstructed upper airway	High-pitched, monophonic; commonly inspiratory	Croup, epiglottitis, post-extubation edema
Pleural friction rub	Inflamed pleural surfaces rubbing together during breathing	Creaking or grating sound heard mainly during inhalation (can occur during both phases of breathing)	Pleurisy
Crackles: inspiratory and expiratory	Excess airway secretions moving with airflow	Coarse; often clear with cough	Bronchitis, respiratory infections
Crackles: early inspiratory	Sudden opening of proximal bronchi	Scanty, transmitted to mouth; not affected by cough	Bronchitis, emphysema, asthma
Crackles: late inspiratory	Sudden opening of peripheral airways	Diffuse, fine; occur initially in the dependent regions	Atelectasis, pneumonia, pulmonary edema, fibrosis

Once you confirm patient-ventilator asynchrony, you should try to identify its underlying cause(s), while simultaneously making efforts to alleviate the patient's respiratory distress:

- Ensure adequate ventilation and oxygenation by disconnecting the patient from the ventilator and providing manual ventilation with 100% O_2 using a BVM device.
- Once the patient is stabilized, perform more detailed assessment and management.
- Removing the patient from the ventilator and manually supporting ventilation and oxygenation can help identify the cause of respiratory distress.
- If the patient's distress resolves upon disconnection, the likely cause of distress is ventilator-related. If the patient's distress continues, it indicates a patient-related problem.

Patient-Related Problems

Airway obstruction (partial or complete) can lead to serious patient-ventilator asynchrony. If airway obstruction is not the problem, you should perform a rapid assessment of the patient to determine other potential causes of distress (e.g., bronchospasm, pulmonary edema, pneumothorax, anxiety, pain). If death appears imminent, you should follow the applicable disease-specific or ACLS protocol before undertaking further patient assessment. Once the patient has been stabilized, you can undertake more detailed assessment and management.

Ventilator-Related Problems

Table 13-15 summarizes the most common ventilator-related problems causing respiratory distress and how to identify them.

Adjust and Check Alarm Systems

Responding properly to ventilatory alarms represents a learned skill that develops fully only with experience. Ventilator alarms indicate ventilator malfunction and changes in patient status that should be corrected by you in an expeditious manner. Alarms can be classified as those set by the ventilator manufacturer (loss of power alarm, gas supply loss, or ventilator malfunction) and those set by you (high/low pressure limit, high/low PEEP, high/low minute ventilation, etc.).

Table 13-16 (see page 406) summarizes some of the most common alarms found in a patient-ventilator system, their recommended settings, and their possible causes.

Alarm systems used by noninvasive positive pressure ventilators (NPPV) vary somewhat according to the manufacturer and device. In general, all NPPV ventilators used in the acute care setting must have a low pressure/disconnect and power failure alarm. Most have a separate apnea alarm and some include high/low volume and high pressure alarms. You generally should respond to these alarms in the same manner as with invasive ventilatory support, with emphasis always on first ensuring that the patient is stable and adequately ventilated and oxygenated. Power failures are a concern with NPPV. When most NPPV ventilators lose power, fresh air is not automatically provided through the circuit, and exhaled air may be rebreathed. Under these circumstances, you must immediately disconnect the patient from the ventilator circuit and provide alternative support for oxygenation and ventilation.

Monitor and Assess Airway Pressures

Airway pressures are key parameters to monitor during mechanical ventilation. Typically, you monitor the peak inspiratory pressure (PIP) and the baseline or PEEP level. Depending on the patient, you also may monitor or manipulate (1) the inspiratory pause (or plateau) pressure, (2) the expiratory pause pressure, and (3) the mean airway pressure (Pmean). Maximum inspiratory and expiratory pressures (MIP/MEP) can also be monitored to assess patient readiness to be weaned during mechanical ventilation. **Figure 13-11** (on page 407) depicts the key pressures you monitor and assess during positive pressure ventilation.

Table 13-15 Identifying Ventilator-Related Problems

Problem/Need	Problem Manifestation
Inadequate F_{IO_2}	• Oxygen analyzer alarm • Low oxygen pressure alarm • Low patient Spo_2 • Clinical signs/symptoms of hypoxemia
Trigger problems	• Auto-PEEP • Patient-ventilator asynchrony • Large drops in pressure at the beginning of inspiration (see ventilator waveforms section) • Increased work of breathing

Flow problems	• During flow-limited ventilation (volume ventilation):
	  • Post-trigger patient effort (flow starvation)
	  • Patient-ventilator asynchrony
	  • Increased work of breathing
	  • "Scooping" of the inspiratory pressure form
	• During pressure-limited ventilation:
	  • Too much flow: spiking of the inspiratory pressure waveform
	  • Insufficient flow: "scooping" of the inspiratory pressure waveform (lack of plateau)

Rate problems	• During CMV
	  • Inverse I:E ratio alarm
	  • Signs of auto-PEEP due to very low I:E ratios
	• During SIMV
	  • Spontaneous rate > 15–20/min
	  • Signs of muscle fatigue/weakness

Tidal volume/pressure limit	• "Beaking" of pressure-volume loop for (indicating overdistention)
Inadequate minute volume	• Hypercapnia/hypocapnia • Minute ventilation < 4–6 L/min for adults
Mode	• Increased work of breathing/respiratory distress • Inability to normalize blood gases, lung mechanics, and other physiology parameters
Auto-PEEP	• Flow not returning to baseline zero at the end of exhalation • Sensitivity problems • Increased work of breathing and/or respiratory distress

Peak Inspiratory Pressure (PIP)

During volume-targeted ventilation the delivered volume is held constant; therefore, PIP and ΔP (PIP-PEEP) will change only if the patient's compliance or resistance changes. Specifically, PIP (and ΔP) will rise if airway resistance increases or lung-thorax compliance falls. Conversely, PIP (and ΔP) will decrease if airway resistance decreases or lung-thorax compliance increases.

However, if the patient's compliance and resistance remain stable, you can cause a change in PIP/ΔP by changing the ventilator's flow, volume, or PEEP settings. PIP rises when you increase either the set flow or volume. Conversely, PIP decreases when you decrease the set flow or volume. Last, adding or removing PEEP raises or lowers the whole airway pressure baseline (and thus PIP) by an equivalent amount. **Table 13-17** (on page 407) summarizes these factors and their effect on PIP during volume-targeted ventilation.

Table 13-16 Common Clinical Alarms During Adult Mechanical Ventilation

Alarm	Recommended Alarm Ventilator Setup (Adults)	Possible Causes
Ventilator Malfunction Alarms		
Loss of power	Preset by manufacturer	• Accidental power cord disconnection • Circuit breakers and fuses • Institutional power failure
Gas supply loss	Preset by manufacturer	• Failure to connect gas hoses • Gas hoses connected to low pressure outlet (e.g., flow meters) • High-pressure line failure
Oxygen analyzer alarm	Usually preset by manufacturer if factory installed (± 5% of setting)	• Gas source failure (air or O_2) • Analyzer needs to be calibrated or replaced • Sudden changes in delivered F_{IO_2} (100% suction)
Patient Status Alarms		
Apnea delay alarm	20 seconds	• Sedation/anesthesia • Low metabolic rate • Low set respiratory rate • Respiratory alkalosis
Low pressure alarm	8 cm H_2O or 5–10 cm below PIP (use spontaneous breaths' PIPs on SIMV)	• Disconnection • Airway/circuit leaks • Alarm set above spontaneous PIP • Improved compliance and/or resistance
High pressure limit	50 cm H_2O or 10–15 cm H_2O above PIP (use mechanical breaths' PIPs on SIMV)	• Increased resistance/decreased compliance • Airway obstruction (partial/complete) • Cough • Secretions, mucous plugs • Patient-ventilator asynchrony • Anxiety, restlessness, pain
Low PEEP/CPAP	3–5 cm H_2O below PEEP	• Disconnection • Airway/circuit leaks
Low exhaled V_T	100 mL or 10–15% below set V_T or spontaneous V_T during SIMV	• Disconnection • Airway/circuit leaks • Pulmonary leaks (broncho-pleural fistula) • Shallow breathing during spontaneous breaths • Coughing • Patient-ventilator asynchrony
Low V_E	4–5 L/min or 10–15% below minimum SIMV or A/C set V_E	• Same as low exhaled V_T • Sedation/anesthesia • Low metabolic rate
High V_E	10–15% above baseline V_E	• Increased metabolic rate (e.g., fever) • Tachypnea • Anxiety, restlessness, pain • Patient waking up from anesthesia/sedation
Temperature	2°C above and below set temperature; not to exceed 37°C	• Dry water chamber • Tubing condensation • Defective wiring, probes, and chamber • Heater malfunctioning • Environmental temperature changes • High minute ventilation and/or high ventilator flow

Adapted from: Shelledy, D. C. Initiating and adjusting ventilatory support. In Wilkins, R. L., Stoller, J. K., & Kacmarek, R. M. (Eds.). *Egan's fundamentals of respiratory care* (9th ed.). St. Louis: Mosby, 2009.

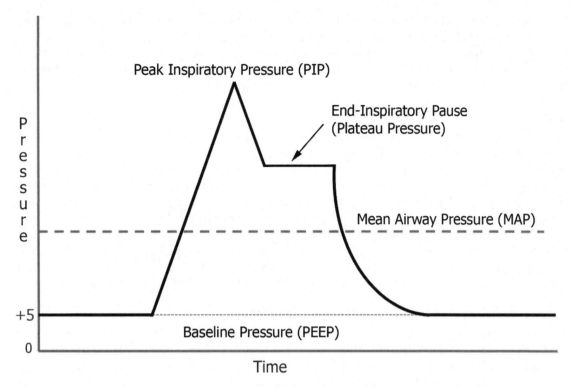

Figure 13-11 Key Pressures That Are Monitored and Assessed During Positive Pressure Ventilation.

Table 13-17 Factors Affecting Peak Pressure During Volume-Targeted Ventilation

	Increases PIP	**Decreases PIP**
Patient factors	Increased airway resistance: • Bronchospasm • Airway edema • Mucous plugging • Kinked tubing	Decreased airway resistance: • Bronchodilator therapy • Resolution of other obstruction (e.g., swelling, secretions, airway edema)
	Decreased compliance: • Pulmonary edema • Surfactant deficiency • Atelectasis • Pneumothorax • Endobronchial intubation • Pneumonia	Increased compliance: • Resolution of pulmonary edema • Re-expansion of lung/lobes • Surfactant instillation • Resolution of pneumonia
Ventilator factors	• Increased flow • Increased V$_T$ • Increased PEEP	• Decreased flow • Decreased V$_T$ • Decreased PEEP

During pressure-limited ventilation, you set the PIP, and ΔP is the only variable held constant during each breath. With ΔP held constant, the VT will change whenever either the patient's compliance or resistance changes. Specifically, VT will tend to decrease when airway resistance increases or lung-thorax compliance falls. Conversely, VT will tend to increase when airway resistance decreases or lung-thorax compliance increases.

Inspiratory Pause (or Plateau) Pressure

During an inspiratory pause or plateau maneuver, flow stops but the exhalation valve remains closed, holding the delivered volume in the lungs. Under these static conditions, any pressure due to flow resistance is eliminated. Thus the PIP drops and holds at a lower level, called the plateau pressure, or Pplat (see Figure 13-11). If a good plateau can be obtained, the resulting pressure is equivalent to the alveolar pressure at that volume. The same factors described in Table 13-17 causing changes in lung compliance and resistance equally apply for plateau pressure changes.

Because the plateau pressure represents the force being applied to stretch the alveoli, it is an important safety measure. In order to prevent ventilator-associated lung injury, you should always try to prevent Pplat from rising above 30 cm H_2O. You can also use Pplat (along with the PIP and PEEP) to calculate the patient's static compliance and airway resistance, as described in the next section.

Measuring Pulmonary Compliance and Airway Resistance

The NBRC hospital expects that you can interpret changes or trends in PIP and Pplat pressures over time, either from flow sheet data or by graphic analysis. The key changes of interest are the difference between PIP and Pplat (airway resistance) and the difference between Pplat and PEEP (compliance):

- Pplat – PEEP = ΔP due to elastic resistance (compliance)
- PIP – Pplat = ΔP due to flow resistance (Raw)

Measuring Compliance

To measure compliance, you institute an inspiratory hold during a volume-targeted breath. If the time is sufficient to ensure equilibration of airway and alveolar pressures, a pressure plateau results. The difference between this plateau pressure (Pplat) and the baseline or PEEP pressure is the force needed to maintain the lungs and thorax at the delivered volume under static conditions. By dividing the corrected tidal volume by this pressure difference, we derive a close estimate of total lung and chest wall compliance (C_{LT}), also called static or effective compliance:

$$C_{LT} = \frac{VT_c}{Pplat - PEEP}$$

When interpreting and assessing static compliance the following must be considered:

- Normal C_{LT} ranges between 60 and 100 mL/cm H_2O (0.06–0.1 L/cm H_2O).
- Diseases of the lung parenchyma such as pneumonia, pulmonary edema, and any chronic diseases causing fibrosis are all associated with decreased compliance.
- Acute changes, such as atelectasis, pulmonary edema, ARDS, or lung compression due to a tension pneumothorax may cause a rapid drop in C_{LT}.
- When C_{LT} is less than 25–30 mL/cm H_2O, as may occur in severe ARDS, the amount of work needed to maintain adequate ventilation is very high and can quickly lead to muscle fatigue and respiratory failure, thus making weaning from ventilatory support difficult.

Measuring Airway Resistance

You also can use Pplat to estimate a patient's airway resistance (Raw). Since PIP reflects total impedance, and Pplat – PEEP corresponds to the pressure needed to overcome elastic recoil (compliance), then the difference between PIP and Pplat must be due to airway resistance. If the inspiratory flow is constant and known with accuracy, then you can estimate airway resistance according to the following formula:

$$\text{Raw} = \frac{\text{PIP} - \text{Pplat}}{\dot{V}(L/sec)}$$

Normal adult airway resistance ranges from about 0.5 to 2.5 cm H_2O/L/sec. An increase in Raw above 10–15 cm H_2O/L/sec in an intubated patient with otherwise normal lungs signals abnormal airway narrowing due to such factors as increased secretions, bronchospasm, pulmonary vascular congestion, or partial occlusion of the artificial airway.

The accompanying box provides an example of these computations, including interpretation of changes over time for an adult patient receiving ventilatory support. Note that in most cases you will need to convert the ventilator flow from L/min to L/sec to obtain an accurate measure of airway resistance (L/min ÷ 60 = L/sec). The mnemonic RCP (Respiratory Care Practitioner *or* Resistance, Compliance, and PEEP) can help you to remember the relationships described in this section. See **Figure 13-12** for a graphic explanation of this mnemonic.

Measuring and Assessing Compliance and Resistance

An adult patient receiving volume-targeted ventilatory support exhibits the following parameters over the designated 4-hour period:

			Time	
Parameter	7:00	8:00	9:00	10:00
V_T (mL)	500	500	500	500
Inspiratory flow (L/min)	40	40	40	40
PIP cm H_2O	50	55	60	65
Pplat cm H_2O	30	30	30	30
PEEP cm H_2O	5	5	5	5

Problems

1. What is the patient's static compliance and airway resistance at 7:00 AM?

2. What major change in this patient's lung mechanics is occurring over these 4 hours?

Solutions

1. Compute static compliance and airway resistance at 7:00 AM:

Compliance:

$$C_{LT} = \frac{V_{T_C}}{\text{Pplat} - \text{PEEP}} = \frac{500}{30 - 5} = \frac{500}{25} = 20 \text{ mL/cm } H_2O$$

Airway Resistance:

First convert L/min to L/sec:

　　L/min ÷ 60 = L/sec

　　40 L/min = 0.67 L/sec

Then compute the airway resistance:

$$\text{Raw} = \frac{\text{PIP} - \text{Pplat}}{\dot{V}(L/sec)} = \frac{50 - 30}{0.67 \text{ L/sec}} = \frac{20 \text{ cm } H_2O}{0.64 \text{ L/sec}} = 29.9 \text{ cm } H_2O/L/sec$$

2. Identify the major change in this patient's lung mechanics over these 4 hours:

- Pplat – PEEP remains constant, so compliance remains unchanged (at 20 mL/cm H_2O)

- PIP – Pplat increases from 20 cm H_2O to 35 cm H_2O, so airway resistance is increasing

---

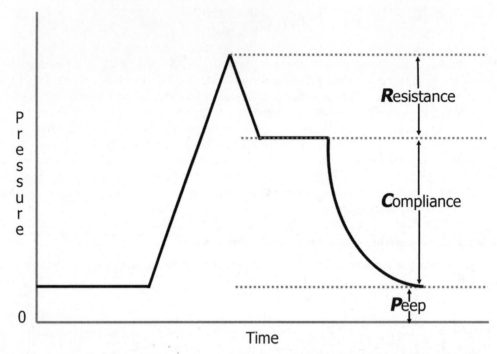

Figure 13-12 RCP (Resistance – Compliance – PEEP) Mnemonic for Relating Airway Pressures During Volume-Targeted Mechanical Ventilation to Lung Mechanics.

End-Expiratory Pause Pressure (Measuring Auto-PEEP)

Like an inspiratory pause, an end-expiratory pause creates a condition of no flow. Under these static conditions, airway and alveolar pressures equilibrate. Thus the end-expiratory pause pressure is also equivalent to alveolar pressure, but in this case measured at the very end of exhalation (just before a new breath is triggered).

Normally, alveolar pressure should be the same as the baseline pressure (or PEEP) at this point in the breathing cycle. However, if any gas remains trapped in the alveoli at end-expiration (dynamic hyperinflation or air trapping), the alveolar pressure at the end of exhalation will exceed the airway pressure baseline or PEEP. As indicated in **Figure 13-13**, if at this point you stop flow and institute a pause, the airway pressure will equilibrate with the higher alveolar pressure, causing a momentary rise in the baseline pressure. This rise in baseline pressure corresponds to the level of residual pressure (and volume) "trapped" in the alveoli that does not fully escape during exhalation. We call this residual pressure *auto-PEEP*. Auto-PEEP can negatively affect ventilator triggering, increase patient-ventilator asynchrony, and impose additional work of breathing on the patient. For causes and management of auto-PEEP, refer to Chapters 14 and 15.

Mean Airway Pressure

The mean airway pressure (Pmean or MAP) is the average pressure applied to the airway over time (refer to Figure 13-11). Factors over which you have control that affect Pmean during mechanical ventilation include all of the following:

- Ventilator mode
- Ventilator rate
- Tidal volume or pressure limit
- Inspiratory pressure waveform
- I:E ratio
- PEEP level

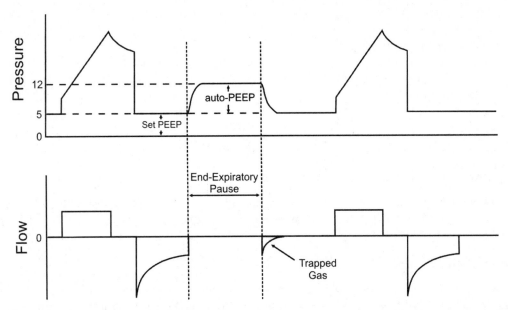

Figure 13-13 Implementation of an End-Expiratory Pause to Measure Auto-PEEP. Occlusion of the expiratory valve toward the end of expiration causes equilibration between the alveoli and airway. A rise in airway pressure rises above the baseline/PEEP level indicates the presence of auto-PEEP. The amount of auto-PEEP is calculated as the difference between the end-expiratory pause pressure and the PEEP pressure, in this case $12 - 5 = 7$ cm H_2O. At the end of the pause, the expiratory valve opens and the remaining trapped gas is exhaled (volume corresponding to the gray area).

All else being equal, you will observe higher Pmean values when there are more machine breaths per minute (higher ventilator rates in control or assist/control modes); larger tidal volumes or pressure limits; "square" inspiratory pressure patterns (including use of inflation hold), higher I:E ratios; and higher PEEP levels. In contrast, you will observe lower Pmean values when there are fewer machine breaths and more spontaneous breaths (e.g., SIMV); lower tidal volumes or pressure limits; nonsquare pressure patterns; lower I:E ratios; and lower PEEP settings.

As Pmean increases, so does the functional residual capacity (FRC). In disease states associated with alveolar collapse and shunting, increases in FRC tend to improve oxygenation and raise the PaO_2. Thus, adjusting Pmean is one more method (in addition to adjusting FIO_2 and PEEP) you can use to alter patient oxygenation. Unfortunately, high Pmean levels can decrease venous return and cardiac output and also increase the risk of pulmonary barotrauma (pneumothorax, pneumomediastinum, subcutaneous emphysema, etc.).

Monitor and Assess I:E Ratios

A more detailed assessment of ventilatory time parameters includes measurement of the inspiratory to expiratory time ratio (I:E ratio) and its components. The I:E ratio is simply the ratio of inspiratory time (I-time) to expiratory time (E-time) during the breathing cycle. You must know how to calculate and adjust time variables when monitoring and assessing patients on mechanical ventilation. Chapter 15 provides details on adjusting time parameters. Our focus here is recognizing normal and abnormal time patterns and performing the needed calculations.

The following key points pertain to the assessment of time parameters:

- In normal individuals the I:E ratio ranges from 1:2 to 1:3.
- In patients with expiratory airflow obstruction (e.g., COPD patients), the E-time is typically prolonged. This results in lower I:E ratios, such as 1:4 or 1:5. A prolonged E-time and low I:E ratio is a cardinal sign of expiratory airflow obstruction!

- Ratios greater than 1:1 (I-time exceeds E-time) are called inverse I:E ratios. Although controversial, inverse I:E ratios are sometimes used during pressure control ventilation to improve oxygenation and lower PEEP levels.
- During flow-limited mechanical ventilation, the delivered volume is a function of the I-time and flow. To compute the required inspiratory flow for a patient receiving flow-limited ventilation, use the following formula:

$$\dot{V}insp = \frac{\dot{V}E}{\%I\text{-time}}$$

where $\dot{V}E$ is the patient's minute volume and %I-time the percent inspiratory time.

Table 13-18 describes some of the most common time parameter calculations you need to master to succeed on the NBRC exam. For examples and good guidance on performing these and other calculations, refer to Chapter 20.

Interpret Airway Graphics

Most mechanical ventilators are equipped with sensors, software, and display equipment that allow graphic visualization of pressure, volume, and flow waveforms during breathing. You can use ventilator graphics to assess or detect:

- Ventilator modes
- Patient-ventilator synchrony
- Adverse events
- Responses to therapy

The most common respiratory waveforms are pressure, flow, and volume over time (scalar graphics) and pressure-volume and flow-volume loops. **Tables 13-19 through 13-22** (on pages 413–416) describe the most common normal configurations and characteristics of these graphs. Chapter 14 provides more detail on using ventilator graphics to modify ventilatory support.

Table 13-18 Time Parameter Calculations

Time Parameter	Description	Formula
Inspiratory time (I-time)	Time in seconds devoted to inspiration	$\dfrac{\text{Total cycle time}}{\text{Sum of I:E ratio parts}}$ or Total cycle time × %I-time
Expiratory time (E-time)	Time in seconds devoted to expiration	Total cycle time − I-time
I:E ratio	Whole number ratio of I-time to E-time, with I-time set to unity (1)	$\dfrac{\text{I-time}}{\text{I-time}} : \dfrac{\text{E-time}}{\text{I-time}}$
Total cycle time	Total breath duration in seconds, from start of one inspiration to another	$\dfrac{60}{f}$ or (I-time + E-time)
Frequency	Number of breaths per minute	$\dfrac{60}{\text{Total cycle time}}$
%I-time ("duty cycle")	Ratio of I-time to total cycle time as a percentage	$\dfrac{\text{I-time}}{\text{Total cycle time}} \times 100$

Table 13-19 Most Common Normal Ventilator Volume-Time Graphics and Their Characteristics

Typical Waveform	Characteristics
Normal volume-time graphic 	• Most often used to detect leaks by comparing inspiratory and expiratory volume. • During volume control mode breath-to-breath variation is minimal (V_T is set and constant). • During pressure control ventilation, breath-to-breath variation can occur due to changes in thoracic-lung compliance.
Volume-time graphic of inflation hold (plateau maneuver) 	Plateau maneuver: • Volume-time waveform during an inspiratory plateau maneuver. • Volume is held on the lungs under static conditions until the inspiratory pause time ends.
Volume-time graphic of SIMV with pressure support 	SIMV with pressure support: • Mechanically controlled breaths are generally larger with a constant mechanical volume. • Spontaneous patient breaths are smaller and vary from breath to breath.
Volume-time graphic during CPAP/PSV (bi-level positive airway pressure) 	CPAP with pressure support: • Note the difference in volume size in comparison with a mechanical breath. • Volume may vary from breath to breath.

Table 13-20 Most Common Normal Ventilator Pressure-Time Waveforms and Their Characteristics

Typical Waveform	Characteristics
Pressure-time graphic during volume-targeted ventilation *(Pressure vs. Time graph showing sawtooth waveforms with "Patient-Triggered" labeled, +5 and 0 marked on Pressure axis)*	• Pressure waveform may vary from breath to breath due to changes in the patient's lung/thoracic compliance and resistance. • Can be used to assess proper sensitivity settings of the assisted breaths if pressure trigger is being used. • During pressure triggering, the absence of a trigger effort indicates a mechanical, time-triggered breath.
Pressure-time graphic with inflation hold (plateau) *(Pressure vs. Time graph with "Peak Inspiratory Pressure (PIP)", "End-Inspiratory Pause (Plateau Pressure)", "Baseline Pressure (PEEP)" labeled, +5 and 0 marked on Pressure axis)*	• During an inspiratory hold maneuver the plateau pressures will reflect true alveolar pressures during static conditions. • Use to calculate patient's resistance and compliance.
Pressure-time graphic of volume-targeted SIMV with pressure support *(Pressure vs. Time graph with "Mechanical Breaths", "Spontaneous Breaths", "Patient-Triggered", "PEEP", "Time-Triggered" labeled, +5 and 0 marked on Pressure axis)*	• Mechanical breath pressures are higher than spontaneous pressure-supported breaths. • Can be used to assess proper sensitivity settings of the assisted breaths if pressure trigger is being used.
Pressure-time graphic of pressure control ventilation (PCV) *(Pressure vs. Time graph showing square waveforms, +5 and 0 marked on Pressure axis)*	• The pressure remains constant throughout inspiration until the breath ends, hence the square shape of the waveform. • Since the pressure limit remains constant for each mechanical breath, all breath will have the same height.

(continues)

Table 13-20 Most Common Normal Ventilator Pressure-Time Waveforms and Their Characteristics (continued)

Typical Waveform	Characteristics
Pressure-time graphic of PCV with different rise times	• Rise time is the time that it takes to reach the set pressure during inspiration. Usually expressed in % of I-time. • Can be use to troubleshoot patient-ventilator asynchrony or fine tune ventilator settings.
Pressure-time graphic of CPAP	• All breaths are spontaneous breaths. • Patient breathes during inspiration *and* exhalation at a baseline airway pressure above zero.

Table 13-21 Most Common Normal Ventilator Flow-Time Waveforms and Their Characteristics

Typical Waveform	Characteristics
Flow-time graphic during volume-targeted ventilation	• During flow-limited volume ventilation, the flow will be a square waveform during inspiration (A). • The rise time can also be adjusted on the flow during volume ventilation to troubleshoot patient-ventilator asynchrony or fine tune ventilator settings (B). • Also use to assess for auto-PEEP or air trapping.
Flow-time graphic during pressure control ventilation (PCV)	• During pressure-limited or pressure-controlled ventilation, the flow is decelerating during inspiration. • Also use to assess for auto-PEEP or air trapping.

Table 13-22 Most Common Mechanical Ventilator Loops and Their Characteristics

Typical Waveform	Characteristics
Pressure-volume loops *(graph: Volume vs Pressure, loops A, B, C labeled with Compliance and Resistance)*	• Graphic representation of the pressure needed to deliver a certain volume. • Helps you assess "at a glance" the patient's resistance and compliance. • Patient's compliance is given by the slope of the curve. The higher the slope (loop A) the less pressure need to deliver the VT (higher compliance). Compare to loop C, where high pressure is required to deliver a smaller VT (low slope indicates low compliance). • Airway resistance is assessed by the width of the loop. The thinner the loop (C), the less airway resistance. A thicker loop (B) indicates increased airway resistance.
Flow-volume loops *(graph: Flow vs Volume, loops A and B, PEFR, PIFR, Reduced Flows; Normal ——, Abnormal ·······)*	• Help you to classify the nature of the airway impairment as either restrictive (reduced volumes), obstructive (reduced flows), or both. • Loop A shows an obstructive patient with reduced expiratory flows and normal volume. • Loop B shows a restrictive process with normal expiratory flows but reduced tidal volume.

Measure FIO$_2$ and/or Liter Flow

According to the AARC, all O$_2$-delivery systems should be checked at least once per day. More frequent checks using a calibrated O$_2$ analyzer should be performed on O$_2$ systems that are:

- Susceptible to variation in O$_2$ concentration
- Applied to patients with artificial airways
- Delivering a heated gas mixture
- Applied to patients who are clinically unstable or require an FIO$_2$ of 0.50 or greater

O$_2$ analysis is particularly important in the care of neonates and infants, due to the risks of oxygen toxicity and retinopathy of prematurity (ROP). To protect against equipment failure causing hypoxemia, you should also monitor FIO$_2$s continuously during mechanical ventilation.

Key points to consider when measuring a patient's FIO$_2$:

- The analyzer probe must be placed proximal to the patient's airway.
- If the goal is continuous monitoring of FIO$_2$ in a ventilator circuit, place the probe proximal to any active humidification systems (before the humidifier). This will avoid the problem of condensation on the sensor, which can cause erroneous readings.
- When analyzing the FIO$_2$ in a pediatric or neonatal oxygen enclosure, place the probe close to the infant's face at the bottom of the enclosure (because oxygen is heavier than nitrogen, it tends to settle).
- If being used for continuous monitoring, set the analyzer's alarms to ±5% of the prescribed FIO$_2$.

For more detail on the proper use and calibration of O$_2$ analyzers, see Chapter 8.

COMMON ERRORS TO AVOID

You can improve your score by avoiding these mistakes:

- Do not perform an Allen test when drawing an ABG from the brachial artery site. There is not collateral circulation to assess for this artery.
- Avoid placing O_2 analyzers distal to a heated humidifier in ventilator circuits; humidity and water vapor pressure may affect the analyzer's readings.
- Avoid performing a capillary blood test in a neonate less than 24 hours old.
- Avoid radial punctures for ABGs if the Allen is negative. Repeat the test on the opposite hand. If still negative, use the brachial artery instead.
- Avoid drawing blood from a distal port of a pulmonary catheter too fast or with the balloon inflated since it may contaminate the sample with arterial blood.
- Do not use pulse oximetry to assess oxygenation in a patient suspected of carbon monoxide (CO) poisoning due to smoke inhalation. The SpO_2 will read falsely high. Recommend CO-oximetry instead.
- Do not evaluate a patient's minute ventilation alone. Always assess for proper VT and rate in conjunction with the minute ventilation.
- Do not use a capillary blood gas test to assess oxygenation status.

SURE BETS

In some situations you can be sure of the right approach to a clinical problem or scenario:

- Always target hemoglobin saturation above 90–92% in order to maintain proper tissue oxygenation.
- Always use pressure monitor alarms for acutely ill patients receiving noninvasive positive pressure ventilation or those requiring long-term 24-hour support.
- During volume control ventilation, an increase in the set flow rate will cause an increase in the peak inspiratory pressure and vice versa. Manipulation of the flow will also affect inspiratory times and I:E ratios.
- Always warm up the site for a capillary blood test before performing the puncture to allow for vasodilation and arterialization of the blood.
- The most efficient breathing pattern is slow, deep breathing.
- During A/C volume-cycled ventilation, changes in the tidal volume, rate, and flow will affect the I:E ratio.
- A healthy adult patient receiving 100% O_2 at sea level should have a PaO_2 of about 650 torr.
- When assessing changes on peak inspiratory pressures during volume-controlled ventilation always evaluate the plateau pressure to determine if a change in resistance or a change in compliance is the primary cause.
- Always set the high/low CPAP/PEEP pressure alarms at ±3–5 cm H_2O above and below set pressure.
- Always confirm SpO_2 accuracy by correlating the heart rate, assessing pulse strength, and evaluating the SpO_2 waveform.
- When interpreting blood gases, always assess ventilation (pH, $PaCO_2$) and oxygenation (PaO_2, SaO_2) separately.
- Always perform an Allen test when drawing an ABG from the radial artery site.
- Normal breath sounds heard at abnormal locations are always an abnormal finding.
- Always use a chest radiograph (or bronchoscopic visualization) to *confirm* proper placement of an endotracheal tube; use bilateral breath sounds and a positive CO_2 colorimetry reading only as a preliminary indicator of proper placement.

PRE-TEST ANSWERS AND EXPLANATIONS

Below are this chapter's pre-test answers and explanations. Be sure to review each answer's explanation thoroughly to help you understand why it is correct. If the explanation is still unclear to you, review the chapter contents or the references and/or refer to this chapter's supplemental resources on the CD.

13-1. Correct answer: B. III, IV, and V. Flat diaphragms and increased radiolucency throughout the lung fields are common in the chest X-ray of a any patient with a COPD condition, as are a *decrease* in peripheral vascular markings, an *increased* retrosternal airspace, and a *narrow* mediastinum.

13-2. Correct answer: A. Patient motion artifact. The most common source of error and false alarms with pulse oximetry is motion artifact. Securing the sensor properly or relocating of the sensor to an earlobe, a toe, or an external naris can help minimize this problem.

13-3. Correct answer: C. Increased work of breathing. Controlled ventilation is poorly tolerated by many patients, often resulting in asynchronous breathing efforts or strenuous attempts to breathe spontaneously. Both conditions can increase the work of breathing, and with it, the oxygen consumption of the respiratory muscles. It is for this reason that sedation or paralysis is often required when controlled ventilation is necessary.

13-4. Correct answer: A. Acute alveolar hyperventilation without hypoxemia. The high pH indicates alkalemia. The low Pa_{CO_2} indicates hyperventilation, consistent with the high pH (respiratory alkalosis). The normal HCO_3 and BE indicate *no* metabolic involvement, hence compensation has *not* begun yet (acute process). The Pa_{O_2} is in the acceptable range at a low F_{IO_2} (no hypoxemia present). Conclusion: acute respiratory alkalosis due to alveolar hyperventilation without hypoxemia.

13-5. Correct answer: C. II, III, and IV. The high-pressure-limit alarm should be set about 10–15 cm H_2O above the peak airway pressure of the mechanical controlled breaths. The low-PEEP/CPAP alarm should always be set 3–5 cm H_2O or 20% below the set baseline pressure. A low exhaled volume alarm should trigger when either the V_T or $\dot{V}_E$ falls 20% below preset values (6 L/min in this question). I:E ratio alarms are used to detect inverse ratios caused by an increased respiratory rate commonly seen during failure of SIMV weaning trials or during patient-ventilator asynchrony.

13-6. Correct answer: D. 90%. Normal Sa_{O_2} should be more than 95% breathing room air. Levels below 90% indicate the need for supplemental O_2 therapy. Drops in oxyhemoglobin content are usually the result of cardiac, pulmonary, or combined cardiopulmonary disease. *Hb saturation data must always be interpreted with knowledge of Hb/Hct levels.* For example, a patient with an Sp_{O_2} of 97% and severe anemia (Hb < 7 g/dL) is still suffering from hypoxemia, due to reduced blood O_2 content.

13-7. Correct answer: B. 35 mL/cm H_2O. Static compliance equals corrected tidal volume divided by the plateau pressure – PEEP. In this instance, static compliance = 700 ÷ (30 – 10) = 700 ÷ 20 = 35 mL/cm H_2O.

13-8. Correct answer: B. Noninvasive pulse oximetry. Besides vital signs, a noninvasive technique like continuous pulse oximetry is the standard of care to monitor the cardiopulmonary status of a patient during moderate sedation procedures. More expensive, invasive techniques such as PFTs or an A-line insertion are required only when more critical, invasive procedures are being done.

13-9. Correct answer: B. 1.00 sec. Given the rate (f) and percent inspiratory time (%I-time), the inspiratory time (I-time) can be computed as: total cycle time × %I-time. Total cycle time = 60/f = 60/12 = 5 sec. I-time = 5 sec × 0.20 = 1.00 sec.

13-10. **Correct answer: B.** Increased cardiac output. Causes of a $PETCO_2$ of zero include (1) a large system leak or disconnection, (2) esophageal intubation, (3) cardiac arrest, and (4) a totally obstructed/kinked artificial airway. Increased cardiac output would cause a *rise* in end-tidal CO_2.

13-11. **Correct answer: D.** The patient is developing atelectasis. The cause of the increased peak inspiratory pressures cannot be increased airway resistance since the (peak – plateau) pressure difference remains constant at ~10 cm H_2O. What is changing is the (Pplat – PEEP) pressure difference, which is increasing due to a gradual rise in plateau pressures. This indicates a decrease in either lung or thoracic compliance. Atelectasis, which causes consolidation, decreases lung compliance. Bronchospasm causes an increase in airway resistance with a widening of the PIP-Pplat difference.

13-12. **Correct answer: A.** Carotid. The radial artery is the preferred site for arterial blood sampling because (1) it is near the skin surface, (2) the ulnar artery provides for good collateral circulation, and (3) the artery is not near any large veins. Other sites include the brachial, femoral, and dorsalis pedis arteries. These sites carry greater risk and should be used only by those with training in alternative site sampling. Carotid arteries are never to be used for arterial puncture.

13-13. **Correct answer: A.** Compensated metabolic acidosis. First, you should recognize that compensation is occurring with this patient because *both* the $PaCO_2$ and BE are abnormally low. Second, because the pH is less than 7.40, you can conclude that the primary problem is the one causing acidosis, in this case the low BE (–10 mEq/L). Therefore, the low $PaCO_2$ must represent compensation for the low BE. Conclusion: the patient has a compensated metabolic acidosis.

13-14. **Correct answer: D.** Proper blood pressure and waveform. The Allen test is indicated only to assess for collateral circulation on the radial artery site *before* performing the procedure. Blood return and ability to flush the line can also occur if the catheter has been inserted on a venous vessel. The best indication that the line has been properly inserted on an artery is the return of arterial blood pressure values accompanied by a good arterial waveform once the line is connected to the transducer and the monitor.

13-15. **Correct answer: C.** I and III only. When obtaining a mixed venous sample, if the balloon is not deflated or the sample is withdrawn too quickly, you may contaminate the venous blood with blood from the pulmonary capillaries (oxygenated blood). The result is always a falsely high oxygen level. Rapid flow of IV fluid can also dilute the blood sample and affect oxygen content measures.

13-16. **Correct answer: C.** Proximal to the heated humidifier. Inaccurate readings can occur with electrochemical oxygen analyzers due to either condensed water vapor or pressure fluctuations. Galvanic cells are particularly sensitive to condensation. To avoid this problem during continuous use in humidified ventilator circuits, place the analyzer sensor proximal (before the humidifer) to any humidification device.

13-17. **Correct answer: B.** It should not be performed in infants less than 72 hours old. A capillary blood puncture should not be performed in infants less than 24 hours old due to the immaturity of the capillary bed after birth. Capillary blood sampling also should be avoided on the heels of infants that have just begun walking; on inflamed, swollen, or edematous tissue; on cyanotic or poorly perfused areas; and when accurate analysis of the oxygenation status is needed.

13-18. **Correct answer: B.** Repeat the test on the right hand. The results of the initial Allen test indicate lack of collateral circulation on the left hand. You should repeat the Allen test on the opposite hand and proceed accordingly. Brachial puncture should be considered if the Allen test fails to show proper collateral circulation in both radial arteries.

13-19. **Correct answer: A.** Decrease the SIMV rate. The blood gas results suggest normal oxygenation with an uncompensated respiratory alkalosis due to hyperventilation. The fact that there is no spontaneous ventilation (total rate = set rate) indicates suppression of the respiratory drive probably due to hypocapnia. In order to stimulate the patient to breathe spontaneously, you need to eliminate the hypocapnia. On the SIMV mode this is best done by decreasing the set respiratory rate on the ventilator.

13-20. **Correct answer: C.** I, II, and IV. During volume-controlled ventilation a sudden fall in peak inspiratory pressure can be caused by any of the following events: (1) improved compliance or resistance; (2) a decrease in either the volume or flow setting; and (3) patient-ventilator system leaks, such as an ET tube cuff leak, a malfunctioning exhalation valve, or tubing disconnection/leak.

13-21. **Correct answer: B.** Pulse oximetry. Due to the patient's involvement in a house fire you should immediately suspect the presence of carbon monoxide poisoning. Carbon monoxide's high affinity for hemoglobin will cause profound hypoxemia. Pulse oximetry is unable to measure carbon monoxide saturations and is contraindicated to assess patients with suspected smoke inhalation. In order to assess for the presence of carbon monoxide in the blood you must run a CO-oximetry blood gas test.

13-22. **Correct answer: D.** Assess for pain. It is very common for a patient after any invasive procedure to develop surgical pain. Since the patient is mechanically ventilated and cannot verbally communicate, abnormal vital signs (usually on the high side of normal) are a common indication of the presence of pain. Asking the patient to indicate if he or she is in pain and providing for proper pain management is the right course of action. Paralytics are indicated for patient-ventilator asynchrony. A chest tube should not be repositioned without assessing a chest X-ray first; asking the patient to relax will not alleviate the pain.

13-23. **Correct answer: B.** Preoxygenate the patient with 100% O_2. Hypoxia and mechanical stimulation of the myocardium are common causes of premature ventricular contractions (PVCs). Several respiratory procedures can cause hypoxia and produce PVCs. Preoxygenating and hyperinflating the patient before suctioning is always required to avoid hypoxia and myocardial irritability, especially in patients suffering from preexisting cardiac diseases. Using a larger catheter, sedating the patient, and suctioning less often will not prevent the hypoxia and the PVCs caused by the hypoxia itself.

13-24. **Correct answer: A.** Thoracic gas volume. Tests that are indicated to assess for the presence and the degree of airway responsiveness are: methacholine bronchoprovocation studies, histamine challenge, and exercise challenge tests. They are also indicated to screen individuals who may be at risk from environmental or occupational exposure to allergens. Thoracic gas volume (via body plethysmography) does not assess for airway responsiveness and reactivity.

13-25. **Correct answer: C.** Liver enzymes. Liver enzymes are indicated to assess suspected liver damage due to infections, alcohol and drug abuse, among others. Cardiac enzymes are indicated when myocardial damage is suspected due to an MI or ischemia. Complete blood count and partial prothrombin time are indicated to evaluate red and white blood cell counts and coagulation status of the blood.

POST-TEST

A post test for this section that includes automated scoring and feedback is available on the accompanying CD. Be sure to complete this additional assessment to confirm your mastery of this section's objectives.

REFERENCES

American Association for Respiratory Care. (1992). Clinical practice guideline. Pulse oximetry. *Respiratory care, 37*, 891–897.

American Association for Respiratory Care. (2001). Clinical practice guideline. Blood gas analysis and hemoximetry. 2001 revision and update. *Respiratory care, 46*, 498–505.

American Association for Respiratory Care. (2001). Clinical practice guideline. Capillary blood gas sampling for neonatal and pediatric patients. *Respiratory care, 46*, 506–513.

American Association for Respiratory Care. (2002). Clinical practice guideline. Oxygen therapy for adults in the acute care facility: 2002 revision and update. *Respiratory care, 47*, 717–720.

American Association for Respiratory Care. (2003). Clinical practice guideline. Capnography/capnometry during mechanical ventilation. 2003 revision and update. *Respiratory care, 48*, 534–539.

Hess, D., & MacIntyre, N. (Eds.). (2002). *Respiratory care: principles and practice*. Philadelphia: W. B. Saunders.

Ruppel, G. L. (2009). *Manual of pulmonary function testing* (9th ed.). St. Louis: Mosby.

Wilkins, R. L., Stoller, J. K., & Kacmarek, R. (Eds.). (2009). *Egan's fundamentals of respiratory care* (9th ed.). St. Louis: Mosby.

Wilkins, R. L., Dexter, J. R., & Heuer, A. J. (2009). *Clinical assessment in respiratory care* (6th ed.). St. Louis: Mosby.

Independently Modify Therapeutic Procedures Based on the Patient's Response

Albert J. Heuer

INTRODUCTION

After respiratory therapy is initiated, your responsibility is to monitor the patient's clinical status regularly, as outlined earlier in this text. Based on the patient's response and changes in clinical status, you often will need to modify or recommend changes in the therapy. This chapter discusses how you can help determine the need to modify therapy, as well as the most common types of changes that you may independently implement in a given situation. Other changes that you may only recommend (because they require a physician's order) are described subsequently in Chapter 15. The following objectives have been established for this chapter to help ensure you are ready for the CRT exam and to sharpen the skills needed to be effective in a clinical setting.

OBJECTIVES

After completion of this chapter, you should be able to demonstrate the knowledge needed to:

1. Terminate treatment based on therapeutic goal attainment, adverse effects, or end-of-life considerations
2. Modify treatment techniques, including IPPB, IS, aerosol therapy, oxygen, and specialty gas (heliox, nitric oxide) therapies; bronchial hygiene; and suctioning
3. Adjust or alter artificial airway management techniques according to patient needs
4. Monitor, modify, and adjust both invasive and noninvasive mechanical ventilation settings in order to optimize oxygenation, ventilation, and patient synchrony
5. Initiate procedures for weaning

WHAT TO EXPECT ON THIS CATEGORY OF THE CRT EXAM

Number of questions: 18
Level of questions: mostly application and analysis, with two recall questions

WHAT'S NEW FOR 2009

As of July 2009, this section of the NBRC CRT examination includes the following *new content areas*:

- Modify specialty gas therapy
  - Heliox (He/O_2)
  - Nitric oxide (NO)

PRE-TEST

Carefully respond to each of the following questions. After completing the pre-test, compare your answers with those provided at the end of this chapter. Then thoroughly review each answer's explanation to help understand why it is correct.

14-1. While suctioning a patient, you observe an abrupt change in the ECG waveform being displayed on the cardiac monitor and a drop in SpO_2. Which of the following actions should you take?
  A. Change to a smaller catheter and repeat the procedure
  B. Stop suctioning and immediately administer oxygen
  C. Decrease the amount of negative pressure being used
  D. Instill 10 mL normal saline directly into the trachea

14-2. After initiating a bronchodilator aerosol via IPPB to an asthmatic, the patient complains of fatigue and shortness of breath. On inspection of the patient, you note increased use of accessory muscles, an increase in heart rate from 90 to 122, and other signs of mild to moderate distress. Which of the following is the appropriate action at this time?
  A. Stop the treatment and immediately chart this untoward reaction
  B. Decrease the flow and have the patient exhale more forcibly
  C. Increase the pressure limit and get the patient to breathe slower
  D. Stop the treatment and stay with the patient until she improves

14-3. A patient is receiving appropriate oxygen therapy via a simple mask at 5 L/min but complains that the mask is confining and interferes with eating. Which of the following oxygen-delivery devices is a suitable alternative?
  A. Nasal cannula at 4–5 L/min
  B. Nasal cannula at 2 L/min
  C. Nonrebreather mask at 10 L/min
  D. A 28% venturi mask at 10 L/min

14-4. During an IPPB treatment being given to a 66-year-old COPD patient, you note signs of further air trapping during exhalation. Which of the following changes in technique should you consider?
  I. Instructing the patient to prolong exhalation
  II. Increasing the inspiratory flow rate
  III. Increasing the preset pressure limit
  IV. Retarding exhalation via a PEEP valve
  A. I, II, and III
  B. II and IV only
  C. II, III, and IV
  D. I, II, and IV

14-5. After initiating nasal CPAP on a patient, you set the prescribed pressure and turn the flow generator on. At this point the mask pressure reading is 0 cm H_2O. The most likely cause of this problem is:
  A. Electrical failure
  B. A large system leak
  C. Patient asynchrony
  D. Too high a flow

14-6. You notice that the air-entrainment ports of a venturi mask are occluded by a patient's bedding. What effect would this have on total flow and FIO_2?
  A. Increase total output flow and decrease FIO_2
  B. Increase both total output flow and FIO_2
  C. Decrease both total flow output and FIO_2
  D. Decrease total output flow and increase FIO_2

14-7. To prevent <u>hypoxemia</u> during suctioning an orally intubated patient, you should do which of the following?
  A. Press alarm silence prior to suctioning
  B. Set vacuum pressure to 100–120 mm Hg before procedure
  C. Administer 100% oxygen through the ventilator for 1–2 minutes before suctioning
  D. Maintain the set FIO_2 and increase PEEP prior to suctioning

14-8. A 48-year-old male is orally intubated, receiving mechanical ventilation with a #7.0 endotracheal tube secured in place. Cuff pressure is found to be 34 cm H_2O during peak inspiration using the minimal occluding volume technique. You should suggest:

A. Replacing the endotracheal tube with a smaller size

B. Performing a minimal leak technique

C. Replacing the endotracheal tube with a larger size

D. Deflating and reinflating the cuff

14-9. An adult patient is being mechanically ventilated on the assist/control mode with a heat and moisture exchanger (HME) being used as humidification. Over the course of 4 hours, you notice that the peak pressure has increased by 12 cm H_2O, but the plateau pressure is unchanged. It also has become more difficult to suction the patient's tracheal secretions. What should you recommend at this time?

A. Switching the patient to the SIMV mode

B. Changing to a heated wick humidifier

C. Instilling normal saline solution before suctioning

D. Switching to a closed catheter suction system

14-10. For a patient who has been weaned from mechanical ventilation but has not been extubated, full ventilatory support should be reinstituted if which of the following occurs?

    I. The blood pressure increases or decreases by 5 mm Hg

    II. The pulse increases by 30 beats per minute

    III. The respiratory rate increases by 10 or exceeds 30 breaths per minute

    IV. The $Paco_2$ increases by 12 torr

A. II and III only

B. III and IV only

C. I, II, and III

D. II, III, and IV

14-11. After initiating assist-control mechanical ventilation, the inverse I:E ratio alarm is triggered. Which of the following should be increased to correct this problem?

A. Inspiratory flow

B. Pressure limit

C. Tidal volume

D. Respiratory rate

14-12. A college student is brought to the emergency department following a motor vehicle accident. He is tachypneic and tachycardic. He is receiving oxygen via a nonrebreathing mask at 10 L/min. You observe that the mask bag fully deflates on each inspiration. What action should you take?

A. Change to a simple mask at 4 L/min

B. Increase the flow rate to 12–15 L/min

C. Change to a nasal cannula at 8 L/min

D. Continue therapy and monitor Spo_2

14-13. A physician orders oxygen per protocol for an otherwise healthy postoperative patient who has a Pao_2 of 52 torr on room air. After initiating a nasal cannula at 2 L/min and repeating an arterial blood gas, the patient's Pao_2 is now 59 torr. What action should you recommend to the physician?

A. Increase the oxygen liter flow and reassess the patient

B. Intubate the patient and institute mechanical ventilation

C. Decrease the oxygen liter flow and reassess the patient

D. Institute continuous positive airway pressure by mask

14-14. A 70-year-old male patient in the emergency department complains of shortness of breath, chest pain, and diaphoresis. The physician with a trauma patient in the room next door asks you to begin an assessment. Your initial action should include all of the following *except*:

A. Monitoring their clinical status, including Spo_2

B. Quickly recommending moderate to high Fio_2

C. Promptly informing the nurse and physician

D. Measuring maximum inspiratory pressure

14-15. You are asked to assess a 16-year-old patient with a severe head cold on 4 L/min of oxygen via nasal cannula. The patient is alert and awake and is complaining that he can't breathe through his nose. His pulse oximeter reads 84% saturation. What action should you take?
   A. Decrease the O_2 flow until the patient is more comfortable
   B. Increase the O_2 flow until the SpO_2 equals or exceeds 90%
   C. Change to a simple mask at 5–7 L/min
   D. Recommend an arterial blood gas before considering any changes

14-16. Soon after a severe asthmatic patient is started on heliox therapy with an 80/20 mix, his SpO_2 drops from 94% to 88%. All of the following actions should be considered *except*:
   A. Checking oxygen analyzer to ensure delivery of prescribed FIO_2
   B. Checking to ensure an adequate seal of the face mask
   C. Recommending a more oxygen-enriched heliox mixture, such as 70/30
   D. Reducing the inspiratory flow

14-17. A physician prescribes incentive spirometry for a postoperative patient who complains of dizziness when performing five inspiratory maneuvers in a row. What action should you take?
   A. Recommend that the therapy be discontinued
   B. Coach the patient to pause before each maneuver
   C. Begin CPR on the patient
   D. Begin oxygen therapy via protocol

14-18. A toddler is receiving volume-controlled ventilation. To minimize volume loss due to compression and tubing expansion, which of the following should you select?
   A. Longer breathing circuit
   B. Low compliance tubing
   C. Large diameter tubing
   D. Smaller-diameter ET tube connector

14-19. A recently intubated 25-year-old female patient has no breath sounds over the left side of her chest. Her SpO_2 on 40% O_2 has dropped from 96% to 90%. At the same time, the peak inspiratory pressure on the ventilator has increased from 35 cm H_2O to 45 cm H_2O. You note a tube length marking of 26 cm at the teeth. What action should you take?
   A. Increase the FIO_2 and the flow rate
   B. Recommend a stat chest X-ray
   C. Administer a bronchodilator
   D. Retract the ET tube up by 3–4 cm

14-20. An 88-year-old patient is having a problem holding the small-volume nebulizer mouthpiece for her bronchodilator treatment. What action should you take?
   A. Change to a dry powder inhaler (DPI)
   B. Change to a metered-dose inhaler (MDI)
   C. Hold the nebulizer for the patient
   D. Change to an aerosol mask

14-21. Each time a patient receiving continuous-flow IMV spontaneously inhales, the pressure drops 6 cm H_2O. Which of the following actions would correct this problem?
   I. Changing to the assist/control mode
   II. Increasing the flow to the IMV reservoir bag
   III. Paralyzing the patient
   A. II only
   B. III only
   C. I and II
   D. II and III

14-22. An infant is placed on continuous-flow CPAP for treatment of hypoxemia. The initial CPAP level is 6 cm H_2O; however, you notice that the pressure falls to 3 cm H_2O with each inspiration. What should you do to correct the problem?
   A. Tell the patient to relax and breathe more slowly
   B. Sedate the patient with diazepam or midazolam
   C. Increase the CPAP to 9 cm H_2O to offset the loss
   D. Increase the system flow to maintain the pressure

14-23. A patient coughs vigorously while receiving postural drainage and percussion on the superior segment of the left lower lobe. You then note that the sputum is mixed with a large amount of bright red blood. You should:
A. Stop the treatment, stabilize the patient, and inform the physician
B. Continue the treatment and make a note of the sputum in the chart
C. Give the patient O_2 by simple mask and continue the treatment
D. Quickly discard the sputum so the patient does not see it and become upset

14-24. Which of the following represents the primary indication for and approved use of inhaled nitric oxide?
A. Hypoxemia associated with obstructive sleep apnea
B. Hypoxemia in neonates with persistent pulmonary hypertension
C. Ventilatory failure in premature neonates
D. Hypoxemia associated with hyaline membrane disease

14-25. A patient is receiving IPPB therapy for atelectasis with a set pressure of 25 cm H_2O. During therapy, the patient's pulse becomes thready and the blood pressure drops from 120/80 mm Hg to 90/50 mm Hg. You should:
A. Decrease the IPPB pressure to 10 cm H_2O and monitor the patient
B. Increase the IPPB pressure to 45 cm H_2O and continue the treatment
C. Discontinue the treatment and notify the physician
D. Change the treatment to intermittent CPAP with 10 cm H_2O PEEP

14-26. Prior to beginning an adrenergic aerosol bronchodilator treatment on an adult patient, you record a resting heart rate of 132 beats/min. Which of the following is the correct action in this case?
A. Double the drug diluent and prolong the administration time
B. Have the patient self-administer the aerosol treatment
C. Postpone therapy until you are able to contact the ordering physician
D. Use half the standard dosage listed in the package insert

14-27. Following administration of a bland aerosol treatment, auscultation reveals rhonchi throughout middle and upper lung fields. You should:
A. Encourage the patient to cough
B. Recommend administration of a bronchodilator
C. Recommend discontinuation of therapy
D. Discontinue the treatment and administer oxygen

14-28. A patient was recently changed from assist/control mode to pressure support ventilation, and the high respiratory rate alarm, which is set at 25, is sounding because the patient is breathing between 25 and 28 breaths per minute. What change should you make to the ventilator alarms?
A. Increase the high respiratory rate alarm to 50
B. Increase the high pressure alarm to 50 cm H_2O
C. Increase the high respiratory rate alarm to 30–35
D. Stop weaning the patient immediately

14-29. While monitoring a patient during a T-tube weaning trial, you note increased patient agitation, increased heart rate (from 85 to 110 beats/min) and respiratory rate (from 15 to 34 breaths/min), and PVCs increasing to an average of 4 per minute. You should:
A. Encourage the patient to relax and continue careful monitoring
B. Request that the patient be given a stat bolus of lidocaine
C. Reconnect the patient to the ventilator with prior settings
D. Request that the patient be given a strong sedative/hypnotic

14-30. After a patient has been on an aerosol from an ultrasonic nebulizer for 5 minutes, she begins to wheeze. What should you do at this time?
A. Recommend that the patient be given IV epinephrine
B. Stop the treatment, monitor the patient, and notify the doctor
C. Add 0.5 mL (2.5 mg) of albuterol to the nebulizer solution
D. Switch the ultrasonic nebulizer source gas to 100% O_2

WHAT YOU NEED TO KNOW: ESSENTIAL CONTENT

Terminating Treatment Based on Patient's Response to Therapy

General Considerations

In general, therapy should be terminated when the patient's safety is in question, the therapeutic objectives have been fully met, the therapy is clearly not achieving the intended goals, or in certain end-of-life situations. During therapy, patient safety is paramount! All patients must be monitored for adverse effects once therapy is initiated, then periodically once therapy is started and after the therapy is complete. A good rule of thumb when a serious adverse effect is suspected is to follow these steps, starting with the "Triple S Rule" (Stop, Stay, Stabilize):

- Stop the therapy.
- Stay with and monitor the patient.
- Stabilize the patient, by providing oxygen therapy, if necessary.
- If in a health care facility, notify the nurse and physician immediately.
- If in an alternate site such as home care, call for help and dial 911.
- If the adverse effect appears life threatening and occurs in a health care facility, call for either a "code blue" or the rapid response team (RRT) as indicated.

Modifying Treatment Techniques

There are a host of other instances when it may be appropriate for you to independently modify therapy based largely on the patient's response. The following sections summarize the most common situations warranting modification of treatment techniques, as well as the recommended actions.

Modifying Incentive Spirometry

Incentive spirometry (IS) involves the use of a simple device to promote lung expansion. The success of this therapy depends heavily on patient cooperation and participation, as well as the effectiveness of your instruction. Incentive spirometry measures and monitors inspired volumes and helps target goals for the patient to achieve. The equipment used is discussed in more detail in Chapter 6. While IS therapy is relatively simple, there are a few situations in which modification is needed in order to achieve clinical objectives. **Table 14-1** summarizes common problems and situations that may occur with IS, the likely causes, as well as modifications helpful in resolving the problems.

Modifying Intermittent Positive Pressure Breathing (IPPB)

IPPB therapy involves the application of positive pressure to the airway during inhalation to hyperinflate the lungs, help treat or prevent atelectasis, and/or aid in secretion clearance. IPPB therapy can also be used to administer and enhance the deposition of aerosolized drugs such as bronchodilators or mucolytics. With IPPB therapy, you decide on the patient interface (e.g., mask, mouthpiece, etc.) and can control and modify the gas source, F_{IO_2}, sensitivity, inspiratory/expiratory flow, and peak pressure. The initiation of IPPB therapy, contraindications, and hazards are discussed in Chapter 12, and the equipment used is described in Chapter 6. **Table 14-2** (see page 429) outlines the common problems that you may experience when administering IPPB, along with their recommended modifications.

Modifying Bland Aerosol Therapy

Bland aerosol therapy is indicated to treat upper airway edema, laryngotracheobronchitis, and subglottic and post-extubation edema. It also may help overcome a humidity deficit in patients with a bypassed upper airway or who are otherwise at risk for retained secretions. Bland aerosol therapy is also used for sputum induction procedures.

Bland aerosol is usually generated by large-volume jet nebulizers; however, you may occasionally use other devices such as ultrasonics. In regard to large-volume jet nebulizers, it is important that you remember the inverse relationship that exists between F_{IO_2} and total flow with air-entrainment devices. Specifically, as you increase the F_{IO_2}, less air is entrained and total output flow decreases. Some of the questions on the CRT exam will likely involve insufficient output flow of these devices at F_{IO_2}s above 40–45%. In other instances, you may need to modify bland aerosol therapy based on either the

Table 14-1 Common Modifications for IS Therapy

Problem/Situation	Possible Cause(s)	Recommended Modification(s)
No volume or flow recorded on IS device, despite inspiratory effort from patient	Equipment assembled incorrectly, flex tube or mouthpiece disconnected, patient exhaling instead of inhaling	Recheck equipment assembly and flex tube/mouthpiece connection, replace unit, and reinstruct patient
Patient cannot generate sufficient inspiratory effort to record volume or flow	Insufficient patient instruction, patient unable to follow directions (e.g., due to sedation, dementia) or generate sufficient inspiratory effort	Reinstruct patient, coach patient to breathe in more deeply, and consider another modality (e.g., IPPB)
Mild dizziness, lightheadedness, and tingling fingers not caused by other factors (e.g., CVA)	Hyperventilation	Coach patient to breathe more slowly (~ 8 breaths per minute) and pause between maneuvers
Patient not showing clinical improvement, despite proper implementation of therapy	Incorrect diagnosis; consider alternative or additional diagnosis other than atelectasis or hypoventilation (e.g., pneumonia)	Call physician and recommend additional or alternative treatment (e.g., antibiotics or IPPB)
Patient cannot achieve enough flow to activate the incentive indicator	An obstructive disorder that prevents the patient from generating the threshold flow needed to use a flow-oriented IS device	Recommend a volume-oriented IS device or one recommended for patients with obstructive disorders

patient's response or a change in the care plan. **Table 14-3** (see page 430) summarizes key problem situations that may warrant adjustments, as well as the specific actions you should to resolve them.

Modifying Aerosol Drug Therapy

In addition to modifying bland aerosol therapy, there are also modifications you can make to optimize the delivery of aerosolized medications. Changes in the drug, dosage, and frequency require a physician's order and are discussed in Chapter 15. However, you can normally modify either the delivery device or the patient's breathing pattern to optimize drug delivery. The most common modifications of this type are described in **Table 14-4** (see page 431).

Modifying Oxygen Therapy

Once O_2 therapy has been ordered by the physician and initiated, there are instances when you should independently modify the mode of delivery and/or the input flow. In certain circumstances, you may even change the FIO_2 in accordance with a preapproved O_2 therapy protocol. Although less common, an oxygen blender may also be used to deliver a desired FIO_2. **Table 14-5** (see page 432) outlines the most common circumstances warranting modification to oxygen therapy.

    Figure 14-1 (see page 433) is an example of an oxygen therapy protocol algorithm (flowchart), which permits you to titrate (or modify) the FIO_2 based on a patient's clinical status and in accordance with the preapproved sequence.

Modifying Specialty Gas Therapy

In addition to oxygen therapy, there are other specialty gases that you may administer in a clinical setting. Most notably, these gases include helium-oxygen or *heliox* and nitric oxide. The NBRC expects you to have a basic understanding of the indications, setup and equipment, troubleshooting, and common modifications involved in administering these two gases.

Table 14-2 Common Modifications for IPPB Therapy

Problem/Situation	Possible Cause(s)	Recommended Modification(s)
Manometer does not increase above zero	Major leak or poor airway seal	Fix any leak in circuit, coach patient for "tight lip seal" with mouthpiece, reposition or switch mask/mouthpiece (e.g., use flanged mouthpiece); if artificial airway, check cuff pressure and tube connection, and adjust terminal flow, if available
The machine does not cycle off at end-inspiration	Major leak or poor airway seal	See above recommended actions
	IPPB valve malfunction	Troubleshoot IPPB valve
Insufficient measured exhaled V_T (< 12–15 mL/kg)	Insufficient pressure setting on the machine	Gradually increase the pressure to achieve V_T of 12–15 mL/kg
Evidence or air trapping, especially with COPD and asthma patients	Increased expiratory airway resistance	Have patient prolong exhalation or mechanically retard it via PEEP valve on the exhalation port
	Insufficient expiratory time	Increase flow or coach patient to breathe slower
Mild dizziness, light-headedness, and parasthesia (tingling in the extremities)	Hyperventilation	Coach patient to breathe slower (< 8–10 breaths/min) and/or pause between breaths; reassess exhaled V_T, and lower set pressure
Clinical evidence of worsening hypoxemia (e.g., decreasing Spo_2, etc.)	Inadequate F_{IO_2}	Switch to device capable of high F_{IO_2} (e.g., Bird Mark 7)
		Provide 100% O_2 (turn off air mix)
	Patient-machine asynchrony	Coach patient to "breathe with the machine"
		Adjust flow for desired I:E ratio
	Excessive mucous	Pause therapy and clear secretions
Patient not responding to drugs aerosolized during IPPB	Insufficient inspiratory time	Decrease the flow
	Dose wasted during expiration	Nebulize drug during inspiration only
Patient not showing clinical improvement, despite proper implementation of therapy	Incorrect diagnosis; consider diagnosis other than atelectasis or hypoventilation (e.g., pneumonia)	Call physician and recommend additional or alternative treatment (e.g., antibiotics)

Table 14-3 Common Situations for Modifying Bland Aerosol Therapy

Problem/Situation	Possible Cause(s)	Recommended Modification(s)
Insufficient aerosol output flow despite an FIO_2 < 40–45%	Insufficient input flow from flow meter	Increase input flow from flow meter
	Condensation in circuit	Drain condensate from circuit and add a water trap
Insufficient aerosol output at FIO_2 > 40–45%	High FIO_2 setting means little air entrainment and low output	Use high-output nebulizer or dual nebulizer setup
Patient hypoxemia, despite nebulizer being properly set up	Insufficient flow output at FIO_2 > 40–45%	Use high-output nebulizer or dual nebulizer setup
		If a T-piece is used, add a reservoir (50 mL of aerosol tubing) to distal end
Risk of infection	Contaminated reservoir	Change nebulizer and do not drain condensate into reservoir
FIO_2 notably higher than setting and output flow decreased	Condensate in tubing	Drain condensate and add a water trap
	Obstructed entrainment port	Remove obstruction from entrainment port
Increase in airway swelling once aerosol therapy initiated	Increase edema due to absorption of moisture	Consider using a humidifier with O_2-delivery device, instead of an aerosol device
Aerosol output irritating to patient	Cold aerosol output may be irritating to patient's airway	Consider changing to heated nebulizer
Despite cool aerosol therapy, patient exhibits signs of retained secretions	Insufficient aerosol delivery	Consider heated aerosol
	Too low a flow	Increase input flow
	Insufficient patient hydration	Recommend increased fluids, if tolerated
Insufficient output of ultrasonic nebulizer for sputum induction	Amplitude setting too low on ultrasonic device	Increase amplitude setting
Excessive aerosol output from ultrasonic nebulizer	Amplitude setting too high	Decrease amplitude setting

Helium–Oxygen (Heliox) Therapy

The value of helium in respiratory care is linked to its low density. Breathing a helium–oxygen mixture decreases the driving pressure needed in ventilation, particularly in the larger airways. Hence, heliox can help decrease the work of breathing associated with large airway obstruction. Some of the major indications for this therapy include:

- Acute upper airway obstruction
- Reversible obstructive disorders such as asthma
- Post-extubation stridor
- Croup

Regarding the equipment and setup, you can mix heliox combinations at the bedside or use commercially available cylinders of either 80% He/20% O_2 or 70% He/30% O_2. One method for mix-

Table 14-4 Common Modifications for Aerosol Medication Therapy

Problem/Situation	Possible Cause(s)	Recommended Modification(s)
Inability to properly actuate or use an MDI, resulting in insufficient drug delivery	Inability to physically activate the device due to functional limitation	Switch to an actuator-assisted device
	Inability to coordinate breathing pattern with device actuation	Coach patient on proper breathing pattern, use a spacer or holding chamber, and consider an SVN
Aerosolized medication ordered via MDI but patient tachypneic (respiratory rate > 20)	Respiratory distress, pain, or anxiety	Use SVN, coach patient to breathe more slowly, with an intermittent breath hold; monitor patient and advise physician and nurse regarding tachypnea
Patient can not hold mouthpiece in place for the SVN, MDI with spacer or trigger a breath-actuated nebulizer	Patient debilitated, cognitively impaired, restrained, has facial weakness, or is otherwise unable to keep mouthpiece in place	If drug is available in other forms, use a mask with the SVN or MDI with spacer and mask
Patient unable to generate sufficient flows to use a dry powder inhaler (DPI)	Patient debilitated, weak, cognitively impaired, or otherwise unable to generate sufficient inspiratory flows	Use an aerosol mask with SVN
Patient receiving supplemental O_2 develops hypoxemia while receiving aerosolized medications via SVN	Inadvertent decrease in F_{IO_2} while receiving aerosolized medication	Maintain F_{IO_2} during therapy, and ensure that SVN tubing is connected to oxygen (not air)
	Parodoxical or other adverse response to therapy	Give supplemental O_2 as appropriate, monitor patient, and advise nurse and physician
Physician orders 3 mL of 20% acetylcysteine mucolytic, but only a strength of 10% is available		Use double the volume (6 mL) of the half-as-potent 10% acetylcysteine to achieve the equivalent dose of the drug
Patient develops severe irritation to the mouth and throat while taking inhaled steroids	Patient develops pharyngitis or oral thrush as a side effect of inhaled steroids	Instruct patient to rinse mouth after receiving inhaled steroids and add a spacer if MDI in use
Patient with low respiratory rate causing wasting of medication	Wasted medication nebulized during prolonged pauses between breaths	Use a breath-actuated nebulizer

ing heliox involves using a nebulizer connected to an O_2 flow meter running at a minimum of 10 L/min, bleeding in 100% helium via a small-bore connection and titrating the flow to achieve the desired F_{IO_2}, which must be continuously monitored via an oxygen analyzer. Another method involves using pre-mixed tanks and flow meters specially calibrated for heliox. A variation of this method involves the use of correction factors in conjunction with standard flow meters. The correction factor for 80/20 heliox is 1.8, which means that for every 10 L/min of indicated flow, the actual heliox flow is 18 L/min (10 L/min × 1.8). Similarly, the factor for 70/30 helium-oxygen mixture is 1.6.

Heliox may be administered using a variety of delivery devices. For spontaneously breathing patients, heliox is generally delivered via a tight-fitting nonrebreathing mask and a flow that is sufficient to meet or exceed the patient's minute ventilation and peak inspiratory flow requirements. Another

Table 14-5 Modifying Oxygen Therapy

Problem/Situation	Possible Cause(s)	Recommended Modification(s)
Patient remains hypoxemic after initiation of nasal O_2 therapy	Patient is a "mouth breather"	Switch to a venturi or simple mask
	Cannula nasal prongs are blocked with secretions	Replace cannula
	Patient needs higher F_{IO_2}	Contact physician for an order to increase or use higher F_{IO_2} as permitted per protocol
	O_2 device connected to air	Ensure that the device is connected to an O_2 flow meter
Patient complains of nasal or mouth dryness	Insufficient humidity causing drying of mucosa	Add a bubble or other type of humidifier, particularly if input flow of nasal cannula is 4 or more L/min
Patient requires a low to moderate F_{IO_2} but has a high/variable minute volume and does not respond to a nasal cannula	Nasal cannula is a low-flow device and not suitable for patients with high/variable minute volume	Switch to a venturi mask that is high flow and suitable for unstable patients with high minute ventilatory needs
Patient has high minute ventilation, needs high F_{IO_2}, and is moderately hypoxemic	Inability to meet high inspiratory flow demands at high F_{IO_2}s	Consider high-flow nebulizer or blender with high-flow flow meter
Non/partial-rebreather mask bag fails to remain inflated	Insufficient input flow	Increase flow meter setting
	Tubing disconnect	Ensure that tubing is correctly connected to flow meter
Patient feels claustrophobic with aerosol mask in use	Confining feeling imposed by mask	Suggest switching to a face tent
Patient has facial injury or burns, but order is for 40% aerosol	Mask may cause irritation or further injury to face	Suggest switching to a face tent
An infant or child in an O_2 enclosure must be removed for a special procedure or transport; a similar moderate F_{IO_2} needs to be maintained outside of the enclosure		Consider a simple mask that can be easily set up but is not easily dislodged
The Sp_{O_2} of an infant receiving CPAP via nasal prongs drops during episodes of crying	Decrease in F_{IO_2} due to mouth breathing associated with crying	Collaborate with nurse to address obvious reasons for crying (e.g., hunger)
		If crying and decrease in Sp_{O_2} continue, consider an enclosure such as an oxyhood (same F_{IO_2})
Air-entrainment mask delivers higher F_{IO_2} than set	Obstruction of entrainment ports with bedding, clothing, etc.	Remove obstructions and monitor patient

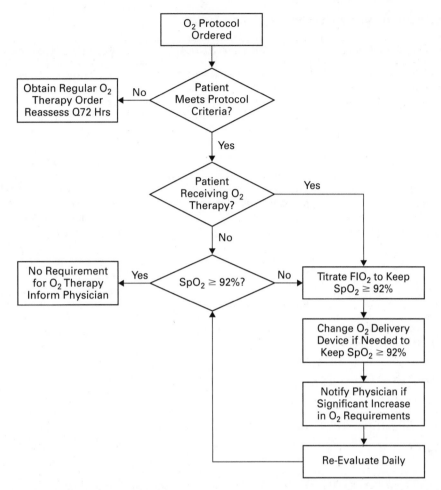

Figure 14-1 Example of an O$_2$ Therapy Protocol. Note that a full O$_2$ therapy protocol also would include patient inclusion criteria and specifications for equipment selection.

approach that has been used to deliver heliox to infants is an oxyhood. However, heat loss and hypothermia associated with the higher thermal conductivity of this gas mixture has limited its use in this way. Heliox mixtures may also be delivered to mechanically ventilated patients with a cuffed artificial airway in place. It should be noted that the performance of ventilators delivering heliox tends to vary significantly by model. As a result, only a ventilator that is FDA approved for delivering heliox, such as the Servo 300 (Maquet), should be used. Even with approved ventilators, you may need to add special modules or use conversion factors to adjust settings. Irrespective of the delivery method, all patients receiving helium-oxygen mixtures should be closely monitored, and an oxygen analyzer with active alarms should always be used to continuously measure the F$_{IO_2}$ of the heliox mixture output to the patient.

You also should note that heliox therapy may be combined with other therapies such as bronchodilators to treat acute obstructive disorders such as status asthmaticus. Heliox may improve deposition of such medications; however, only certain nebulizers have been approved for such use, and output may vary due to the characteristics of heliox.

Once heliox is in use, you may need to modify or troubleshoot the therapy. **Table 14-6** summarizes the major situations where such changes may be appropriate.

Inhaled Nitric Oxide (INO) Therapy

Inhaled nitric oxide (INO) is a potent pulmonary vasodilator. Because it relaxes the capillary smooth muscle of the pulmonary vessels, it has been shown to reduce intrapulmonary shunting, improve arterial oxygenation, and decrease both pulmonary vascular resistance and pulmonary artery pressures.

Table 14-6 Common Modifications for Heliox Therapy

Problem/Situation	Possible Cause(s)	Recommended Modification(s)
Patient receiving 80/20 heliox mixture has signs and symptoms of mild to moderate hypoxemia (Sp_{O_2} about 88–92%)	Insufficient F_{IO_2} delivery to patient	Analyze the F_{IO_2} to ensure prescribed oxygen concentration is being delivered, and if prescribed F_{IO_2} is confirmed, consider recommending a more oxygen-enriched mixture, such as 70/30 heliox
Patient receiving 80/20 heliox via nonrebreathing mask 10 L/min, but the reservoir bag completely collapses during inspiration	Insufficient seal and/or missing or malfunctioning one-way valves	Ensure adequate seal of mask and that one-way valves are functioning properly; use an input flow adequate to keep reservoir bag inflated throughout breathing cycle, and if set up with a standard (oxygen) flow meter, ensure proper conversion factor (1.8 for 80/20) being used
	Insufficient input flow	
Less effective cough and spontaneous secretion clearance	Lower-density heliox inhibits expulsive phase of coughing	Wash out helium with air-oxygen mixture before therapeutic coughing
Excessive heat loss and hypothermia for infant receiving heliox via oxyhood	Higher thermal conductivity associated with helium	Warm and humidify heliox gas and closely monitor patient
Variability in medication (bronchodilator) delivery via helium-oxygen mixture	Variability in particle size and deposition associated with the lower density of heliox	Use only nebulizers approved for heliox and monitor patient response to therapy
Patient receiving heliox through cuffed artificial airway/ventilator setup with signs of volume loss and/or ventilatory insufficiency	Excessive volume loss from insufficient air in airway cuff or failure to use conversion factors to adjust ventilator settings	Add air to artificial airway cuff to ensure adequate seal (MOV), and if airway seal adequate, use conversion factors to adjust settings and account for lower density; use only a ventilator approved for heliox therapy
Evidence of lung over distention ("beaked" pressure-volume graphic) on patient receiving heliox through a ventilator	Excessive volume delivery and lung distension because of failure to account for lower-density gas	Use conversion factors to adjust settings, confirm use of ventilator approved for heliox therapy, and closely monitor patient

After several years of testing, INO was approved for the treatment of term and near-term (> 34 weeks) neonates with hypoxemic respiratory failure associated with persistent pulmonary hypertension of the newborn (PPHN). INO has also been used in adults to treat pulmonary hypertension associated with acute respiratory distress syndrome (ARDS), although no significant improvement in longer-term clinical outcomes has been shown in such patients.

Though INO can be administered to spontaneous-breathing patients via a nasal cannula or a mask, it is more commonly used for mechanically ventilated patients. The equipment setup includes the INOvent (Ikaria) delivery system and special cylinders, which may be interfaced with many commercially available ventilators. The cylinders contain nitric oxide in concentrations of either 100 or 800 ppm, which is then further diluted before delivery to the patient. The INOvent delivery system uses a nitric oxide injector and a flow sensor that are placed in the inspiratory side of the ventilator circuit, near the ventilator outlet. Nitric oxide is then injected into the ventilator circuit in proportion to the inspiratory gas flow to achieve the desired dose. The recommended initial dose of INO is 20 ppm but can often be quickly reduced to 5–6 ppm.

Note that when nitric oxide comes in contact with oxygen, a toxic by-product known as nitrogen dioxide (NO_2) is produced. INO equipment is designed to limit the contact time between these two gases and thus minimize the production of NO_2. Nitric oxide and NO_2 levels, as well as FIO_2, are continuously analyzed through a sampling line connected near the distal end of the circuit near the patient's airway. Active alarms are used to detect excessive levels of nitric oxide and NO_2, or undesired changes in FIO_2. NO_2 levels should not exceed 2–3 ppm.

In many cases, the benefits of increased oxygen saturation and decreased pulmonary artery pressure may be seen within minutes or hours of initiating such therapy. Treatment should be continued for up to 14 days, or until underlying oxygenation desaturation has resolved. Factors to consider when preparing to withdraw therapy are as follows:

- Reduce INO to lowest effective dose, ideally 5–6 ppm or less.
- Ensure patient is hemodynamically stable.
- Verify patient tolerance of FIO_2 of 40% or less and PEEP 5 cm H_2O or less.
- Monitor patient closely during withdrawal of therapy.
- Prepare to provide hemodynamic support if required.

At the recommended doses, INO has been shown to have minimal toxicity and adverse side effects. However, though quite rare, hazards have been reported that include excessive methemoglobin levels, worsening of congestive heart failure, and rebound effect (reoccurrence of hypoxemia/pulmonary hypertension) soon after withdrawal of therapy. INO is also contraindicated in some patients, most notably neonates with certain cardiovascular anomalies such as coarctation of the aorta. In order to maximize patient safety and the overall effectiveness of therapy, there may be instances when you, as the respiratory therapist, may recommend modifications. **Table 14-7** summarizes these situations.

Modifying Bronchial Hygiene Therapy

Bronchial hygiene therapy includes a variety of techniques designed to help mobilize and remove secretions. These techniques include the following:

- Manual and mechanical chest percussion and vibration
- Postural drainage
- Directed coughing
- Positive expiratory pressure (PEP)
- Intrapulmonary percussive ventilation (IPV)
- Mechanical insufflation-exsufflation

These therapies are described in more detail in Chapter 11. Often, one or more of these techniques can be combined with other therapies to help clear secretions, including bland aerosol administration or inhaled medications (e.g., mucolytics and bronchodilators). When several techniques are employed to clear secretions, the recommended sequence should generally be followed:

- Open them up (with bronchodilators)
- Thin them out (with bland aerosol and/or mucolytic agents)
- Clear them out (by bronchial hygiene techniques)

While these techniques may be effective in helping clear secretions, there are instances when you should modify the position, duration, or technique or recommend a different bronchial hygiene strategy. **Table 14-8** (see page 437) summarizes common problems and situations that may warrant modifying bronchial hygiene therapy, as well as specific changes to consider.

Modifications Relating to the Management of Artificial Airways

Artificial airways are used in clinical practice in a variety of situations and are primarily indicated to:

- Correct impending or actual airway obstruction
- Facilitate ventilation
- Protect the airway
- Remove secretions

Table 14-7 Common Modifications Involving Nitric Oxide Delivery

Problem/Situation	Possible Cause(s)	Recommended Modification(s)
Immediately after initiating INO therapy, NO_2 levels steadily rise above 2–3 ppm	Failure to flush system during setup	Flush system with 100% oxygen before initiating therapy
INO initiated at 20 ppm but no clinical improvement is seen	Improper equipment setup	Ensure equipment is properly set up and functioning
	Poor or paradoxical response	Recommend alternative (pharmacological) therapy
INO therapy is started with an initial dose of 6 ppm, but no clinical improvement is seen	Initial dose is too low	Recommend an increase in the initial dose, up to 20 ppm, and monitor patient closely
Analyzed nitric oxide (NO) level drops to 0	NO supply tank is empty	Check NO tank pressure and switch or replace NO cylinder
NO, NO_2, and O_2 analyzer readings suddenly drop to 0	Obstructed or disconnected sample line	Check/reconnect gas sampling line, and replace in-line sampling line filter
NO, NO_2, and O_2 analyzer readings altered during bronchodilator therapy via SVN	Alternation of prescribed gas mixture by nebulizer flow	Recommend bronchodilator therapy via MDI
	Disruption of circuit to place nebulizer in line	Add MDI adaptor to circuit
NO_2 level noted above 2–3 ppm	NO_2 analyzer malfunction	Check and recalibrate NO_2 analyzer
	Excessive contact time between INO and O_2	Check proper setup of all equipment
During weaning or immediately after withdrawing INO, patient becomes hemodynamically unstable and/or hypoxemic	Patient not tolerating weaning of INO at this time	If weaning, recommend patient be returned to original INO dosage
	Rebound effect	If INO recently withdrawn, recommend increased F_{IO_2} and hemodynamic support (vasopressors), consider reinstituting INO, and closely monitor patient

Table 14-8 Common Modifications to Bronchial Hygiene Therapy

Problem/Situation	Possible Cause(s)	Recommended Modification(s)
Patient has pain when you perform directed coughing or chest physical therapy	Post abdominal or thoracic surgery or injury (trauma)	Coordinate coughing and therapy sessions with pain mediation, assist patient in splinting the operative site, and use "huff" coughing (FET) instead of regular cough
Patient cannot generate sufficient cough to clear secretions	Patient has paralysis or neuromuscular weakness	Implement manually assisted exhalation via application of pressure to the thoracic cage or epigastric region (chest compression or "quad cough");[a] also consider mechanical insufflation-exsufflation (see Chapter 11) or suctioning
Patient coughs violently while in head-down position	Mobilization of secretions or other stimulation of cough mechanism	Discourage strong coughing in head-down position since this can increase ICP, sit patient up until the cough subsides, and coach patient to "huff" cough to clear secretions
Postural drainage of certain lung segments requires head-down (Trendelenberg) position, but such positions may not be tolerated or may be contraindicated in some patients.	Head-down position may cause vomiting/aspiration, dyspnea, cerebral bleeding, cardiovascular compromise or worsening of other conditions	Approximate the position as closely as possible and consider postural drainage in a lateral decubitus or supine position; consider alternative therapy not requiring positional change, such as mechanical insufflation-exsufflation or PEP; apply therapy for shorter time interval than ideal period of 10–15 minutes per position; and monitor patient closely
Patient complains of pain or discomfort during CPT therapy	Percussion or vibration being applied too rigorously or too near an incision or injury	Reduce intensity of percussion or vibration or consider another device (electric or pneumatic percussor); do not apply percussion or vibration too near incision or injury; and coordinate coughing sessions with pain medication.
Patient cannot cooperate with postural drainage or other bronchial hygiene therapy	Patient is aged or confused	Consider alternative therapy not requiring patient cooperation such as mechanical insufflation–exsufflation
Patient develops excessive secretions in throat and mouth during bronchial hygiene therapy	Secretions being mobilized as a result of therapy	Place patient in upright position, encourage them to cough, and consider suctioning or mechanical insufflation–exsufflation to assist secretion clearance

(continues)

Table 14-8 Common Modifications to Bronchial Hygiene Therapy (continued)

Problem/Situation	Possible Cause(s)	Recommended Modification(s)
Patient requires percussion and vibration but has had recent thoracic surgery or injury, which means there is the potential for disturbing incision or injury and thus causing bleeding, pain, or infection		Consider using an electrically or pneumatically powered percussor/vibrator; apply percussion and vibration a safe distance from incision/injury or to posterior chest; and coordinate coughing sessions with pain medication
Postural drainage sessions frequently conflict with meals (e.g., ordered 3 times a day), which carries the potential for vomiting and/or aspiration of recent meal		Time the administration of therapy at least 30–60 minutes before or after meals
Patient with, or at risk for, hypoxemia, but for whom bronchial hygiene is indicated	Underlying condition resulting in chronic and/or acute hypoxemia (e.g., COPD)	Provide additional supplemental O_2 and monitor the SpO_2 throughout procedure
	Movement of secretions or mucous plug to larger airways impeding ventilation	Consider 100% O_2 during therapy for critically ill patients, and shorten the administration time
Patient on PEP therapy is having difficulty keeping mouthpiece in place	Neuromuscular weakness or difficulty following commands	Coach patient on proper technique, and consider PEP via mask or another technique such as postural drainage
a. Chest compression or "quad cough" is contraindicated for patients with osteoporosis, flail chest, unconscious patients with unprotected airways, in pregnant women, and in those with acute abdominal pathology.		

Artificial airways (discussed in more detail in Chapter 6) include oral and nasal pharyngeal airways (nasal trumpet), laryngeal mask airway (LMA), endotracheal tubes, and tracheostomy tubes. Once an artificial airway is in place, there may be instances when it may be appropriate for you to make modifications in order to better achieve the goals of the care plan and/or to minimize the likelihood of unwanted hazards and side effects. **Table 14-9** outlines the most common situations of this type along with recommended actions.

Modifying Suctioning Technique

Suctioning the airway is an effective means of secretion clearance, which can be applied alone or in combination with bronchial hygiene therapy and aerosolized medications. As previously noted in this text, patients should be suctioned with the smallest effective size (a maximum of 12–14 Fr for adults), using the lowest suction pressure (not to exceed −100 to −120 mm Hg for adults) for not more than 10–15 seconds. As with other therapies, there are times when you should independently adjust the suctioning technique, as noted in **Table 14-10** (see page 441).

Modifications in Mechanical Ventilation

Once mechanical ventilation is initiated, it is often necessary to make changes. Many changes require a physician's order such as those relating to the mode of ventilation or "primary" settings including tidal volume, rate, FIO_2, and PEEP. You cannot make these modifications independently (unless they are covered under a preapproved therapy protocol). You can, however, suggest modifications to the treatment plan; see Chapter 15. In most institutions, including the NBRC hospital, the changes that you can make without a physician's order generally are limited to "secondary" settings such as inspiratory flow,

Table 14-9 Common Modifications in the Management of Artificial Airways

Problem/Situation	Possible Cause(s)	Recommended Modification(s)
Nasal discomfort associated with nasopharyngeal airway	Too large a nasopharyngeal in use given the patient's size	Use a smaller-size airway (e.g., switch from 32 to 28 FR)
	Device in place for too long	Switch to the opposite naris, and change every 8 hours and use water-soluble jelly
Intubated patient has an oropharyngeal airway in place that is excessively moving around the mouth	Too small or large an oropharyngeal airway in use	Switch to an appropriately sized airway, measuring from earlobe to corner of mouth (do *not* tape an oropharyngeal airway in place)
Awake intubated patient with an oropharyngeal airway is gagging and trying to spit it out	Discomfort associated with oropharyngeal airway	Consider removing the airway and using a bite-block device to secure the ET tube
		Recommend sedation (avoid oropharyngeal airway in conscious patients)
Difficult intubation	Glottis is located anteriorly or there is excessive epiglottic tissue due to swelling or obesity	Reposition patient; consider laryngeal mask airway (LMA) or fiberoptic intubation
	Incorrect laryngoscope blade/endotracheal tube (ETT) size	Ensure correct-size ETT and laryngoscope blade
	Patient agitated or anxious	Recommend sedation, and request that an anesthesiologist perform the procedure
Adult who has an ET tube secured at 26-cm mark has absent breath sounds and insufficient chest rise on the left side, high peak pressures, and poor oxygenation	Intubation of the right mainstem bronchus likely	Retract ET approximately 2–3 cm; after bilateral breath sounds are heard, resecure tube, monitor patient, and recommend a chest X-ray
Gurgling sound is heard around the mouth of an orally intubated, but otherwise stable patient	Most likely insufficient air in ET tube cuff	Add air to cuff using minimal leak or MOV technique to maximum pressure of 25 cm H_2O
	Cuff may be blown or the pilot balloon tubing may have a leak	If cuff does not hold pressure, consider an ET tube exchanger or recommending reintubation
ET tube cuff pressure measured at a pressure in excess of 25 cm H_2O	Excessive air in cuff	Remove air from cuff using minimal leak or MOV to maximum pressure of 25 cm H_2O
	Too small an ET tube	Recommend reintubation (or use ET tube exchanger) with appropriate-sized ET tube

(continues)

439

Table 14-9 Common Modifications in the Management of Artificial Airways (continued)

Problem/Situation	Possible Cause(s)	Recommended Modification(s)
Evidence of mucous plugging, retained or very thick secretions for a *spontaneous-breathing* patient with an artificial airway	Humidity deficit due to a bypassed upper airway	Consider continuous or intermittent heated, bland aerosol via tracheostomy collar or T-piece
Evidence of retained or very thick secretions for a *mechanically ventilated* patient with an artificial airway	Humidity deficit due to a bypassed upper airway	If HME or cool humidity system in use, switch to alternative system, such as a heated-wick humidifier
Patient with an artificial airway has coarse rhonchi on auscultation; secretions can be seen or vibrations from them can be felt in airway	Excessive airway secretions	Suction airway using proper-size catheter (12–14 Fr for adult) and vacuum pressures (–100 to –120 mm Hg for adult), for no more than about 10–15 seconds
Redness and excessive green or brown foul-smelling secretions noted around the stoma of a tracheostomy patient	Infected and irritated tracheostomy stoma	Ensure that trach stoma is cleaned and that the inner cannula and dressing/drain sponge changed at least every 8 hours, and notify nurse and physician that stoma may be infected
Mechanical ventilator for an intubated and appropriately sedated patient suddenly sounds a high pressure alarm, no return tidal volume	Mucous plug in ET tube	Attempt to pass a suction catheter, lavage, and suction, and recommend immediate extubation and reintubation, or inner cannula change, if tracheostomy tube in place
Patient has an artificial airway but a suction catheter cannot be passed	Partial airway obstruction	Lavage and attempt to suction; if obstruction persists, recommend extubation and reintubation (ET tube) or change inner cannula (tracheostomy tube)
	Suction catheter too large	Use smaller suction catheter (12–14 Fr for adult)

sensitivity, I:E ratio, and alarms. Changes in mechanical ventilation settings covered by a protocol are described more thoroughly elsewhere in this text.

In making changes to ventilator settings, it is generally best to do so one parameter at a time, especially when making adjustments to either oxygen (e.g., FIO_2 or PEEP) or ventilation (e.g., tidal volume or respiratory rate). Several simultaneous changes make it difficult to determine the impact of any single adjustment. Additionally, in cases of patient-ventilator asynchrony or problems with ventilator alarms, it is best to promptly determine whether the origin is related mainly to the patient or to a ventilator setting.

Table 14-11 (see page 442) summarizes the most common changes that you can make independently, related to invasive positive pressure ventilation.

Chapter 13 provides guidance on procedures for the initial setting of ventilator alarms. **Table 14-12** (see pag 443) outlines some of the common problems and situations involving ventilator alarms that are most likely to appear on the CRT exam, including needed alarm adjustments.

Table 14-10 Common Modifications for Suctioning

Problem/Situation	Possible Cause(s)	Recommended Modification
Suction catheter does not advance during nasotracheal suctioning	Deviated septum or nasal polyps	Use opposite naris
	Suction catheter too large	Use smaller catheter and more lubricant
Suction catheter does not advance through an appropriately sized artificial airway (ET or trach tube)	Suction catheter too large	Use a smaller catheter, generally a maximum of a 12 or 14 Fr for most adults
Small amount of blood or streaks noted in secretions	Nasal or airway trauma due to repeated suction attempts	Use smallest effective suction catheter size and consider (1) more liberal use of lubricant or soft red-rubber catheters, (2) a nasopharyngeal airway if there is need for repeated suctioning, and (3) noninvasive airway clearance such as mechanical insufflation–exsufflation
Patient becomes hypoxemic during suctioning procedure	Hypoventilation or underinflation due to airway suctioning	Pre- and postoxygenate and ventilate with 100% F_{IO_2} and BVM; apply suction for no more than 10–15 seconds, and, for ventilator patients, use closed suction system
Patient suddenly becomes bradycardic during suctioning	Vasovagal response due to suction catheter stimulating airway	Stop suctioning, apply supplemental O_2, monitor patient, and notify nurse and physician; consider shorter suctioning time.
Patient has evidence of loose or mobile secretions that cannot be suctioned	Suction pressure set too low	Increase suction pressure to a maximum of –80 to 120 mm Hg
	Suction catheter too small	Use appropriate-size catheter to a maximum of 12–14 Fr for adults
	Secretions too thick	Consider saline lavage, ensure adequate humidification, and consider aerosolized mucolytics with bronchodilators
Intubated and mechanically ventilated patient has evidence of copious secretions in the *left lung*	Left-sided bronchitis or pneumonia	Use a Coudé (angled tip) suction catheter to aid insertion into the left mainstem bronchus
No vacuum pressure	System leak, vacuum off, obstruction or kinking in tubing	Fix system leak, turn vacuum on, fix obstruction or kinked tubing

Table 14-11 Modifications in Invasive Positive Pressure Ventilation

Problem/Situation	Possible Cause(s)	Recommended Modification(s)
Patient-ventilator asynchrony (patient origin)	Patient respiratory distress due to excessive secretions, bronchospasm, hypoxemia, or air trapping	Assess patient to help determine if *patient or machine* origin; if the cause is patient-related (e.g., mucus, bronchospasm, hypoxemia), address cause (e.g., suction, bronchodilators, increased FIO_2/PEEP), and if not promptly resolved, consider a period of manual ventilation with FIO_2 100%, advise nurse and physician
	Inadequate sedation	Recommend sedation and advise nurse and physician
Patient-ventilator asynchrony (ventilator-setting origin)	Inappropriate trigger sensitivity	Adjust sensitivity: –0.5 to –2.0 cm H_2O or 1–3 L/min
	Insufficient inspiratory flow	If flow-limited ventilation, increase flow to eliminate post trigger effort or consider an adaptive flow setting, if available; if pressure-limited ventilation, adjust rise-time to eliminate multiple spiking at plateau
	Excessive inspiratory time resulting in 1:1 or inverse I:E ratio	If *intentionally* set to achieve clinical objectives (e.g., increase oxygenation), consider recommending sedation; if *unintentional*, consider increasing inspiratory flow or decreasing set rate to achieve an I:E ratio of 1:2 or 1:3
Auto-PEEP, detected via flow and/or volume waveform not returning to zero (patient origin)	Increase in airway resistance or tachypnea	Suction airway; recommend bronchodilators or sedation
Auto-PEEP, detected via flow and/or volume waveform not returning to zero (ventilator-setting origin)	Inadequate expiratory time and/or excessive inspiratory time	Increase inspiratory flow, and consider other measures such as reduction in respiratory rate setting or reduce/eliminate pause time
Insufficient returned tidal volume or sudden decrease in ventilating pressure	Leak in circuit or patient interface	Fix leak in circuit or add air to artificial airway cuff
Patient on mechanical ventilation has HME, and thick secretions and peak pressures have increased while plateau pressures have been constant	Increase in peak airway pressures with constant plateau pressures suggests increase in airway resistance, which may be due to humidity deficit resulting in thick secretions or an HME partially obstructed with secretions	Switch to a heated humidifier capable of providing higher relative/absolute humidity; suction airway to help remove secretions, particularly once humidifier replaced

(continues)

Table 14-11 Modifications in Invasive Positive Pressure Ventilation (continued)

Problem/Situation	Possible Cause(s)	Recommended Modification(s)
Excessive condensation (rain-out) in tubing	Cooling of saturated gas during delivery of breath through ventilator tubing	Use heated wire circuit or add a water trap
Volume loss from a ventilator circuit for a neonatal or young pediatric patient	Volume loss due to circuit tubing expansion (circuit compliance) and gas compression	Use a low compliance (stiff) circuit and low volume innards (humidifier) to minimize volume loss
While weaning on pressure support, patient develops high respiratory rate, hypoxemia, and other signs of mild to moderate distress	Patient not tolerating weaning attempt	Place patient back on full ventilator support (assist/control mode) and monitor closely, and recommend changes in settings, such as F_{IO_2}, as appropriate

Table 14-12 Adjustments to Ventilator Alarms Settings and Monitoring

Problem/Situation	Possible Cause(s)	Recommended Modification(s)
Excessive ventilator alarm activation (primarily patient origin)	*High pressure*: mucous plug, kinked tube, decreased compliance, or bronchospasm	Suction, reposition ET tube, or provide bronchodilator therapy
	Low pressure: disconnect, improved compliance, or leak	Reconnect patient or fix leak (e.g., in nebulizer)
	High rate: patient distress, weaning failure, or agitation	Assess patient, cease weaning attempt, recommend sedation
	Low minute volume: leak, hypoventilation, apnea, or weaning failure	Fix leak, place patient back on full ventilator support
	High minute ventilation: hypermetabolic state, hypoxemia, hypercarbia, agitation, or brain injury	Recommend ABG, sedation, chemically paralyze patient, add deadspace
Excessive ventilator alarm activation caused by inappropriate settings	A high respiratory rate alarm set at 20 is sounding for an adult who is weaning	Adjust ventilator to appropriate settings; the high respiratory rate alarm should be set at 5–10 above the actual rate to a maximum of 30–35/min
	High pressure alarm for an adult is set at 25 cm H_2O and is sounding	Increase the high pressure alarm to 5–10 cm H_2O above the patient's actual pressure, subject to a maximum of 45–50 cm H_2O
	Low minute ventilation alarm for an adult is set at 2.0 L	Low minute ventilation alarm should be set at approximately 2.0 L below actual, but never below 4.0–5.0 L for an adult
	Low pressure alarm is set at 3 cm H_2O	Low pressure should always be set at approximately 5–10 cm H_2O below peak pressures but never lower than 5 cm H_2O, to ensure that leak or patient disconnect is promptly detected

Beyond general guidelines for adjusting ventilator alarms, the NBRC expects you to be able to apply these concepts to specific clinical situations. The accompanying box describes several common problems involving ventilator alarm adjustments and discusses the appropriate action in such cases.

Case Summaries: Adjusting and Responding to Ventilator Alarms

Case 1: The weaning patient

Problem: An adult patient was recently switched from full ventilatory support (AC-550-12-50%-+5 PEEP) to pressure support of 12 cm H_2O and appears to be tolerating weaning well. However, several alarms are sounding, including alarms for low tidal volume (set at 450 mL) and high respiratory rate (set at 25).

Discussion: Alarm settings that were appropriate for original settings may not be reflective of a modest drop in tidal volume and an increase in respiratory rate, which may be expected during weaning. In this situation, you should modify alarms to recognize the expected changes in tidal volume and respiratory rate during weaning. In this instance, the low tidal volume alarm can be safely decreased to approximately 250–300 mL, and the high respiratory rate can be safely changed to 30–35.

Also note that if and when it becomes necessary to switch from pressure support back to full ventilatory support (assist/control) for such reasons as an overnight rest period or failed weaning attempt, it is often necessary to modify the alarms accordingly. In general, high respiratory rate should be decreased to about 10 above the total respiratory rate (set plus additional), and low tidal volume should be about 100 mL below that which is set. In this instance, the high respiratory rate alarm should be decreased back to about 25 breaths per minute and the low tidal volume back to 450 mL.

Case 2: Changing between pressure control and volume control ventilation

Problem: An adult patient on pressure control ventilation, with a ΔP (pressure differential) of 20 cm H_2O and +5 cm H_2O PEEP, is switched to volume control (AC-550-12-50%-+5 PEEP). The high pressure alarm, which is set at 30 cm H_2O, is sounding, and you see that the pressure manometer on the ventilator is reading a peak airway pressure of 35 cm H_2O.

Discussion: The high pressure alarm should be increased to recognize the somewhat higher ventilating pressure of 35 cm H_2O associated with switching to volume ventilation. In this instance, you should increase the high pressure alarm to 5–10 cm H_2O above actual peak airway pressure, subject to a maximum of 45–50 cm H_2O.

Keep in mind that if and when you make the opposite change—that is, move this patient from pressure to volume control—the peak airway pressure alarm setting may be too high, given the ventilating pressure of 25 cm H_2O. In such an instance, you should lower the peak airway pressure alarm setting to 30–35 cm H_2O (5–10 cm H_2O above peak airway pressures).

Case 3: Change in set volume

Problem: A 5-foot, 10-inch adult ventilator patient is initially set up on the settings AC-750-12-60%-+5 cm H_2O. Due to ABG results and a subsequent comprehensive assessment, V_T is reduced to 550 mL. However, tidal volume on the apnea (backup) remains at 750 mLs. Later, during weaning, the patient becomes apneic, the apnea alarm is activated, and the patient is ventilated at a tidal volume of 750 mLs.

Discussion: The tidal volume on the apnea parameters is inappropriately high. Without a reduction in the "apnea" V_T, the patient is at risk for being overventilated and his lungs overdistended, especially if he becomes apneic on a spontaneous or weaning mode. Any time a significant change is made to the settings (such as a switch to pressure support ventilation), the apnea alarms and settings should be checked and changed, if appropriate, to maximize patient safety. In this instance, the patient's "apnea" tidal volume should be reduced to 550 mL.

In this instance, it is very likely that the low V_T alarm may be in need of adjustment to about 450 mL or 100 mL below the new V_T.

Case 4: Artificial airway obstruction

Problem: For a ventilator patient, you note that suddenly both the low V_T and high pressure limit alarm are sounding on each inspiration and that the patient's Spo_2 is 85% and the heart rate is 148.

Discussion: The sudden decrease in V_T and increase in ventilating pressures strongly point to an apparent acute airway obstruction (e.g., kinked or clogged ET tube). If the patient shows signs of distress and there is a question about the functioning of the ventilator and/or airway, disconnect the patient from the ventilator and ventilate with 100% oxygen via a manual

---

(continues)

resuscitator and troubleshoot the ventilator. If you are still unable to manually ventilate the patient, quickly try to pass a suction catheter; if this is not successful, extubate the patient and manually ventilate with a mask.

Case 5: Remote alarm problem

Problem: Ventilator alarm is sounding, but remote alarm monitor is not activated.

Discussion: This problem appears to be rooted in either the remote alarm cable not being connected or a remote alarm equipment problem. To identify such problems, remote alarms should be tested each shift to ensure they are properly functioning. This involves ensuring that the cable is connected and the alarms are functional. Faulty cables or remote alarm units should be immediately replaced and/or repaired.

In addition to the changes related to invasive positive pressure ventilation and alarms, you will need to be familiar with the most likely modifications involving noninvasive positive pressure ventilation (NPPV). These modifications are described in **Table 14-13**.

Ventilator Waveform Evaluation

In addition to the above modifications for mechanically ventilated patients, a review and interpretation of ventilator graphics may help identify the need to make certain changes independently. Below are the most commonly found waveforms that would warrant independent action by you as the respiratory therapist.

Patient–Ventilator Asynchrony

Asynchrony between the patient and ventilator can be seen as irregularly spiked flow and/or irregular pressure waveform, as displayed in **Figure 14-2**. As discussed in Table 14-11, patient asynchrony may originate from the patient or the ventilator setting. If patient related, you should independently troubleshoot and address the most common patient causes, including suctioning a patient with excessive mucous or mucous plugging, recommending bronchodilators for bronchospasm, or recommending sedation for agitated patients. If the problem is related to ventilator settings, consider inappropriate trigger sensitivity and inadequate inspiratory flow as the most frequent causes. Usually, increasing the flow or adjusting the sensitivity to a proper level will solve the problem.

Table 14-13 Modifications in Noninvasive Positive Pressure Ventilation

Problem/Situation	Possible Cause	Recommended Modification
Patient's clinical status suggests the need for only nocturnal ventilation or intermittent ventilation	A variety of conditions resulting in hypoventilation, including neuromuscular conditions and sleep apnea	Consider recommending NPPV
Patient on NPPV objects to discomfort or major leak from nasal mask or other interface	Mask or interface too tight, ill fitting, or otherwise unsuitable	Loosen interface to use minimum pressure to achieve a seal or consider alternative mask or interface, including nasal pillows
Patient on NPPV complains of extreme airway dryness	Inadequately humidified gas	Consider adding heated humidity
Patient is on NPPV with 15 L/min O_2 bleed-in to circuit, but remains mildly hypoxemic	Inability of certain NPPV ventilators to deliver high F_{IO_2} due to significant dilution with room air	Consider a device which is capable of delivering high F_{IO_2}s (BiPAP Vision), and bleed additional O_2 directly into BiPAP mask and closely monitor patient
A patient's mouth is wide open during NPPV via nasal mask, and the pressure manometer fails to reach the set inspiratory pressure	Major leak through the mouth	Consider adding a chin strap or using a full-face mask

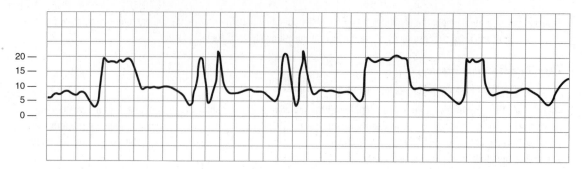

Figure 14-2 A Graphical Display of Patient–Ventilator Asynchony Showing Irregular Pressure Waveform.

Source: Burns, S.M. (Ed.). (2006). *AACN protocols for practice: noninvasive monitoring* (2nd ed.). Sudbury, MA: Jones and Bartlett Publishers.

Inappropriate Sensitivity

The sensitivity setting is inappropriate when the patient must exert excessive negative pressure or excessive inspiratory flow to initiate a breath, as reflected in **Figure 14-3**. An inappropriate sensitivity setting can impose additional work of breathing on adult patients and cause patient-ventilator asynchrony. In general, the solution to this problem is to adjust the sensitivity to an appropriate level, usually less than –1.5 to 2.5 cm H_2O for a pressure trigger or about 3.0 L/min for a flow trigger.

Volume Loss

Volume loss means that the set (or intended) tidal volume was not delivered to and/or returned from the patient. The volume-time waveform, such as that shown in **Figure 14-4**, reveals this situation in that the exhaled volume does not return to zero. The problem most often is a leak in the patient–ventilator interface. Leaks usually occur around the artificial airway or a connection in the ventilator circuit. If you determine the leak is due to the artificial airway and the airway is properly positioned, the best fix usually involves readjusting the cuff pressure using either the minimal leak or minimal occluding volume technique (see Chapter 10). If you determine that the leak is in the ventilator circuit, either fix the loose connection or replace the circuit.

Auto-PEEP

Auto-PEEP occurs when the patient is still exhaling as the next breath is delivered. This causes excessive gas to remain trapped in the lungs of a mechanically ventilated patient. Auto-PEEP may occur for a variety of reasons but is most commonly caused by insufficient exhalation time, patient asynchrony,

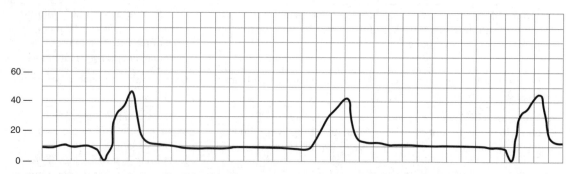

Figure 14-3 Ventilator Graphic Showing Inappropriate Sensitivity Requiring a Patient to Exert Excessive Negative Pressure to Trigger the Ventilator (Below –1.5 to –2.0 cm H_2O).

Source: Burns, S.M. (Ed.). (2006). *AACN protocols for practice: noninvasive monitoring* (2nd ed.). Sudbury, MA: Jones and Bartlett Publishers.

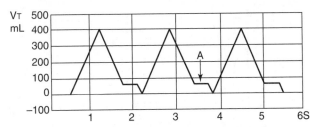

Figure 14-4 Volume–Time Graphic Showing Volume Loss. Note that the expired volume does not return to baseline.

Source: Burns, S.M. (Ed.). (2006). *AACN protocols for practice: noninvasive monitoring* (2nd ed.). Sudbury, MA: Jones and Bartlett Publishers.

or increased airway resistance. The problem can manifest in several ways, most commonly as an expiratory flow waveform that does not return to zero before the next breath, as shown in **Figure 14-5**. To measure the amount of auto-PEEP, perform an end-expiratory hold maneuver, as described in Chapter 13. Once you confirm its presence, you will need to manage it according to its cause. If the cause is insufficient exhalation time, you should either increase the inspiratory flow, decrease the inspiratory time, or increase the expiratory time. If auto-PEEP is associated with excessive airway resistance, you can often reduce or eliminate it by suctioning or administering bronchodilators. Managing auto-PEEP associated with patient–ventilator asynchrony is discussed in Chapter 15.

Overdistention

When using excessive ventilating pressures, a patient may be predisposed to overdistention of the lung that can lead to barotrauma. On a pressure–volume curve, such as that shown in **Figure 14-6**, overdistention becomes apparent when the pressure–volume curve flattens significantly beyond the upper inflection point. Due to its resemblance to a bird, this is sometimes called a "beaked" pressure–volume curve. When you observe this problem, you generally can resolve it by reducing either the volume (in volume ventilation) or the pressure setting, in accordance with existing mechanical ventilation protocols. In the absence of a protocol, a change in a volume or pressure setting usually requires a physician's order and thus would be achieved by recommendation, not independent action.

Weaning from Ventilatory Support

In order to initiate weaning from ventilatory support, you generally need a physician's order. However, the specific means of weaning often is governed by preapproved protocols, which give you some discretion as to the methods used, including the speed with which the patient may be weaned. Chapter 12 provides details on weaning procedures, including implementation of protocol-based spontaneous breathing trials and weaning ALI/ARDS patients using the NHLBI ARDS protocol.

Other Modifications in Mechanical Ventilation

There are other circumstances when modifications are appropriate in mechanical ventilation. Whether or not you can independently make such alterations depends on factors such as the type of change

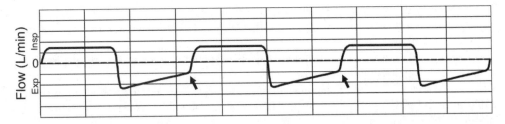

Figure 14-5 A Flow–Time Graphic Showing Auto-PEEP. Expiratory flow does not return to zero baseline before next machine breath, indicating gas-trapping (arrows).

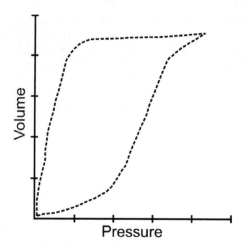

Figure 14-6 Pressure–Volume Loop Indicating Overdistention During a Positive Pressure Breath. Beyond the upper inflection point, small changes in volume result in very large increases in pressure, making the loop appear like the "beak" of a bird.

and use of protocols in your workplace. One example is the addition of mechanical deadspace in a ventilator circuit to address a respiratory alkalosis due to hyperventilation. In such a circumstance, a protocol may permit you to add mechanical deadspace near the circuit Y connector to cause CO_2 re-breathing and thus help normalize ABG results. However, it is more common for modifications of this type to require a physician's order, and hence you should normally only *recommend* this action. The use of mechanical deadspace and other changes that usually require a physician's order are described in detail in Chapter 15.

COMMON ERRORS TO AVOID

You can improve your score by avoiding these mistakes:

- Never continue therapy on a patient who exhibits severe adverse reactions. Instead, if you note adverse reactions, stop the therapy, monitor the patient closely, and notify the physician and nurse.
- Never apply percussion or vibration too close to surgical incisions or chest injury or trauma. Instead, apply the therapy a safe distance (6–12 inches) from incision or injuries.
- Never use incentive spirometry on an uncooperative patient or one who can not follow commands. Instead, consider recommending IPPB, which can be used to treat or prevent atelectasis regardless of mental status.
- In general, do not use a standard air-entrainment device to deliver a high FIO_2 (greater than 45–50%) to a spontaneously breathing patient. Instead, consider (1) a nonrebreathing mask, (2) a high-flow cannula, (3) two large-volume nebulizers connected in parallel, or (4) a high-output nebulizer.
- Never use an electronically powered (air compressor) device to deliver IPPB therapy to a patient requiring high FIO_2s. Instead, consider pneumatically powered devices like the Bird Mark 7 or Bennett PR-II, which can deliver a high FIO_2.
- Never drain tubing condensate back into a nebulizer. Rather, place a water trap in line to capture the condensate.
- Never use an MDI or a DPI on a patient who is in tachypneic or in severe respiratory distress. Instead, use a small-volume nebulizer.
- Never use a standard nasal cannula on a patient requiring a low FIO_2 but who has a high or unstable minute ventilation. Instead, use a high-flow device such as an air-entrainment (venturi) mask or high-flow cannula should be used instead.
- During postural drainage, never keep a nauseous patient or one coughing violently in a head-down position. Instead, sit the patient up, monitor closely, and notify the physician and nurse.

- Never keep a nasopharygeal airway in place (in the same naris) for more than one day.
- Never use low-flow systems, like nasal cannulas, to administer heliox therapy to spontaneously breathing patients. Instead, administer heliox using a tight-fitting nonrebreathing mask at a minimum flow of 10–15 L/min (you might also consider a high-flow cannula).
- Avoid tracheal damage by never inflating endotracheal tube cuffs to pressures above 25 cm H_2O. Instead, aim for lower pressures or use either the minimal occluding volume (MOV) or minimal leak technique (MLT).
- Never use oropharyngeal airways in fully conscious patients.
- To avoid the potential for tracheal tissue damage or an airway leak, never keep an undersized ET tube in place for a long time period. Instead, recommend that an appropriate-size tube be put in place via either reintubation or a tube exchanger.
- Never use excessive suctioning pressure or application time. Instead, suction adult patients with the lowest effective negative pressure for no longer than 10–15 seconds.
- When making changes to primary ventilator settings, never make more than one change at a time that affects either oxygen (e.g., FIO_2 or PEEP) or ventilation (e.g., tidal volume or respiratory rate).
- Never continue using a heat and moisture exchanger (HME) for a patient who develops thick, bloody, or copious secretions. In these cases, switch to a heated humidifier.
- Never set the low minute ventilation alarm on adults receiving ventilator support below 4.0–5.0 L/min.
- When using a CPAP or BiPAP™ mask, minimize tissue damage by avoiding too tight a fit.

SURE BETS

In some situations you can be sure of the right approach to a clinical problem or scenario:

- When you suspect a serious adverse effect, *always* follow these steps:
  - Stop or pause the therapy.
  - Stay with the patient and monitor him or her.
  - Notify the nurse and physician, if the patient is at a health care facility.
  - If the adverse effect appears life threatening, initiate a "code blue" if the patient is in a health care facility or activate EMS if the patient is in an alternate site such as home care.
- Always ensure a good lip seal during IS or IPPB hyperinflation therapy. If a good lip seal is not possible (neuromuscular weakness) but patient is at risk for atelectasis, consider IPPB via mask.
- When administering heliox therapy, always use an oxygen analyzer with active alarms to continuously measure the FIO_2.
- Always remember to use the appropriate conversion factor (1.8 for 80/20 and 1.6 for 70/30 mixture) when using a standard flow meter to administer heliox therapy.
- If you suspect insufficient drug delivery with an MDI, always review the technique and consider adding a holding chamber or spacer or adding an actuator assist device for patients unable to activate the device.
- Always consider adding humidity for patients on a nasal cannula with flows greater than 4 L/min or for those who may be at risk for retained secretions (e.g., patients with bronchitis or pneumonia) but who need moderate- to high-flow O_2 therapy.
- If the tubing is correctly set up to a nonrebreathing mask and the bag fails to remain at least partially inflated during inspiration, always increase the flow.
- Always preoxygenate and hyperinflate patients with 100% O_2 before suctioning and ensure that the appropriate-size catheter is used.
- Always consider using a Coudé suction catheter when attempting to target the left lung in suctioning.
- Always ensure that the tracheal stoma is cleaned and the inner cannula and dressing are changed at least every 8 hours to minimize the chance of infection.
- To avoid ventilator self-cycling or imposing excessive work on the patient, always ensure that the triggering sensitivity is properly set at –0.5 to –2.0 cm H_2O (pressure trigger) or –1.0 to –3.0 L/min (flow trigger).

- If the ventilator pressure manometer fluctuates widely during inspiration or if the inspiratory flow waveform is "scalloped," always consider increasing the inspiratory flow.
- When administering nitric oxide (NO) to a mechanically ventilated patient, always ensure that NO, nitrogen dioxide (NO_2), and F_{IO_2} levels are continuously analyzed and are at acceptable levels.
- Always consider increasing the flow if you observe an unintended inverse I:E ratio during flow-limited ventilation.
- To maximize patient safety and avoid unnecessary alarm activation, always set, check, and adjust ventilator alarms several times during each shift. Pay special attention to low pressure (disconnect) and low minute ventilation alarms.
- Always check and appropriately adjust ventilator alarms when making major ventilator settings changes, such as switching to pressure support to begin weaning.

PRE-TEST ANSWERS AND EXPLANATIONS

Below are this chapter's pre-test answers and explanations. Be sure to review each answer's explanation thoroughly to help you understand why it is correct. If the explanation is still unclear to you, review the chapter contents or the references and/or refer to this chapter's supplemental resources on the CD.

14-1. **Correct answer: B.** Stop suctioning and immediately administer oxygen. If you observe any major change in a patient's heart rate or rhythm or other adverse effect during suctioning, immediately stop the procedure and give oxygen to the patient, while providing manual ventilation as necessary.

14-2. **Correct answer: D.** Stop the treatment and stay with the patient until she improves. Depending on the goals of therapy and the condition of the patient, IPPB treatments typically vary in duration from 10 to 20 minutes. Should you observe any untoward effects, or should the patient exhibit signs of tiring or other adverse effects, immediately stop the treatment and stay at the bedside until the patient is stabilized.

14-3. **Correct answer: A.** Nasal cannula at 4–5 L/min. A simple mask with an input flow delivers an oxygen concentration of about 35–40%. A nasal cannula with an input flow of 4–5 L/min would yield an F_{IO_2} of 36–40% and is therefore the best answer. All other choices would result in a substantial change in the F_{IO_2}, and the choice involving a mask would not address the issues of confinement and difficulty eating.

14-4. **Correct answer: D.** I, II, and IV. Increased expiratory times may be appropriate during IPPB therapy given to patients with certain forms of COPD. This can be achieved by (1) coaching the patient to prolong the expiratory phase, (2) increasing the inspiratory flow, or (3) mechanically retarding exhalation via a PEEP valve placed distal to the expiratory port.

14-5. **Correct answer: B.** A large system leak. After a patient is fitted with a nasal CPAP mask and has the prescribed pressure valve attached, the unit is turned on and checked for leaks. An inability to generate any pressure indicates that a large system leak is present.

14-6. **Correct answer: D.** Decrease total output flow and increase F_{IO_2}. Occlusion of the entrainment port would decrease (or eliminate) the entrainment of air. Because the entrainment of air accounts for a significant amount of output, the total flow of the device would drop. The decrease in entrained air would also mean that less air would be available to dilute the oxygen. Hence, the F_{IO_2} would increase.

14-7. **Correct answer: C.** Administer 100% oxygen through the ventilator for 1–2 minutes before suctioning. To prevent hypoxemia during suctioning of an intubated patient, you should hyperinflate and hyperoxygenate the patient with 100% oxygen via resuscitation bag or through the ventilator.

14-8. **Correct answer: C.** Replacing the endotracheal tube with a larger size. You should use a "tube exchanger" to change the endotracheal tube or recommend reintubating the patient with a larger endotracheal tube in order to prevent excessive cuff pressures and mucosal damage.

14-9. **Correct answer: B.** Changing to a heated wick humidifier. An increase in the peak pressure without an increase in the plateau pressure indicates an increase in airway resistance. Difficulty in suctioning secretions suggests that the increase in resistance is caused by retained secretions. Since thick or bloody secretions are contraindications to using a heat and moisture exchanger, you should switch the patient over to a humidifier capable of providing higher absolute humidity, such as a heated wick-type device.

14-10. **Correct answer: D.** II, III, and IV. The significant increase in pulse, respiratory rate, and $Paco_2$ indicate that the patient is having significant problems and needs to be placed back on the ventilator. The change in blood pressure is not significant.

14-11. **Correct answer: A.** Inspiratory flow. During routine assist-control ventilation, I:E ratios are normally maintained in the 1:2 to 1:4 range. An inverse I:E ratio alarm indicates that the I-time exceeds the E-time. This is often due to a peak flow setting that is too low. You should either increase the flow, decrease the volume, or decrease the respiratory rate to give more time for exhalation.

14-12. **Correct answer: B.** Increase the flow rate to 12–15 L/min. Reservoir bag deflation on inspiration is a sign of inadequate flow; increase the flow rate to prevent room air entrainment and Fio_2 reduction.

14-13. **Correct answer: A.** Increase the oxygen liter flow and reassess the patient. Based on the data given, O_2 has been prescribed per protocol to correct arterial hypoxemia on an otherwise healthy patient. The initial response indicates that this objective is not being fully met because the Pao_2 is still below the normal range of 80–100 torr. In light of this patient's hypoxemic state and the use of an oxygen therapy protocol, the Fio_2 should be gradually increased and the patient reassessed until the targeted Pao_2 or 80–100 torr or an Spo_2 of greater than 92–95% is achieved. When assessment reveals that supplemental O_2 is no longer needed, most protocols permit it to be discontinued or placed on standby.

14-14. **Correct answer: D.** Measuring maximum inspiratory pressure. All of the above actions except maximum inspiratory pressure (MIP) measurement are indicated in this emergency situation.

14-15. **Correct answer: C.** Change to a simple mask at 5–7 L/min. An Spo_2 of 84% is substantially below normal. However, the nasal oxygen therapy is probably not effective because this patient is probably breathing through his mouth. The oxygen therapy should therefore be switched to a mask capable of approximating the Fio_2 of nasal cannula at 4 L/min.

14-16. **Correct answer: D.** Reducing the inspiratory flow. Oxygenation can be a problem for some patients receiving heliox therapy, particularly an 80/20 mixture, which has about the same Fio_2 as room air. After checking the seal of the mask and confirming the Fio_2, you may consider recommending a more oxygen-enriched heliox mixture such as 70/30. In such instances, you may also need to increase the inspiratory gas flow to prevent collapse of the reservoir bag. However, decreasing the inspiratory flow would be inappropriate in this situation.

14-17. **Correct answer: B.** Coach the patient to pause before each maneuver. To avoid light-headedness or dizziness associated with hyperventilation, a patient using incentive spirometry should be coached to perform one or two maneuvers and then to breathe normally for 30–60 seconds before initiating another maneuver.

14-18. **Correct answer: B.** Low compliance tubing. "Compressed volume" is machine-delivered volume that the patient does not receive due to gas compression (following Boyle's law) and circuit expansion. Compressed volume is most critical when delivering small volumes to infants and toddlers. The larger the volume and more compliant the full gas delivery system is (including ventilator "innards," humidifier volume, and delivery tubing), the greater the compressed volume loss will be. Therefore, to minimize compressed volume loss in infants and toddlers, you should use small-diameter, stiff delivery tubing and humidifiers and ventilators with low internal volumes.

14-19. **Correct answer: D.** Retract the ET tube up by 3–4 cm. The most likely problem is right-sided mainstem bronchus intubation, as suggested by the clinical findings including decreased ventilation to the left chest and a reduction in Pao_2. Given that the tube is secured at 26 cm, which is quite deep for this patient, the ET tube should be retracted by about 3 cm.

14-20. **Correct answer: D.** Change to an aerosol mask. Changing to a mask will eliminate the need for the patient to hold the mouthpiece in place, thus benefiting the patient and saving you time.

14-21. **Correct answer: A.** II only. A drop in pressure below baseline that coincides with the patient's inspiration with a continuous-flow system indicates inadequate flow. In general, a drop in pressure of 2 cm H_2O is acceptable; any greater decrease in pressure means that system flow should be increased.

14-22. **Correct answer: D.** Increase the system flow to maintain the pressure. A fall in inspiratory pressure during continuous-flow CPAP suggests that the patient's flow is exceeding the system flow (insufficient flow). To overcome this problem, increase the flow until the pressure drop is no more than 1–2 cm H_2O.

14-23. **Correct answer: A.** Stop the treatment, stabilize the patient, and inform the physician. Hemoptysis or coughing up blood is one potentially rare but serious side effect of postural drainage, percussion, and vibration. As with all serious side effects, the treatment should be stopped, the patient stabilized and monitored closely, and the physician notified.

14-24. **Correct answer: B.** Hypoxemia in neonates with persistent pulmonary hypertension. The primary indication and approved use of inhaled nitric oxide is for the treatment of term and near-term neonates with hypoxemic respiratory failure due to persistent pulmonary hypertension of the newborn (PPHN).

14-25. **Correct answer: C.** Discontinue the treatment and notify the physician. Positive pressure can adversely affect the hemodynamic status of a patient. When that occurs, you should stop the treatment, stabilize the patient, and then notify and suggest alternative therapies to the physician.

14-26. **Correct answer: C.** Postpone therapy until you are able to contact the ordering physician. In general, an adrenergic bronchodilator should not be given if a patient is already experiencing tachycardia. Moreover, once a treatment is begun with an adrenergic drug, it should be terminated if the pulse rate increases more than about 20 beats/min.

14-27. **Correct answer: A.** Encourage the patient to cough. Rhonchi is caused by air moving through secretions in the lungs. Patients with rhonchi after receiving a bland aerosol should be encouraged to cough to clear the loose secretions.

14-28. **Correct answer: C.** Increase the high respiratory rate alarm to 30–35. When weaning on pressure support, a modest increase in respiratory rate is common and generally should be tolerated up to a maximum of 30–35 breaths per minute. In this instance, the high respiratory rate alarm should be increased to 30–35 breaths per minute.

14-29. **Correct answer: C.** Reconnect the patient to the ventilator with prior settings. Development of severe agitation, tachypnea, tachycardia, bradycardia, hypotension, asynchronous or paradoxical breathing, angina, or cardiac arrhythmias during a T-tube weaning trial usually indicate that the patient is not tolerating it well and that ventilatory support should be reinstituted.

14-30. **Correct answer: B.** Stop the treatment, monitor the patient, and notify the doctor. A patient who starts wheezing during an ultrasonic nebulizer treatment is likely developing a bronchospasm in response to the high-density aerosol (an adverse reaction). In general, when a patient experiences an adverse reaction to therapy, you should stop the therapy, monitor the patient closely, and then contact the physician.

POST-TEST

A post-test for this chapter that includes automated scoring and feedback is available on the accompanying CD. Be sure to complete this additional assessment to confirm your mastery of this chapter's objectives.

REFERENCES

Burns, S. M. (Ed.). (2006). *AACN Protocols for practice: Noninvasive monitoring* (2nd ed.). Sudbury, MA: Jones & Bartlett.

Butler, T. J. (2009). *Laboratory exercises for competency in respiratory care* (2nd ed.). Philadelphia: FA Davis.

Kasmarek, R. M., Dimas, S., & Mack, C. W. (2005). *The essentials of respiratory care* (4th ed.). St. Louis: Mosby.

Wilkins, R. L., Stoller, J. K., & Kacmarek, R. M. (Eds.) (2009). *Egan's fundamentals of respiratory care* (9th ed.). St. Louis: Mosby.

Wilkins, R. W., Sheldon, E. L., & Heuer, A. J. (2009). *Clinical assessment in respiratory care* (6th ed.). St. Louis: Mosby.

Wyka, K. A., Mathews, P. J., & Clark, W. F. (2002). *Foundations of respiratory care*. Albany: Delmar.

15 Recommend Modifications in the Respiratory Care Plan

Albert J. Heuer
Narciso E. Rodriguez

INTRODUCTION

Beyond providing initial respiratory care to patients, you often must recommend modifications to the care plan based on the patient's response and changes in a patient's clinical status. This chapter reviews both the criteria for determining the need for a care plan modification as well as the implementation of such changes. By learning the following objectives, you will help ensure your readiness as a candidate for the NBRC CRT exam and position yourself to be safe and effective in a clinical setting.

OBJECTIVES

After completion of this chapter, you should be able to demonstrate knowledge needed to recommend modifications to the respiratory care plan, including the following:

1. Initiation of procedures such as bronchopulmonary hygiene, artificial airway insertion, and mechanical ventilation
2. Selecting medications, including bronchodilators, anti-inflammatories, mucolytics, sedatives, paralyzing agents, and diuretics
3. Removing and discontinuing therapies related to mechanical ventilation (i.e., recommending weaning, extubation, and decannulation)
4. Changes related to mechanical ventilation involving invasive versus noninvasive ventilation, the mode, and alarms settings, in addition to other changes intended to enhance patient synchrony, oxygenation, ventilation, and I:E ratio
5. Based on mechanical ventilation waveform interpretation, recommend changes related to eliminating auto-PEEP and flow starvation, as well as reducing plateau pressure
6. Other modifications related to patient position and oxygen therapy as well as drug dosages, concentration, and frequency

WHAT TO EXPECT ON THIS CATEGORY OF THE CRT EXAM

Number of questions: 17
Level of questions: about 15% recall, 60% application, 25% analysis

WHAT'S NEW FOR 2009

As of July 2009, this section of the NBRC CRT examination includes the following *new content areas*:

- Recommend:
  ○ Treatment of pneumothorax
  ○ Adjustment of fluid balance
  ○ Adjustment of electrolyte therapy
- Recommend pharmacologic interventions, including use of:
  ○ Hypertonic saline
  ○ Analgesics
  ○ Paralytic agents
  ○ Surfactants
  ○ Vaccines (e.g., pneumovax 23, influenza)

PRE-TEST

Carefully respond to each of the following questions. After completing the pre-test, compare your answers with those provided at the end of this chapter. Then, thoroughly review the explanation for each answer to help you understand why it is correct.

15-1. A patient with acute bronchitis is receiving mechanical ventilation. Wheezing is heard over all lung fields, and rhonchi are heard over the central airways. Previously suctioned secretions have been quite thick. The patient's peak pressure is 45 cm H_2O, and plateau pressure is 20 cm H_2O. All of the following would be useful to treat the patient's condition *except*:
   A. Albuterol (Proventil)
   B. Ipratropium bromide (Atrovent)
   C. Acetylcysteine (Mucomyst)
   D. Pancuronium bromide (Pavulon)

15-2. A 75-year-old female patient with a fractured hip has been bedridden for at least one week. The patient has clear breath sounds, but they are diminished slightly in the bases. The patient has normal pulmonary function based on bedside spirometry. Which of the following should you recommend?
   I. Bronchodilator therapy
   II. Deep suctioning
   III. Incentive spirometry treatments
   IV. Coughing and deep breathing
   A. I and III only
   B. II and IV only
   C. III and IV only
   D. I, II, and IV

15-3. An intubated patient in the ICU needs to undergo bedside bronchoscopy and is in need of short-term moderate sedation. Which of the following agents would you recommend for this procedure?
   A. Propofol (Diprivan)
   B. Haloperidol (Haldol)
   C. Lorazepam (Ativan)
   D. Cisatracurium (Nimbex)

15-4. You are assisting a medical resident performing an emergent intubation on a somewhat combative patient. The resident wants to briefly paralyze the patient to facilitate this procedure. Which drug would you recommend for this purpose?
   A. Pancuronium (Pavulon)
   B. Succinylcholine (Anectine)
   C. Vecuronium (Norcuron)
   D. Cisatracurium (Nimbex)

15-5. A physician is having difficulty visualizing the airway of an obese patient during an emergency intubation procedure. He asks for your recommendation to quickly secure the airway and provide ventilation. You should recommend:
   A. A cricothyrotomy
   B. Inserting an LMA
   C. Sedating the patient
   D. Using a double-lumen ET tube

15-6. A 90-kg male patient with a flail chest injury is being mechanically ventilated in the assist/control mode with an F_{IO_2} of 0.5, a set rate of 18, and a tidal volume of 600 mL. He is involuntarily breathing above the set rate for a total respiratory rate of 28–30 breaths/min. Results of an arterial blood gas analysis are as follows:

pH	7.52
$Paco_2$	27 torr
HCO_3	21 mEq/L
BE	–2 mEq/L
Pao_2	81 torr
Sao_2	96%

On the basis of these results, the most appropriate action is to:
A. Increase the F_{IO_2}
B. Add mechanical deadspace
C. Increase the ventilator rate
D. Increase the tidal volume

15-7. A 87-year-old nursing home patient is admitted with pneumonia. On assessment the patient presents with a 103.2°F temperature, dry mucous membranes, urine output of 10 mL/hr for the past two hours, mild hypotension, and increased hematocrit on his CBC. You should recommend to the ER physician all of the following *except*:
A. Initiating IV fluids immediately
B. Beginning diuretic therapy
C. Minimizing insensible water loss
D. Documenting fluid intake/output every hour

15-8. Which of the following airway routes would you recommend to immediately ventilate a trauma patient in a neck brace with a suspected cervical spine injury who was admitted to the emergency department?
   I. Orotracheal intubation
   II. Nasotracheal intubation
   III. Laryngeal mask airway
A. II only
B. III only
C. II or III only
D. I, II, or III

15-9. A COPD patient being mechanically ventilated appears to be developing auto-PEEP. Which of the following should you recommend to improve this situation?

A. Decreasing the I:E ratio
B. Adding an inspiratory hold
C. Using an inverse I:E ratio
D. Using a decelerating flow pattern

15-10. You are managing a 49-year-old male patient, who weighs about 80 kg (175 lbs.), who is on a mechanical ventilator with the following settings and blood gases:

Ventilator Settings		Blood Gases	
V_T	750 mL	pH	7.42
Rate	12/min	$Paco_2$	36 torr
F_{IO_2}	0.35	Pao_2	58 torr
Mode	Assist/control	HCO_3	23 mEq/L
PEEP	5 cm H_2O		

What changes should you now recommend to the physician?
A. Increasing the F_{IO_2} to 0.45
B. Changing the mode to SIMV
C. Adding 150 mL of deadspace
D. Increasing the rate to 16/min

15-11. A patient with heart failure is receiving volume-cycled ventilation and has a pulmonary artery catheter in place. The ventilator peak pressure is 45 cm H_2O, and plateau pressure is 25 cm H_2O. The patient's pulmonary artery pressure is 42/33 mm Hg, and pulmonary capillary wedge pressure (PCWP) is 28 mm Hg. Lung sounds indicate dependent crackles and wheezing. Which of the following should you recommend?
A. Administering albuterol (Proventil)
B. Decreasing the mean airway pressure
C. Administering furosemide (Lasix)
D. Removing the PA catheter—it is malfunctioning

15-12. A patient is receiving a treatment with 2.5 mg of albuterol and 3.0 mL of normal saline in the emergency department. The heart rate prior to therapy is 80 beats/min, and at the end of therapy is 128 beats/min. You should recommend:
A. Adding acetylcysteine (Mucomyst) to the treatment
B. Decreasing the dosage of albuterol
C. Increasing the amount of saline per treatment to 5 mL
D. Changing to ipratropium bromide (Atrovent)

15-13. An adult patient who suffered a cerebral contusion and resulting cerebral edema from an automobile accident has just been placed on volume-cycled mechanical ventilation while in the emergency department. Initial ABG values are as follows:

pH	7.39
$Paco_2$	42 torr
HCO_3	25 mEq/L
BE	0 mEq/L
Pao_2	92 torr
Sao_2	95%

What should you recommend for the management of this patient?
A. Maintaining the present settings and monitor the patient
B. Increasing the minute volume on the ventilator
C. Increasing the inspired O_2 percentage
D. Changing to pressure control ventilation

15-14. Which of the following drugs would be most appropriate to recommend as a substitute for albuterol (Proventil) for a patient who has bronchospasm and whose cardiac rate increases by 50 beats/min with each treatment?
A. Isoetharine (Bronkosol)
B. Isoproterenol (Isuprel)
C. Racemic epinephrine
D. Ipratropium bromide (Atrovent)

15-15. A patient with neuromuscular disease has been on ventilatory support for 4 months via tracheostomy. At this point, she requires only nighttime ventilator support. Which of the following artificial airways should you recommend?
A. Tracheostomy button
B. Bivona tracheostomy tube
C. Cuffed, fenestrated tracheostomy tube
D. Uncuffed, standard tracheostomy tube

15-16. A physician orders 3 L/min O_2 via simple mask to a 33-year-old post-op female patient with moderate hypoxemia breathing room air (Pao_2 = 52 torr). The correct action at this time is to:
A. Carry out the physician's prescription exactly as written
B. Recommend a flow of at least 5 L/min to wash out CO_2
C. Recommend that the mask be changed to a cannula at 2 L/min
D. Not apply the oxygen until contacting the medical director

15-17. A patient in combined hypoxemic and hypercapnic respiratory failure due to an acute restrictive disorder is placed on a ventilator in the SIMV mode at a rate of 12 breaths/min and a PEEP of 10 cm H_2O. Soon thereafter, she begins to exhibit a paradoxical breathing pattern with intercostal retractions. Which of the following changes should you recommend?
A. Decreasing the PEEP level to 5 cm H_2O
B. Decreasing the rate to 8 breaths/min
C. Switching over to the pure CPAP mode
D. Providing supplemental pressure support

15-18. You are asked to assess whether a 65-kg (143-lb.) patient with a neuromuscular disorder being mechanically ventilated in the SIMV mode is ready for weaning. After obtaining the following data during a bedside spontaneous breathing assessment, what would you recommend?

Spontaneous tidal volume	250 mL
Minute ventilation	10 L/min
Vital capacity	650 mL
Max inspiratory pressure (MIP)	–20 cm H_2O

A. Beginning a spontaneous breathing T-piece trial
B. Postponing weaning and reevaluating the patient
C. Beginning weaning using a pressure support protocol
D. Beginning weaning by decreasing the SIMV rate

15-19. An adult patient started on cool mist therapy after extubation begins to develop stridor. Which of the following actions should you recommend?
  A. Changing from cool mist to heated aerosol
  B. Administering a racemic epinephrine treatment
  C. Reintubating the patient immediately
  D. Drawing and analyzing an arterial blood gas

15-20. An 8-hour-old, 28-week gestational age neonate is being maintained in an oxygen hood with an F_{IO_2} of 0.65. The neonatologist believes that the patient has infant respiratory distress syndrome (IRDS). Based on the following results, what should you recommend?

pH	7.36
$Paco_2$	44 torr
HCO_3	24 mEq/L
BE	0 mEq/L
Pao_2	52 torr

  A. Increasing the O_2 hood concentration to 100%
  B. Beginning inhaled nitric oxide (INO) therapy
  C. Administering pulmonary surfactant with Beractant (Survanta)
  D. Starting high-frequency ventilation

15-21. A physician asks your recommendation regarding sedation for a mechanically ventilated patient in the ICU. You would consider recommending all of the following to calm this patient *except*:
  A. Pentobarbital (Nembutal)
  B. Propofol (Diprivan)
  C. Lorazepam (Ativan)
  D. Cisatracurium (Nimbex)

15-22. A ventilator patient is admitted with atelectasis and a lower than predicted functional residual capacity (FRC). This has caused hypoxemia. What should you recommend to correct the atelectasis and improve the FRC?
  A. Adding PEEP
  B. Increasing the F_{IO_2}
  C. Suctioning the patient more frequently
  D. Starting pressure support ventilation

15-23. A 25-year-old asthma patient has continual symptoms that limit her physical activity. Along with frequent exacerbations of her condition, her FEV_1/FVC is less than 60% of predicted. Which of the following drugs should you recommend to help control her condition over the long term?
  I. Albuterol (Proventil) MDI 2 puffs 3 times a day (tid)
  II. Fluticasone (Flovent) MDI 2 puffs 4 times a day
  III. Salmeterol (Serevent) 2 puffs twice a day (bid)
  A. II only
  B. III only
  C. II and III only
  D. I and II only

15-24. Which of the following four adult patients receiving ventilatory support is the best candidate for weaning?

Patient	VC (L)	$\dot{V}_E$ (L/min)	Spon Rate breaths/min	MVV (L/min)	MIP (cm H_2O)	%Shunt
A	0.5	4.1	14	6.3	−21	16%
B	1.5	4.6	15	9.7	−33	17%
C	0.9	12.1	40	14.3	−28	12%
D	1.3	6.3	28	16.7	−42	28%

  A. Patient A
  B. Patient B
  C. Patient C
  D. Patient D

15-25. While reviewing the lab chemistry of a patient in metabolic acidosis due to renal failure, you would expect the following electrolyte to be abnormally high:

A. Glucose

B. Bicarbonate

C. Chloride

D. Potassium

WHAT YOU NEED TO KNOW: ESSENTIAL CONTENT

Recommending Changes in Bronchial Hygiene Therapy

The primary indication for bronchial hygiene therapy is to assist in removing retained secretions from a patient's airway. The indications, proper performance, and other details related to the removal of bronchopulmonary secretions are detailed in Chapter 11. Often, this therapy is initiated because it was deemed appropriate and ordered by the physician. However, there are instances when you will recommend that bronchial hygiene therapy be added to the care plan or modified based on changes in the patient's condition or response to therapy.

Clinical findings that suggest the presence of retained secretions include the following:

- Visible secretions in the airway
- Coarse breath sounds/rhonchi
- Increased work of breathing
- Ineffective spontaneous coughing
- Deterioration of arterial blood gas values
- X-ray changes indicating retained secretions
- Ventilator changes (increased PIP during VCV; decreased V_T during PCV)
- Changes in monitored flow and pressure graphics
- Suspected aspiration of gastric or upper airway secretions

Modifying Bronchial Hygiene Therapy

Chapter 14 covers many of the situations that would warrant modifying bronchial hygiene therapy. In general, modifications may be appropriate in light of preexisting conditions (e.g., increased intracranial pressure), recent procedures (e.g., surgery), and patient demographics (e.g., age) or an adverse reaction to the therapy (e.g., hypoxemia). In general, modifications involve one or more of the following (1) altering the duration of therapy, (2) altering the positions used, or (3) using a different bronchial hygiene strategy. The accompanying box gives some examples of recommended modifications for bronchial hygiene therapy.

Bronchial Hygiene Modification

- Shorten the duration for a given postural drainage position for patients who become anxious or otherwise do not tolerate the therapy.

- Avoid a head-down position for patients with elevated ICP and instead rotate the patient laterally to approximate the position as closely as possible.

- Discourage strenuous coughing for stroke patients or those otherwise predisposed to increased ICP. Instead, instruct these patients to use a "huff" cough or sit them up until the cough subsides.

- If you think a patient might become hypoxemic during the procedure, provide appropriate supplemental O_2 and monitor the Spo_2 throughout the procedure.

- If bronchospasm occurs, stop therapy, return patient to original position, monitor him or her closely, administer supplemental O_2, contact physician, and recommend bronchodilators.

- If complications or adverse events occur during the therapy (e.g., hypoxemia, arrhythmias), stop the therapy, return the patient to the original position, monitor him or her closely, administer oxygen as necessary, and promptly contact the physician.

Recommending Changes in Patient Positioning

Proper positioning can play an important role in optimizing patient care by enhancing oxygenation and ventilation (spontaneous or via mechanical ventilation), assisting with secretion removal and other therapeutic procedures, as well as facilitating diagnostic procedures. The patient positions used in postural draining of specific lung segments and lobes are outlined in Chapter 11. **Table 15-1** summarizes when it may be appropriate for you to recommend a change in the patient's position.

Recommending Insertion and/or Modifications of Artificial Airways

There are instances when you should recommend the insertion or modification of an artificial airway based on your assessment of the patient. **Table 15-2** summarizes the major indications for insertion of an artificial airway. The equipment used for the insertion of an artificial airway and the care of such devices are discussed in Chapters 5, 10, and 18.

Chapter 14 discusses the common adjustments in artificial airway management that you can perform independently. However, some changes involving artificial airways require a physician's order. Such changes often relate to the size, type, or other major feature of the artificial airway. **Table 15-3** (see page 462) outlines the most common situations warranting such recommendations.

Table 15-1 Recommending Modifications in Patient Position

Clinical Situation	Recommended Position Change
General dyspnea	Semi-Fowler's position (consider recommending other therapy such as supplemental O_2)
Orthopnea (dyspnea while supine) generally associated with CHF	Semi-Fowler's or high Fowler's position (consider recommending other therapy such as supplemental O_2)
Perform postural drainage on patient with increased ICP or at risk for aspiration	Avoid Trendelenburg (head-down) position Recommend rotating patient laterally to approximate position
Perform postural drainage on an immobile, bedridden patient	Recommend rotation/vibration bed
To perform IPPB/IPV therapy	Semi-Fowler's or Fowler's (avoid slouching); supine is acceptable for patients unable to tolerate an upright position
Mechanically ventilated patient with unilateral disease (e.g., consolidation, atelectasis)	Place patient in "good lung down" position
Mechanically ventilated patient with poor oxygenation despite high F_{IO_2} and PEEP	Consider recommending prone positioning or kinetic therapy bed
Positioning for chest tube insertion	Involved side should be slightly elevated with arm flexed over head
Positioning for thoracentesis	Patient sitting on the edge of the bed, leaning forward over pillow-draped bedside table, arms crossed with assistant in front for stability
Immobile patient at risk for bed sores	Recommend position change (side to side) every 2–4 hours
Performing CPR on a patient in bed	Place a "compression board" under the patient's back or put bed in "CPR" mode

Table 15-2 Indications for Artificial Airways

Artificial Airway	Indications
Oropharyngeal airway	Stabilize tongue to facilitate ventilation
Nasopharyngeal airway	Facilitate frequent nasal suctioning and ventilation
Laryngeal mask airway (LMA)	Facilitate short-term artificial ventilation; an alternative during difficult intubations
Endotracheal tube (oral)	Facilitate airway protection, artificial ventilation (up to 2 weeks), and secretion clearance
Endotracheal tube (nasal)	In the presence of oral or mandibular trauma or pathology, facilitate airway protection, artificial ventilation, and secretion clearance; improve access for oral care when artificial airway is indicated
Tracheostomy tube (cuffed, unfenestrated)	Facilitate long-term airway protection, artificial ventilation, and secretion clearance; improve access for oral care when artificial airway is indicated; potential for improved weaning prospects
Tracheostomy tube (cuffed, fenestrated)	Above indications with added benefit of permitting phonation (speaking)
Tracheostomy tube (uncuffed)	Maintain patent airway (e.g., in obstructive sleep apnea) and permit supplemental oxygenation and humidification for patient with bypassed upper airway
Tracheostomy button	Maintain patent airway (e.g., obstructive sleep apnea) and permit supplemental oxygenation and humidification for patient with bypassed upper airway

Recommending Treatment of a Pneumothorax

A tension pneumothorax is a serious condition that may be life threatening if not recognized and treated accordingly. If you suspect the presence of a pneumothorax, you can recommend the following: (1) placing the patient in 100% oxygen therapy, (2) ordering a stat chest X-ray, and (3) doing a needle decompression in the appropriate side if the patient's condition becomes life threatening. If the patient is on mechanical ventilation you can recommend ventilator changes aimed to minimize peak inspiratory airway pressures and barotrauma (e.g., decrease or eliminate PEEP, decrease flow, or lower VT). Signs and symptoms of a tension pneumothorax include:

- Increased work of breathing
- Decreased chest excursion on the affected site
- Decreased or absent breath sounds in the affected site
- Tracheal deviation away from the affected site
- Hyperresonant percussion note on the affected side
- Absence of lung markings and radiolucency on the chest X-ray
- Sudden increase in ventilator pressures during mechanical ventilation accompanied by sudden respiratory distress

For treatment of a small tension pneumothorax (< 25%) you can recommend placing the patient on a 100% nonrebreathing mask to help reabsorption of the pneumothorax. Treatment of a large tension pneumothorax requires a thoracotomy procedure, which is described in more detailed in Chapter 17.

Recommending Adjustment in Fluid Balance

As mentioned in Chapter 3, the normal fluid intake and output (I/O) for adults is 1–2 liters/day, or 25–50 mL/hr. Maintaining the balance between intake and output is essential to maintain proper metabolic functions. **Table 15-4** (see page 463) lists the most common signs associated with alteration of fluid balance and some common management strategies you could recommend.

Table 15-3 Recommending Modifications for Artificial Airways

Problem/Situation	Possible Cause(s)	Recommended Modification(s)
Clinical evidence (e.g., SpO_2) of impending respiratory failure	Inadequate oxygenation (e.g., pneumonia) and/or ventilation (e.g., neuromuscular disease)	Recommend immediate intubation
Clinical evidence or inadequate airway protection	Diminished neurologic function (e.g., drug overdose); airway injury, facial trauma, or burns	Recommend immediate intubation
Difficult intubation	Glottis located anteriorly or excessive epiglottic tissue; incorrect laryngoscope blade/ET tube size; patient agitated or anxious	Reposition patient's airway and recommend laryngeal mask airway (LMA) or fiberoptic intubation; recommend correct-size ET tube and laryngoscope blade or sedation
Excessive ET tube cuff leak despite adequate pilot balloon pressure	Blown ET tube cuff; broken/defective pilot balloon or pilot tube; too small an ET tube	Recommend reintubation with proper-size tube (e.g., 8.0–9.0 for average adult male)
Intubation indicated in the presence of facial or mandibular trauma or pathology	Oral intubation contraindicated	Recommend nasal intubation or tracheostomy tube
Oral ET tube in place but need for long-term ventilation exits	Failed weaning attempts	Recommend tracheostomy
Unfenestrated tracheostomy tube in place but patient wishes to talk	Improvement in patient condition	Recommend fenestrated trach tube with Passy-Muir speaking valve
Need to maintain an airway without an indication for artificial ventilation	Obstructive sleep apnea or upper airway pathology (tumor or scarring); chronic, excessive secretion production	Recommend uncuffed trach tube or tracheostomy button
Patient has an artificial airway but a suction catheter can't be passed	Partial airway obstruction Suction catheter too large	Lavage airway and attempt to suction Use smaller suction catheter (12–14 Fr for adult); if patient compromised, recommend immediate extubation if ET tube or change inner cannula for trach tube
Artificial airway no longer indicated	Improvement in patient condition per weaning protocol or procedures	Recommend extubation or decannulation
Need for mechanical ventilation in a patient with unilateral lung disease	Unilateral lung infections, localized tumors, lobectomies, or pneumonectomies	Recommend a double-lumen ET tube

Recommending Adjustment of Electrolyte Therapy

Monitoring electrolyte concentrations is also very important in critically ill patients and in patients with abnormal fluid balance. Three electrolyte concentrations commonly measured in these patients are: sodium (Na^+), potassium (K^+), and chloride (Cl^-). For normal electrolyte values, refer to Chapter 3. **Table 15-5** lists the most common causes of low (hypo) and high (hyper) serum levels of these electrolytes as well as some suggested actions you can recommend for their treatment.

Table 15-4 Common Signs of Fluid Balance Alteration and Management Strategies

Alteration	Common Signs	Recommended Management Strategies
Dehydration (negative I/O)	• Dry mucous membranes • Hypotension • Diminished urine output • Decreased skin turgor • Increased hematocrit • Thick and tenacious secretions • Decreased central venous pressure (CVP) • Decreased pulmonary capillary wedge pressures (PCWP)	• Increase IV fluid intake rate • Minimize sensible and insensible water loss • If patient on mechanical ventilation, provide for active humidification • If thick secretions are present, recommend mucolytics • In critically ill patients, recommend the insertion of a CVP or PA catheter to closely monitor fluid status • Avoid the use of diuretics
Overhydration (positive I/O)	• Pedal edema • Pulmonary edema • Hepatomegaly • Jugular venous distension • Decreased hematocrit • Increased CVP • Increased PCWP	• Restrict and closely monitor fluid intake (IV and orally) • Recommend diuretic therapy • Recommend inotropic agents if heart failure is suspected • Recommend dialysis if renal failure is present • In critically ill patients, recommend the insertion of a CVP or PA catheter to closely monitor fluid status

Table 15-5 Causes of Abnormal Electrolytes and Recommendations for Their Treatment

Electrolyte	Causes of LOW Serum Levels (Hypo)	Causes of HIGH Serum Levels (Hyper)	Recommendations
Sodium	• Diuresis • Overhydration • Antidiuretic hormone abnormalities	• Fluid loss • Diabetes • Antidiuretic hormone abnormalities	• Treat the underlying cause • Monitor fluid balance • Recommend IV replacement of electrolyte if necessary
Potassium	• Vomiting • Nasogastric suction • Diarrhea • Diuretics • Renal disease • Metabolic alkalosis	• High-potassium diet • Renal failure • Metabolic acidosis • Red blood cell hemolysis	• Treat the underlying cause • Monitor fluid balance • If low, recommend IV replacement of electrolyte if necessary • If low and using diuretics, recommend potassium-sparing diuretics • If high, recommend high-dose aerosolized albuterol treatment or a potassium diuretic medication
Chloride	• Severe vomiting • Chronic respiratory acidosis • Renal disease • Burns • Nasogastric suction • Metabolic alkalosis	• Prolonged diarrhea • Metabolic acidosis • Respiratory alkalosis • Renal disease • Thyroid gland disease	• Treat the underlying cause • Monitor fluid balance • Recommend IV replacement of electrolyte if necessary

Recommending the Initiation and Modification of Pharmacologic Therapy

Based on a patient's clinical status or response to therapy, it is often appropriate for you to recommend that respiratory medications be initiated, modified, or discontinued. **Table 15-6** summarizes the most common clinical situations when you should recommend that medications be initiated, and **Table 15-7** indicates those situations in which pharmacology therapy should be modified. For ACLS drugs indications and recommendations refer to Chapter 17.

Table 15-6 Recommending the Initiation of Medications

Clinical Situation	Recommended Medication(s)
Acute airway obstruction associated with asthma or similar condition	Adrenergic bronchodilators, including levalbuterol or albuterol; consider continuous nebulization, and systemic steroids such as prednisone
Maintenance (prophylactic) medication for asthma management	Recommend any one or a combination of: • An inhaled steroid (e.g., fluticasone) • A long-acting beta-agonist (e.g., Salmeterol) • A leukotriene inhibitor (e.g., montelukast [Singulair]) • Mast cell stabilizer (cromolyn sodium) • Advair (salmeterol and fluticasone) discus
Chronic airway obstruction associated with COPD	Recommend an anticholenergic bronchodilator such as ipratropium bromide or tiotropium bromide with an adrenergic bronchodilator such as albuterol; long-acting beta agonist such as salmeterol (Serevent) plus an inhaled steroid
Retained, thick/tenacious secretions	Recommend acetylcysteine (Mucomyst) or dornase alpha (Pulmozyme) if cystic fibrosis or bronchiectasis is present
Need to increase the volume of secretions for sputum induction	Recommend an aerosolized nebulizer treatment with 3 to 10% hypertonic normal saline solution
Physician orders acetylcysteine but patient at risk for bronchospasm	Recommend that a bronchodilator be added to acetylcysteine, to prevent bronchospasm
Post-extubation stridor and airway edema	Recommend 0.5 mL of 2.25% racemic epinephrine with 3 mL normal saline solution
Physician asks for recommendations to anesthetize a patient's airway before a bronchoscopy	Recommend the administration of lidocaine (1%, 2%, or 4%) or cetacaine via aerosol prior to the procedure
Severe patient agitation or ventilator-patient asynchrony	Recommend sedation such as propofol (Diprivan) and possibly a non-depolarizing paralyzing agent such as cisatracurium (Nimbex)
Respiratory depression induced by natural and synthetic opioid narcotics such as heroin	Recommend an opioid antagonist like naloxone (Narcan) to reverse respiratory depression from narcotics
Difficult intubation	Recommend sedation with midazolam (Versed) and possibly a depolarizing paralyzing agent such as succinylcholine (Anectine)
Pulmonary edema associated with CHF and/or peripheral edema due to right heart failure	Recommend a diuretic such as furosemide (Lasix) and possibly an inotropic medication such as digoxin

(continues)

Table 15-6 Recommending the Initiation of Medications (continued)

Clinical Situation	Recommended Medication(s)
Diuretic indicated for a patient with marginally low serum potassium (3.5 mEq/L)	Recommend a potassium-sparing diuretic such as amiloride
Refractory Gram-negative infections of the respiratory tract	Recommend inhaled tobramycin (Tobi) or gentamycin
Premature newborn having difficulty breathing or with clinical signs of infant respiratory distress syndrome (IRDS)	Recommend surfactant administration as a prophylactic in newborn prematurity or to treat IRDS; common surfactant agents are Beractant (Survanta), calfactant (Infasurf), and poractant alfa (Curosurf)
To treat or prevent influenza	Recommend anti-influenza agents such as oseltamivir (Tamiflu) or zanamivir (Relenza)
To prevent pneumococcal pneumonia and pneumococcal infections in elderly and immunocompromised patients	Recommend pneumococcal vaccine polyvalent (Pneumovax 23); recommend revaccination every 5 years for very high risk populations

Recommending Sedation and Neuromuscular Blockade

Although you cannot independently initiate sedation or muscle relaxant therapy, you may recommend that such medications be added to the care plan. These medications fall into four categories: sedatives, neuroleptics/antipsychotics, analgesics, and paralytics (neuromuscular blocking agents). **Table 15-8** includes the major indications for these drugs, followed by a discussion of the major features of each class of medication.

Table 15-7 Recommending Modifications to Drug Dosage or Concentration

Clinical Situation	Recommended Modification(s)
Patient heart rate increases significantly (by more than 20% of baseline) or other unwanted side effect occurs during or after a short-acting beta$_2$ agonist bronchodilator treatment	Stop the treatment, monitor the patient, notify the nurse and doctor, and recommend that: • The dose be reduced or • A drug with minimal beta$_1$ side effects (e.g., levalbuterol) be considered
A short-acting beta$_2$ agonist bronchodilator is prescribed and indicated, but patient has a recent history of uncontrolled atrial fibrillation, significant tachycardia, or other dysrhythmias	Recommend a drug with minimal beta$_1$ side effects (e.g., levalbuterol) be considered or an anticholinergic bronchodilator be considered
A physician orders an incorrect drug dosage (e.g., 25 mg albuterol or 0.5 mL Atrovent) to be given via SVN every 6 hours	Contact the physician and recommend the correct dose (e.g., Atrovent dose of 0.5 mg with 3 mL normal saline); note: the physician should be contacted immediately for order clarifications whenever a medication dosage appears incorrect
Prophylactic asthma management in patients ≤ 2 years old	Recommend either: • Montelukast (Singulair), the only leukotriene inhibitor approved for young children, or • Cromolyn sodium (Intal), mast cell stabilizer
2 mL of 20% acetylcysteine is ordered, but only 10% acetylcysteine is available	Recommend that 4 mL (twice the volume) of the more dilute 10% acetylcysteine be administered

Table 15-8 Classification and Indications of Major Muscle Relaxants and Neuromuscular

Drug Category	Indication
Sedatives	
Barbiturates: • Thiopental (Pentothal) Benzodiazepines: • Diazepam (Valium) • Lorazepam (Ativan) • Midazolam (Versed) Others: • Etomidate (Amidate) • Ketamine (Ketalar) • Propofol (Diprivan)	• Facilitate minor invasive procedures • Decrease patient-ventilator asynchrony • Increase overall patient comfort • Reduce symptoms of "ICU psychosis" • For moderate sedation required in certain ambulatory procedures
Analgesics	
Opioids: • Morphine • Codeine • Fentanyl (Sublimaze) • Heroin • Hydrocodone • Hydromorphone (Dilaudid) • Meperidine (Demerol) • Oxycodone (OxyContin)	• Treatment and management of pain • Any surgical procedures likely to generate pain and suffering • Long-term control of chronic pain • Facilitate patient-ventilator synchrony
Paralytics/Neuromuscular Blocking Agents	
Depolarizing: • Succinylcholine (Anectine) Non-depolarizing: • Cisatracurium (Nimbex) • Pancuronium (Pavulon) • Rocuronium (Zemuron) • Vecuronium (Norcuron)	• Facilitate "control mode" ventilation • Facilitate intubation • Muscle relaxation during surgery • Facilitate patient-ventilator synchrony • Help to decrease ICPs • Reduce oxygen consumption
Neuroleptics/Antipsychotics	
• Haloperidol (Haldol) • Chlorpromazine (Thorazine) • Lithium (Lithobid)	• Hallucinations • ICU psychosis • Dementia

Sedatives

- Common sedatives used in the ICU setting include benzodiazepines, barbiturates, and propofol. These drugs decrease anxiety and produce amnesia, *but don't alleviate pain.*
- Concerns related to sedatives use include:
  - Long half-lives
  - Drug accumulation, with resultant prolonged effects
  - Cardiac depression
- Drug accumulation is a common problem with midazolam (Versed), especially if used for longer than 48 hours or in obese patients (due to high lipid solubility).
- Cardiac depression is seen mainly with midazolam or propofol (Diprivan).
- Benzodiazepine action can be quickly reversed with flumazenil (Romazicon).
- Propofol (Diprivan) is often the sedative of choice for rapid induction of anesthesia in the ICU for minor invasive procedures. It has a rapid onset and a half-life of less than 30 minutes.

- A single IV dose (2–5 mg) of midazolam (Versed) may be used to facilitate other respiratory procedures such as intubation and bronchoscopy.
- Diprivan and Versed should be used with caution because they often cause hypotension and respiratory depression.

Table 15-9 summarizes the most common sedatives given via IV infusion.

Neuroleptics/Antipsychotics

- In addition to sedation, neuroleptics and antipsychotics may be given to patients who are experiencing delirium or "ICU psychosis."
- Symptoms of delirium include disorganized thinking, hallucinations, and disorientation.
- The neuroleptic drug of choice for delirium/psychosis is haloperidol (Haldol).
- Haldol is usually given intravenously in 2–10 mg doses every 2–4 hours.
- Prolongation of the QT interval on the EKG is a possible side effect of Haldol, so it should be used cautiously in patients who are at risk for QT prolongation.

Analgesics

- Analgesics should be prescribed for every patient receiving mechanical ventilation who may be experiencing pain.
- Morphine is the drug of choice for patients with stable cardiovascular status.
- For patients with unstable cardiovascular status, the histamine-associated hypotension that morphine may cause can be avoided by using fentanyl (Sublimaze) or hydromorphone (Dilaudid).
- A patient receiving large or continuous doses of narcotics must be monitored for the development of ileus. Tolerance of tube feedings and bowel movements should be assessed frequently.

Paralytics/Neuromuscular Blocking Agents

- Paralytics or neuromuscular blocking agents are used to paralyze a patient in order to allow controlled mechanical ventilation.
- Paralytics should never be used unless the patient is receiving full ventilatory support with properly set disconnect alarms tested to confirm their function.
- *Paralytics have no sedative or analgesic effects.* For this reason, paralytics must always be administered with a sedative and, in the presence of pain, an analgesic.
- There are two classes of neuromuscular blocking agents: nondepolarizing (inhibit acetylcholine) and depolarizing (prolong depolarization of the postsynaptic receptors).
- The depolarizing agents have a short duration of action and are used for short-term paralysis during intubation. Succinylcholine (Anectine) is the model depolarizing agent.
- The nondepolarizing agents produce prolonged paralysis and are used for controlled mechanical ventilation. Examples include pancuronium (Pavulon), vecuronium (Norcuron), and cisatracurium (Nimbex).

Table 15-9 Common IV Sedative Dosages and Responses

	Lorazepam	Midazolam	Propofol
Trade name	Ativan	Versed	Diprivan
Loading dose	0.05 mg/kg	0.03 mg/kg	0.5 mg/kg
Infusion rate	0.5–5 mg/hr	1–20 mg/hr	0.5–3 mg/kg/hr
Onset of action	5–15 minutes	1–3 minutes	1 minute
Half-life	6–15 hours	1 hour	< 30 minutes

Recommending Changes in Oxygen Therapy

Chapter 6 describes the features and appropriate uses of various oxygen-delivery devices. Chapter 14 also contains an example of an O_2 therapy protocol that would allow you to modify therapy independently based on preapproved clinical criteria. However, in the absence of such protocols, you may be limited to recommending changes in input flow, delivery device, or FIO_2 to meet the patient's needs. **Table 15-10** outlines the most common clinical situations that would warrant recommended changes in oxygen therapy.

Recommending Changes in Mechanical Ventilation

While patients are mechanically ventilated, a host of changes are generally appropriate to best achieve clinical objectives and maximize tolerance of this life-supporting measure. Some changes to mechanical ventilation settings require a physician's order and may only be recommended by you. Such recommended modifications relate to the type and mode of ventilation, as well as an array of settings changes aimed at enhancing oxygenation and ventilation, and improving patient synchrony and comfort.

Table 15-10 Recommending Changes in Oxygen Therapy

Clinical Situation	Recommended Modification(s)
A COPD patient becomes lethargic and disoriented soon after being placed on a nasal cannula at 5 L/min	Recommend to the physician that the input flow be reduced to 2 L/min or switch to a air-entrainment mask at 24 to 28% O_2; continue to closely monitor patient and notify the nurse
Physician orders oxygen via simple mask with input flow of 3 L/min for an adult patient	Recommend that the input flow be increased to a minimum of 5 L/min to ensure "washout" of CO_2
A patient on a simple mask at 5 L/min complains that the mask is confining and interferes with his ability to eat	Recommend the device be switched to a nasal cannula with a flow of 4–6 L/min, which will deliver a FIO_2 (0.35–0.40) similar to that of the mask
Nasal cannula at 2 L/min is in use on a patient with a high or unstable minute ventilation who requires an FIO_2 of 0.28	Recommend a high-flow device such as a 28% air-entrainment mask, which can meet the patient's minute ventilation and maintain an stable FIO_2
A patient on a 40% air-entrainment mask has a SpO_2 of 89%	Recommend that the FIO_2 be increased to 0.5 and monitor patient's response closely
A patient on a simple mask at 10 L/min has a PaO_2 of 212 torr	Recommend a reduction in FIO_2, either by decreasing the input flow to 5 L/min or switching to a nasal cannula at about 5 L/min (FIO_2 of about 0.40)
A patient's SpO_2 increases from 85% to 87% only after the FIO_2 is increased from 0.40 to 0.50	Recommend CPAP of at least 5–10 cm H_2O and supplemental O_2 (FIO_2 of approximately 0.50) or consider recommending intubation
A physician orders a nonrebreather mask for a "code blue" patient in respiratory arrest	Immediately recommend a BVM that can provide an FIO_2 of 1.0 and can be used to effectively ventilate the patient
A patient in the ER is apparently having a myocardial infarction and is on a nasal cannula at 4 L/min	Recommend a nonrebreathing mask with an input flow sufficient to keep the reservoir bag from collapsing through the breathing cycle
The aerosol mist intermittently disappears from the end of the T-piece of an intubated patient performing an spontaneous breathing trial	Recommend adding a second aerosol nebulizer in tandem or bleeding oxygen accordingly to increase the total output flow of the system

Improving Patient–Ventilator Synchrony

Because asynchrony may interfere with a patient's treatment plan and ultimate recovery, it is very important for you to promptly recognize its presence, identify its causes, and recommend measures to remedy it. Refer to Chapter 14 for a more detailed discussion on ventilator asynchrony. If you notice patient-ventilator asynchrony, you must take the following into consideration:

- Patient–ventilator asynchrony may be caused by problems with either the patient or the ventilator.
- Patient-related problems generally stem from respiratory distress. Consequently, if the source of distress is quickly identified and remedied, the issue of asynchrony will be alleviated.
- If the ventilator patient is in severe distress, the first step should be to ensure adequate ventilation and oxygenation by following these steps:
  - Disconnect the patient from the ventilator
  - Manually ventilate the patient with 100% oxygen
  - Rapidly assess the patient
  - Initiate or recommend action to address the distress and asynchrony, according to **Table 15-11**

After patient-related causes of asynchrony have been ruled out, you should then consider ventilator-related problems, keeping in mind the following:

- The first step in addressing machine-related problems should be to perform an operational verification procedure (OVP), also known as a self-test.
- Successful completion of the OVP rules out ventilator malfunction or circuit problems and shifts focus on the appropriateness of ventilator settings.

Table 15-12 outlines the most common machine-related causes of ventilator-patient asynchrony and the corresponding recommended actions.

Enhancing Oxygenation

During mechanical ventilation, oxygenation can be affected mainly by two parameters—the F_{IO_2} and the PEEP level. In general, the higher the F_{IO_2} and PEEP level, the higher the Pa_{O_2}/Sa_{O_2}.

The following guidelines should be considered:

- If hyperoxia is present (usually $Pa_{O_2} > 100$ torr), you should lower the parameter (F_{IO_2} or PEEP) that is potentially most dangerous to the patient at that moment.
- If the Pa_{O_2} or Sa_{O_2} is low (< 60 torr or < 90%), hypoxemia is present, and either the F_{IO_2} or the PEEP level should be increased.

Table 15-11 Recommended Actions in Patient-Related Ventilator Asynchrony

Clinical Situation	Recommended Action
Partial or complete airway obstruction	Attempt to pass suction catheter or otherwise clear occlusion, change inner cannula (if trach tube), or recommend extubation/reintubation
Pneumothorax likely	Recommend stat chest X-ray and chest tube, if necessary
Bronchospasm	Administer prescribed bronchodilators or recommend them if not prescribed
Increased secretions	Suction airway and recommend mucolytics as appropriate
Pain	Recommend pain medication (e.g., morphine)
Anxiety	Recommend sedatives (e.g., Ativan, Versed)
Seizures	Recommend anti-seizure medication (e.g., Dilantin)
ICU psychosis or delirium	Recommend antipsychotics (e.g., Haldol)

Table 15-12 Recommended Actions in Machine-Related Ventilator Asynchrony

Clinical Situation	Recommended Action
Improper trigger sensitivity	Adjust pressure trigger level to –0.5 to –2 cm H_2O or recommend a flow trigger at 1–3 L/min
Inadequate FIO_2 or PEEP	Recommend increase in FIO_2 up to 0.60 for SpO_2 90–92%, and consider recommending PEEP $\geq$ 10 cm H_2O if inadequate response to high FIO_2
Flow starvation	If flow-limited ventilation, increase flow, use a ventilator that provides flow compensation, or recommend pressure-limited ventilation
Rate problems	If using CMV, set rate to ensure adequate expiratory time, and if using SIMV, increase mandatory rate or pressure support until spontaneous rate decreases accordingly with the patient's status
Inappropriate tidal volume or pressure limit	Ensure appropriate tidal volume setting or pressure change to achieve tidal volume in the range of 5–8 mL/Kg, and inspect pressure-volume curve for overdistention (see Chapter 14)
Inadequate minute ventilation	Ensure minimum minute ventilation of at least 4–6 L/min, or higher if appropriate
Mode problems	Give preference to pressure-limited modes and/or those that provide compensation during ventilation Recommend placing the patient back to previous mode after a mode change if current mode is not tolerated
Auto-PEEP	Check for and eliminate auto-PEEP as described in Chapters 13 and 14

According to these guidelines, if a patient on 10 cm H_2O PEEP and 75% oxygen has a PO_2 of 150 torr, the high FIO_2 is of most concern (O_2 toxicity) and should be lowered. In contrast, if a patient on 18 cm H_2O PEEP and 45% oxygen has a PO_2 of 150 torr, the high PEEP level is of most concern (barotrauma) and should be lowered.

Likewise, which parameter you choose to raise depends on the cause of the hypoxemia. If the problem is a simple V/Q imbalance (indicated by a PaO_2 > 60 torr on a FIO_2 < 0.6), increasing the FIO_2 will probably do the job. However, if the problem is shunting (indicated by a PaO_2 < 60 torr on a FIO_2 > 0.6), simply raising the FIO_2 won't help. Instead, PEEP must be added or increased.

In order to decide between adding PEEP or increasing the FIO_2, you should follow the "60-60 Rule" to determine the cause and treatment of hypoxemia:

- If the PO_2 is greater than 60 torr on an FIO_2 less than 0.6, the problem is mainly a V/Q imbalance that will respond to a simple increase in FIO_2.
- If the PO_2 is less than 60 torr on an FIO_2 greater than 0.6, the problem is shunting and PEEP/CPAP must be added or increased.

Methods to determine the "best" or optimum PEEP levels are discussed in detail in Chapter 12.

Improving Alveolar Ventilation

You confirm the presence of abnormal alveolar ventilation via a blood gas report showing an abnormal pH due to an abnormal $PaCO_2$. A low $PaCO_2$ can be normalized by recommending a decrease in the minute volume. Conversely, a high $PaCO_2$ can be restored to normal levels by recommending an increase in the minute volume. To estimate how much you should increase or decrease the minute volume, use the following formula:

$$\text{new } \dot{V}_E = \text{current } \dot{V}_E \times \frac{\text{current } PaCO_2}{\text{desired } PaCO_2}$$

For example, if a mechanically ventilated patient with a minute volume of 6 L/min has a pH of 7.25 and a $Paco_2$ of 60 torr, you can restore a normal $Paco_2$ by increasing the minute volume. The new minute volume would be 6.0 L/min × 60/40 = 9.0 L/min, with 40 torr being the desired normal $Paco_2$.

Exactly how you change the minute volume depends on the mode of ventilation being used. **Table 15-13** indicates the best ways to increase or decrease minute volume for the most common modes of ventilatory support. Note that rate changes are the preferred method to alter minute volume, as long as the patient's tidal volume is properly set up (4–12 mL/kg of PBW with a plateau pressure < 30 cm H_2O).

Adjusting the Inspiratory to Expiratory Time Ratio (I:E) Settings

I:E Ratio

The I:E ratio is simply the ratio of inspiratory time (I-time) to expiratory time (E-time):

$$I:E = \frac{I\text{-time}}{E\text{-time}}$$

For example: If a patient has an I-time of 1.5 seconds and an E-time of 4.5 seconds, her I:E ratio is 1.5 to 4.5, or 1:3. In normal individuals, the I:E ratio ranges from 1:2 to 1:3. In patients with expiratory airflow obstruction (e.g., COPD patients), the expiratory time is typically prolonged. This results in *lower* I:E ratios, such as 1:4 or 1:5. A prolonged expiratory time combined with a low I:E ratio is a cardinal sign of expiratory airflow obstruction. Expiratory airflow obstruction is a major cause for auto-PEEP and the problems it causes, including asynchrony and increased work of breathing. Measures you can recommend to treat severe expiratory flow obstruction causing auto-PEEP include:

- Administering bronchodilator therapy
- Keeping the airway clear/removing secretions
- Increasing the ET/trach tube size (if too small)

Table 15-13 Changes in Minute Volume Depending on Ventilatory Mode

Mode	To Increase V̇E	To Decrease V̇E
Volume-Targeted Ventilation		
CMV (control)	Increase VT	Decrease rate[a]
CMV (assist/control)	Increase VT	Decrease rate[a] Add deadspace
SIMV	Increase rate[a] Add pressure support	Decrease rate[a]
Pressure-Targeted Ventilation		
PCV	Increase ΔP Increase rate[a]	Decrease ΔP Decrease rate[a]
PSV	Increase ΔP	Decrease ΔP
BiPAP™	Increase ΔP (IPAP – EPAP)	Decrease ΔP (IPAP – EPAP)
APRV	Increase ΔP Increase release frequency[a]	Decrease ΔP Decrease release frequency[a]

a. Rate changes (within the adult limit of 8–26/min) are the preferred method to change minute volume. Adjust rates to achieve optimum total cycle time, while keeping VT between 4 to 12 mL/kg of predicted body weight (PBW) while maintaining plateau pressure < 30 cm H_2O.

- Decreasing the I:E ratio (decrease rate, increase flow, etc.)
- Decreasing tidal volume/minute volume, within safe limits
- Allowing patient to breathe spontaneously
- Applying extrinsic PEEP, pressures up to 80% of auto-PEEP level

Total Cycle Time

During time-triggered/time-cycled modes of ventilator support (such as flow-limited CMV and pressure control ventilation), you can set and manipulate time parameters on the ventilator. The key parameter under clinician control in these modes is the total cycle time. The total cycle time is computed as either (1) the simple sum of I-time plus E-time or (2) the frequency of breathing (f) divided into 60 (second/min):

$$\text{Total cycle time} = \frac{60}{f} = \text{I-time} + \text{E-time}$$

For example, if a patient is receiving PCV with an I-time of 2 seconds and an E-time of 3 seconds, his total cycle time = 2 + 3 = 5 seconds. Alternatively, if a patient is receiving flow-limited control-mode CMV at a preset rate of 15 per minute, her total cycle time = 60/15 = 4 seconds. Any recommendations you make regarding a change in respiratory rate will affect the total cycle time. Decreasing the rate will lengthen the cycle time, and increasing the rate will shorten it.

Percent Inspiratory Time (%I-time or "Duty Cycle")

Another key time parameter used in mechanical ventilation is the percent inspiratory time (%I-time), also called the duty cycle (time during which the ventilatory is doing its "duty" of delivering a breath). To compute the %I-time, one needs to know both the inspiratory time and total cycle time:

$$\%\text{I-time} = \frac{\text{I-time}}{\text{total cycle time}} \times 100$$

Using the above example again, if a patient is receiving PCV with an I-time of 2 seconds and an E-time of 3 seconds, his percent inspiratory time = 2/5 × 100 = 40%. You may want to recommend changes in %I-time in situations where the I:E needs to be changed, as when managing auto-PEEP or when instituting inverse ratio ventilation.

Relationship of %I-time to I:E ratio

Obviously, the %I-time and I:E ratio are related to one another. In the above example, the %I-time is 40%, while the I:E ratio is 2:3 (which reduces to 1:1.5). In both equations, the numerator (on top) is the inspiratory time. The difference lies in the denominators (bottom) of the equations. For the I:E ratio, the denominator is simply the expiratory time. For the %I-time, the denominator is the total cycle time (sum of inspiratory and expiratory times). **Table 15-14** translates the common I:E ratios into their %I-time equivalents.

Note in the above table some I:E ratios greater than 1:1. Since these are the reverse (or inverse) of normal (inspiratory time exceeds inspiratory time), they are called reverse (or inverse) I:E ratios. Although controversial, reverse or inverse I:E ratios can be recommended during pressure control ventilation to improve oxygenation and lower PEEP levels.

Relationship of %I-time to Flow and Minute Ventilation

During flow-limited CMV, the delivered volume is a function of the inspiratory time and flow. To compute the required inspiratory flow for a patient receiving flow-limited CMV, apply the following formula:

$$\dot{V}(\text{L/min}) = \frac{\dot{V}_E(\text{L/min})}{\%\text{I-time(decimal)}}$$

Table 15-14 Converting I:E ratios Into %I-time

I:E ratio	%I-Time
1:4	20%
1:3	25%
1:2	33%
1:1.5	40%
1:1	50%
1.5:1 or 1: 0.66	60%
2:1 or 1: 0.5	67%
3:1 or 1: 0.33	75%

where $\dot{V}$ is the patient's minute volume and %I-time the percent inspiratory time. The accompanying box provides an example of a calculation using this formula as it might appear on the CRT exam. **Table 15-15** outlines the most common situations that may warrant adjustments in I:E ratio, as well as some recommended changes.

Determination of Ventilator Flow Setting (Flow-Limited CMV)

Example: A patient receiving flow-limited CMV at a rate of 15 breaths/min has a tidal volume of 600 mL. The doctor specifies an I:E ratio of 1:4. What flow should you set to achieve these parameters?

First, compute the minute volume:

$\dot{V} = 15 \times 600 = 9.0$ L/min

Next, compute or look up the percent inspiratory time:

%I-time = 20% (Table 15-14)

Last, compute the inspiratory flow needed (be sure to use the decimal equivalent for %I-time)

$$\dot{V} = 9.0/0.20 = 45 \text{ L/min}$$

Modify Ventilator Techniques

Chapter 12 covers the initiation of mechanical ventilation, including the selection of the mode of ventilation. However, as a result of changes in a patient's condition and the ultimate goal of successfully weaning patients from ventilatory support, it is common for you to recommend ventilator technique changes, including modifications to the mode of ventilation. **Table 15-16** summarizes the most common situations that warrant a recommendation to changes in the mode of ventilation during volume-targeted ventilation. **Table 15-17** (see page 475) provides similar guidance for recommending changes during pressure-targeted ventilation.

Table 15-15 Recommended Changes Affecting I:E Ratio in Mechanically Ventilated Patients

Clinical Situation	Recommended Modification(s)
Acute (asthma) or chronic (COPD) airway obstruction resulting in air trapping	Decrease inspiratory time (or %I-time) by increasing inspiratory flow or by directly decreasing I-time or increasing E-time, and decrease respiratory rate to increase E-time or if in a control mode, switch patient to SIMV if possible
Auto-PEEP	Decrease inspiratory time (or %I-time) by increasing inspiratory flow or by directly decreasing I-time or increasing E-time, and decrease respiratory rate to increase E-time or if in a control mode, switch patient to SIMV if possible
Increase oxygenation in patient suspected of shunting	Consider recommending reverse or inverse I:E ratios with pressure control ventilation to improve oxygenation and lower PEEP levels
Prolonged inspiratory time coupled with evidence of flow starvation per waveform graphic analysis	Increase flow to normalize flow wave graphic and maximize patient comfort
Patient ventilator asynchrony coupled with 1:1 or inverse I:E ratio	Review the rationale for a 1:1 or inverse I:E ratio and consider recommending a more physiologic I:E ratio of 1:2 or 1:3

Monitoring and Adjusting Alarm Settings

Procedures for setting ventilator alarm limits are described in Chapter 13. **Table 15-18** summarizes the most common alarms and recommended actions.

Table 15-16 Recommending Changes to the Mode of Ventilation (Volume Targeted)

Clinical Situation	Recommended Modification(s)
Full ventilatory support needed but rate and/or breathing pattern must be controlled (e.g., hyperventilation syndrome or brain injury)	Recommend CMV control mode
Full ventilatory support upon ventilator initiation without need for full rate control; failed weaning attempt	Recommend CMV assist-control (A/C) mode
Full ventilator support is needed, but total respiratory rate results in hyperventilation (respiratory alkalosis) on assist-control mode	Recommend SIMV
To provide incremental lowering of ventilatory support, such as during weaning or to improve spontaneous tidal volume	Recommend SIMV with consideration to also using pressure support for spontaneous breath augmentation
To overcome imposed work of breathing caused by artificial airways or ventilator circuit	Recommend pressure support ventilation (PSV)
To boost spontaneous tidal volume of patients with muscle weakness in SIMV (low rate) or spontaneous modes	Recommend PSV
Tachypnea or low tidal volume during SIMV with signs of increased work of breathing	Recommend adding or increasing the PSV level or switching patient back to previous mode

Table 15-17 Recommended Changes to the Mode of Ventilation (Pressure Targeted and Other Types)

Clinical Situation	Recommended Modification(s)
To reduce airway pressures (plateau pressure) in patients with low lung compliance (ARDS) on volume-targeted ventilation	Recommend pressure control ventilation (PCV)
To improve oxygenation and eventually lower PEEP and FIO_2 levels in ventilator patients with refractory hypoxemia	Recommend PCV with inverse I:E ratio or high-frequency oscillation or jet ventilation
To ventilate and oxygenate patients with extremely low compliance and poor oxygenation (shunting) associated with ARDS	Recommend high-frequency oscillation or jet ventilation
To avoid intubation of patients requiring short-term ventilatory support due to exacerbations of CHF or COPD	Recommend noninvasive positive pressure ventilation (NPPV), such as bi-level ventilation
To avoid reintubation of patients who develop mild to moderate hypercapnia after extubation	Recommend noninvasive positive pressure ventilation (NPPV), such as bi-level ventilation
To avoid or minimize atelectasis associated with lung-protection strategies	Consider recommending airway pressure release ventilation (APRV) or "open lung" strategies such as lung recruitment maneuvers

Table 15-18 Common Ventilator Alarms and Recommended Adjustments or Actions

Ventilator Alarm Activated	Recommended Action(s)[a]
Ventilator inoperative/loss of power	Manually ventilate patient and troubleshoot ventilator, replace ventilator if necessary
Low pressure, low PEEP/CPAP	Check for and fix circuit or airway leaks or disconnections
Low exhaled minute ventilation	Check and fix leaks or disconnections; consider failed weaning attempt
High pressure limit	If sudden rise in PIP, suction secretions, alleviate mucous plug, place bite block, recommend sedation (if patient agitated), assess for pneumothorax; if gradual rise in PIP, consider bronchodilators (if due to increased resistance) or recommend PCV (if due to decreased compliance), check for condensation in the circuit
High exhaled minute ventilation	If on CMV, consider recommending SIMV mode or sedation; consider adding mechanical deadspace, if there is accompanying respiratory alkalosis
High respiratory rate	Assess for pain or any other cause of respiratory distress; during weaning attempts, consider failure to wean and return to previous settings or add PSV if on SIMV
FIO_2	Analyze FIO_2 with calibrated oxygen analyzer, calibrate ventilator cell, and recommend replacing ventilator cell
Temperature	Check settings, water feed, and temperature sensors, and replace heater, circuit and sensors
Apnea	Recommend return to CMV, if weaning in progress or reduction in sedation, if warranted
a. The recommended action anticipates that with any ventilator alarm activation that either exceeds approximately 30–60 seconds or is accompanied by patient distress, you will conduct a quick but thorough assessment of the patient-ventilator interface before taking any of the proposed actions.	

The first rule in monitoring and responding to a ventilator alarm is to ensure patient safety. If there are any signs of patient distress while a ventilator alarm is sounding, be sure to follow these steps:

- Remove the patient from the ventilator.
- Manually ventilate the patient.
- Ask for help if necessary.
- Assess and monitor the patient.
- If patient-related problem, treat and/or recommend treatment:
  - Suction airway
  - Administer bronchodilators
  - Check artificial airway and recommend reintubation if necessary
- Troubleshoot ventilator-related problem:
  - Fix circuit leak
  - Readjust alarm parameters to correct level
- Once patient is stabilized and/or ventilator problem fixed, reconnect patient.
- Monitor patient-ventilator interface to ensure no repeat of episode.

Another important consideration regarding ventilator alarm is to ensure that a functional remote monitoring system is in place wherever clinicians might be outside "sight and sound" range of the patient.

Adjusting Ventilator Settings Based on Graphics

Chapter 14 describes situations in which you should independently modify ventilator settings based on waveform assessment. Several ventilator graphics depicting these scenarios are also included in the same chapter. In addition to remedies that you may independently initiate, such as correcting inappropriate sensitivity, there are other changes that you may only recommend to the physician, such as initiating sedation for asynchrony. **Table 15-19** summarizes the most common situations and the likely recommended solutions.

Changing Type of Ventilator and Breathing Circuit

Selecting and Changing Ventilators

As a therapist you are responsible for selecting among or switching between ventilators, including pneumatic, electric, fluidic, and noninvasive devices. Chapter 6 outlines general criteria for selecting

Table 15-19 Recommending Adjustment of Ventilator Settings Based on Graphics

Clinical Situation	Recommended Action(s)
Patient-Ventilator Asynchrony: Seen on graphical waveform as irregularly spiked flow and/or irregular pressure waveform	Recommend bronchodilators for bronchospasm or chest X-ray if pneumothorax is suspected, or appropriate medication in the presence of agitation, pain, seizures, or delirium
Auto-PEEP: Manifested in several ways on ventilator graphics, including an expiratory flow waveform that does not return to baseline before the next breath	Suction or recommend bronchodilators for airway resistance problems and increase expiratory time either by increasing the inspiratory flow or directly changing the inspiratory time
Overdistention: As evidenced on the waveform graphic by a "beak" at the upper inflection point in the volume/pressure loop	Appropriately reducing the volume (in volume ventilation) or the pressure setting, in accordance with existing protocols or recommending such in the absence of a protocol
Airway leaks: Seen on a failure of the expiratory volume waveform to return to baseline	Check for leaks and/or disconnections on the patient-ventilator system; if chest tube present, check for water-seal chamber leak and consider broncho-pulmonary fistula

ventilators based on patient variables, application settings, and needed capabilities. **Table 15-20** takes those criteria a step further and outlines recommendations for ventilator selection based on specific clinical scenarios likely to appear on the CRT exam.

Selecting and Changing Ventilator Circuits

Chapter 6 provides details on the design and selection of ventilator circuits. In general, a ventilator circuit should be selected based on its compatibility with the ventilator. For example, microprocessor-controlled ventilators used in an acute care setting usually employ *dual-limb* circuits. Ventilators used at home or for transport generally use a *single-limb* circuit equipped with an external exhalation valve. Most bi-level pressure ventilators used in noninvasive ventilation also use a single-limb circuit. Once the ventilator is in use, you may have to change a soiled or malfunctioning circuit. In addition, you may occasionally need to change or modify a ventilator circuit in order to help meet your patient care objectives. The most common changes in ventilator circuitry likely to appear on the CRT exam include:

- Using low-compliance circuit for neonates and young pediatric patients to minimize volume loss
- Changing or modifying a single-limb circuit by adding PEEP capabilities to the exhalation valve
- Adding an additional exhalation port to a bi-level pressure ventilator circuit (e.g., whisper swivel valve) for patients at risk for CO_2 retention
- Adding 50–100 mL mechanical deadspace between the ventilator circuit's Y-connector and the patient's airway to raise the $Paco_2$ and manage acute respiratory alkalosis (generally limited to ventilator modes that do *not* include spontaneous breaths)

Other Recommendations Related to Ventilator Settings

Other ventilator modifications that you may recommend involve those designed to minimize ventilator-induced lung injury. Chapter 12 details the most common approach to ventilator strategies as applied

Table 15-20 Recommending, Selecting, and Changing Ventilator Type

Clinical Scenario	Recommended Ventilator Type and Characteristics
Critical care setting	Microprocessor-controlled ventilator with a variety of modes, alarms, and settings, as well as graphical display capabilities
Profoundly ill patient with ARDS or any type of hypoxic failure not responding to conventional ventilation	Ventilator capable of inverse ratio pressure control or APRV; high-frequency oscillator or jet ventilator
Patient with an artificial airway who may be or become candidate for weaning	Ventilator capable of pressure support, bi-level pressure ventilation, or other potential weaning capabilities and monitoring alarms
Intermittent ventilation, cooperative patient without an artificial airway	Noninvasive positive pressure (BiPAP™) or negative pressure (cuirass) ventilator
Home setting or similar alternate site	Small and light electrically powered ventilator with A/C and IMV modes and alarm functions
General transport	Sufficiently small and light, pneumatically powered, electronically controlled ventilator, with battery backup
Air transport (unpressurized)	Volume ventilator with correction for decreased atmospheric pressure and Po_2
MRI testing	Small and light pneumatically powered and controlled ventilator
Hyperbaric therapy	Pneumatically powered and controlled ventilator

to acute respiratory failure patients. Other related lung-protective strategies you may recommend include:

- Volume-targeted ventilation with low tidal volumes (4–6 mL/kg of PBW)
- Volume-targeted ventilation with low plateau pressures (< 30 cm H_2O)
- Pressure-controlled ventilation with PIP less than 30 cm H_2O
- "Dual-mode" ventilation (e.g., pressure-regulated volume control)
- Airway pressure release ventilation (APRV)

You may recommend these techniques in conjunction with *permissive hypercapnia*. Permissive hypercapnia is a ventilation strategy in which a higher than normal $Paco_2$ is accepted in exchange for the lower risk of lung injury associated with smaller tidal volumes or peak airway pressures. In the National Heart, Lung, and Blood Institute (NHLBI) ARDS protocol, you can accept hypercapnia/respiratory acidosis until the pH falls below 7.3, at which point you would recommend either an increase in rate or administration of sodium bicarbonate.

A final area to recommend special ventilator settings involves specific clinical conditions. Patients with a clinically significant bronchopulmonary fistula who do not ventilate or oxygenate well on other settings may respond well to high-frequency oscillation or jet ventilation. Likewise, ventilator patients who are particularly at risk for developing atelectasis may be candidates for "open-lung" techniques such as recruitment maneuvers involving periodic use of PEEP levels as high as 20–30 cm H_2O.

Recommending Weaning from Mechanical Ventilation and Extubation

Once mechanical ventilation is initiated, your treatment plan should focus on successfully removing the patient from the ventilator as soon as possible. Before you recommend trying to do so, you first need to determine whether the patient is ready for weaning. According to the AARC, patients receiving mechanical ventilation for respiratory failure are ready to undergo weaning assessment whenever the following criteria are met:

1. Evidence for some reversal of the underlying cause of respiratory failure
2. Adequate oxygenation, e.g.,
   a. Pao_2/Fio_2 > 150–200
   b. PEEP ≤ 5–8 cm H_2O
   c. Fio_2 ≤ 0.4–0.5
3. pH ≥ 7.25
4. Hemodynamic stability (no myocardial ischemia or significant hypotension)
5. The capability to initiate an inspiratory effort

Table 15-21 describes related weaning measures and their threshold values that are likely to appear on the CRT exam.

The following must be considered when interpreting weaning parameters:

- Weaning parameters should be assessed collectively; if most or all of them are favorable, weaning should be recommended.
- A variety of weaning methods have been deemed effective in a clinical setting.
- One of the most widely accepted methods involves using pressure support ventilation (PSV) to obtain a V_T of 10–12 mL/kg, then titrating it downward, as tolerated by the patient, to a level of 5–6 cm H_2O.
- Unwanted physiological changes, such as a respiratory rate greater than 30 or a heart rate greater than 130–140, may signal that the patient is not tolerating the weaning process and should be returned to full ventilatory support.
- If the patient tolerates a "T-piece trial" and has good airway protective reflexes, you should recommend that the patient also be extubated.
- Once a patient is extubated, you should recommend that the patient be placed on an oxygen-delivery device with an Fio_2 slightly higher (10% increase in Fio_2) than that which he or she was on during mechanical ventilation.

Table 15-21 Weaning Parameters and Their Thresholds

Parameter	Threshold Suggesting Readiness to Wean
Negative inspiratory force (NIF/MIP)	$\geq$ –20 to –25 cm H_2O
Tidal volume (mL/kg of PBW)	$\geq$ 5 mL/kg
Vital capacity (mL/kg of PBW)	$\geq$ 10–15 mL/kg
Respiratory rate	< 30 breaths/min
Minute volume	< 10 L/min
Rapid shallow breathing index (rate/V_T)	$\leq$ 100

Extubated patients should be closely monitored for signs that mechanical ventilation should be reinitiated. These signs may include:

- Unstable vital signs (significant increase in respiratory rate and/or hear rate, hypo/hypertension)
- Stridor
- Decrease in Sp_{O_2}
- Pa_{O_2} less than 60 torr or Pc_{O_2} greater than 50 torr
- Prolonged accessory muscle use or paradoxical breathing
- Altered mental status
- Hemodynamic instability

COMMON ERRORS TO AVOID

You can improve your score by avoiding these mistakes:

- When performing postural drainage, avoid recommending a head-down position for patients with increased ICP and instead rotate the patient laterally to approximate the desired position.
- Never recommend sedatives, such as benzodiazepines, to relieve pain. These drugs are often helpful in decreasing anxiety but don't alleviate pain.
- Never recommend weaning a patient from mechanical ventilation who is hemodynamically compromised, has unstable vital signs, or requires Fi_{O_2}s in excess of 0.50–0.60 or PEEP level greater than 10 cm H_2O.
- Never attempt to perform CPR on a patient who is in bed unless a "compression board" is placed under their back or the bed is in "CPR mode."
- Never recommend prophylactic or maintenance medications such as cromolyn sodium or long-acting beta-agonist bronchodilators such as salmeterol for patients experiencing a severe asthmatic episode or in status asthmatics.
- To prevent oxygen-induced hypoventilation, never recommend Fi_{O_2} much above 0.28 for COPD patients suspected of also being CO_2 retainers.
- Never recommend PEEP levels in excess of 5 cm H_2O for ventilator patients who are hemodynamically unstable or at risk for developing a pneumothorax.
- Never recommend 1:1 or inverse I:E ratios for mechanically ventilated patients who are not sedated or who are hemodynamically unstable.
- Never initiate low inspiratory flows or short expiratory times on ventilator patients who are at risk for air trapping and auto-PEEP.
- Never recommend a conventional ventilator with iron-based metals and microprocessors for use in an MRI room. Instead, recommend a pneumatically powered and controlled ventilator.
- Never simply recommend sedation for patient-ventilator asynchrony before ruling out other patient causes such as bronchospasm, airway obstruction and pneumothorax, or ventilator-related causes such as insufficient inspiratory flow or inappropriate pressure support.
- Never set a low-pressure (disconnect) alarm much below 5–8 cm H_2O.
- Never use a standard high-compliance circuit for neonates or young pediatric patients.

SURE BETS

In some situations you can be sure of the right approach to a clinical problem or scenario:

- Always stop postural drainage in the head-down position if the patient begins to cough vigorously. Sit up and stabilize the patient before continuing with therapy.
- To facilitate a difficult intubation, always consider recommending a depolarizing paralyzing agent such as succinylcholine (Anectine), which has a rapid onset and short duration.
- Always recommend rapid-sequence intubation for patients with clinical signs of impending respiratory failure or inadequate airway protection.
- Always consider a laryngeal mask airway (LMA) when an immediate intubation is indicated but not easily achievable or in the presence of a difficult airway.
- Always recommend the use of the correct-size ET tube when assisting with intubation. In general, recommend the following tube sizes: average adult male: 8.0–9.0 mm, average 16-year-old: 7.0; average 3-year-old: 4.5 mm (uncuffed).
- Always recommend placing a spontaneous-breathing patient who is dyspneic in a Fowler's or high Fowler's position, to help promote chest excursion and lung expansion.
- Always recommend a fast-acting adrenergic bronchodilator for a patient with severe bronchospasm associated with asthma or a similar condition.
- For patients with unstable or high minute ventilation who need a low to moderate FIO_2 (0.24–0.50), always recommend a high-flow device such as an air-entrainment mask.
- For patient-ventilator asynchrony, always consider and recommend measures to address both patient-related causes, such as airway obstruction and anxiety, as well as machine-related causes, such as inappropriate trigger sensitivity or inspiratory flow.
- Always recommend increasing PEEP above 5–10 cm H_2O for ventilator patients who are hemodynamically stable but hypoxemic despite an FIO_2 in excess of 0.50–0.60.
- Always recommend increasing either the ΔP (IPAP – EPAP) or the respiratory rate when seeking to increase the $\dot{V}E$ for a patient on BiPAP™.
- Always ensure that there is appropriate full ventilatory support backup before recommending that a patient be placed on a weaning mode, such as SIMV with pressure support, CPAP or pressure support alone.
- Always consider recommending a pressure-targeted mode or dual mode of ventilation when attempting to reduce a ventilator patient's peak and/or mean airway pressure.
- When a patient in ARDS does not respond well to conventional volume and pressure modes of ventilation, consider recommending high-frequency oscillation or jet ventilation.
- When responding to a ventilator alarm, always start by checking patient causes such as disconnect or airway leak (low pressure) or bronchospasm or secretions (high pressure).
- Always disconnect a patient from the ventilator and manually ventilate him or her with 100% oxygen if a ventilator alarm can not be fixed within 15–30 seconds, especially if the patient is in distress.
- Always insert an oropharyngeal airway if you are unable to ventilate a patient with any bag-valve-mask device.

PRE-TEST ANSWERS AND EXPLANATIONS

Below are this chapter's pre-test answers and explanations. Be sure to review each answer's explanation thoroughly to help you understand why it is correct. If the explanation is still unclear to you, review the chapter contents or the references and/or refer to this chapter's supplemental resources on the CD.

15-1. **Correct answer: D.** Pancuronium bromide (Pavulon). Based on the clinical presentation, the immediate problem appears to be bronchospasm (wheezing) and thick secretions (rhonchi) causing an increase in airway resistance (increased PIP – plateau). A bronchodilator (albuterol or ipratropium) *and* a mucolytic (acetylcysteine) are indicated to treat this situation. Suctioning this patient will also be helpful in removing excessive secretions. Pancuronium bromide (Pavulon) is a non-depolarizing neuromuscular blocking agent that will not achieve bronchodilation or clear the airways. In fact, Pavulon can cause release of histamine, which can cause bronchospasm.

15-2. **Correct answer: C.** III and IV only. At this point, the patient is at high risk for developing atelectasis due to retained secretions and immobility. An initial regimen of incentive spirometry and deep breathing and coughing may well prevent atelectasis and aid secretion clearance.

15-3. **Correct answer: A.** Propofol (Diprivan). Propofol is the agent of choice for rapid sedation of patients undergoing minor invasive procedures. It has a quick and short half-life (< 30 minutes). Haloperidol (Haldol) is a neuroleptic/antipsychotic agent, not a sedative. Lorazepam (Ativan) is a sedative used for long-term sedation. Cisatracurium (Nimbex) is a neuromuscular blocking agent, not a sedative.

15-4. **Correct answer: B.** Succinylcholine (Anectine). For relatively short-term paralysis during procedures such as endotracheal intubation, a depolarizing agent like succinylcholine (Anectine) is recommended. Non-depolarizing agents such as pancuronium (Pavulon), vecuronium (Norcuron), and cisatracurium (Nimbex) produce prolonged paralysis and are generally used for long-term management of mechanically ventilated patients.

15-5. **Correct answer: B.** Inserting an LMA. You should recommend a laryngeal mask airway (LMA) when the physician is unable to properly visualize the vocal cords and needs to secure the airway quickly. An emergency cricothyrotomy is a surgical procedure indicated only when the oral and nasal routes are unavailable. Sedation may help, but agitation is not the problem with this patient. Likewise, changing the type of ET tube used will not help with visualizing the airway either.

15-6. **Correct answer: B.** Add mechanical deadspace. Adding mechanical deadspace will cause rebreathing of CO_2, and thus $PaCO_2$ will increase. Another potential answer would have been to switch to the SIMV mode or to sedate the patient, but these are not given as a choice.

15-7. **Correct answer: B.** Beginning diuretic therapy. Dehydration is very common in the elderly due to improper fluid intake and altered fluid metabolism. Common signs of dehydration are: dry mucous membranes, hypotension, diminished urine output, decreased skin turgor, increased hematocrit, thick and tenacious secretions, decreased central venous pressure (CVP), and decreased pulmonary capillary wedge pressure (PCWP).

15-8. **Correct answer: C.** II or III only. Generally, patients with cervical spine injuries cannot be intubated via the oral route. For these patients, either nasotracheal intubation or insertion of a laryngeal mask airway are good alternatives, with the nasotracheal route preferred if the need for positive pressure ventilation is likely to be long term.

15-9. **Correct answer: A.** Decreasing the I:E ratio. Due to their high expiratory flow resistance, COPD patients are more likely to develop auto-PEEP during mechanical ventilation. If the problem is associated with bronchospasm, you should recommend a bronchodilator. If not, you can recommend decreasing the I:E ratio by (a) shortening inspiration (by using higher flows and/or lower tidal volumes) or (b) lengthening the expiratory time by using lower rates or switching to SIMV mode. Another alternative is to apply external PEEP in an amount less than the auto-PEEP level. This helps prevent the small airway closure during exhalation that can cause air trapping.

15-10. **Correct answer: A.** Increasing the FIO_2 to 0.45. The blood gas analysis indicates normal ventilation and acid-base balance with moderate hypoxemia. With an FIO_2 below 0.50, the hypoxemia is most likely due to a V/Q imbalance. In this instance, you should increase the FIO_2 to 0.45. If this does not adequately address the problem, you may need to consider an increase in PEEP.

15-11. **Correct answer: C.** Administer furosemide (Lasix). The diagnosis of heart failure and the increased PA and PCWP suggest that this patient is in congestive heart failure. In order to alleviate the backup of fluid in the lungs, the therapy plan should generally include a rapid-acting diuretic such as furosemide (Lasix) as well as positive inotropic agents as Digoxin and Dopamine.

15-12. **Correct answer: B.** Decreasing the dosage of albuterol. The significant increase in heart rate (above 20 from baseline) indicates that this dosage of albuterol (Proventil) is provoking systemic side effects in this patient. Before considering a different drug, you should recommend trying a reduced dosage of albuterol and monitor carefully for both desired effects and side effects.

15-13. **Correct answer: B.** Increasing the minute volume on the ventilator. Although the ABG values are within normal range, some evidence suggests that hyperventilating closed-head trauma patients may be beneficial during the first 24–48 hours of their management. Typically, the target is a $Paco_2$ of approximately 25–30 torr. This causes cerebral vasoconstriction, resulting in a reduction in intracranial pressure and swelling.

15-14. **Correct answer: D.** Ipratropium bromide (Atrovent). Most sympathetic bronchodilators will result in some $beta_1$ stimulation, causing an increase in heart rate. Though albuterol has fewer $beta_1$ effects than earlier adrenergic bronchodilators, it may result in a significant increased heart rate in some patients. In this instance, a therapist might recommend an anticholinergic bronchodilator such as ipratropium bromide (Atrovent). An alternative may have been to recommend one of the newest sympathetic bronchodilators, levalbuterol (Xopenex) with fewer $beta_1$ effects, but that was not a choice.

15-15. **Correct answer: C.** Cuffed, fenestrated tracheostomy tube. For a patient with a tracheostomy on long-term mechanical ventilation who still requires intermittent support, a cuffed, fenestrated tracheostomy tube is the ideal airway. With the inner cannula in place and cuff inflated, a fenestrated trach tube performs like a standard tube and can be used for positive pressure ventilation. However, fenestrated trach tubes have one or more openings in their posterior curvature that permits air movement through the tube (from trachea to larynx) when the inner cannula is removed. This air flow allows phonation (talking) and facilitates communication. In addition, by removing a fenestrated tube's inner cannula, plugging the outer cannula, and deflating its cuff, you can test the patient's ability to resume normal upper airway function.

15-16. **Correct answer: B.** Recommend a flow of at least 5 L/min to wash out CO_2. With this level of hypoxemia, this patient should immediately receive moderate O_2 concentrations, as available by simple mask. However, a simple mask requires a flow of at least 5 L/min in order to replenish the O_2 and prevent CO_2 rebreathing.

15-17. **Correct answer: D.** Providing supplemental pressure support. SIMV with PEEP is an appropriate choice for a patient in combined hypoxemic and hypercapnic respiratory failure due to an acute restrictive disorder. Coexisting respiratory muscle fatigue in these patients may necessitate the addition of pressure support ventilation to supplement the spontaneous breaths during SIMV and overcome the resistance imposed by the artificial airway.

15-18. **Correct answer: B.** Postponing weaning and reevaluating the patient. Although the patient's vital capacity and MIP are borderline adequate, the tidal volume is very low (3.8 mL/kg). The (missing) spontaneous breathing rate calculated by 10 L/min ÷ 0.250 L/breath = 40 breaths/min is too high. This yields a rapid shallow breathing index of 40/0.25 = 160, far above the threshold of 100. You should recommend postponing weaning and reevaluating the patient at a later date.

15-19. **Correct answer: B.** Administering a racemic epinephrine treatment. The development of stridor after extubation indicates glottic edema. When you hear stridor, you should be wary of further problems, as the swelling can dramatically worsen. If stridor is present, a racemic epinephrine treatment may be given to lessen the swelling. In children, post-extubation edema is often subglottic and may require reinsertion of the airway.

15-20. **Correct answer: C.** Administering pulmonary surfactant with Beractant (Survanta). The acid-base balance for this infant is within normal range; hence mechanical ventilation is not warranted. However, the patient has refractory hypoxemia ($PaO_2 \leq 60$ with $FIO_2 \geq 0.60$), probably due to shunting from the IRDS. Surfactant administration is indicated for premature babies (25–34 weeks) for the prevention and treatment of RDS since their ability to produce their own surfactant is not fully developed. Lack of mature surfactant in premature babies is a major contributor to IRDS. Increasing the FIO_2 to 100% is not warranted at this time, and it may increase the risk of retinopathy of prematurity (ROP). INO therapy is indicated only for persistent pulmonary hypotension of newborn (PPHN).

15-21. **Correct answer: D.** Cisatracurium (Nimbex). Common sedatives used to calm patients in the ICU include benzodiazepines like lorazepam (Ativan), barbiturates like pentobarbital (Nembutal), and propofol (Diprivan). Cisatracurium (Nimbex) is a neuromuscular blocking agent, not a sedative.

15-22. **Correct answer: A.** Adding PEEP. In mechanically ventilated patients with atelectasis and hypoxemia, PEEP is indicated. PEEP increases the FRC by recruiting collapsed alveoli, which improves oxygenation by decreasing shunting.

15-23. **Correct answer: C.** II and III only. Based on the symptoms and PFT results, the patient has severe persistent asthma. Long-term control of severe persistent asthma is best achieved by combining both an inhaled corticosteroid (like fluticasone) and a long-acting adrenergic bronchodilator (such as salmeterol). This combination is available as the Advair discus, but that is not one of the choices. Short-acting inhaled beta$_2$-agonists like albuterol are also prescribed but are indicated for quick relief of exacerbations, not long-term control.

15-24. **Correct answer: B.** Patient B. Assuming all else is equal, Patient B (with a VC > 15 mL/kg, a resting VT of > 300 mL, an NIF > −20 cm H_2O, and a shunt fraction of 17%) is the most viable candidate for weaning.

15-25. **Correct answer: D.** Potassium. Metabolic acidosis increases H^+ levels outside the cells. In an effort to buffer this acidosis, intracellular K^+ ions are exchanged with extracellular H^+, producing hyperkalemia. Correcting the metabolic acidosis usually corrects the hyperkalemia

POST-TEST

A post-test for this chapter that includes automated scoring and feedback is available on the accompanying CD. Be sure to complete this additional assessment to confirm your mastery of this chapter's objectives.

REFERENCES

Butler, T. J. (2009). *Laboratory exercises for competency in respiratory care* (2nd ed.). Philadelphia: FA Davis.

Irwin, R. S., Rippe, J. M., Lisbon, A., & Heard, S. (2008). *Procedures, techniques and minimally invasive monitoring in intensive care medicine* (4th ed.). Philadelphia: Lippincott, Williams & Wilkins.

Kasmarek, R. M., Dimas, S., & Mack, C. W. (2005). *The essentials of respiratory care* (4th ed.). St. Louis: Mosby.

Wilkins, R., & Dexter, J. R. (2009). Clinical laboratory studies. In Wilkins, R. L., Sheldon, R. L., & Heuer, A. J. (Eds.) *Clinical assessment in respiratory care* (6th ed.). St. Louis: Mosby.

Wilkins, R. L., Stoller, J. K., & Kacmarek, R. M. (2009). *Fundamentals of respiratory care* (9th ed.). St. Louis: Mosby.

Wyka, K. A., Mathews, P. J., & Clark, W. F. (2002). *Foundations of respiratory care*. Albany: Delmar.

16

Determine Appropriateness of the Prescribed Respiratory Care Plan and Recommend Modifications When Indicated

Louis M. Sinopoli

INTRODUCTION

The ability to determine appropriate therapy and recommend modifications when needed is an important part of a good respiratory therapist's job and is found on the NBRC CRT exam. This part of the exam is difficult for many students and clinicians because it requires integration of the basics, such as indications and treatment options for most respiratory conditions, with analysis and decision making, key parts of the NBRC CRT exam skill set. This requires you to analyze detail in the test item you are given and provide a rationale, or logical reasoning, as the basis for recommending modifications in therapy to the physician. In addition, if you practice in a hospital where you are rarely given the opportunity to use such thinking skills, you may need to spend a larger portion of your exam preparation time on this topic. To be successful on this part of the exam, you must focus on: (1) collection and assessment of patient data, (2) analysis of the data, and (3) selection of the appropriate course of therapy for your patient.

OBJECTIVES

After completion of this chapter, you should demonstrate the knowledge needed to:

- Analyze available information to determine the pathophysiological state
- Review planned therapy for appropriateness
- Determine appropriateness of prescribed therapy and goals for identified pathophysiological state
- Recommend changes in therapeutic plan when indicated
- Develop, perform, and monitor outcomes of respiratory care quality assurance activities
- Develop, apply, and monitor outcomes of respiratory care protocols

WHAT TO EXPECT ON THIS CATEGORY OF THE CRT EXAM

Number of questions: 4
Level of questions: 25% recall, 75% application

WHAT'S NEW FOR 2009

As of July 2009, this section of the NBRC CRT examination includes *no new content areas*. In fact, the number of items in this category for 2009 has been reduced from 9 to 4 by elimination of all analysis items.

PRE-TEST

Carefully respond to each of the following questions. After completing the pre-test, compare your answers with those provided at the end of this chapter. Then thoroughly review each answer's explanation to help understand why it is correct.

16-1. A patient who is breathing room air and in a coma as a result of acute carbon monoxide poisoning has a Pao_2 of 95 torr and $Paco_2$ of 30 torr. Which of the following changes in the treatment plan would you recommend?
 A. Administer high concentrations of oxygen
 B. Initiate mechanical ventilation
 C. Initiate chest percussion and postural drainage
 D. Administer mask CPAP

16-2. IPPB treatments are sometimes given to patients with emphysema to:
 A. Lower the diaphragm
 B. Abolish the cough reflex
 C. Improve alveolar ventilation
 D. Increase FRC

16-3. Which of the following conditions is an indication for the use of CPAP?
 A. Tension pneumothorax
 B. Pulmonary embolism
 C. Pulmonary edema
 D. Asthma

16-4. The primary aim in treating cardiogenic pulmonary edema is to:
 A. Increase venous return to the heart
 B. Decrease right heart and systemic venous pressures
 C. Decrease left heart and pulmonary vascular pressures
 D. Increase pulmonary fluid and blood volume

16-5. Despite an intensive regimen of incentive spirometry, chest percussion, and nasotracheal suctioning, a postoperative patient continues to exhibit clinical manifestations of atelectasis due to large airway obstruction. The best treatment approach in this case is:
 A. Intubation and mechanical ventilation
 B. Bedside therapeutic bronchoscopy
 C. Transtracheal aspiration
 D. Aerosol therapy with acetylcystine

16-6. You would initiate O_2 therapy in all of the following cases *except*:
 A. Treating carbon monoxide poisoning
 B. Decreasing myocardial work
 C. Treating absorption atelectasis
 D. Treating arterial hypoxemia

16-7. A patient who just suffered a severe closed head injury is being supported in the CMV mode of ventilatory support. Which of the following goals should you recommend for the initial 24–48 hours of ventilatory support?
 A. Allow as much spontaneous breathing as possible (IMV)
 B. Maintain a high mean pressure using PEEP at 10–15 cm H_2O
 C. Maintain a $Paco_2$ of 50–60 torr (deliberate hypoventilation)
 D. Maintain a $Paco_2$ of 25–30 torr (deliberate hyperventilation)

16-8. You are reviewing a postoperative patient's care plan. The physician has changed the patient's therapy from incentive spirometry to IPPB. The most likely goal for this change is to:
 A. Deliver aerosolized bronchodilators
 B. Improve inadequate alveolar oxygenation
 C. Prevent lower lobe atelectasis
 D. Treat progressive respiratory muscle weakness

16-9. Which of the following would you recommend for a patient that has emphysema with chronic $Paco_2$ retention who experiences hypoxemia at rest?
 A. CPAP
 B. Incentive spirometry
 C. Oxygen via nonrebreathing mask
 D. Low-flow oxygen

16-10. Which of the following would be considered objective data to use in the assessment of the patient in order to formulate possible causes of respiratory distress and a respiratory care plan?
A. Laryngeal edema
B. Inspiratory stridor
C. Bronchodilator
D. Bronchoscopy

16-11. Which of the following is the first step in respiratory care protocol application?
A. Observe universal precautions at all times
B. Review medical records
C. Check physician order for respiratory care protocol
D. Perform initial patient evaluation

16-12. All of the following are potential sources of data for identifying patient care–related problems in a comprehensive quality improvement program *except*:
A. Analysis of department budgeting
B. Audit of patient medical records
C. Examination of incident reports
D. Review of patient ratings and complaints

16-13. Which of the following could be used as quality assurance outcome criteria to assess the effectiveness of bronchial hygiene therapy?
   I. Change in sputum production
  II. Change in chest X-ray
  III. Patient subjective response to therapy
  IV. Change in ABG values or oxygen saturation

A. I and II only
B. II and IV only
C. I, III, and IV
D. I, II, III, and IV

16-14. As part of your department's quality improvement program, you identify an infection control problem. Which of the following should be investigated as potential causes of this problem?
   I. Lack of proper training
  II. Equipment or supply deficiencies
  III. Failure to follow set procedures
A. II only
B. III only
C. I and III only
D. I, II, and III

16-15. Which of the following mechanisms is the best way to objectively assess the effectiveness of therapy in a quality assurance program?
A. Assess the post-treatment status of patients on one or more pre-defined criteria
B. Survey a sample of patients who received the specified therapy to determine their satisfaction
C. Compare pre- and post-treatment patient status on one or more pre-defined criteria
D. Analyze morbidity and mortality statistics for patients receiving the specified therapy

WHAT YOU NEED TO KNOW: ESSENTIAL CONTENT
Analyzing Available Data to Determine Pathophysiological State

It is essential that you are well informed on all the indications, contraindications, and modifications needed for common respiratory problems. You'll need to do much more than just memorize these facts, however. Only one of the nine items on this section of the exam is at the recall or memorization level, which means that you must be able to pay attention to key data and analyze it in the context presented to determine appropriate therapy.

    A good respiratory care plan begins with careful identification and assessment of the patient's condition. Once you identify the patient's problem(s), you should plan to provide or recommend the most appropriate therapies. For example, if assessment indicates that wheezing and a reduced FEV_1

respond to bronchodilator therapy, your plan should include aerosolized beta-agonists. **Table 16-1** summarizes common findings in patients undergoing respiratory care (Objective Data), the problem or problems that these findings usually indicate (Assessment), and the types of therapy that should be provided or recommended (Considerations for Care Plan).

Reviewing Planned Therapy to Establish Therapeutic Plan

In reviewing planned therapy, it is important to pay attention to the specifications in the order as well as the logical use of the therapy given the patient's problem. A typical plan should specify:

- Therapeutic objectives
- Specifics of equipment type and settings
- Drug names, dosages, and frequency of administration
- Relevant cautions or protocols to follow

In addition, interdisciplinary and family plans should also specify:

- Interdisciplinary requirements, conflicts, and solutions
- Family requirements for education, communication, and monitoring

Determining Appropriateness of Prescribed Therapy and Goals for Identified Pathophysiological State

On the exam, you must first recall specific information about the identified pathophysiological state, such as respiratory failure (Table 16-1). Then, you must analyze the data provided in order to determine the appropriate course of action. For example, if a patient suffering from a drug overdose is in ventilatory failure, then mechanical ventilation to prevent hypoventilation will be needed. However, if the problem is hypoxemic respiratory failure caused by shunting (as in ARDS), then mechanical ventilation with PEEP and a focus on oxygenation will be most appropriate.

Recommending Changes in Therapeutic Plan When Indicated Based on Data

If the data indicate the therapeutic plan is not meeting the desired objectives, then you should recommend appropriate changes. For example, if a patient with a weak cough is having problems with secretion clearance and the problem persists after a regimen of directed coughing, you should recommend either mechanical insufflation-exsufflation or nasotracheal suctioning (Table 16-1).

Performing Respiratory Care Quality Assurance

Respiratory care quality improvement activities usually focus on identifying and resolving problems related to patient care and clinical performance. Usually, a departmental committee develops and carries out its quality improvement plan under the supervision of the medical director and/or quality assurance department. According to the AARC, the goals of a respiratory care quality improvement plan should include at least the following:

- To provide ongoing monitoring of both the quality and appropriateness of respiratory care
- To ensure that respiratory care methods and procedures are cost efficient
- To ensure that respiratory care methods and procedures are effective
- To identify, rank, and resolve patient care–related problems

Nine key steps are needed to systematically implement a quality improvement plan. As depicted in **Figure 16-1**, these steps include: the identification of problems, the determination of problem causes, the ranking of problems, the development of strategies for problem resolution, the development of appropriate measures, the implementation of problem resolution strategies, the compilation of results, the evaluation of outcomes, and the reporting of results.

Table 16-1 Common Findings of Objective Data, Assessment, and Planning in Respiratory Care Patients

Objective Data	Assessment	Considerations for Care Plan
Airways		
Wheezing	Bronchospasm and inflammation	Bronchodilator therapy Inhaled corticosteroids
	Congestive heart failure (CHF)	Diuretic (e.g., Lasix[a])
Stridor	Laryngeal edema	Cool bland aerosol/racemic epinephrine
	Tumor/mass	Bronchoscopy
Rhonchi/tactile fremitus	Secretions in large airways	Directed coughing; PEP/vibratory PEP therapy; suctioning
Cough		
Weak cough	Poor secretion clearance	Directed coughing; mechanical insufflation-exsufflation; suctioning
Secretions		
> 30 mL/day	Excessive secretions	Bronchial hygiene therapy; systemic hydration; bland aerosol therapy; suctioning
Mucopurulent (yellow/thick) sputum	Acute airway infection	Treat underlying cause[a]; antibiotic therapy[a]
Pink, watery, frothy secretions	Pulmonary edema	Treat underlying cause[a] (e.g., CHF); CPAP or BiPAP™, oxygen
Lung Parenchyma		
Dull percussion note, bronchial breath sounds	Infiltrates, atelectasis, consolidation	Incentive spirometry, IPPB, O_2 therapy; consider therapeutic bronchoscopy[a] for atelectasis due to large airway obstruction
Opacity on chest X-ray	Infiltrates, atelectasis, consolidation	Incentive spirometry, IPPB, O_2 therapy; consider therapeutic bronchoscopy[a] for atelectasis due to large airway obstruction
Pleural Space		
Hyperresonant percussion	Pneumothorax	Evacuate air[a]; lung expansion therapy
Dull percussion	Pleural effusion	Evacuate fluid[a]; lung-expansion therapy
Acid–Base Disorders		
Acute respiratory acidosis	Acute ventilatory failure	Mechanical ventilation (consider NPPV initially)[a]
Compensated respiratory acidosis	Chronic ventilatory failure	Low-flow O_2; bronchial hygiene therapy
Metabolic alkalosis	Hypokalemia	Treat underlying cause[a]; give potassium[a]
	Hypochloremia	Treat underlying cause[a]; give chloride[a]

(continues)

Table 16-1 Common Findings of Objective Data, Assessment, and Planning in Respiratory Care Patients (continued)

Objective Data	Assessment	Considerations for Care Plan
Metabolic acidosis	Shock/lactic acidosis	O_2 therapy; restore circulation; administer $NaHCO_3$[a]
	Ketoacidosis (diabetes)	Treat underlying cause[a]; administer $NaHCO_3$[a]; hyperventilate
	Renal failure	Treat underlying cause[a]; dialysis[a]
Oxygenation		
$Pao_2 < 60$ torr $Fio_2 < 0.60$ V/Q imbalance	Moderate hypoxemia	O_2 therapy; treat underlying cause
$Pao_2 < 60$ torr $Fio_2 > 0.60$ Shunting	Severe hypoxemia	PEEP/CPAP, oxygen

a. Physician ordered.

Adapted from: Des Jardins, T., Burton, G. G., & Tietsort, J. (1997). *Respiratory care case studies: The therapist driven protocol approach.* St. Louis: Mosby-Yearbook.

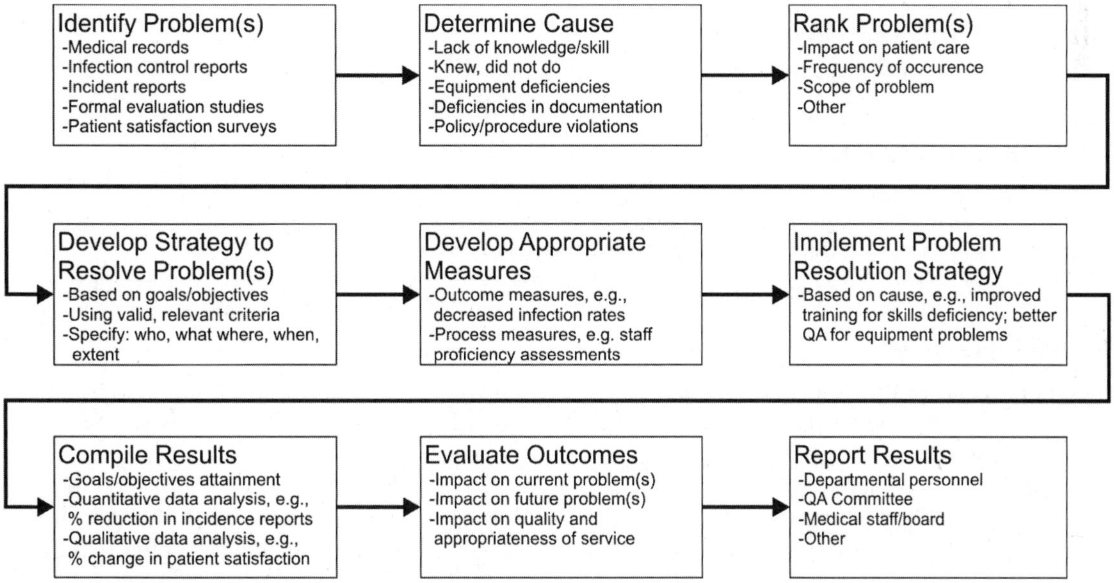

Figure 16-1 Respiratory Care Quality Assurance Flow Chart.

Modified from: Hastings, D. (1988). The AARC's model quality assurance plan. *AARC Times, 12(2),* 25.

Successful implementation of the quality improvement plan demands that the respiratory care service develop criteria addressing the therapeutic goals, appropriateness, and means of evaluating the effectiveness of each specific high-utilization and high-risk procedure. The following box provides an example of such criteria for oxygen therapy, followed by an example application of the quality improvement protocol.

Quality Assurance Criteria for Oxygen Therapy

Therapeutic Goals

1. To prevent or reverse hypoxemia and tissue hypoxia

2. To decrease myocardial work

3. To decrease the work of breathing

Appropriateness of Care

1. The patient must be diagnosed as having or being at risk of developing hypoxemia and/or tissue hypoxia; or

2. The patient must be diagnosed as having suffered a myocardial infarction within the last 72 hours; and

3. Oxygen dosing and mode of therapy will follow the criteria specified in the Respiratory Care Policy and Procedure Manual.

Evaluation of the Effectiveness of Therapy

Effectiveness of therapy is evaluated by comparing the pre-treatment and post-treatment status of the patient according to the following criteria. To be considered effective, at least one item from the following list must apply:

- Increase in Pao_2 or Spo_2
- Reversal or absence of cyanosis
- Decrease in heart rate
- Decrease in blood pressure
- Resolution of cardiac dysrhythmias
- Decrease in respiratory rate
- Increase in level of consciousness
- Decrease in %HbCO
- Relief of dyspnea

Adapted from: Larson, K. (1988). The well-defined quality assurance plan. *AARC Times, 12*(2):1524.

Identifying Problems

Using the quality improvement process just described, various data sources, including patients' medical records, would be used to determine the extent to which oxygen-therapy services are being appropriately used.

Normally, an objective problem indicator, such as "90% of all patients receiving oxygen therapy will meet the appropriateness of care criteria," is helpful in problem identification. If the indicator is not being met (e.g., if only 70% of the patients meet the appropriateness of therapy criteria), a problem exists.

Determining Causes

Once a problem has been identified, its cause must be determined. For example, the fact that only 70% of the patients receiving oxygen therapy meet the specified criteria may result from such factors as the ordering physicians' lack of knowledge of the criteria, their failure to follow known criteria, or their failure to discontinue therapy when indicated.

Resolving Identified Problems

Once the underlying cause is identified, a strategy to resolve the problem must be developed, implemented, and evaluated. For example, if the problem with oxygen therapy use is based on the new medical residents' failure to follow the appropriateness of care criteria, proper orientation and/or in-service education may be needed. Once conducted, the impact of the selected strategy on the desired outcome should be assessed. Ideally, evaluation of the outcomes of intervention should be based on the initial problem indicator. For example, we would want to know whether the in-service education program for the medical residents increased the percentage of patients who receive oxygen therapy and meet the appropriateness criteria.

Reporting and Ongoing Monitoring

Problem identification and resolution activities, including the relative success of intervention strategies, must be documented and reported regularly. Moreover, even successful interventions must be monitored over time to ensure that a given problem does not recur. Only in this manner can the respiratory care service ensure that its services are appropriately utilized and effective in meeting patient needs.

Developing, Monitoring, and Applying Respiratory Care Protocols

The NBRC CRT exam requires that candidates be proficient in applying treatment protocols. Physicians have traditionally written orders for respiratory care services that were specific and allowed no variation by the therapist providing the treatment. Protocols have been developed that allow properly trained respiratory therapists to independently initiate and adjust therapy, within guidelines previously established by the medical staff. According to the American College of Chest Physicians (ACCP), key elements required in a medically acceptable respiratory care protocol include the following:

- Clearly stated objectives
- Outline of the protocol, including a decision tree or algorithm
- Description of alternative choices at decision and action points
- Description of potential complications and corrections
- Description of end-points and decision-points where the physician must be contacted

The accompanying box outlines the general steps in respiratory care protocol application, as recommended by the AARC.

Guidelines for Preparing a Respiratory Care Protocol

I. Perform initial patient evaluation
  A. Check physician order for respiratory care protocol
  B. Review medical records
    1. Admitting (and consulting) physician assessment
    2. All admitting and working diagnoses
    3. Pertinent pulmonary history
    4. Pertinent reports of diagnostic evaluations
      a. Laboratory tests (including blood, urine, and sputum)
      b. Radiographs
      c. Arterial blood gases, including specific F_{IO_2} or oxygen liter flow
      d. Pulmonary function tests
      e. Vital signs
      f. Oxygen saturation by pulse oximetry, including specific F_{IO_2} or oxygen liter flow
  C. Initiate patient contact
    1. Introduction to patient
    2. Verification of patient
    3. Explanation of purpose of visit by therapist
  D. Observe universal precautions at all times

(continues)

E. Perform pertinent physical examination
    1. Vital signs
    2. Chest inspection, palpation, percussion, auscultation
    3. Spirometry
    4. Pulse oximetry
    5. Other diagnostic evaluations (e.g., arterial blood gas)

II. Formulate appropriate management plan
  A. Indications
  B. Therapeutic objectives
  C. Therapy
  D. Precautions/contraindications
  E. Delivery method
  F. Frequency
  G. Medication dose
  H. Patient/family education where appropriate
  I. Monitor therapy (including adverse effects)
  J. Assess efficacy of therapy (patient outcomes)
  K. Modify plan to achieve optimal efficacy and outcome
  L. Discontinue therapy
  M. Identify physician and other appropriate health care personnel
  N. Integration of respiratory care protocol into overall patient management
  O. Management plan basis
    1. AARC Clinical Practice Guidelines
    2. Other appropriate medical literature
    3. Specific institutional preferences (including inventory of available protocols)

III. Documentation of respiratory care protocol application in medical record
  A. Date and time of protocol initiation
  B. Pertinent medical history and physical examination
  C. Pertinent diagnostic results
  D. Management plan details (as outlined in section II)
  E. Physician notification criteria—guidelines for physician notification of patient status change (as directed by respiratory care medical director, appropriate hospital committee, and medical staff)
  F. Adverse reaction, if any, and remedial steps taken
  G. Notification of physician, nurse, and other appropriate health care professionals
  H. Required departmental documentation
  I. Signature with credential

IV. Reevaluation
  A. Assess management plan with each treatment or at a pre-established frequency based on patient acuity
  B. Modify therapy based on:
    1. AARC Clinical Practice Guidelines
    2. Other appropriate medical literature
    3. Specific physician orders
    4. Patient report (evaluation of care by therapist, based on patient's current status and assessed at shift report)
  C. Adjustments in therapy will be:
    1. Documented in the patient record, including reasons for change
    2. Communicated to the patient's physician, nurse, and other appropriate health care professionals

V. Discontinuation
  A. Upon discontinuation of therapy, the therapist will refer to all indications for therapy as being resolved and/or addressed, via documentation in the patient record
  B. Communicate discontinuation to the patient's physician, nurse, and other appropriate health care professionals

Source: American Association for Respiratory Care. (n.d.). *Guidelines for preparing a respiratory care protocol (RC protocol).* Courtesy of the American Association for Respiratory Care. Reprinted with permission.

Examples of Protocol Algorithms

It is a good idea to be familiar with the most common protocols used in respiratory care. In its Resources section, the AARC provides a selection of nationally developed and approved protocols on its website (www.aarc.org), with access limited to active members. Currently, the AARC provides model protocols in the following areas:

- Adult cute care:
  - Aerosol therapy protocol
  - Oxygen protocol
  - Hyperinflation (lung volume expansion) protocol
  - Bronchopulmonary hygiene protocol
  - Adult patient assessment form
- Adult ICU:
  - Mechanical ventilation
- Pediatric acute care:
  - Aerosol therapy protocol and algorithm
  - Oxygen protocol and algorithm
  - Hyperinflation/lung volume–expansion protocol and algorithm
  - Bronchopulmonary hygiene protocol and algorithm
  - Pediatric assessment tool
  - Pediatric assessment (neurological)
- Pediatric ICU:
  - Ready to extubate
  - Bronchiolitis ventilator management protocol
  - Neonatal ventilator management protocol
  - Guidelines for surfactant administration
  - Pediatric normal lung ventilator guidelines
  - Acute lung injury ventilator guidelines

Figure 16-2 provides the basic algorithm for the AARC aerosol therapy bronchodilator (BD) model protocol. The full online protocol is supplemented by a comprehensive list of references and the applicable AARC Clinical Practice Guidelines. Links to other representative protocols are provided on the accompanying CD.

Protocol Monitoring and Quality Assurance

Successful implementation of respiratory care protocols requires ongoing quality monitoring to assess their effectiveness. Elements of protocol implementation that should be monitored include therapist competency, medical and therapist compliance, protocol outcomes, participant feedback, and patient satisfaction. Relevant protocol outcome measures can include the following:

- Physician protocol orders (appropriateness and duration)
- Comparison of protocol patients to those receiving care by standard order (e.g., by DRG, case-mix index, etc.)
- Costs (direct costs, number of procedures, duration of treatment, missed treatments)
- Clinical outcomes (changes in physiologic measures such as SpO_2, $FEV_1\%$; adverse responses; length of stay; readmissions)
- Effect on staff (productivity, satisfaction)
- Miscellaneous (percentage of protocol patients vs. percentage of physician-directed patients)
- Number of patients on protocols by DRG, case-mix index for severity score, assessment scoring system for severity of respiratory illness, patient satisfaction scores

AEROSOL THERAPY PROTOCOL

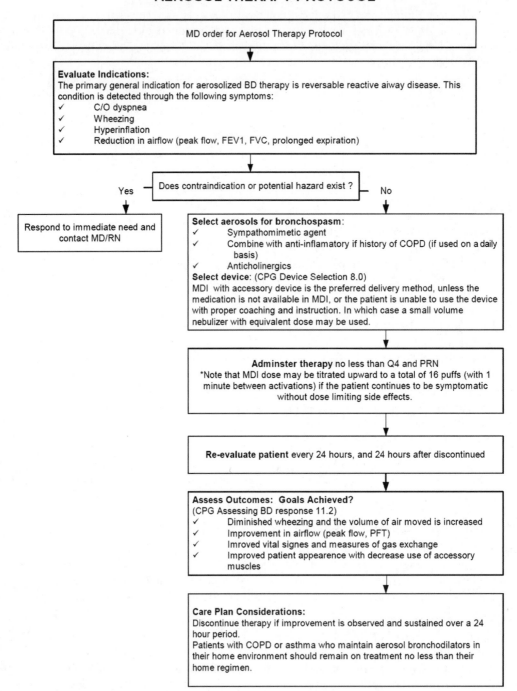

Figure 16-2 Algorithm for Aerosol Therapy Bronchodilator (BD) Model Protocol.

Source: Courtesy of the American Association for Respiratory Care; Phillips-Clar, J., Ford, R., Tietsort, J., Peters, J., & Vines, D.

COMMON ERRORS TO AVOID

You can improve your score by avoiding these mistakes:

- Never assume that all wheezing is due to bronchospasm or asthma; congestive heart failure (CHF) can cause similar symptoms but requires different treatment (a fast-acting diuretic).
- Never recommend mechanical ventilation for chronic ventilatory failure when the blood gas indicates compensated respiratory acidosis; instead, recommend conservative management (e.g., low-flow O_2, bronchial hygiene therapy) and careful monitoring.
- Never recommend raising the F_{IO_2} above 0.60 in the presence of severe hypoxemia due to shunting; instead, recommend adding PEEP/CPAP.
- Never proceed with a protocol beyond a defined end-point or when a notification criterion requires you to contact the physician.

SURE BETS

In some situations you can be sure of the right approach to a clinical problem or scenario:

- Always differentiate atelectasis/consolidation from pleural effusion before recommending the appropriate treatment.
- Always recommend oxygen, circulatory support, and $NaHCO_3$ when metabolic acidosis is due to shock.
- Always recommend CPAP/PEEP in the presence of severe hypoxemia due to shunting ($Pa_{O_2} < 60$ torr on $F_{IO_2} > 0.60$).
- Always assess the patient's pathophysiological state before recommending any course of action.
- Whenever evaluation data indicate that a therapeutic plan is not meeting the desired objectives, always consider or recommend appropriate changes in respiratory care.
- When formulating respiratory care plans, always consider family requirements for education, communication, and monitoring.
- When participating in quality assurance efforts, always try to identify the cause(s) of problems before developing corrective strategies.
- Always conduct a comprehensive initial patient evaluation (e.g., chart review, physical assessment) before developing a respiratory care plan or implementing a protocol.
- Always include multiple methods to assess the efficacy of therapy (patient outcomes) in your care plans.
- Always document any adjustments in therapy (including reasons for change) in the patient record.

PRE-TEST ANSWERS AND EXPLANATIONS

Below are this chapter's pre-test answers and explanations. Be sure to review each answer's explanation thoroughly to help you understand why it is correct. If the explanation is still unclear to you, review the chapter contents or the references and/or refer to this chapter's supplemental resources on the CD.

16-1. **Correct answer: A.** Administer high concentrations of oxygen. In this case, the Pa_{O_2} is misleading because it represents only dissolved oxygen (CO alters oxyhemoglobin saturations but not Pa_{O_2}). The immediate history and finding of coma is a sufficient basis to recommend administration of high concentrations of oxygen to eliminate the carbon monoxide. In addition, notice that a ventilator is not needed, since the patient is able to breathe well enough to have a Pa_{CO_2} of 30. If work of breathing does not appear overwhelming (no data to support), then high O_2 should be your immediate therapy of choice. Also, because the patient is currently on room air, due to time your first of the choices given should be to give high O_2—otherwise the patient may expire before you can start any of the other choices in the question.

16-2. **Correct answer: C.** Improve alveolar ventilation. IPPB is used on patients who can not (due to the increased work of breathing) or will not take a deep breath. Its primary function is to increase alveolar ventilation by taking over the work of breathing through assisted IPPB.

16-3. **Correct answer: C.** Pulmonary edema. CPAP can help overcome the shunting and hypoxemia common in both cardiogenic and noncardiogenic pulmonary edema. In cardiogenic pulmonary edema, CPAP can help decrease venous return and thus decrease pulmonary blood flows and pressures. In non-cardiogenic pulmonary edema (e.g., ARDS), CPAP (or PEEP) opens collapsed alveoli and improves the V/Q ratio.

16-4. **Correct answer: C.** Decrease left heart and pulmonary vascular pressures. The primary aim in treating cardiogenic pulmonary edema is to decrease left heart and pulmonary vascular pressures. Note that one key to the correct answer is to identify the therapeutic goal for a patient with the given condition.

16-5. **Correct answer: B.** Bedside therapeutic bronchoscopy. Should conservative measures fail in treating atelectasis due to large airway obstruction, therapeutic bronchoscopy is indicated. This procedure can usually be performed at the bedside with conscious sedation. Note that data are collected and analyzed in the item, and you are expected to pick the plan that best matches the data and analysis provided.

16-6. **Correct answer: C.** Treating absorption atelectasis. Indications for O_2 therapy include: documented hypoxemia, acute care situations in which hypoxemia is common (e.g., shock, trauma, CO poisoning), acute myocardial infarction (to decrease myocardial workload), and short-term therapy for patients likely to develop hypoxemia (e.g., during post-anesthesia recovery). Absorption atelectasis is a potential *hazard* of supplemental O_2 therapy. Note that with this type of question, being familiar with clinical practice guidelines for O_2 therapy and O_2 therapy protocols would provide the content needed to answer a question about indications for therapy.

16-7. **Correct answer: D.** Maintain a Pa_{CO_2} of 25–30 torr (deliberate hyperventilation). In patients with recent closed head trauma and increased intracranial pressures, deliberate 25–30 torr during the first 24–48 hours of care is indicated to help reduce intracranial pressure. Note the focus on the goal in this question. You are expected to analyze the data and recognize that two answers are measure-able (good) goals, but only one is consistent with the therapeutic objective of decreasing ICP. Besides looking for a goal that can be best monitored and measured objectively, knowing the effects of Pa_{CO_2} on cerebral blood flow is required to select the best answer.

16-8. **Correct answer: D.** Treat progressive respiratory muscle weakness. IPPB is used instead of incentive spirometry when a patient can not (physically) or will not take a deep breath. The only scenario that fits this indication for IPPB is progressive respiratory muscle weakness, which would lead to a patient being unable to take a deep breath. Note that in most situations the therapist would probably initiate this order change; you are being tested to see if you know the primary indication for suggesting a modification of the deep breathing therapy from incentive spirometry to IPPB.

16-9. **Correct answer: D.** Low-flow oxygen. Patients with emphysema may hypoventilate when given moderate to high concentrations of oxygen (due to elimination of their hypoxic drive). It is therefore recommended that hypoxemic COPD patients receive no more oxygen than needed to raise their Pa_{O_2} to the 55–60 torr range. Normally, this can be achieved using low-flow (1–2 L/min) oxygen or an air-entrainment mask that will control the F_{IO_2}. Note that when the question asks you to "recommend" something, analyzing the data presented and *matching* it to the best therapy answer of the choices offered is the winning strategy.

16-10. **Correct answer: B.** Inspiratory stridor. Inspiratory stridor is a symptom, whereas laryngeal edema is part of the assessment (possible problems). A bronchodilator or bronchoscopy (drugs and diagnostic test) would be part of the plan (see Table 16-1). Note that when you are asked for objective data to use in making an assessment and plan, the key is to look for the choice that has the most objective data in the choices offered.

16-11. **Correct answer: C.** Check physician order for respiratory care protocol. See respiratory care protocol outline provided in this chapter.

16-12. **Correct answer: A.** Analysis of department budgeting. Department budget should not have much consideration when investigating the causes of patient care–related issues. Note that in this question, you must analyze the list and look for the answer that is least important in uncovering the causes of patient care–related problems.

16-13. **Correct answer: D.** I, II, III, and IV. All of these data could be used as quality assurance outcome criteria. Remember, outcome criteria for quality assurance must always fit one of the data collection categories of subjective or objective data. In this question, subjective patient data were placed there because we usually put emphasis on objective data, but most experts agree that even though patient data are subjective data, they should not be discounted completely when assessing the effectiveness of therapy. If objective data support improvement, but the patient does not feel any better, that is valuable information that must be considered in the analysis and plan.

16-14. **Correct answer: D.** I, II, and III. All three items in this list should be investigated as potential causes of an infection control problem. Training can impact how procedures are carried out, supply deficiencies can make therapists not change equipment as often as recommended, and failure to follow set infection control procedures for whatever reason will result in a failed quality assurance program.

16-15. **Correct answer: C.** Compare pre- and post-treatment patient status on one or more pre-defined criteria. Comparison of pre- and post-treatment status on pre-defined criteria ensures you don't jump to therapeutic conclusions without the data to support such conclusions.

POST-TEST

A post-test for this chapter that includes automated scoring and feedback is available on the accompanying CD. Be sure to complete this additional assessment to confirm your mastery of this chapter's objectives.

REFERENCES

American Association for Respiratory Care. (n.d.). Guidelines for preparing a respiratory care protocol (RC protocol). Retrieved April 15, 2009, from http://www.aarc.org (Protocol Resources; members only area).

American College of Chest Physicians. Respiratory Care Section Steering Committee. (1992). *Position paper: Respiratory care protocols*. Chicago: American College of Chest Physicians. Retrieved April 15, 2009, from http://www.aarc.org (Protocol Resources; members only area).

Des Jardins, T., Burton, G. G., & Tietsort, J. (1997). *Respiratory care case studies: The therapist driven protocol approach*. St. Louis: Mosby-Yearbook.

Orens, D., Kester, L., Ford, R., Salyer, J. Acevedo, R., & Stewart, K. (n.d.). Strategies for measuring protocol outcomes. Retrieved April 15, 2009, from http://www.aarc.org (Protocol Resources; members only area).

Vines, D. (2003). Quality in acute care protocols. Retrieved April 15, 2009, from http://www.aarc.org (Protocol Resources; members only area).

Wilkins, R. L., Stoller, J. K., & Kacmarek, R. M. (Eds.). (2009). *Egan's fundamentals of respiratory care* (9th ed.). St. Louis: Mosby.

CHAPTER 17

Initiate, Conduct, or Modify Respiratory Care Techniques in an Emergency Setting

Albert J. Heuer

INTRODUCTION

Respiratory therapists play a vital role in providing prompt and appropriate care in emergency settings. After all, the "A" and "B" in the ABCs of CPR involve effective management of the airway and breathing. Additionally, there have been changes to the American Heart Association CPR guidelines, and providing proper emergency care is extremely important in a clinical setting. As a result of this and because providing respiratory care in emergency settings remains a content area included in NBRC exams, you should review this area carefully when preparing for the CRT exam. By learning the material in this chapter, you will be able to fulfill the objectives noted below and help enable yourself to pass the CRT exam.

OBJECTIVES

After completion of this chapter, you should be able to demonstrate knowledge needed to:

1. Treat cardiopulmonary collapse by being able to:
   a. Recognize cardiopulmonary emergencies
   b. Initiate appropriate respiratory care in emergency settings
   c. Understand and apply basic life support and elements of advanced life support
   d. Assist in the initial diagnosis and treatment of a tension pneumothorax
   e. Appropriately monitor such patients and modify care if necessary
2. Participate in safe and effective intra-hospital and external ground and air patient transport
3. Participate as a member of the medical emergency team (MET)
4. Prepare for and assist with disaster management

WHAT TO EXPECT ON THIS CATEGORY OF THE CRT EXAM

Number of questions: 3
Level of questions: about 1/3 each from the recall, application, and analysis categories

WHAT'S NEW FOR 2009

As of July 2009, this section of the NBRC CRT examination includes the following *new content areas*:

- Treat a tension pneumothorax
- Participate in:
  - Land/air patient transport
  - Medical emergency team (MET), e.g., rapid response team

PRE-TEST

Carefully respond to each of the following questions. After completing the pre-test, compare your answers with those provided at the end of this chapter. Then thoroughly review each answer's explanation to help understand why it is correct.

17-1. During a "code blue" or other medical emergency, a physician is having trouble starting an intravenous line. Which of the following drugs can be placed down an endotracheal tube during emergency life support?
  I. Naloxone
  II. Lidocaine
  III. Atropine
  IV. Epinephrine
  A. II and IV only
  B. I, II, and III
  C. III and IV only
  D. I, II, III, and IV

17-2. Which of the following techniques can be used to determine effectiveness of ventilation?
  I. Looking for the rise and fall of the victim's chest
  II. Feeling for air exchange near the victim's mouth and nose
  III. Listening for audible breathing efforts from the victim
  A. I and II only
  B. II and III only
  C. I and III only
  D. I, II, and III

17-3. At the onset of adult mouth-to-mouth or mouth-to-mask ventilation, you should provide:
  A. Two normal breaths, then assess the pulse
  B. Four fast, shallow breaths, then assess the pulse
  C. Four slow, deep breaths, then immediately start compressions
  D. One very slow breath, then immediately start compressions

17-4. After two attempts of ventilating an infant in respiratory arrest, you still cannot deliver breaths. At this point you should:
  A. Apply back blows, followed by chest thrusts
  B. Try to ventilate again with smaller puffs
  C. Apply six to ten strong abdominal thrusts
  D. Go on to provide external cardiac compressions

17-5. The ideal ratio of chest compressions to rescue breaths that should be given by a single rescuer during a cardiopulmonary resuscitation (CPR) attempt on an adult is:
  A. 5:1
  B. 15:2
  C. 2:15
  D. 30:2

17-6. When transporting critically ill patients who are receiving supplemental oxygen in unpressurized aircraft, it is often necessary to make which adjustment in F_{IO_2} in order to maintain adequate oxygenation?
  A. Increase the F_{IO_2}
  B. Decrease the F_{IO_2}
  C. Increase ventilation
  D. No change to ventilation or F_{IO_2} is needed

17-7. The proper rate and depth of external chest compressions for an adult is a rate of:
  A. 80–100/min with a depth of 1 inch
  B. 70–80/min with a depth of 1 to 1½ inches
  C. 100/min with a depth of 1½ to 2 inches
  D. 60–80/min with a depth of 1½ to 2 inches

17-8. The initial energy level for defibrillation for ventricular fibrillation is:
- **A.** 100 joules
- **B.** 200 joules
- **C.** 300 joules
- **D.** 360 joules

17-9. All of the following monitoring equipment is mandatory when transporting a critically ill patient within or outside of the hospital *except*:
- **A.** End-tidal CO_2 monitor
- **B.** An oxygen source/delivery device
- **C.** Blood pressure monitor/cuff
- **D.** Cardiac monitor/defibrillator

17-10. If the number of ventilators needed to support patients in respiratory failure after a chemical disaster is insufficient to meet the need, your *initial* response should be to:
- **A.** Contact other local facilities and arrange for patient transfers
- **B.** Call and order additional backup ventilators from the vendor
- **C.** Enlist non-respiratory personnel to perform manual ventilation
- **D.** Assign patients without needed equipment to triage priority Black

WHAT YOU NEED TO KNOW: ESSENTIAL CONTENT

Basic Life Support (BLS)

Basic life support (BLS) is the foundation for most emergency care. You should fully expect that concepts related to BLS will be included on the CRT exam.

BLS support can help restore ventilation and circulation to victims of airway obstruction, and respiratory and cardiac arrest without the use of specialized equipment. These procedures should be applied until the victim is revived or until advanced life support equipment and personnel are available.

In sequence, the key steps in BLS are:

1. Assess the victim for unresponsiveness ("tap and shout").
2. Open the airway: head tilt/chin lift or jaw thrust (obstructed airway maneuvers if needed).
3. Check for breathing: look, listen, feel for breathing 5–10 seconds.
4. If breathing, place in recover position.
5. If not breathing, give two normal breaths, each lasting 1 second.
6. If breaths go in, check for pulse up to 10 seconds.
7. If no pulse, begin CPR: cycles of chest compression and breaths for 2 minutes (5 cycles); reassess after every 5 cycles.
8. If pulse is present but no breathing, provide rescue breaths only.
9. If a breath does not make the chest rise, reposition (retilt) the head and try another breath.
10. If breath still does not make chest rise, assume obstructed airway, give cycles of 30 chest compressions, look for object in mouth, remove object if visible, give 2 breaths.

Note that the last three steps are the traditional "ABCs" of resuscitation: Airway, Breathing, and Circulation. **Table 17-1** outlines the key differences in these basic life support steps as applied to adults, children (1–8 years old), and infants (< 1 year old). Techniques for health care professionals (HCPs) are noted as such.

Advanced Cardiac Life Support (ACLS)

In addition to demonstrating competency in basic life support, the NBRC expects that you will be able to treat cardiopulmonary collapse according to the American Heart Association (AHA) ACLS protocols. These protocols are summarized in clinical algorithms for specific cardiopulmonary and medical emergencies.

Adult Resuscitation Protocols

The most common adult cardiopulmonary emergencies stem from one of four cardiac arrhythmias that produce pulseless cardiac arrest. These rhythms include ventricular fibrillation (VF), rapid ventricular

Table 17-1 Summary of Basic Life Support

	Adult and Older Child (> 8 years)	Child (1–8 years)	Infant (< 1 year)
When to activate EMS/call a "code blue"	Call immediately after determining unresponsiveness and get defibrillator	Call after providing 2 minutes of care, if alone; get defibrillator	Call after providing 2 minutes of care, if alone
Pulse check	Carotid/femoral	Carotid/femoral	Brachial
Compression location	2 hands on breastbone between nipples	1 or 2 hands on breastbone between nipples	2 fingers on breastbone just below the nipple line; use 2-thumb technique for neonates
Compression depth	1½ to 2 inches	⅓ to ½ depth of chest or 1–1½ inches	⅓ to ½ depth of chest or ½ to 1 inch
Compression-to-breaths ratio (single HCP)	30:2	30:2	30:2 (3:1 for neonates)
Compression-to-breaths ratio (two HCPs)	30:2*	15:2	15:2 (3:1 for neonates)
Compression rate	Approx. 100/minute	Approx. 100/minute	Approx. 100/minute
Breathing method	*Lay personnel:* Mouth-to-mouth Barrier device if available *HCP:* Bag-mask ventilation and O_2 ASAP	*Lay personnel:* Mouth-to-mouth Barrier device if available *HCP:* Bag-mask ventilation and O_2 ASAP	*Lay personnel:* Mouth-to-mouth and nose Mouth-to-nose as alternative Barrier device if available *HCP:* Bag-mask ventilation and O_2 ASAP
Foreign body airway obstruction in a *responsive* victim	Abdominal thrusts (Heimlich maneuver)	Abdominal thrusts (Heimlich maneuver)	Alternate 5 back blows with 5 chest thrusts
Automatic external defibrillator (AED) use	Yes	Yes (only if pediatric pads available)	*No AED for infants!*
	Deliver 1 shock, followed immediately by 2 minutes of CPR, then reassess	Deliver 1 shock, followed immediately by 2 minutes of CPR, then reassess	

Abbreviation: HCP, health care provider. *Once an advanced airway in place, give on breath every 8 sec simultaneously with compressions.

tachycardia (VT), pulseless electrical activity (PEA), and asystole. Electrocardiography (ECG) tracings for both VF and VT are displayed and summarized in **Figure 17-1** and **Figure 17-2**, respectively.

In addition, the ACLS algorithms for responding to VF and pulseless VT, as well as that for asystole and PEA, are shown in **Figure 17-3** (see page 503) and **Figure 17-4** (see page 503), respectively. For practical purposes, in preparing for the CRT exam you should be able to first quickly recognize these rhythms and then promptly apply the appropriate steps in these algorithms.

Medications

ACLS also involves the use of an array of medications that may be indicated in cases of cardiopulmonary collapse. In general, as a CRT exam candidate, you are not expected to know all of these drugs,

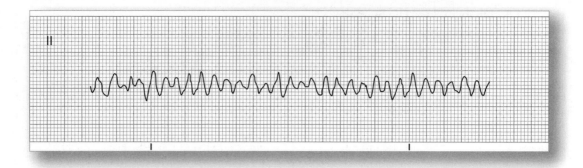

Figure 17-1 Example of Ventricular Fibrillation.

Source: Garcia, T., and Miller, G.T. (2004) *Arrhythmia recognition: the art of interpretation.* Sudbury, MA: Jones and Bartlett Publishers.

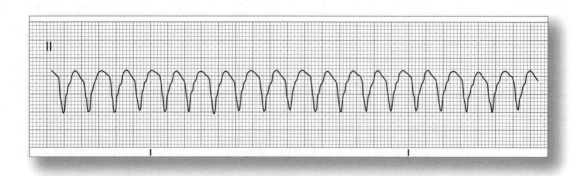

Figure 17-2 Example of Ventricular Tachycardia.

Source: Garcia, T., and Miller, G.T. (2004) *Arrhythmia recognition: the art of interpretation.* Sudbury, MA: Jones and Bartlett Publishers.

dosages, and indications. However, you are expected to have knowledge of selected emergency medications. **Table 17-2** (see page 504) summarizes the most common ACLS medications administered via intravenous (IV) infusion for adults. In the absence of IV access, those medications that may be instilled through an ET tube are noted accordingly.

Equipment

In preparing for the CRT exam, you should be familiar with indications for, and proper use of, respiratory equipment used in emergency settings, including manual resuscitation devices described in Chapter 6, as well as selected artificial airways (e.g., ET tubes and laryngeal mask airways) and oxygen-delivery devices (e.g., nonrebreathing masks), also covered in Chapters 6 and 10.

You also will be expected to know how to properly use an automated external defibrillator (AED) and have general knowledge of standard defibrillator use. Consequently, candidates should be familiar with the AARC Clinical Practice Guideline on Resuscitation and Defibrillation in the Health Care Setting, as revised in 2004.

Monitoring and Assessment

Once a prompt clinical assessment has identified the presence of a cardiopulmonary emergency and appropriate interventions have begun, it is imperative that the patient be monitored. You are expected to know the major ways in which a patient should be assessed during CPR and immediately following a successful resuscitation of a patient. This may range from periodic pulse and breathing checks, generally after five cycles of CPR, to more advanced assessment methods, including electrocardiography, pulse oximetry, end-tidal CO_2 monitoring, and arterial blood gas monitoring. These monitoring and assessment methods are also covered in more detail in Chapter 13.

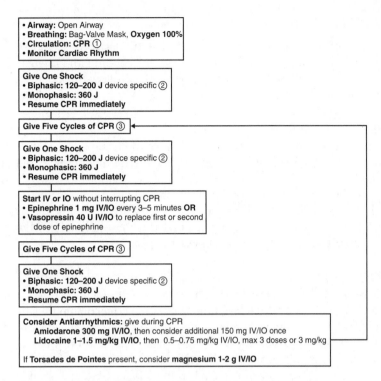

- **Airway:** Open Airway
- **Breathing:** Bag-Valve Mask, **Oxygen 100%**
- **Circulation: CPR** ①
- **Monitor Cardiac Rhythm**

Give One Shock
- **Biphasic: 120–200 J** device specific ②
- **Monophasic: 360 J**
- **Resume CPR immediately**

Give Five Cycles of CPR ③

Give One Shock
- **Biphasic: 120–200 J** device specific ②
- **Monophasic: 360 J**
- **Resume CPR immediately**

Start IV or IO without interrupting CPR
- **Epinephrine 1 mg IV/IO** every 3–5 minutes **OR**
- **Vasopressin 40 U IV/IO** to replace first or second
   dose of epinephrine

Give Five Cycles of CPR ③

Give One Shock
- **Biphasic: 120–200 J** device specific ②
- **Monophasic: 360 J**
- **Resume CPR immediately**

Consider Antiarrhythmics: give during CPR
   Amiodarone 300 mg IV/IO, then consider additional 150 mg IV/IO once
   Lidocaine 1–1.5 mg/kg IV/IO, then 0.5–0.75 mg/kg IV/IO, max 3 doses or 3 mg/kg

If **Torsades de Pointes** present, consider **magnesium 1-2 g IV/IO**

1 When caregiver does not witness the arrest, may give 5 cycles of CPR before attempting to defibrillate.
2 If you are not certain of the device's effective dose range, deliver 200 J.
3 If **spontaneous pulse** present, begin post-resuscitation care.

Figure 17-3 ACLS Algorithm for Adult Ventricular Fibrillation and Pulseless Ventricular Tachycardia.

Source: Porter, W. (2007). *Porter's pocket guide to emergency and critical care.* Sudbury, MA: Jones and Bartlett Publishers.

Asystole and PEA

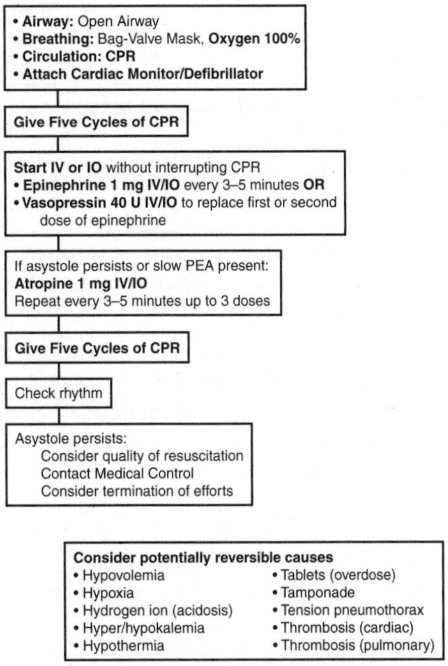

- **Airway:** Open Airway
- **Breathing:** Bag-Valve Mask, **Oxygen 100%**
- **Circulation: CPR**
- **Attach Cardiac Monitor/Defibrillator**

Give Five Cycles of CPR

Start IV or IO without interrupting CPR
- **Epinephrine 1 mg IV/IO** every 3–5 minutes **OR**
- **Vasopressin 40 U IV/IO** to replace first or second
   dose of epinephrine

If asystole persists or slow PEA present:
Atropine 1 mg IV/IO
Repeat every 3–5 minutes up to 3 doses

Give Five Cycles of CPR

Check rhythm

Asystole persists:
   Consider quality of resuscitation
   Contact Medical Control
   Consider termination of efforts

Consider potentially reversible causes
- Hypovolemia
- Hypoxia
- Hydrogen ion (acidosis)
- Hyper/hypokalemia
- Hypothermia
- Tablets (overdose)
- Tamponade
- Tension pneumothorax
- Thrombosis (cardiac)
- Thrombosis (pulmonary)

Figure 17-4 ACLS Algorithm for Asystole and Pulseless Electrical Activity.

Source: Porter, W. (2007). *Porter's pocket guide to emergency and critical care.* Sudbury, MA: Jones and Bartlett Publishers.

Pediatric and Neonatal Emergencies

Although the CRT exam tends to emphasize concepts related to adults, some exam content relates to pediatric and neonatal patients. Variations of BLS techniques for children and infants are detailed in Table 17-1. In terms of children, the NBRC will expect that you can follow the key pediatric advanced life support (PALS) and neonatal resuscitation protocols.

Pediatric Resuscitation

The most likely CRT exam scenarios involving pediatric advanced life support are those for pulseless arrest algorithm. As depicted in **Figure 17-5** (see page 505), the PALS algorithm for pulseless arrest is similar to that for adults, with the exception that the strength of the defibrillation shock and the dosage of medications like epinephrine vary by patient weight. It should also be noted that one of the most common medical emergencies associated with pediatric patients is airway obstruction by foreign body. Consequently, as a CRT exam candidate, you should be familiar with responding to obstructed airways in both conscious (see Table 17-1) and unconscious pediatric patients.

Neonatal Resuscitation

In addition to pediatric resuscitation, you must be familiar with the resuscitation protocol for neonates, as shown in **Figure 17-6** (see page 506). Note that if the baby is pink, meconium-free, breathing or crying, and has good muscle tone, only routine care is needed. Babies that are flaccid, cyanotic, or apneic normally require stimulation and supplemental O_2. If color, heart rate, and breathing are not restored within 30 seconds, you should provide manual positive pressure ventilation via face mask. *Heart rates below 60 always require chest compressions in neonates*. If the infant does not respond to these measures, epinephrine should be administered and intubation and mechanical ventilation considered.

Table 17-2 ACLS Medication Summary

Medication	Initial Adult IV Dosage	Classification/Indication
Epinephrine[a]	1 mg every 3–5 minutes up to 0.2 mg/kg	Vasoconstrictor; may improve cerebral perfusion
Vasopressin (ADH)	40 units × 1	Vasoconstrictor; may improve cerebral perfusion
Atropine[a]	0.5–1.0 mg every 3–5 minutes, up to 0.04 mg/kg	Cardiac stimulant: for selected bradycardias, PEA, or asystole
Lidocaine[a]	1.0–1.5mg/kg, every 5–10 minutes, up to 3 mg/kg	Anti-arrhythmic: for VF and VT
Amiodarone (Cordarone)	300 mg rapid infusion followed by 150 mg in 3–5 minutes and every 10 minutes, up to 2.2 g/day	Anti-arrhythmic: for VF and VT

a. Denotes a medication that may be instilled via ET tube if IV access is not established. In such cases, it is recommended that the dose be doubled and it be followed with the instillation of 10 mL normal saline.

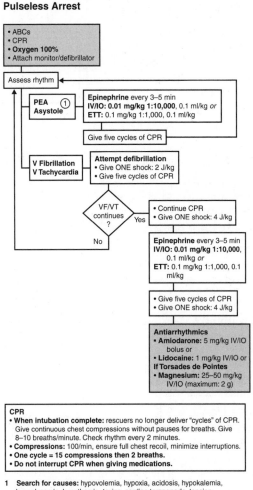

Figure 17-5 Pediatric Pulseless Arrest Algorithm.

Source: Porter, W. (2007). *Porter's pocket guide to emergency and critical care.* Sudbury, MA: Jones and Bartlett Publishers.

Treat a Tension Pneumothorax

A cardiopulmonary emergency that is likely to appear in some form on the CRT exam is a tension pneumothorax. You should be familiar with the most common signs and symptoms, as well as emergency treatment, of this acute, potentially life-threatening disorder.

A pneumothorax occurs when a hole or tear in lung tissue permits air to escape into pleural space. A simple pneumothorax may occur spontaneously (during vigorous coughing) and generally involves a small amount of air leaking into the pleural space at atmospheric pressure. Spontaneous pneumothoraces may actually go unnoticed and resolve without treatment. A *tension* pneumothorax, in contrast, occurs when a sizable amount of air under pressure enters the pleural space. This condition is even more serious for patients receiving positive pressure ventilation, which invariably causes a rapid buildup of pleural pressure, thus compressing the heart and lungs, as well as key vessels such as the vena cava and aorta. Such patients will often deteriorate quite rapidly due to compromised cardiac output and oxygenation. For this reason, prompt detection and treatment of this condition are essential.

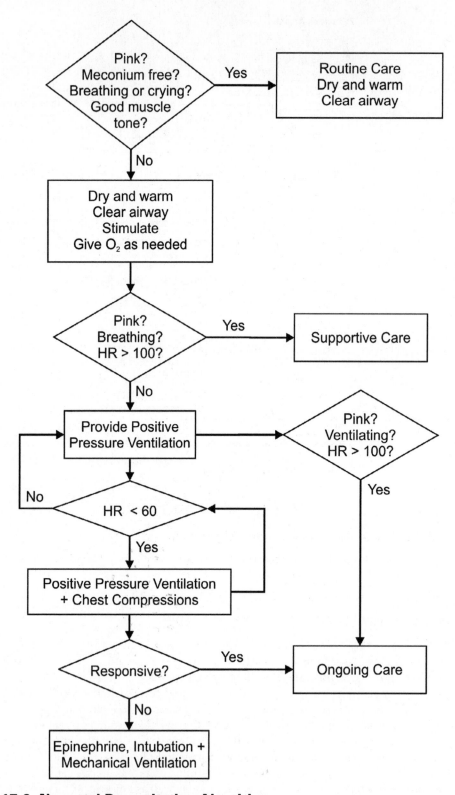

Figure 17-6 Neonatal Resuscitation Algorithm.

Diagnosis

Factors that may predispose patients to a tension pneumothorax include: mechanical ventilation with high airway pressures (> 40–45 cm H_2O), chest trauma, and conditions associated with excessively high compliance such as advanced emphysema. When any of these factors is coupled with a rapid decline in clinical status, you should consider the possibility of a tension pnuemothorax. While such a diagnosis is generally confirmed via a chest X-ray, you should be mindful of the following clinical manifestations:

- Rapid decline in cardiopulmonary status (hypotension, hypoxemia)
- Decreased or absent breath sounds on the affected side
- Hyperresonance when percussing the affected side
- Possible subcutaneous emphysema
- Tracheal shift away from the affected side (severe cases)
- Rapid increase in ventilator pressures (if mechanical or manual ventilation in use)
- Shock and/or PEA in severe, untreated cases

A chest X-ray confirming the diagnosis of a tension pneumothorax will typically show an underinflated lung on the affected side, flattening of the diaphragm, expansion of the rib spaces, and a mediastinal shift to the opposite side.

Initial Treatment

Once diagnosis is confirmed, the treatment is emergency decompression of the chest, also known as a *needle thoracostomy*. As outlined in the accompanying box, needle thoracostomy involves insertion of a large-bore angiocath (14-gauge in an adult, 18-gauge or 20-gauge in an infant) into the second intercostal space over the top of the third rib in the midclavicular line. This procedure should be done using sterile technique, and proper placement should elicit a rush of air through the catheter, often followed by rapid improvement in blood pressure and cardiovascular status. However, since needle thoracostomy simply converts a tension pneumothorax into a simple pneumothorax, full resolution of the problem usually requires lung reexpansion, via insertion of a conventional chest tube, as discussed in Chapter 18.

Basic Procedure for Needle Thoracostomy

1. Place patient in upright position if tolerated
2. Locate puncture site (second intercostal space in the midclavicular line)
3. Prepare site with Betadine and/or alcohol scrubs
4. Insert angiocath over the top of the third rib until the catheter hub is against the chest wall
5. Listen for a rush of air
6. Assess for immediate improvement in cardiorespiratory status
7. Remove the needle
8. Secure the angiocath in place and attach a flutter (Heimlich valve)
9. Immediately prepare for tube thoracostomy (chest tube insertion)

Patient Transport

In addition to knowing the essentials of adult, pediatric, and neonatal resuscitation, as well as addressing other cardiopulmonary emergencies, the NBRC expects you to be competent in transporting critically ill patients. The main focus is on ensuring patient safety during transport, through appropriate planning and proper execution by competent staff utilizing all necessary equipment. Our focus here is on both intra-hospital transport as well as external transport via land or air. In reviewing this material, keep in mind that concepts covered elsewhere in this text, including airway management and O_2 cylinder duration of flow, may be included in this portion of the exam.

Also keep in mind that whether engaged in transport within or outside the hospital, you may be responsible for determining that the patient is stable enough to be moved. This preassessment should include vital signs, hemodynamic values, oxygenation, ventilation, and any other relevant clinical parameters needed to determine if a patient can be transported. According to the AARC, patient transport is contraindicated when any of the following cannot be reasonably ensured during transport:

- Provision of adequate oxygenation and ventilation
- Maintenance of acceptable hemodynamic performance
- Adequate monitoring of the patient's cardiopulmonary status
- Maintenance of airway control

Intra-Hospital Patient Transport

Most patient transports take place within a hospital or health care facility. For this reason, you can be relatively sure that the CRT exam will include one or more questions related to transporting critically ill patients within the hospital.

According to the Society of Critical Care Medicine (SCCM), proper patient transport must address the following four areas: communication, personnel, equipment, and monitoring. Regarding communication, SCCM recommends the following:

- Members of the transport team should communicate with the team at the receiving location.
- Before transport, the receiving location confirms that it is ready to receive the patient.
- Members of the health care team are notified as to the timing of the transport and needed equipment.
- Documentation includes the physician's order, indications for transport, and patient status throughout.

In regard to accompanying personnel, the SCCM recommends that at least two people accompany all critically ill patients; usually a critical care nurse and a respiratory therapist. An ACLS-trained physician should also accompany unstable patients.

The SCCM recommends the following equipment to support the patient during transport:

- Blood pressure monitor (or standard blood pressure cuff)
- Pulse oximeter
- Cardiac monitor/defibrillator
- Equipment for airway management and secretion clearance (appropriately sized)
- O_2 source with sufficient duration of flow, plus a 30-min reserve
- BVM (with mask) or portable ventilator
- Basic resuscitation drugs, including epinephrine and antiarrhythmic agents
- Supplemental medications, such as sedatives and narcotic analgesics
- Ample supply of appropriate IV fluids and medications
- Fully charged, battery-operated infusion pump

Basic quality assurance demands that all equipment is checked for proper operation prior to transport. In terms of airway management, the position of the patient's ET tube should be noted and resecured before transport. In regard to support for ventilation and oxygenation, hospital protocols usually dictate whether you use a BVM portable transport ventilator. If you use a transport ventilator, it must be capable of providing 100% O_2 and PEEP; have both disconnect and high-pressure alarms, and sufficient portable power supply for the duration of transport. An HME generally is satisfactory for providing humidification via the ventilator circuit. Unless precise F_{IO_2} levels are required, you should default to providing 100% O_2 during transport. If the patient being transported requires a ventilator mode or settings that a portable ventilator cannot duplicate, you should ensure that the parameters to be used during transport are well tolerated by the patient by a trial run in the originating unit.

Basic physiologic monitoring during transport should to the extent possible duplicate that provided for the patient in the originating unit and includes at least the following:

- Continuous ECG monitoring
- Continuous pulse oximetry
- Periodic measurement of blood pressure, pulse rate, and respiratory rate
- Periodic assessment of breath sounds

If the patient is receiving ventilatory support during transport, you should also monitor airway pressures (PIP, PEEP) and tidal volumes. If using a BVM, this may require attaching a pressure manometer and respirometer. According to the SCCM, some patients being transported also may require monitoring of expired CO_2 (capnography), as well as intra-arterial blood pressure and ICP.

There are many hazards and complications to be on guard for during patient transport. These problems may involve equipment misuse or malfunction or a change in patient status. Equipment misuse or malfunction includes hyperventilation associated with overzealous manual BVM ventilation, accidental extubation, loss of IV access, loss of PEEP/CPAP, loss of O_2 supply, and ventilator, monitor, or IV pump failure. You can avoid most of these problems by (1) proper pre-planning (including equipment prechecks), (2) always having a backup BVM with mask and PEEP/CPAP valve ready to go, and (3) carefully monitoring the patient and "plumbing" during movement or position changes. Ensuring proper pre-planning and provision of appropriate equipment, supplies, and support personnel is also the best way to address any potential changes that might occur in patient status during transport.

Air and Land Transport

Many special considerations pertain to transporting critically ill patients outside the hospital. Some of these issues are similar to those for intra-hospital transport, such as the need to ensure that the patient is stable enough to be moved, the training and personnel involved, the need for good pre-planning and communication, as well as equipment issues, including an adequate O_2 supply.

However, there are some unique aspects of ground and air transport, most of which fall into the following categories:

- Choosing among ground and air transport modes
- Managing increased patient movement and stimulation
- Accommodating the need for special personnel and equipment
- Addressing the effects of altitude on PaO_2 and closed air spaces

Factors involved in selecting the mode of external transportation include the distance to be traveled, the condition of the patient, input from medical personnel, availability of ambulance or aircraft, as well as weather conditions. **Table 17-3** summarizes the major advantages and disadvantages of transporting patients via ground, helicopter, and fixed-wing aircraft, all of which need to be considered when choosing the mode of transportation.

Once the mode of transport is selected, it is important to secure the patient and all equipment to prevent unwanted movement. You also should be aware that patient overstimulation and stress can occur during ground transportation, due to the frequent stops, starts, turns, bumps, and "road noise." Air transport also can stress a patient, especially when there is excessive vibration and/or insufficient temperature control during flight. These problems are particularly serious when transporting infants and children, who are most vulnerable to such stimuli. For these reasons, all patients being externally transported should be properly positioned and secured, with appropriate sound protection and temperature control.

In addition, you should closely monitor the vital signs and general clinical status of all patients being transported so that any untoward distress can be quickly identified and addressed. Due to the high background noise in some aircraft, you may need to use an automated noninvasive system to monitor blood pressure and an amplified stethoscope to listen to breath sounds. Moreover, because most audible medical equipment alarms cannot be heard in noisy aircraft, you often will have to depend on visual alarms and good patient assessment.

As with intra-hospital transport, highly skilled clinicians and appropriate equipment are essential. Most commonly, the air/land transport team includes a physician, respiratory therapist, and nurse or paramedic. In combination, these personnel should have the applicable advanced life support certification and experience, as well as proficiency in administering IV, intramuscular (IM), subcutaneous (SC), and inhaled medications; artificial airway management; and mechanical ventilation.

Table 17-3 Advantages and Disadvantages of Patient Transport via Ground and Air

Mode	Advantages	Disadvantages
Ground/ambulance	1. Generally most efficient within 100-mile distance 2. Often usable when inclement weather (fog) prevents air travel 3. Provides more work area for transport team 4. Less vibration and noise than helicopter 5. Usable in the absence of landing sites for air travel	1. Generally slower than air travel 2. Not practical in difficult terrain
Helicopter	1. Most efficient for distances between 100 and 250 miles 2. Faster than ground methods 3. May be faster for short distances in difficult terrain 4. Does not require landing strip and often can land near hospital	1. High noise and vibration resulting in overstimulation 2. May be grounded in inclement weather 3. Small work area 4. Expensive to maintain and operate 5. *Hypobaric* effects, which must be understood by crew
Fixed-wing aircraft	1. Fastest and most efficient for distances in excess of 250 miles 2. Less vibration and noise than helicopter 3. Able to travel at high altitudes, perhaps over inclement weather	1. May be grounded in inclement weather 2. Must be landed at an airport, requiring further patient transport 3. Small work area 4. Expensive to maintain and operate 5. *Hypobaric* effects, which must be understood by crew

As the respiratory therapist on the team, you are responsible for ensuring that properly functioning and age-specific equipment is available during transport. Equipment needs for air and land transport are essentially the same as those previously described for intra-hospital transport. Ideally, the transport ventilator should be able to function using either 110-volt AC (supplied by a generator or inverter in the ambulance or aircraft) or 12-volt DC power (the typical voltage provided by a vehicle battery/alternator). If the portable ventilator is to be used for air transport, you'll want to ensure that its volume, pressure, and flow settings can be adjusted either manually or automatically for variations in altitude and barometric pressure. In addition, you'll want to include a calibrated polarographic or fuel cell O_2 analyzer, and an SVN with applicable drugs for inhalation (e.g., bronchodilators, racemic epinephrine).

For air transport, you must understand the effects of altitude on oxygenation and closed air spaces. As a transport helicopter or airplane climbs to cruising altitude, the atmospheric and cabin pressures decrease. As demonstrated in **Table 17-4**, in unpressurized cabins this creates a *hypobaric* condition, which lowers the inspired, alveolar, and arterial partial pressure of oxygen. At 2,000 feet, the reduction in partial pressures is minimal, but at altitudes above 5,000 feet, even a patient with normal lung capacity can suffer hypoxemia unless supplemental O_2 is provided.

To compute a patient's equivalent F_{IO_2} needs at cruising altitude compared with sea level, you should apply the following formula (based on Dalton's law):

$$F_{IO_2} \text{ at altitude} = F_{IO_2} \text{ at sea level} \times \frac{760}{P_B \text{ altitude}}$$

Table 17-4 Effect of Altitude on Oxygenation with $F_{IO_2} = 0.21$

Altitude (ft)	P_B[a]	P_{IO_2}	P_{AO_2}	P_{aO_2}[b]
0	760	160	100	95
2,000	706	148	88	80
5,000	632	133	73	68
8,000	565	119	59	54
10,000	523	110	50	45

a. All pressures in torr/mm Hg.
b. Assumes a $P_{(A-a)O_2}$ of 5 torr and no compensation.

where "P_B altitude" equals the barometric pressure in torr at the cruising altitude used for transport. For example, assume you will be transporting a patient receiving 50% at sea level in an airplane that will be cruising at 8,000 feet (P_B = 565 torr). You would compute the needed F_{IO_2} as:

$$F_{IO_2} \text{ at altitude} = 0.50 \times \frac{760}{565} = 0.67$$

Note that at 8,000 ft or higher, you cannot provide an F_{IO_2} equivalent to 0.80 or more at sea level. For this reason, patients requiring 80% or more oxygen at sea level will likely have to either be placed on PEEP/CPAP or have their PEEP levels raised to ensure adequate oxygenation.

Some transport aircraft provide pressurized cabins (especially some fixed-wing jets). However, most pressurized cabins are maintained at only about 75% sea level pressure, which is nearly the same as being in an unpressurized cabin at 8,000 ft. In theses cases, you still need to compute an equivalent F_{IO_2}, but you should substitute the known cabin pressure for the P_B at altitude.

Of course, the goal of O_2 supplementation should generally be to achieve a SpO_2 of 90% or greater, regardless of F_{IO_2} or altitude. Fortunately, pulse oximetry readings are not affected by altitude and should therefore be the final criteria for judging the adequacy of patient oxygenation during transport.

A second factor that you need to consider during air transport is the relationship between gas volume and pressure. This effect is well known to anyone who has flown on a commercial airline and felt their inner ears "pop" as the plane climbs or descends. The principle involved is Boyle's law, whereby the volume of a gas varies inversely with its pressure. Based on this principle, as altitude increases and atmospheric pressure drops, gas volume increases, and vice versa. Consequently, there are a few special considerations, especially with mechanically ventilated patients. These include changing the set tidal volume, pressure limit, and/or PEEP to maintain proper ventilation and lung expansion, and then adding or removing air from ET or tracheostomy tube cuff to maintain a proper seal without damaging the tracheal mucosa.

In terms of cuff pressures, as altitude increases, so too does the volume of gas in the cuff. Because the tube cuff is restricted in its ability to expand within the trachea, small increases in volume can result in a large increase in pressure. Indeed, some studies have reported a doubling of cuff pressures at altitudes as low as 3,000 ft. The only good way to accommodate these changes (and those associated with descent from altitude) is to readjust the cuff pressure using the minimal leak or occluding volume technique every few minutes when the altitude is changing.

A more difficult problem occurs when using a transport ventilator that does not provide adjustments to compensate for changes in altitude and barometric pressure. The difficulty arises from the fact that different ventilators perform differently at altitude. For example, volume-limited ventilators that use turbines or blowers will tend to deliver *lower* than set volumes at altitude, whereas pneumatically powered systems that use differential pressure transducers to measure flow will tend to deliver *higher* than set volumes at altitude. One approach to this problem with microprocessor-controlled ventilators is to temporarily disconnect the patient (and support with BVM + O_2) and recalibrate the device once you reach cruising altitude. Another solution is to follow the ventilator manufacturer's recommendation for adjusting settings at various barometric pressures. Last, you can empirically adjust delivered volume or pressure according to end-tidal CO_2 levels as monitored by capnography. Unfortunately, capnometers also are affected by altitude, with the PETCO$_2$ reading directly proportional to the barometric pressure (causing a falsely low PETCO$_2$ reading at altitude). This error can be overcome by recalibrating the capnometer's high reading at the cruising altitude with a standard known concentration of CO_2 (usually 5%). Unfortunately, this adds equipment and weight to the aircraft, which may not be desirable.

Other complications are associated with "trapped" gas volume changes—i.e., gas in an enclosed space that cannot equilibrate with the ambient pressure. This is a common problem in patients with a pneumothorax and/or excessive gas in the stomach or bowel, but it can also occur in patients after skull trauma or neurosurgery (pneumocephalus) or those suffering from penetrating eye wounds (intraocular gas). Such problems should be identified and managed prior to transport—e.g., via insertion of a chest or nasogastric tube. Last, if a patient suffering from decompression sickness (the "bends") has to be transported to a hyperbaric facility, you should try to ensure that the cabin pressure is maintained as near to sea level as possible. In this condition, the lower the ambient pressure, the worse the morbidity and mortality.

Medical Emergency Teams

In an effort to enhance the quality of patient care, most hospitals have established medical emergency teams (METs), also known as *rapid response teams*. Their purpose is to intervene and help stabilize patients who are rapidly deteriorating outside of the ICU setting. The team is often composed of an ICU nurse, a physician or physician assistant, and a respiratory therapist.

The MET is generally activated via overhead page and/or beeper when a patient exhibits signs and symptoms of physiologic instability prior to cardiopulmonary arrest. For adults, the specific criteria for doing so often include one or a combination of the following:

- Acute change in mental status or overall clinical appearance
- Heart rate < 40 or > 130, or respiratory rate < 8/min or > 30/min
- Systolic blood pressure < 90 torr
- Spo$_2$ < 90%, especially with supplemental O_2
- Acute change in urinary output to < 50 ml over 4 hours

While the MET functions as a consultant regarding staff education and patient assessment, it often provides direct care. The most common interventions performed or assisted by respiratory therapists include: suctioning, adjusting the FIO$_2$, providing noninvasive ventilation, administering bronchodilators, and intubating. Other procedures performed by the MET may include IV or arterial line insertion, CVP or PAP line placement, and the administration of fluid or medications such as furosemide (Lasix).

Once the MET has responded, the event should be recorded in the patient's medical record. Many institutions have implemented a separate MET record form for such purposes. In general, the documentation should reflect the time and duration, patient's vital signs and clinical status (before, during, and after the event), any interventions and procedures applied, the clinical outcome (transferred to ICU or stepdown unit), and the names and disciplines of the team members who responded.

Disaster Management

It is not unusual for the CRT exam to contain a question or two on disaster management and response. Unfortunately, given the various types of disasters, this is a very broad topic. The good news is that there is a central theme to much of what is expected of you in this area. Most of the clinical proficiencies relate to either hospital and respiratory care department preparedness planning or implementation of triage and decontamination/isolation procedures.

In terms of hospital and respiratory care department preparedness planning, all health care facilities are expected to have in place large-scale emergency plans. Such plans must take into account not only patient care during disasters but also how the facility itself can manage direct damage or loss of resources during a catastrophe. For the respiratory care department, preparedness planning involves consideration of at least the following elements:

- Patient needs
  - Estimate numbers of patients who may require:
    - Ventilatory support
    - Medical gas therapy (O_2 or air)
    - Suction (vacuum)
- Personnel
  - Determine number of staff required to meet patient needs.
  - Have in place a staff emergency call-back procedure.
  - Have a plan in place to enlist non-respiratory personnel to perform manual ventilation.
- Equipment
  - Maintain inventory of available ventilators.
  - Maintain adequate number of disposable BVMs to meet needs.
  - Determine backup equipment to meet needs.
  - Have plan in place to acquire additional backup equipment.
  - Have plan in place to transfer patients if backup equipment unavailable.
  - Have plans in place for failure of gas supply systems:
    - Estimate quantity of backup required for each gas (air, O_2)
    - Estimate ancillary equipment needs (regulators, portable suction, etc.)
    - Have deployment plan for distribution/maintaining backup gas sources

In regard to responding to external emergencies, **Table 17-5** outlines several of the most common types of disasters, most common associated patient conditions, and the primary roles of respiratory therapists in such incidents.

Due to the large number and variable type of casualties that may present to a health care facility after a disaster, rapid triage is essential. Personnel assigned triage responsibilities evaluate each patient and quickly prioritize their management according to the basic scheme outlined in **Table 17-6**. If the disaster involves a suspected chemical, biological, radiological, or nuclear incident (CBRN), triage should take place *outside the facility* and be conducted in conjunction with decontamination.

Table 17-5 Role of the Respiratory Therapist (RT) in Disaster Response

Category	Resulting Patient Conditions	Clinical-Related Roles for RT
Natural catastrophe (e.g., earthquake, flood, fire, tornado)	Trauma (chest/head), near-drowning, thermal burns, hypovolemic or septic shock, dehydration	Initial assessment/triage, infection control, cleaning, disinfection, sterilization, barrier and isolation, PPE, ongoing monitoring
Chemical (e.g., chlorine gas)	Inhalation injury, ventilatory/ oxygenation respiratory failure, chemical burns, pneumonia, sepsis, ARDS	Prompt recognition and initial assessment, triage and decontamination, airway management, ventilation and oxygenation, common antidote therapy (e.g., atropine for nerve agents), patient monitoring
Biological (natural [e.g., SARS] or bioterrorist [e.g., anthrax])	Inhalation injury, ventilatory/ oxygenation respiratory failure, pneumonia, sepsis, ARDS	Prompt recognition and initial assessment, triage, airway management, ventilation and oxygenation, infection control, isolation techniques, antimicrobial therapy, patient monitoring
Radiologic/nuclear	Trauma, blast injuries, profound thermal burns, inhalation injury, radiation poisoning, dehydration	Prompt recognition and initial assessment, triage and decontamination, airway management, ventilation and oxygenation, isolation, and barrier techniques specific to ionizing radiation

Table 17-6 Disaster Triage Priorities

Triage Priority	Meaning	Action (After Decontamination if CBRN Incident)
Red	Critical patients in need of immediate life-saving care	Move to emergency department
Yellow	Relatively stable patients needing prompt medical attention	Move to emergency department
Green	Patients with minor injuries that can wait for appropriate treatment	Move patients with minor trauma to emergency department; move those with minor medical issues to waiting area
Black	Deceased patients and those who have no chance of survival	Move to morgue

Triage, decontamination, and treatment usually proceed in sequence through specific "zones," each requiring a different level of personal protective equipment (PPE) for health care personnel. Given its potentially high risk of hazardous contamination, initial triage is termed the "Hot Zone," in which National Institute for Occupational Safety and Health (NIOSH)-approved self-contained breathing apparatus (SCBA) should be employed. Decontamination occurs in the "Warm Zone," where NIOSH-approved hooded powered air-purifying respirators (PAPR) with FR57 filters are recommended. After decontamination, patients are received in the treatment area, where standard PPE precautions are normally satisfactory.

Triage often identifies patients who require immediate life support before undergoing decontamination. Also, in some cases, decontamination and initial medical treatment may occur simultaneously. For these reasons, you may need to be proficient in the use of all types and levels of personal protective equipment during the management of a disaster.

In terms of managing large outbreaks of respiratory infections due to natural epi-/pandemics or biological terrorism, the following key considerations apply:

1. All persons with signs or symptoms of a respiratory infection (cough, labored breathing, etc.) should be instructed to maintain good respiratory hygiene/cough etiquette:
   a. Cover the nose and mouth when coughing or sneezing.
   b. Use tissues to contain respiratory secretions.
   c. Dispose of tissues in the nearest waste receptacle after use.
   d. Wash hands after contact with respiratory secretions and contaminated objects and materials.
2. Health care facilities should ensure that tissues, hands-free receptacles, and hand hygiene facilities are provided to patients and visitors in waiting areas.
3. Health care facilities should offer surgical masks to persons who are coughing and encourage them to sit at least three feet away from others in waiting areas.
4. Health care workers should practice droplet precautions, in addition to standard precautions, when examining a patient with symptoms of a respiratory infection.
5. Once a likely infectious agent is suspected, appropriate infection control measures need to be activated, to include:
   a. Placement of the patient in a negative pressure isolation room (where available).
   b. Use of standard, contact, and droplet precautions.
   c. Use of airborne precautions (including N95 respirators for all persons entering the room).
   d. Restriction of patient movement (and use of a surgical mask for transport).
   e. Avoiding droplet-producing procedures (e.g., nebulizers, chest physiotherapy, bronchoscopy).

COMMON ERRORS TO AVOID

You can improve your score by avoiding these mistakes:

- Never use an AED on an infant (< 1 year old).
- Avoid compressions in excess of ½ to 1 inches during infant CPR to help prevent injury to the patient.
- Don't treat the monitor!!! If the monitor shows asystole but the patient appears awake, alert, and in no apparent distress, don't begin CPR.
- Never treat a pneumothorax with a needle decompression (needle thoracostomy) or a chest tube until the diagnosis has been confirmed with a chest X-ray.
- Never forget a manual resuscitator bag *and a mask* when you are transporting intubated and ventilated patients so you will be able to ventilate them if they become inadvertently extubated.
- Never use an adult or pediatric manual resuscitator bag/mask to ventilate a neonate. Use the appropriate age-specific equipment.
- Don't forget that during air transport, it is often appropriate to increase the F_{IO_2} in order to maintain adequate oxygenation, and it may also be necessary to temporarily adjust tidal volume and artificial airway cuff pressure to ensure the safety of mechanically ventilated patients.
- Never wait for a physician to arrive to begin assessing a patient as part of a medical emergency team (MET).
- During management of respiratory epidemics, avoid droplet-producing procedures (e.g., nebulizers, chest physiotherapy on patients with suspected infections).

SURE BETS

In some situations you can be sure of the right approach to a clinical problem or scenario:

- Always remember the ABCDs (Airway, Breathing, Circulation, Defibrillation) of CPR.
- Always look, listen, and feel before starting CPR; the patient may simply be sleeping!
- Always give a compression-to-breath ratio of 30:2 in single-rescuer CPR, regardless of the victim's age.
- Always give compressions at a depth of 1½ to 2 inches for an adult patient.
- If the chest doesn't rise with the first breath in CPR, don't panic—always reposition the head first and try another breath!
- Always have an appropriate-sized manual resuscitator bag and proper mask when transporting a critically ill patient.
- Always suspect a tension pneumothorax when a patient is rapidly deteriorating in the presence of any of the following: a unilateral decrease in breath sounds and chest expansion, hyperresonance when percussing affected side, shifting of the trachea away from affected side, and subcutaneous emphysema.
- When assisting a physician with a needle thoracostomy for the emergency treatment of a tension pneumothorax, always recommend that the needle be placed over the second rib in the midclavicular line.
- Always apply chest compressions to a neonate whose heart rate is less than 60.
- When assisting in the transport of a critically ill patient, always ensure that you have an adequate oxygen supply and delivery device, as well as an array of age-appropriate respiratory equipment, including a manual resuscitator bag, transport ventilator/circuits, and intubation equipment.
- Always practice droplet precautions, in addition to standard precautions, when examining a patient with symptoms of a respiratory infection.

PRE-TEST ANSWERS AND EXPLANATIONS

Below are this chapter's pre-test answers and explanations. Be sure to review each answer's explanation thoroughly to help you understand why it is correct. If the explanation is still unclear to you, review the chapter contents or the references and/or refer to this chapter's supplemental resources on the CD.

17-1. **Correct Answer: D.** I, II, III, and IV. Naloxone, lidocaine, atropine, and epinephrine all can be administered via the endotracheal tube during emergency life support.

17-2. **Correct Answer: D.** I, II, and III. Once an airway has been opened and ventilation started, you should assess its effectiveness by looking for the rise and fall of the victim's chest and listening for breathing efforts, which should be audible. You can also feel for air exchange by placing a check near the victim's mouth and nose.

17-3. **Correct Answer: A.** Two normal breaths, then assess the pulse. According to the American Heart Association guidelines, at the onset of adult mouth-to-mouth or mouth-to-mask ventilation, once the airway is open, you should give two normal breaths, each lasting about 1 second, then assess the pulse for up to 10 seconds.

17-4. **Correct Answer: A.** Apply back blows, followed by chest thrusts. After two failed attempts to ventilate an infant in respiratory arrest, there is most likely an obstruction. For older patients, an obstructed airway is addressed via abdominal thrusts (the Heimlich maneuver). However, for infants back blows are combined with chest thrusts. Chest thrusts may also be used for pregnant women and in markedly obese persons. Both procedures are normally followed by checking the airway and removal of any obstruction.

17-5. **Correct Answer: D.** 30:2. In accordance with AHA guidelines, in one- and two-rescuer CPR for adults, the ratio for chest compressions to breaths is 30 compressions to every two breaths, with a re-assessment after five cycles.

17-6. **Correct Answer: A.** Increase the FIO_2. In accordance with Dalton's law, the partial pressure of oxygen at sea level is 160 torr, versus only 134 torr at the increased altitude. As a result, in order to maintain acceptable oxygenation, it is often necessary to increase the FIO_2 during air transport. For example, a patient on room air would need an FIO_2 of approximately 31% to maintain the same PaO_2 at an altitude of 10,000 feet.

17-7. **Correct Answer: C.** 100/min with a depth of $1\frac{1}{2}$ to 2 inches. For adult resuscitation, a chest compression rate of approximately 100/min with a depth of $1\frac{1}{2}$ to 2 inches should be achieved.

17-8. **Correct Answer: D.** 360 joules. The initial energy level for defibrillation (via typical monophasic device) is 360 joules, not 200 joules per the old AHA ACLS guidelines. Individual subsequent shocks are given after each five cycles, also at 360 joules.

17-9. **Correct Answer: A.** End-tidal CO_2 monitor. A blood pressure monitor (or standard blood pressure cuff), an oxygen source and delivery device, as well as a cardiac monitor/defibrillator should accompany every critically ill patient on transport.

17-10. **Correct Answer: C.** Enlist non-respiratory personnel to perform manual ventilation. Preparedness planning for the respiratory care department includes estimating the number of patients who may need ventilatory support, determining number of staff members required to meet patient needs, and having in place a staff emergency call-back procedure. Should the available equipment and personnel not be able to meet patient needs, the first step would be to enlist non-respiratory personnel to perform manual ventilation using disposable BVMs. Once adequate immediate patient support is ensured, you can attempt to get additional backup equipment and/or make arrangements to transfer patients to other facilities.

POST-TEST

A post-test for this chapter that includes automated scoring and feedback is available on the accompanying CD. Be sure to complete this additional assessment to confirm your mastery of this chapter's objectives.

REFERENCES

American Association for Respiratory Care. (1995). Clinical practice guideline. Management of airway emergencies. *Respiratory Care, 40,* 749–760.

American Association for Respiratory Care. (2002). In-hospital transport of the mechanically ventilated patient. 2002 revision and update. *Respiratory Care, 47,* 721–723.

American Association for Respiratory Care. (2004). Resuscitation and defibrillation in the health care setting. 2004 revision and update. *Respiratory Care, 49,* 1085–1099.

American Heart Association. (2005). Adjuncts for airway control and ventilation, *Circulation,* 112 (Suppl I), IV 51–57.

American Heart Association. (2005). Electrical therapies: Automated external defibrillators, defibrillation, cardioversion, and pacing. *Circulation,* 112 (Suppl I) IV 35–46.

American Society of Anesthesiologists. (2003). Practice guidelines for management of the difficult airway. *Anesthesiology, 98,* 1269–1277.

Butler, T. J. (2009). *Laboratory exercises for competency in respiratory care* (2nd ed.). Philadelphia: FA Davis.

Field, J. M., Hazinski, M. F., Gilmore, D. (2006). *Handbook of emergency cardiovascular care.* Dallas: American Heart Association.

Kaveh, J., Bradford, B. W., McDonald, K. M., & Wachter, R. M. (2001). *Making health care safer: A critical analysis of patient safety practices.* Evidence report/technology assessment #43 (AHRQ Publication 01-E058). Rockville, MD: Agency for Healthcare Research and Quality.

Warren, J., Fromm, R. E., Orr, R. A., Rotello, L. C., & Horst, H. M. (2004). Guidelines for the inter- and intrahospital transport of critically ill patients. *Critical Care Medicine, 32,* 56–62.

Act As an Assistant to the Physician Performing Special Procedures

Albert J. Heuer

INTRODUCTION

In addition to directly providing respiratory care to patients, you may assist physicians with a host of therapeutic and diagnostic procedures. Though there are several such procedures, the NBRC will expect you to be especially familiar with your role when assisting with intubation and bronchoscopy. In addition, you must have a basic understanding as to how you may assist with thoracentesis, tracheostomy, chest tube insertion, and cardioversion. You also should know how moderate sedation and ultrasound can facilitate some of these procedures. Because competency in these areas is important, you should review this material carefully when preparing for the CRT exam. By fulfilling the following objectives, you will help demonstrate your mastery of this material and your readiness regarding these content areas.

OBJECTIVES

After completion of this chapter, you should be able to demonstrate knowledge needed to act as an assistant to the physician performing the following special procedures:

1. Intubation
2. Bronchoscopy
3. Thoracentesis
4. Tracheostomy
5. Chest tube insertion
6. Cardioversion
7. Other procedures, including moderate sedation and ultrasound

WHAT TO EXPECT ON THIS CATEGORY OF THE CRT EXAM

Number of questions: 2
Level of questions: generally 1 recall and 1 application question

WHAT'S NEW FOR 2009

As of July 2009, this section of the NBRC CRT examination includes the following *new content areas*:

- Thoracentesis
- Tracheostomy

- Chest tube insertion
- Moderate (conscious) sedation
- Ultrasound

PRE-TEST

Carefully respond to each of the following questions. After completing the pre-test, compare your answers with those provided at the end of each chapter. Then, thoroughly review the explanation for each answer to help you understand why it is correct.

18-1. You are assisting a physician performing a bronchoscopy on a spontaneously breathing patient who is alert, awake, and anxious. Which of the following medications should you recommend for the patient's anxiety prior to the procedure?
 A. Lidocaine HCI (Xylocaine)
 B. Vecuronium bromide (Norcuron)
 C. Epinephrine 1:10,000 solution
 D. Midazolam HCI (Versed)

18-2. While performing a fiberoptic bronchoscopy, a patient's SpO$_2$ drops from 91% to 84%. Which of the following actions would be appropriate?
 I. Applying suction through the scope's open channel
 II. Delivering O$_2$ through the scope's open channel
 III. Increasing the cannula or mask O$_2$ flow
 A. I and II
 B. II and III
 C. I and III
 D. I, II, and III

18-3. What initial energy level would you recommend to a physician preparing to perform cardioversion on a patient in atrial flutter?
 A. 50 joules
 B. 150 joules
 C. 200 joules
 D. 360 joules

18-4. In what position should you place an unconscious patient in order to facilitate a thoracentesis procedure?
 A. Lying flat, supine, head on pillow
 B. Lying flat, prone, feet raised 12 inches
 C. Sitting up and leaning slightly forward and supported in front
 D. Semi-Fowler's with knees raised

18-5. You are assisting a physician performing oral intubation of a 45-kg (98-lb.) adult female patient. Which of the following endotracheal tube sizes should you select for this patient?
 A. 6.0–6.5 mm
 B. 7.0–7.5 mm
 C. 8.0–8.5 mm
 D. 9.0–10.0 mm

18-6. You are caring for a mechanically ventilated patient who has been orally intubated for 2 weeks and has failed multiple weaning attempts over the past 2 days. What should you recommend at this time?
 A. Immediate extubation
 B. Placing a smaller oral ET tube
 C. Performing a tracheostomy
 D. Placing a nasopharyngeal airway

18-7. Which of the following statements regarding cardioversion are *false*?
 A. It is indicated for atrial fibrillation and atrial flutter
 B. Synchronized shock helps prevent the procedure from causing an arrhythmia
 C. It is the primary electrical therapy for ventricular fibrillation
 D. Direct current discharges of 50–100 joules are applied to adults

18-8. The physician asks for your input regarding chest tube placement for a patient with a pneumothorax. In what anatomic location should you recommend that the tube be inserted?
 A. The second intercostal space at the midaxillary line
 B. The second or third intercostal space at the anterior axillary line
 C. The fourth or fifth intercostal space at the midclavicular line
 D. The fourth or fifth intercostal space at the anterior axillary line

18-9. A physician is about to perform cardioversion on a patient with unstable atrial flutter who is receiving oxygen via a nonrebreather mask. After the initial shock has been delivered, the patient's SpO_2 drops to 85%, respirations become slow and shallow, and heart rate is now 82 beats/minute with normal sinus rhythm. The next immediate action should be:
  A. Open the airway, assist with a manual ventilator bag at 100% oxygen
  B. Administer 2 mg of naloxone (Narcan)
  C. Deliver another synchronized shock
  D. Intubate and place on mechanical ventilation

18-10. You are assisting a physician with an elective intubation. In addition to auscultation, what methods should you recommend to confirm proper tube placement?
  I. Capnometry
  II. Esophageal detection device
  III. Pulse oximetry
  IV. CO_2 colorimetry
  A. I, II, and IV
  B. II, III, and IV
  C. I, II, and III
  D. I, III, and IV

WHAT YOU NEED TO KNOW: ESSENTIAL CONTENT

Endotracheal Intubation

Endotracheal intubation involves properly placing an ET tube into a patient's mouth or nose, through the glottis and into the trachea, to facilitate oxygenation and/or ventilation. This procedure is generally performed as a potentially life-saving measure. Though at some hospitals you will be trained to actually perform this procedure, it is more common for you to assist a physician with either a standard bedside endotracheal intubation or a rapid sequence intubation. As a result, the CRT exam includes questions that relate to this procedure, including the indications, hazards, and proper equipment. The emphasis in this chapter is on the procedure and selected use of equipment necessary when assisting with an endotracheal intubation. For more detail on the selection, assembly, use, and troubleshooting of key equipment used in this procedure, see Chapter 6.

Indications

Major indications for intubation include impending or actual (1) airway compromise, (2) respiratory failure, or (3) the need to protect the airway. Specific conditions include but are not limited to the following:

- Obstruction of the artificial airway
- Apnea
- Acute traumatic coma
- Penetrating neck trauma
- Cardiopulmonary resuscitation
- Surfactant instillation in premature infants
- Severe allergic reactions
- Sedative or narcotic drug effect
- Foreign body airway obstruction
- Severe laryngospasm
- Severe bronchospasm

Contraindications

General contraindications that apply to intubation, as well as the other procedures in this chapter, include lack of adequate facilities or trained personnel. In addition, the major contraindication specific to intubation in the case of an immediate life-threatening condition is a do-not-resuscitate (DNR) order or other properly documented evidence of the patient's desire not to be resuscitated.

Role of the Respiratory Therapist

Table 18-1 summarizes your role in assisting with a standard bedside intubation, followed by some elaboration of several of these steps.

Before intubation, you or another clinician should ensure that there are no orders that would contraindicate intubation, such as a valid DNR or do-not-intubate (DNI) order. However, in the absence of a DNR or DNI order, the physician orders for an emergency intubation and associated procedures such as sedation administration may initially be done verbally. However, it is imperative for you to ensure that a physician's order to intubate is written in the medical record either before or promptly after the procedure (if a verbal order was initially given). After the intubation has been successfully performed and the patient stabilized, you also should make sure that the physician orders a chest X-ray to confirm tube placement and writes orders for initial ventilator settings, as appropriate.

Required Equipment

The following list specifies the equipment needed for routine endotracheal intubation. Those marked with an asterisk (*) are typically included on an intubation tray.

- CDC barrier precautions (gloves, gowns, masks, eyewear)
- Towels (for positioning)
- Stethoscope
- Oxygen flow meter and connecting tubing
- Bag-valve-mask (BVM) manual resuscitator
- Vacuum source/suction apparatus (regulator, portable pump, etc.)
- Suction catheters (flexible suction catheters, Yankauer [tonsillar] tip, etc.)
- Local anesthetic (spray)*
- Lubricating jelly*
- Laryngoscopes (2) with assorted blades, batteries, and bulbs*
- Endotracheal tubes (at least 3 different sizes)*
- Stylet(s)*
- Magill forceps*
- Syringe*
- Devices used to confirm placement (EDD, CO_2 detector, light wand, etc.)
- Tape and/or ET tube holders(s)*
- Oropharyneal airways and/or bite blocks*
- Monitoring equipment, such as pulse oximetry and ECG

Note: A fiberoptic bronchoscope and equipment may be needed for difficult intubations.

Selecting and Testing the Equipment

Once the intubation tray is opened and other equipment obtained, you should begin assembling and testing the equipment. This will initially involve selecting the appropriate type and size of laryngoscope blade. The choice of a straight (Miller) or a curved (MacIntosh) blade is largely a matter of clinician preference. However, blade size is governed by the patient's age and size. In general, you select a size 4 for a large adult, a size 3 for a small adult or adolescent, and a size 2 for a pediatric patient. The blade should then be connected to the handle to confirm illumination. If the blade light does not illuminate, you should first recheck the connection between the handle and blade, and then either try another blade or replace the bulb or batteries. On fiberoptic scopes, if you cannot obtain light through the blade channel with a good handle connection, you need fresh batteries.

Once you have assembled the laryngoscope and confirmed its function, an appropriate-sized ET tube should be obtained and tested. Guidelines for ET tube size selection are provided in Chapter 10. In general, you should recommend using the following tube sizes: average adult male, 8.0–9.0 mm; adult female, 7.0–8.0 mm; average 16-year-old, 7.0 mm; and a 3-year-old, 4.5 mm. The ET tube cuff patency should then be checked by connecting a syringe to the pilot balloon and then inserting approximately 5–10 mL of air into the cuff and checking for leaks. If no leaks are detected, the cuff should be completely deflated. It is generally appropriate to leave the syringe connected to the pilot balloon with the plunger pulled back, to inflate the cuff upon successful intubation.

Table 18-1 Respiratory Therapist's Role When Assisting with Intubation

Therapist's Function	Purpose
Before the Procedure	
Verify, interpret, and evaluate doctor's order or protocol	To ensure there is a written or verbal physician's order and that there is no DNR order
Wash hands and apply standard transmission-based precautions	To minimize the spread of infection
Select and gather equipment, including multiple ET tube sizes and laryngoscope blades, as well as a syringe and stylet	To minimize delays and to ensure patient well-being
Assemble and checks equipment, including laryngoscope light, ET tube cuff, and BVM	To minimize delays from equipment failure and to ensure patient well-being
Lubricate ET tube and stylet	To help ensure easy insertion
Ensure oral suction device is set up and functional	To ensure secretion clearance and better visualization of glottis
During the Procedure	
Assess patient and ensure monitoring equipment (pulse oximetry, ECG)	To minimize the likelihood of adverse reaction or patient harm
Monitor patient vital signs and clinical status, including his or her response to moderate sedation, if given	To ensure patient safety throughout procedure
Check and remove patient dentures, if applicable	To facilitate insertion of laryngoscope and better visualization of glottis
Position patient in sniffing position, unless contraindicated (e.g., cervical neck injury)	To facilitate visualization of glottis
Anesthetize the airway, if appropriate	To minimize patient discomfort
Preoxygenate patient with F_{IO_2} of 100%	To ensure adequate oxygenation
Assist in intubation with patient positioning, oral suctioning, laryngoscope insertion, applying cricoid pressure, etc.	To help ensure a prompt and safe intubation
Inflate the cuff, manually secure tube, ventilate and oxygenate via BVM	To ensure patient safety
Assess ET tube placement through auscultation of chest and stomach and use of detection device	To ensure tube placement and patient safety
If ET tube placement is in question, deflate cuff, remove ET tube, and begin manual ventilation and oxygenation	To ensure patient safety
After the Procedure	
Note and mark tube markings and secure tube	To ensure proper tube placement and patient safety
Reassess patient's clinical status	To ensure patient safety
Suction patient if necessary	To ensure airway patency
Ensure appropriate ventilation and oxygenation	To ensure patient safety

(continues)

Table 18-1 Respiratory Therapist's Role When Assisting with Intubation (continued)

Therapist's Function	Purpose
Ensure chest X-ray is performed and reposition tube if necessary	To confirm tube placement and ensure patient safety
Record results in chart and other pertinent records	To maintain medical and legal record of procedure and patient response
Verify that intubation order has been written, if initial order was verbal	To ensure appropriate legal record of physician order

Many physicians prefer using a stylet, which adds rigidity to the ET tube and aids in oral insertion. Therefore, you should make sure one is available. When preparing for a nasal intubation, you should have Magill forceps ready for the physician.

You also should ensure that there is a properly functioning vacuum/suction source, and that a suction canister, connection tubing, and Yankauer (tonsillar) tip have been set up. A variety of flexible suction catheters should be available. Personal protective equipment, such as a mask, eye protection, and gloves, should also be available.

Preparing and Monitoring the Patient

When assisting with an intubation, you need to position the patient properly. The patient may need to be pulled up to the head of the bed. Unless an unstable neck injury is suspected, you should then place the patient in a "sniffing" position, as depicted in **Figure 18-1**. In the presence of an unstable

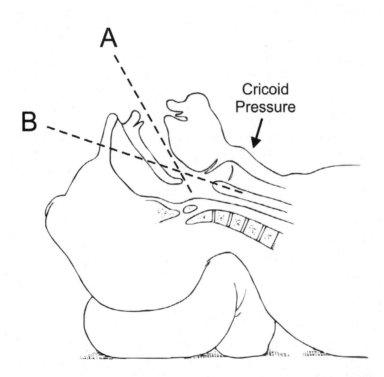

Figure 18-1 Sniffing Position for Intubation. The neck is slightly flexed, and the is head extended. Place a pillow or towels under the head and neck, but not under the shoulders. Compared to the angle with no flexion or extension (A), this position provides a straighter line of vision from the mouth to the vocal cords (B). External pressure applied to the cricoid cartilage (Sellick maneuver) can provide even better alignment of the anatomic structures for intubation.

cervical spine, the sniffing position should be avoided. In such instances, it may be necessary for the physician to modify this procedure, perhaps using a fiberoptic bronchoscope to aid in tube placement.

Once the patient is positioned, you may find it necessary to clear secretions or vomitus from the oropharynx using a Yankauer tip. In addition, in conscious or semiconscious patients, a local anesthetic such as an aerosolized 2% tetracaine spray (Cetacaine) aids intubation by blocking the gag reflex. You can use a tongue depressor to help spray the posterior pharynx. For nasal intubation, spray Cetacaine into the nasal passages and coat the tube with lidocaine jelly. For elective procedures, you can nebulize a 4% lidocaine solution via SVN. In order to help prevent hypoxemia, you should also preoxygenate the patient with 100% oxygen via a BVM with an O_2 reservoir.

The patient's vital signs and pulse oximetry should be monitored before, during, and immediately following intubation. For patients who have received moderate sedation, special attention should be paid for the presence of adverse reactions to such medications, including hypotension and nausea. In addition, it is also highly desirable to assess heart rhythm via ECG throughout the procedure. You should frequently communicate the patient's vital signs and overall clinical status to the physician performing the intubation, especially if the patient's condition deteriorates prior to, during, or immediately following the procedure.

Assisting with Tube Insertion

When assisting with this procedure, there are measures you can take to help the physician promptly and properly insert the ET tube. For oral intubations, you can suggest the use of a stylet, which adds rigidity and maintains the shape of an ET tube during oral intubation. Stylets come in various sizes and are usually constructed of malleable metals. Ideally, the distal tip of the stylet should be rounded and/or soft. *To prevent airway trauma during oral intubation, the stylet tip must never extend beyond the ET tube tip.*

If you are assisting a physician with a nasal intubation, ensure that Magill forceps are available to help advance the ET tube through the glottis under direct visualization. The ET tube should also be well lubricated to aid passage through the nose. *Do not use a stylet for nasal intubation!* The tube is directed inferiorly and posteriorly. Once the tip of the tube is in the oropharynx, you may help open the mouth so the physician can insert the laryngoscope and visualize the glottis. The physician will then use the Magill forceps to grasp the tube just above the cuff and direct it between the cords. Unless contraindicated, flexion of the neck will help advance the tube past the cords. In assisting with tube insertion, you should ensure that the proper-size ET tube is used and that the tube be lubricated to ease with its insertion. For oral or nasal intubation, you may apply moderate pressure on the cricoid cartilage, known as a Sellick maneuver, to help the physician visualize the glottis and close off the esophagus.

In general, intubation attempts should not exceed 30 seconds, and you should keep the physician informed of the elapsed time, as well as the patient's vital signs and SpO_2 during the procedure. In case the physician is having difficulty with tube insertion, you should be prepared to do the following:

- Resume ventilating the patient with 100% oxygen via BVM.
- Suction the oral pharynx or airway.
- Have at least one smaller-size ET tube readily available.
- Where available, suggest the insertion of a laryngeal mask airway (LMA).
- Suggest that the procedure be done by an anesthesiologist, perhaps with the use of a fiberoptic bronchoscope.

Once the ET tube has been passed through the vocal cords and properly positioned in the trachea, you should promptly inflate the cuff with about 10 mL of air, temporarily secure the tube with your hand or tape, and then immediately begin manual ventilation with 100% O_2.

Assessing Tube Placement

Immediately following the intubation and artificial ventilation, successful placement of the ET tube into the trachea may be initially assessed through auscultation and patient's overall clinical status. However, a more reliable means to quickly assess ET tube placement is by using an *esophageal detection device* (EDD). With the squeeze bulb–type EDD, you first squeeze the bulb to create a negative pressure, *then* attach it to the ET tube. Quick reexpansion of the bulb upon release indicates positioning in an open airway (usually the trachea). If the tube is in the esophagus, it will *not* reinflate. This is because the esophagus lacks cartilaginous support, which causes it to collapse around the tube and obstructs in distal openings.

A syringe-type EDD (with a 15-mm adapter) is also available. With this device, if the ET tube is in the esophagus, you will feel strong resistance when you try to aspirate air (the barrel will actually tend to recoil if released); if in an open airway, you can freely aspirate air into the syringe. EDDs are not recommended for detecting esophageal intubation in children under 1 year old.

A *colorimetric CO_2* detector functions like pH paper, with an indicator that changes color when exposed to different CO_2 levels. To use the device, you place it *between* the patient's ET tube connector and the BVM. If the ET tube is in the trachea, the device should change color from purple to tan (or possibly yellow) with each exhalation. You can estimate the %CO_2 based on the following color ranges:

- Range A (purple): < 0.5% CO_2
- Range B (tan): 0.5–2.0% CO_2
- Range C (yellow): > 2.0% CO_2

Two different versions are available: one for patients more than 15 kg (33 lb.) and a pediatric model for patients weighing between 1 and 15 kg. The device can be used for up to 3 hours.

CO_2 detectors are effective in detecting most esophageal intubations. In cardiac arrest victims, however, expired CO_2 levels may be near zero due to poor pulmonary blood flow, yielding a false-negative result. Generally, expired CO_2 levels increase with the return of spontaneous circulation. Unfortunately, CO_2 analysis is not a reliable indicator of mainstem bronchial intubation.

After preliminary assessment of proper tube placement via auscultation, EDD, and CO_2 detector, you should initially secure the ET tube to the skin using tape and record the depth of insertion to the incisors using the centimeter markings on the tube. After confirming proper placement via chest X-ray, you should consider securing the tube using a commercially available device designed for this purpose.

Rapid Sequence Intubation

Certain situations may warrant a special intubation procedure called *rapid sequence intubation*. This procedure is the preferred method for intubating conscious patients who have not fasted and are thus at high risk for aspiration. To facilitate intubation, the patient immediately is rendered unconscious using a short-acting anaesthetic, such as etomidate, and is paralyzed using either succinylcholine or a non-depolarizing neuromuscular blocking agent like rocuronium. The goal is to rapidly intubate without having to use BVM ventilation. **Figure 18-2** details the rapid sequence intubation procedure used in such situations. Note that rapid sequence intubation generally should not be used for "crash" airway management of unconscious and apneic patients. In these cases, you should proceed with or recommend immediate BVM ventilation and intubation without anesthesia induction or paralysis.

Bronchoscopy Assisting

Bronchoscopy involves direct visual examination of upper airway, vocal cords, and tracheobronchial tree to the fourth to sixth bronchial generations. Therapeutic indications include secretion and foreign body removal. Diagnostic use involves obtaining fluid or tissue specimens for microbiologic or cytologic assessment via bronchial washings, brush biopsy, bronchoalveolar lavage, and endobronchial and transbronchial biopsy.

Indications

Specific indications for flexible fiberoptic bronchoscopy include the following:

- The presence of lesions of unknown etiology on the chest X-ray film or the need to evaluate recurrent or persistent atelectasis or pulmonary infiltrates
- To investigate hemoptysis, persistent unexplained cough, localized wheeze, or stridor
- The need to obtain lower respiratory tract secretions, cell washings, and biopsies for cytologic, histologic, and microbiologic evaluation
- The need to determine the location and extent of injury from toxic inhalation or aspiration

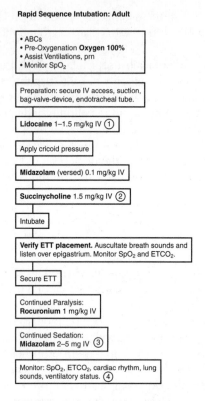

Rapid Sequence Intubation: Adult

- ABCs
- Pre-Oxygenation **Oxygen 100%**
- Assist Ventilations, prn
- Monitor SpO₂

Preparation: secure IV access, suction, bag-valve-device, endotracheal tube.

Lidocaine 1–1.5 mg/kg IV ①

Apply cricoid pressure

Midazolam (versed) 0.1 mg/kg IV

Succinylcholine 1.5 mg/kg IV ②

Intubate

Verify ETT placement. Auscultate breath sounds and listen over epigastrium. Monitor SpO₂ and ETCO₂.

Secure ETT

Continued Paralysis: **Rocuronium** 1 mg/kg IV

Continued Sedation: **Midazolam** 2–5 mg IV ③

Monitor: SpO₂, ETCO₂, cardiac rhythm, lung sounds, ventilatory status. ④

1 **Lidocaine:** is indicated when ICP is elevated. May consider premedicating with **fentanyl** 200 mcg IV to decrease sympathetic response.
2 **Succinylcholine:** obtain history. **Do not give succinylcholine if familial history of malignant hyperthermia is noted. Succinylcholine is contraindicated in penetrating eye injury, severe burns or crush injuries that are 2–5 days old or in the presence of hyperkalemia or in patients with chronic muscular conditions (i.e., muscular dystrophy).** The onset of **succinylcholine** is 30–60 seconds, duration is 8–10 minutes.
3 **Consider pain control measures. Neither paralytics nor sedatives provide pain control.**
4 **Keep the patient warm.** Paralyzed patients lose much of their ability to generate body heat.

Figure 18-2 Rapid Sequence Intubation Algorithm.

Source: Porter, W. (2007). *Porter's pocket guide to emergency and critical care.* Sudbury, MA: Jones and Bartlett Publishers.

- To evaluate problems associated with ET or tracheostomy tubes (tracheal damage, airway obstruction, or tube placement)
- The need for aid in performing difficult intubations
- The suspicion that secretions or mucous plugs are responsible for atelectasis
- To remove abnormal endobronchial tissue or foreign material by forceps, basket, or laser
- To retrieve a foreign body (although rigid bronchoscopy may be preferred)

Contraindications

As is the case with most invasive procedures, the absence of either a documented patient consent or a physician's order represents an absolute contraindication. Other major contraindications for performing fiberoptic bronchoscopy are summarized in **Table 18-2**.

Role of the Respiratory Therapist

Table 18-3 (see page 528) is a summary of the potential roles for you as the respiratory therapist in assisting a physician who is performing a bronchoscopy.

Table 18-2 Contraindications for Bronchoscopy

Absolute	Relative
• Absence of consent from the patient or his or her representative unless a medical emergency exists • Absence of an experienced clinician to perform or closely and directly supervise the procedure • Lack of adequate facilities and personnel to care for such emergencies as cardiopulmonary arrest, pneumothorax, or bleeding • Inability to adequately oxygenate the patient during the procedure • Coagulopathy or uncontrolled bleeding • Severe obstructive airway disease • Severe refractory hypoxemia • Unstable hemodynamic status including dysrhythmias	• Lack of patient cooperation • Recent myocardial infarction or unstable angina • Partial tracheal obstruction • Moderate-to-severe hypoxemia or any degree of hypercapnea • Uremia and pulmonary hypertension • Lung abscess • Superior vena cava obstructions • Debility, malnutrition • Respiratory failure requiring mechanical ventilation • Disorders requiring laser therapy, biopsy of large obstructing lesions or multiple transbronchial biopsies • Known or suspected pregnancy (because of radiation exposure)

Note: The safety of bronchoscopic procedures in asthmatic patients is a concern, but the presence of asthma does not preclude the use of these procedures.

Patient Preparation

You should ensure that the patient takes nothing by mouth (NPO) after midnight for a morning bronchoscopy and NPO after light breakfast for afternoon procedures. Routine medications (especially antiasthmatic drugs) may be taken at any time with a small amount of water. Routine lab work, including clotting times, BUN, CBC, and platelet count, is essential to exclude a bleeding disorder—especially if a biopsy is to be performed. Some measure of pulmonary function is useful (spirometry, blood gases) to assess pulmonary reserve and document bronchospasm. Moderate sedation (described later in this chapter) with a narcotic (meperidine 25–75 mg) or an anxiolytic/sedative (diazepam 10 mg) is given parenterally 15–30 minutes before the procedure. Atropine 0.4 mg is given intramuscularly as a vagolytic agent at the same time unless contraindicated by the presence of arrhythmia, narrow angle glaucoma, or urinary retention.

Equipment

A fiberoptic bronchoscope (see **Figure 18-3** on page 529) and halogen or xenon light source are needed for this procedure. The bronchoscope is equipped with a thumb lever that allows angulation of the distal end of the instrument. A 2- to 2.6-mm channel runs the length of the scope. This channel is used to (1) inject medications or lavage fluid, (2) aspirate secretions, and (3) obtain fluid or tissue specimens. Tissue specimens are obtained using specialized instruments, such as bronchial brushes and forceps.

Procedure

Bronchoscopy may be performed with the patient in supine or sitting position. The patient gargles with 2% lidocaine solution or tetracaine 2% aerosolized spray (Cetacaine), or aerosolized 4% lidocaine is used to anesthetize the pharynx. The bronchoscope tip is lubricated with Xylocaine jelly and introduced transnasally or transorally with the use of a bite block. Lidocaine 2% solution is then injected through the bronchoscopic channel in 2-mL aliquots for anesthesia of the vocal cords and entire tracheo-bronchial tree. Because lidocaine can cause seizures and respiratory arrest, the total dosage should generally not exceed 400 mg. The duration of action generally lasts 20–30 minutes. Once adequate anesthesia has been obtained, a detailed visual examination is performed. Subsequently, other procedures such as biopsies, washings, and brushings can be carried out.

Table 18-3 Respiratory Therapist's Role When Assisting with Bronchoscopy

Therapist's Function	Purpose
Before the Procedure	
Help identify potential need for a bronchoscopy such as retained secretions or foreign body removal	To determine which patients may benefit from the procedure in order to maximize clinical outcomes
Review chart to confirm: physician order, signed consent form, no contraindications (e.g., coagulopathy), special precautions	To confirm physician's order, that the patient has agreed to it, and that it isn't contraindicated, and to determine any special infection control procedures
Prepare/ensure proper function of equipment, including bronchoscope, light source, TV monitor, video recorder, medications, specimen traps	To minimize unnecessary delay and likelihood of patient harm from procedure
Prepare patient, providing patient education and pre-medication	To minimize untoward delays and patient well-being
Ensure "time out" to confirm correct patient and procedure	To minimize patient harm and medical errors
During the Procedure	
Ensure proper function of all equipment (bronchoscope, light source, TV monitor) needed during procedure	To minimize unnecessary delay from equipment failure
Assist physician in obtaining specimens; help with medication preparation (e.g., mucomyst, epinephrine)	To minimize unnecessary delay and likelihood of patient harm from procedure
Monitor patient vital signs and overall clinical status; respond to adverse reactions	To minimize patient harm from adverse reactions
After the Procedure	
Monitor patient vital signs and clinical status	To ensure the patient has tolerated procedure and detect adverse reactions
Ensure specimens are properly labeled and sent to lab	To help ensure accurate diagnosis and treatment
Clean, disinfect/sterilize equipment, then ensure it is properly stored	To minimize nosocomial infection risk and potential damage to equipment
Record results in chart and other pertinent records	To maintain medical and legal record of procedure and patient response

Patient Screening and Monitoring

It is imperative that all patients for whom a bronchoscopy is planned be prescreened for contraindications (Table 18-2) and that they be closely monitored immediately before, during, and after the procedure. After the procedure, the patient should remain NPO for 2 hours or longer until the gag reflex is fully restored. Because of the premedication, outpatients should not allowed to drive until the following day. Transient fever and mild hemoptysis may be noted for the next 24 hours (bleeding is most common after transbronchial biopsy).

Clinical Information Acquired from Procedure

Bronchoscopy provides information regarding the patency and condition of the central airways. It is also used to obtain cell and tissue specimens via washings, brushing, or biopsy techniques. Typically, you place tissue specimens in a fixing agent such as formalin, while mucous and lavage fluids are aspirated into empty sterile collection bottles for additional analysis.

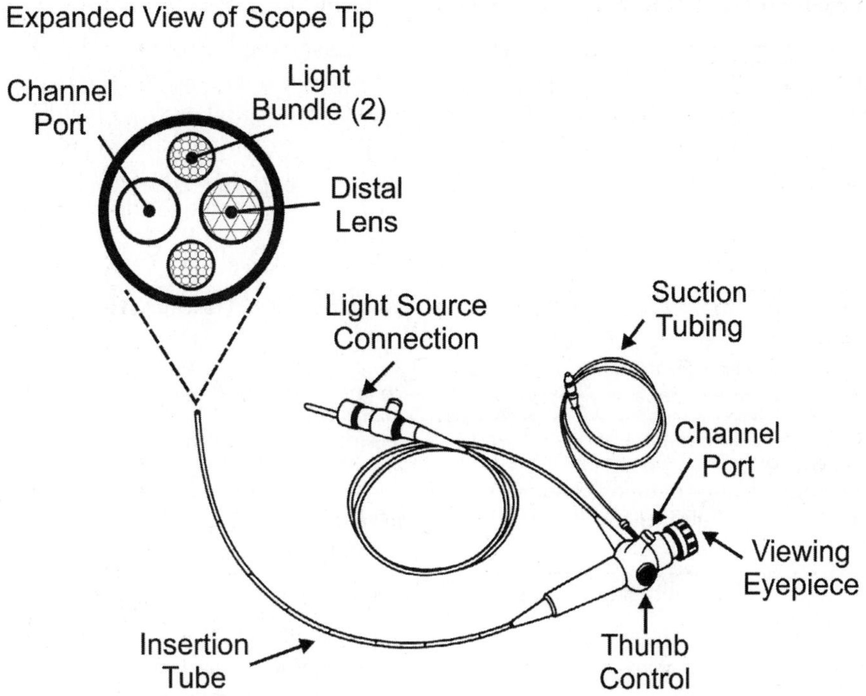

Expanded View of Scope Tip

Figure 18-3 Fiberoptic Bronchoscope.

Additional Considerations

Bronchoscopy is relatively safe. The risks are highest in patients with underlying cardiac disease and the elderly. Patients with asthma or hyperreactive airways are prone to bronchospasm and laryngospasm, and thus require especially careful preparation and monitoring. Because a drop in PaO_2 of about 20 torr is common during bronchoscopy, supplemental O_2 should always be administered, either via a nasal cannula (for the oral route) or a mask modified to allow introduction of the scope through the nose. If the patient is intubated, FIO_2 should generally be increased by 10% or more during the procedure to minimize the likelihood of hypoxemia.

Tracheotomy

Tracheotomy involves gaining access to the trachea through an opening in the neck. The opening can be created by surgical incision or using a special dilator kit. Once the opening has been established, a tracheostomy tube is placed into the trachea and properly secured. While tracheotomy may be performed as an emergency procedure on patients with upper airway trauma or obstruction, in most instances it is carried out electively by a skilled physician or surgeon after the patient's airway has been established. When this procedure is done electively at the bedside on an intubated patient, you may be asked to assist.

Indications and Contraindications

While there are a variety of specific clinical scenarios where tracheotomy may be indicated, all fall under the following general categories:

- To bypass a partial or complete upper airway obstruction
- To provide access for secretion removal
- To facilitate prolonged mechanical ventilation

There are essentially no absolute contraindications for this procedure. However, because it can cause bleeding, elective tracheotomy should not be performed until severe coagulopathies are corrected. In addition, critically ill patients should be stabilized as much as possible beforehand.

Role of the Respiratory Therapist

In general, the physician performing tracheotomy will receive some assistance from a clinician with surgical training, such as another physician, a nurse, or a surgical technician. They will be responsible for helping gather and set up equipment, as well as acting as "another set of hands" for the physician performing the procedure. However, you can perform a vital role in assisting with this procedure. **Table 18-4** summarizes the key elements involved in assisting with tracheotomy. Postprocedure and ongoing care of a patient with an established tracheostomy is discussed in Chapter 10.

Table 18-4 Respiratory Therapist's Role When Assisting with Tracheostomy

Therapist's Function	Purpose
Before the Procedure	
Confirm physician order and signed "informed consent" and help identify contraindications (coagulopathy) and special precautions	To ensure physician's order, that the patient has consented, and that procedure is not contraindicated; to identify special infection control procedures
Ensure that a crash cart and intubation equipment are readily available	To enhance patient safety and address potentially life-threatening responses to this procedure
Gather equipment, as noted below *Note:* The therapist must ensure that a tracheostomy tube that is one size smaller than that being inserted is always available	To ensure equipment necessary to remove old ET tube, monitor the patient, and oxygenate/ventilate
Patient/caregiver education	To ensure that patient and/or caregiver(s) understand procedure
Ensure "time out" to confirm correct patient and procedure	To minimize patient harm and chance of medical errors
Monitor patient clinical status, including vital signs, SpO_2, overall appearance	To obtain baseline data and ensure that patient can tolerate the procedure
During the Procedure	
Continue to monitor clinical status and respond to adverse reaction or deterioration	To ensure patient is tolerating procedure; to identify adverse response
Ensure adequate airway at all times	To ensure patient safety
Prepare for ET tube withdrawal according to physician's instructions (partially deflating ET tube cuff), as appropriate	To ensure an adequate airway and transition to tracheostomy tube
Per physician's instructions, deflate the ET tube cuff, remove tape, and slowly withdraw ET tube *Note:* The ET tube should be removed just before insertion of the tracheostomy tube	To ensure an adequate airway and transition to tracheostomy tube
Ensure proper placement via breath sounds, $ETCO_2$	To ensure patient ventilation and safety
Secure tracheostomy tube and continue ventilating through it	To ensure an adequate airway and prevent accidental decannulation
After the Procedure	
Monitor patient vital signs and clinical status	To ensure patient safety
Ensure a chest X-ray is ordered	To ensure proper tube placement
Clean up and document in patient record	To maintain medical and legal record of procedure and patient response

Equipment

In general, the physician will ensure that he or she has the necessary surgical equipment to perform the tracheotomy procedure itself. You need to identify and gather the equipment needed to maintain the airway, monitor the patient, and support ventilation and oxygenation. In general, you should obtain the following equipment:

- Gown and gloves, mask, and cap
- Sterile towels, drapes, sponges (for patient)
- Extra tracheostomy tube that is one size smaller than that being inserted
- 10-mL syringe, for removing air from the endotracheal tube cuff
- Scissors for removing tape or other securing device
- Manual resuscitation bag (BVM)
- Flow meter and O_2 source
- Intubation equipment (should be readily available)
- Hazardous waste receptacle

Hazards and Complications

Because tracheotomy is an invasive and stressful procedure, there are several hazards and complications you need to be on guard for, as summarized in **Table 18-5**. Should you note or suspect any of these problems either during the procedure or when subsequently caring for the patient, be sure to immediately communicate your concern to the physician and nurse. If the problem appears life-threatening, try to stabilize the patient and call for help.

Thoracentesis

Thoracentesis involves the insertion of a needle into the pleural space, usually to remove accumulated fluid, as occurs in pleural effusion. A lateral chest X-ray can help identify the presence and amount of pleural fluid. In addition, diagnostic ultrasound is typically used to determine the specific location of the fluid and to identify the proper insertion site for the thoracentesis needle. Ultrasound also may be used to guide needle insertion.

Indications and Contraindications

Diagnostically, thoracentesis is used to gather pleural fluid for analysis to help determine the presence of underlying conditions such as infection, malignancy, CHF, or cirrhosis. Therapeutically, thoracentesis is performed whenever excessive pleural fluid interferes with lung expansion and impairs oxygenation and/or ventilation. Major contraindications for thoracentesis include the following:

- Absence of a properly signed physican's order or informed consent (except in the case of a medical emergency)
- Absence of an experienced clinician to perform or supervise the procedure
- Inadequate facilities or personnel to handle hazards such as pneumothorax or bleeding

Table 18-5 Tracheostomy Hazards and Complications

Procedural	Post-Procedure
Adverse reaction to sedation	Infection
Tissue trauma at incision site	Bleeding
Airway compromise or loss of patient airway	Pain or discomfort
Excessive bleeding	Tracheal stenosis
Hypoxemia	
Aspiration	

- An uncooperative patient
- Inability to identify the top of the rib
- Severe coagulopathy (platelet count < 50,000/mm^3)
- Severe bullous lung disease
- Mechanical ventilation with PEEP
- Status post pneumonectomy (lung removal)
- Markedly elevated hemidiaphragm

Role of the Respiratory Therapist

You may assist the physician before, during, and immediately following thoracentesis. *Prior* to the procedure, your assessment of the patient may actually help determine the need for the procedure. Your bedside assessment may reveal that the patient has a dullness to percussion and decreased breath sounds in the affected region. When such findings are combined with the presence of predisposing factors such as malignancy, CHF, or respiratory infection, you should suspect a pleural effusion and you should inform the nurse and physician. In preparing for the procedure, you may also provide assistance by ensuring the chart contains the physician's order and signed informed consent, identifying the patient and any contraindications, helping gather the equipment, and educating the patient. *During* the procedure, you may assist with the equipment, in monitoring, as well as in stabilizing and positioning the patient. The patient should generally be positioned sitting up and leaning slightly forward and supported in front by medical personnel or a height-adjusted bedside table. *After* the procedure, you should help monitor the patient, ensure that any pleural fluid specimens are properly labeled and/or processed, and that the results are documented in the patient chart. In some institutions, the thoracentesis protocol also requires that a chest X-ray be performed after the procedure to rule out a pneumothorax.

Equipment

Table 18-6 lists the key equipment used for thoracentesis according to its purpose.

Table 18-6 Thoracentesis Equipment

Purpose	Equipment
Skin preparation	• Sterile gloves, sponges, and drape(s) • Iodophor solution
Local anesthesia	• Local anesthesia (2% lidocaine) with small-gauge (25 gauge) needle • Large needle (18–22 gauge, 2-in. long) with 5-mL syringe
Pleural access	• Two 2-mL syringes and one 50-mL Luer-lok syringe • 4-gauge needle with 16-gauge catheter *or* 20-gauge, 1.5-in. needle • Three-way stopcock, 1-liter container, and tubing • Sterile clamp • Adhesive tape and bandage
Specimen collection	• Two 15-mL (red-top) tubes • 5-mL heparinized glass syringe with ice slush bag for transportation • Sterile anaerobic transport media bottle • Heparin solution (1:1000) for cytology and cell block specimens • Other containers (7-mL purple-top), as appropriate

Hazards and Procedural Considerations

The thoracentesis procedure itself has many steps that will be performed by the physician. It is highly likely that your role will include only those functions mentioned above and that the NBRC will focus primarily on those items. However, you also need to understand the major hazards associated with this procedure, which include the following:

- Hypoxemia
- Pneumothorax and hemothorax
- Hemorrhage/bleeding
- Puncture of the liver or spleen
- Infection

Based on knowledge of these hazards, when assisting with thoracentesis you should ensure that supplemental O_2 as well as equipment needed for chest tube insertion and intubation are available. In addition, you should closely monitor the overall clinical status of the patient undergoing thoracentesis, via both vital signs and pulse oximetry.

Chest Tube Insertion (Tube Thoracostomy)

Chapter 17 describes the use of needle thoracostomy for the emergency treatment of a tension pneumothorax. For long-term management of pneumothorax and/or for removal of pleural fluid or blood, a chest tube needs to be inserted.

Chest tube insertion involves placement by a physician of a sterile tube (24–36 Fr) into the pleural space. For pneumothorax, the tube is generally inserted into the fourth or fifth intercostal space at the anterior axillary line, while for fluid drainage native sites may be used. Once secured, the tube is generally connected to a pleural drainage system, to which 15–20 cm H_2O of suction is applied. The use of pleural drainage systems is described in more detail in Chapter 6.

Indications and Contraindications

There are several indications for chest tubes, including pneumothorax, hemothorax, empyema, chytlothorax (collection of lymphatic fluid), and pleural effusion. Chest tubes may also be used to administer drugs or chemicals into the pleural space, including antibiotics for infection and agents to prevent the recurrence of a pleural effusion.

In addition to the general contraindications that apply to many of the procedures described in this chapter (lack of an order or patient consent), the major contraindication for this procedure is the absence of significant air or fluid in the pleural space. Also, because this procedure involves making a small incision, coagulopathy and an uncooperative patient may contraindicate a chest tube insertion.

Role of the Respiratory Therapist

In addition to helping gather and set up the equipment, your role when assisting with chest tube insertion mainly involves correctly identifying the patient, monitoring the patient and equipment, as well as helping identify and respond to any adverse reactions. Proper setup and monitoring of the chest tube drainage system is discussed in Chapter 6 of this text. In addition, the patient's overall clinical status should be monitored and documented prior to, during, and immediately following the procedure. In fact, your routine assessment may have uncovered the presence of a pneumothorax and hence the need for a chest tube. In addition, patient monitoring during or after the procedure may reveal an adverse response such as excessive bleeding or hemodynamic instability, requiring special measures or even resuscitative efforts. In addition, you may help secure the chest tube and prevent inadvertent or premature removal of the chest tube.

Equipment

When assisting the physician with chest tube insertion, one of your primary roles may be to gather equipment. Listed below is the equipment most commonly used for this procedure, some of which may be included in many standard chest tube insertion kits.

- Sterile gown and gloves, mask, and cap (for physician/clinician)
- Sterile towels, drapes, and sponges (for patient)
- 10-mL syringe, 18-, 21-, and 25-gauge needles and 1% lidocaine
- 2 Kelly clamps
- Mayo scissors
- Tissue and towel forceps
- Suture set
- Scalpel and #10 blade
- Chest tubes (24–36 Fr)
- Chest tube drainage system
- Petroleum gauze and tape

Hazards and Procedural Considerations

Given that your major role when assisting with this procedure is patient monitoring and assessment, you should know the major hazards and complications of chest tube insertion, which include the following:

- Bleeding
- Tissue trauma
- Secondary pneumothorax

In general, a chest tube should be removed once the condition that led to its insertion has resolved. During the first one or two days after removal, you should help monitor the patient's cardiopulmonary status with particular emphasis on the recurrence of the pneumothorax or underlying pathology, as well as any other adverse response. Crepitus at the site of insertion always suggests recurrence of air leakage into the pleural space.

Cardioversion

Synchronized cardioversion involves the application of an electrical shock to the heart that is *synchronized* to occur generally during the R wave of an ECG. This procedure is used to treat several different arrhythmias, which generally are not immediately life threatening. The indications, equipment, and major aspects of the procedure are described below.

Indications and Contraindications

Table 18-7 lists the arrhythmias for which synchronized cardioversion is indicated along with the recommended energy level recommended for each. In general, *immediate cardioversion is needed if a ventricular rate greater than 150 persists despite efforts to control it with applicable drugs.*

Table 18-7 Arrhythmias and Energy Levels for Synchronized Cardioversion

Arrhythmia	Incremental Energy Levels in Joules (Monophasic)[a]
Atrial fibrillation	100 J → 200 J → 300 J → 360 J
Atrial flutter	50 J → 100 J → 200 J → 300 J → 360 J
Other supraventricular tachycardia (due to reentry)	50 J → 100 J → 200 J → 300 J → 360 J
Monomorphic ventricular tachycardia (if stable)	100 J → 200 J → 300 J → 360 J
Polymorphic ventricular tachycardia (irregular form and rate) and unstable	Treat as ventricular fibrillation with high-energy shock (360 J)
a. Biphasic waveforms using lower energy are acceptable if documented to be clinically equivalent or superior to reports of monophasic shock success. Consult the device manufacturer for specific recommendations.	

In the presence of applicable arrhythmias, the only major contraindications for cardioversion are lack of properly trained personnel or the patient's desire not to be treated. It should also be noted that certain conditions such as severe chest trauma or recent thoracic surgery may require modification to standard procedures.

Role of the Respiratory Therapist

Your role in cardioversion mainly involves helping correctly identify the patient, as well as monitoring and responding to any adverse reactions. In rare instances, patients receiving cardioversion worsen and require cardiopulmonary resuscitation. Thus, you should monitor patients closely and ensure that suction, intubation and O_2 equipment, as well as a bag-valve-mask are readily available. The basic cardioversion procedure is outlined in the accompanying box.

Basic Cardioversion Procedure

Equipment and Patient Preparation

1. Premedicate whenever possible with sedative (e.g., Versed) with or without analgesia (e.g., fentanyl).
2. Turn on defibrillator.
3. Attach monitor leads to the patient ("white to right, red to ribs, what's left over to the left shoulder") and ensure proper display of the patient's rhythm.
4. Engage the synchronization mode by pressing the "sync" control button.

Assessment and Implementation

5. Look for markers on the R waves indicating sync mode.
6. If necessary, adjust R wave gain until sync markers occur with each ORS complex.
7. Select appropriate energy level for the identified arrhythmia (refer to Table 18-7).
8. Position conductor pads on patient (or apply gel to paddles).
9. Position paddles on patient (sternum/apex).
10. Announce to the team members: "Charging defibrillator—stand clear!"
11. Press "charge" button on apex paddle (right hand).
12. When the defibrillator is charged, begin the final "clearing chant." State firmly in a forceful voice the following chant before each shock:
    - "I am going to shock on three. One, I'm clear." (Check to make sure you are clear of contact with the patient or the stretcher and equipment.)
    - "Two, you are clear." (Make a visual check to ensure that no one continues to touch the patient or stretcher. In particular, do not forget about the person providing ventilation. That person's hands should not be on the ventilatory adjuncts, including the ET tube!)
    - "Three, everybody is clear." (Check yourself one more time before pressing the shock buttons.)
13. Apply about 25 lbs. of pressure on both paddles.
14. Press the "Shock" button(s).
15. Check the monitor. If tachycardia persists, increase the joules according to Table 18-7.
16. Activate the "sync" mode after delivery of each synchronized shock. Most defibrillators default back to unsynchronized mode after delivery of a synchronized shock.

Follow-up

17. Remove paddles and clean site.
18. Record pertinent data in chart.
19. Notify appropriate personnel and make any necessary recommendations or modifications to the patient care plan.

Table 18-8 Moderate Sedation Medications

Drug	Classification	Key Side Effects	Reversing Agent
Midazolam (Versed)	Benzodiazepine	Hypotension, sleepiness and confusion, impaired reflexes	Flumazenil (Romazicon)
Lorazepam (Ativan)	Benzodiazepine	See above	Flumazenil (Romazicon)
Diazepam (Valium)	Benzodiazepine	See above	Flumazenil (Romazicon)
Propofol (Diprivan)	Sedative	Hypotension, transient apnea	
Fentanyl (Fentanyl Citrate)	Opioid/narcotic	Respiratory depression, confusion, nausea	Naloxone (Narcan)
Mederidine (Demerol)	Opioid/narcotic	Confusion, hypotension, histamine release, nausea	Naloxone (Narcan)

Moderate (Conscious) Sedation

Without some form of sedation, many of the procedures described in this chapter, particularly intubation, bronchoscopy, and cardioversion, would be uncomfortable or even intolerable for the patient. As a result, selected medications may be administered to patients to induce a "twilight sleep" state of consciousness known as *moderate sedation*. Moderate sedation helps minimize patient discomfort during such procedures, including rapid sequence intubation.

When moderately sedated, the patient should be arousable and their respiratory drive completely intact. Once the sedation is administered, your assessment of the patient should include vital signs, cardiopulmonary and airway status, pulse oximetry, and any adverse side effects from the procedure or the medications. Hence, it is imperative that you are familiar with the most common medications used in conscious sedation and their major side effects and hazards. It is also important to note that several of the drugs used to moderately sedate patients may be reversed if unwanted side effects occur, such as respiratory depression or hypotension. **Table 18-8** summarizes medications most commonly used for moderate sedation, including the classification, key side effects, and reversing agents, if applicable.

COMMON ERRORS TO AVOID

You can improve your score by avoiding these mistakes:

- To minimize tissue trauma during intubation, never permit the tip of the stylet to extend beyond the end of an endotracheal tube.
- Never perform bronchoscopy in the presence of absolute contraindications such as refractory hypoxemia, unstable hemodynamic status, or inability to oxygenate patient.
- Never attempt potentially uncomfortable procedures such as cardioversion, chest tube insertion, or bronchoscopy unless the patient has been premedicated with a medication such as Versed to achieve moderate sedation.
- When assisting with a tracheostomy procedure, never remove the endotracheal tube until just before the insertion of the tracheostomy tube.
- Never attempt to assist with an intubation unless you have a complete intubation tray that includes a fully functional laryngoscope with multiple blades, several different-size endotracheal tubes, a stylet, suction source and catheter(s), and a device to confirm tube placement.
- Never only one means of verifying successful intubation. Instead, confirm success with at least two methods, including auscultation of the lungs and epigastric region, end-tidal capnography, colorimetry, esophageal detector device, and chest X-ray.
- Never place patients with neck trauma in a "sniffing position" for intubation.

- Never use a stylet for nasal intubation.
- Never use more than 100 joules for initial attempts at synchronized cardioversion; initial energy levels of 50 joules are appropriate for A-flutter and supraventricular tachycardia (SVT).

SURE BETS

In some situations you can be sure of the right approach to a clinical problem or scenario:

- Always announce "clear" several times and verify that no one is in contact with the patient before attempting cardioversion.
- When positioning patients for a thoracentesis procedure, always ensure that they are adequately supported in front to help prevent them from falling and being injured.
- Always confirm proper functioning of endotracheal tube cuff, pilot balloon, and valve by first inflating the cuff with a syringe prior to intubation.
- After each attempt of cardioversion, always activate "sync" mode again, in addition to selecting the appropriate change in energy level.
- Always recommend a tracheostomy for an orally intubated patient who is expected to remain mechanically ventilated for some time.
- Always recommend an immediate chest tube insertion (or needle decompression) for a patient with a tension pneumothorax.
- Always recommend the use of the correct-size endotracheal tube when assisting with intubation. In general, recommend using the following tube sizes: adult male, 8.0–9.0 mm; adult female, 7.0–8.0 mm; average 16-year-old, 7.0 mm; and a 3-year-old, 4.5 mm.
- Always suggest diagnostic ultrasound prior to a thoracentesis to determine the specific location of the fluid and to identify the ideal insertion site for the needle or catheter.
- Always closely monitor patient's vital signs, pulse oximetry, and EKG/ECG before, during, and immediately following cardioversion or bronchoscopy.
- Always monitor a patient's vital signs, pulse oximetry, and other clinical indicators during procedures such as tracheostomy, chest tube insertion, bronchoscopy, and cardioversion. If necessary, administer supplemental oxygen to address or prevent hypoxemia during or immediately following such procedures.
- Always ensure that a manual resuscitator bag-valve-mask and oxygen source are nearby in case a patient experiences severe adverse effects of procedures such as bronchoscopy, chest tube insertion, thoracentesis, or cardioversion.
- Always make sure that the patient is NPO for at least 8–12 hours prior to bronchoscopy to minimize aspiration risk.
- Always recommend that an X-ray be ordered after certain special procedures such as intubation and chest tube insertion.

PRE-TEST ANSWERS AND EXPLANATIONS

Below are this chapter's pre-test answers and explanations. Be sure to review each answer's explanation thoroughly to help you understand why it is correct. If the explanation is still unclear to you, review the chapter contents or the references and/or refer to this chapter's supplemental resources on the CD.

18-1. **Correct Answer: D.** Midazolam HCI (Versed). Benzodiazepines like midazolam (Versed) are usually recommended for the treatment of anxiety prior to and during conscious (moderate) sedation procedures. The effects of medication such as Versed are also reversible, if the need arises.

18-2. **Correct Answer: B.** II and III. During bronchoscopy, the patient's oxygenation should be monitored continuously via pulse oximeter. If desaturation occurs, the F_{IO_2} should be increased during the procedure, or the procedure can be halted and O_2 can be given through the bronchoscope's open channel.

18-3. **Correct Answer: A.** 50 joules. In accordance with AHA guidelines, the initial energy level for performing cardioversion for a patient in atrial flutter should be 50 joules. Energy levels may be increased to 100, 200, or more joules if initial attempts are unsuccessful.

18-4. **Correct Answer: C.** Sitting up and leaning slightly forward and supported in front. When helping position a conscious patient for a thoracentesis, you should sit the patient up and leaning slightly forward with adequate support in front.

18-5. **Correct Answer: B.** 7.0–7.5 mm. For adult females, an ET tube between 7.0 and 8.0 mm is usually selected. Since a 45-kg (98-lb.) woman is small, a 7.0–7.5 mm tube is generally appropriate.

18-6. **Correct Answer: C.** Performing a tracheostomy. A tracheostomy should be performed because recent weaning has been unsuccessful and it is likely that the patient will remain mechanically ventilated for some time. In addition, trachestomy tubes may actually facilitate weaning because they are much shorter than ET tubes and therefore impose less resistance on the patient during weaning.

18-7. **Correct Answer: C.** It is the primary electrical therapy for ventricular fibrillation. Cardioversion is the application of a QRS-synchronized shock to the myocardium. Synchronization helps avoid causing a cardiac arrhythmia. Cardioversion is the primary electrical therapy when the arrhythmia features distinct QRS complexes, as in all supraventricular arrhythmias and ventricular tachycardia. Generally, discharges of 50–100 joules are sufficient to restore a normal cardiac rhythm in adults. Larger energy levels generally of 360 joules are often indicated for ventricular fibrillation.

18-8. **Correct Answer: D.** The fourth or fifth intercostal space at the anterior axillary line. In most instances, a chest tube is generally inserted through the fourth or fifth intercostal space at the anterior axillary line.

18-9. **Correct Answer: A.** Open the airway, assist with a manual ventilator bag at 100% oxygen. The next immediate action should be to open the patient's airway and provide for proper oxygenation and ventilation. The patient's airway might have obstructed during the procedure due to oversedation or the patient's own anatomy.

18-10. **Correct Answer: A.** I, II, and IV. Besides auscultation of chest and stomach, other methods like observation of chest movement, tube length (cm to teeth), esophageal detection devices, capnometry, colorimetry, and fiberoptic laryngoscopy can be used to confirm ET tube position at bedside. In addition, a chest X-ray should also be ordered, which can help determine proper tube placement.

POST-TEST

A post-test for this chapter that includes automated scoring and feedback is available on the accompanying CD. Be sure to complete this additional assessment to confirm your mastery of this chapter's objectives.

REFERENCES

American Association for Respiratory Care. (1995). Clinical practice guideline. Management of airway emergencies. *Respiratory Care, 40,* 749–760.

American Association for Respiratory Care. (2004). Resuscitation and defibrillation in the health care setting. 2004 revision and update. *Respiratory Care, 49,* 1085–1099.

American Association for Respiratory Care. (2007). Clinical practice guideline. Bronchoscopy Assisting. 2007 revision and update. *Respiratory Care, 52,* 74–80.

American Heart Association. (2005). Adjuncts for airway control and ventilation. *Circulation,* 112 (Suppl I), IV: 51–57.

American Heart Association. (2005). Electrical therapies: Automated external defibrillators, defibrillation, cardioversion, and pacing. *Circulation, 112* (Suppl I) IV: 35–46.

American Society of Anesthesiologists. (2003). Practice guidelines for management of the difficult airway. *Anesthesiology, 98*, 1269–1277.

Butler, T. J. (2009). *Laboratory exercises for competency in respiratory care* (2nd ed.). Philadelphia: FA Davis.

Field, J. M., Hazinski, M. F., & Gilmore, D. (2006). *Handbook of emergency cardiovascular care*. Dallas: American Heart Association.

Irwin, R. S., Rippe, J. M., Lisbon, A., & Heard, S. O. (2008). *Intensive care medicine* (4th ed.). Philadelphia: Lippincott, Williams & Wilkins.

Wilkins, R. L., Stoller, J. K., & Kacmarek, R. M. (2009). *Fundamentals of respiratory care* (9th ed.). St. Louis: Mosby.

Initiate and Conduct Pulmonary Rehabilitation and Home Care

Kenneth A. Wyka
Albert J. Heuer

INTRODUCTION

Pulmonary rehabilitation and home care are important specialties within the respiratory care profession. However, because practice in these areas is limited, the NBRC includes only a relatively small number of related test items. Fortunately, most questions on these topics can be answered based on general clinical knowledge, much of which is covered elsewhere in this text. Here, we focus on specific skills unique to those settings that will help you do well on this section of the exam.

OBJECTIVES

After completion of this chapter, you should demonstrate the knowledge needed to:

1. Monitor and maintain home respiratory equipment
2. Explain the planned therapy and associated goals of pulmonary rehabilitation and home care to patients and their family/caregivers to achieve therapeutic outcomes
3. Educate patients and family in disease management as it pertains to pulmonary rehabilitation and home care
4. Interact with a case manager
5. Counsel both patient and family concerning smoking cessation
6. Instruct patient and family to ensure safety and infection control
7. Modify respiratory care procedure for home use
8. Qualify patients for home oxygen reimbursement
9. Properly document pulmonary rehabilitation and home care plan and outcomes

WHAT TO EXPECT ON THIS CATEGORY OF THE CRT EXAM

Number of questions: 2
Level of questions: 50% recall, 50% application

WHAT'S NEW FOR 2009

As of July 2009, this section of the NBRC CRT examination includes the following *new content areas*:

- Monitor and maintain home respiratory equipment
- Interact with a case manager
- Modify respiratory care procedures for use in home

PRE-TEST

Carefully respond to each of the following questions. After completing the pre-test, compare your answers with those provided at the end of this chapter. Then thoroughly review each answer's explanation to help understand why it is correct.

19-1. The essential goals of pulmonary rehabilitation include all of the following *except*:
  A. Improve exercise tolerance
  B. Reduce perceived dyspnea
  C. Improve health related quality of life
  D. Reverse lung damage

19-2. In order to meet the goals of pulmonary rehabilitation and return the patient to the highest level of functional capacity, all of the following approaches may be used *except*:
  A. Multidisciplinary approach
  B. Education and related counseling
  C. Mandatory participation for all COPD patients
  D. Flexible approaches to meet varied patients' needs

19-3. Pulmonary rehabilitation programs should include which of the following components:
  I. Patient education
  II. Breathing techniques and exercises
  III. Physical reconditioning
  IV. Smoking cessation and related counseling
  A. III and IV only
  B. I, II, and III
  C. II, III, and IV
  D. I, II, III, and IV

19-4. Patients in pulmonary rehabilitation can perform physical conditioning exercises safely if they exercise to what percent of their target heart rate?
  A. 50%
  B. 75%
  C. 90%
  D. 100%

19-5. What is the primary purpose of patient documentation in pulmonary rehabilitation?
  A. Demonstrate patient involvement and note outcomes
  B. Insurance reimbursement
  C. Investigative research
  D. Patient documentation is not required in pulmonary rehabilitation

19-6. Emergency situations that home mechanical ventilation caregivers must be trained to recognize and manage include all of the following *except*:
  A. Ventilator or power failure
  B. Tension pneumothorax
  C. Artificial airway obstruction
  D. Ventilator circuit problems

19-7. You have been asked to organize a patient/family education program as part of a discharge plan for a patient requiring home ventilatory support. Which of the following methods would be best for training the family in operation of the ventilator chosen?
  A. Put the patient on the selected device while still hospitalized
  B. Set up and review the ventilator after the patient gets home
  C. Show the family the ventilator in a full-day session
  D. Give the family the operating manual for the ventilator

19-8. Which of the following are acceptable indicators of hypoxemia for purposes of justifying home oxygen therapy?
  I. A resting PaO_2 of 55 torr (room air)
  II. A nocturnal fall in SaO_2 from 95% to 91%
  III. A resting arterial Hb SaO_2 of 84% (room air)
  A. I and II only
  B. II and III only
  C. I and III only
  D. I, II, and III

19-9. Basic principles of infection control in the home care setting include which of the following?

    I. Avoiding visits by friends with respiratory infections

    II. Having caregivers follow proper handwashing technique

    III. Incinerating all disposable equipment and supplies

  A. I and II only

  B. II and III only

  C. I and III only

  D. I, II, and III

19-10. In addition to counseling, all of the following prescription medications may be effective as smoking cessation aids, *except*:

  A. Buproprion SR

  B. Varenicline (Chantix)

  C. Inhaled steroids

  D. Nicotine replacement medications

WHAT YOU NEED TO KNOW: ESSENTIAL CONTENT

Pulmonary Rehabilitation

As a CRT exam candidate, you should familiarize yourself with selected aspects of pulmonary rehabilitation. These areas include the purpose and goals, patient selection, the key components of such programs, and the documentation, as outlined in several of the following sections of this chapter.

According to the American College of Chest Physicians and American Association of Cardiovascular and Pulmonary Rehabilitation, the essential therapeutic goals for pulmonary rehabilitation include:

- Improving a patient's exercise tolerance
- Reducing level of perceived dyspnea
- Improving health-related quality of life
- Reducing emergency department visits and hospital admissions
- Reducing the overall costs of health care

Consistent with these goals, the primary benefits to participants in pulmonary rehabilitation programs are increased ability to perform activities of daily living (ADLs), including daily hygiene, cooking, and possibly selected social activities. In addition, many participants report an improved sense of well-being. *However, pulmonary rehabilitation will not reverse the disease process or increase life expectancy.*

In order to meet these goals and return the patient to the highest level of functional capacity, most effective approaches to pulmonary rehabilitation use the following strategies:

- Multidisciplinary approach, including respiratory care
- Education and related counseling
- Multiple forms of treatment, including breathing retraining and physical conditioning
- Flexible specific approaches to meet the patient's varied needs
- Medical direction and involvement

Patient Selection

Impairments in the cardiopulmonary system can reduce a patient's capacity to exercise or perform physical activities in four major ways:

1. Abnormal pulmonary mechanics (changes in chest/lung compliance and airway resistance)
2. Abnormal gas exchange resulting in hypoxemia and arterial desaturation
3. Reduced cardiac output
4. Sensation or perception of dyspnea

Patients with the following chronic pulmonary diseases or conditions are candidates for pulmonary rehabilitation:

- COPD
- Asthma
- Bronchiectasis
- Cystic fibrosis
- Interstitial lung diseases, including pulmonary fibrosis and sarcoidosis
- Those undergoing lung volume reduction surgery

In terms of selection, the physician initially assesses the patient for the presence of one or more of these conditions. Patients should be further screened to verify that they are motivated to participate in their care, perhaps by pursuing a smoking cessation plan, if appropriate. Additional medical screening generally includes the following:

- Complete patient history consisting of medical and surgical history, occupational history, family history, and social activities (nicotine, alcohol, and/or drug use)
- Physical examination
- Laboratory testing (complete blood count, blood chemistry, theophylline level and alpha-1 antitrypsin titer)
- Electrocardiogram
- Arterial blood gas analysis
- Pulmonary function testing
- Chest X-ray

Cardiopulmonary Exercise Testing

In addition to these assessments, an essential aspect of enrollment screening, monitoring progress, and measuring rehabilitation outcomes is the cardiopulmonary exercise test. This testing is particularly important in patients with COPD because these patients tend to have a high degree of intolerance for physical activity due to a proportionately high CO_2 production, dyspnea, and development of respiratory acidosis. This is the most complex and important test in terms of the patient data and information. It provides for the following:

- Differentiation between pulmonary and cardiac causes of dyspnea
- Determination of the degree of oxygen desaturation that occurs with physical exertion
- Establishment of baselines for patient's levels of physical conditioning
- Determination of a patient's target heart rate, to be used in the physical reconditioning
- Enabling physicians and practitioners to follow patient progress
- Possibly excluding patients from pulmonary rehabilitation

Chapter 4 provides more detail on the indications for, procedures for performing, and interpretation of cardiopulmonary exercise tests.

Program Components

In addition to properly screening the patients, you should be familiar with the following major components of pulmonary rehabilitation programs.

Patient Education

The education component of pulmonary rehabilitation programs includes selected topics and instructional principles designed to maximize participant learning. Educational topics may relate to the basics of respiratory disease, pulmonary anatomy, respiratory medications and equipment, nutrition and hydration, and stress management. **Table 19-1** includes a listing of educational topics we recommend be covered in these programs.

Table 19-1 Educational Topics for a Pulmonary Rehabilitation Program

Topic	Key Points
Purpose of pulmonary rehabilitation and the patient's role	Return the patient to the highest level of functioning and tolerance for activities of daily living (ADLs); active participation by the patient is required to achieve goals
Cardiopulmonary anatomy and physiology	Structure of the heart and lungs and how they work
Cardiopulmonary pathophysiology	Major differences between obstructive and restrictive lung diseases
Breathing techniques and retraining	Diaphragmatic and pursed-lip breathing techniques, inspiratory resistance breathing
Stress management and relaxation	Ways to cope with stress, proper breathing techniques, and avoidance of panic breathing
Physical reconditioning	Exercises to promote agility, strength, and endurance
Cardiopulmonary pharmacology	Major cardiopulmonary medications and their effects on the body and proper use
Home care	Use and maintenance of oxygen and other respiratory care devices including small-volume nebulizers
Chest physiotherapy	Postural drainage positions and other bronchopulmonary hygiene methods
Nutrition and diet	Key elements of good nutrition, weight control, and hydration
Specific strategies for maximizing ADLs	Vocational counseling focusing on activities that promote a more active and productive lifestyle

In terms of instructional strategies useful in teaching pulmonary rehabilitation patients, we recommend that you:

- Be prepared and knowledgeable about topic(s).
- Create a comfortable learning environment.
- Encourage family and caregiver participation.
- Appeal to varied learning styles (visual, hands-on).
- Encourage questions.
- Keep sessions short, break it down into brief segments.
- Use understandable (lay) terms.
- Distribute written supplemental material.
- Reinforce concepts and follow up.

Breathing Techniques and Exercises

Breathing techniques used in pulmonary rehabilitation include pursed-lip breathing, diaphragmatic or abdominal breathing, coughing techniques, and use of breathing devices for positive expiratory pressure (PEP) therapy and sustained maximal inspiration (SMI). See **Table 19-2** for a description of the more common techniques and exercises used in pulmonary rehabilitation. In addition, Chapters 6, 11, and 12 describe several major breathing aids and coughing devices used by patients for breathing retraining.

Physical Reconditioning Exercises

Exercises used in pulmonary rehabilitation fall into three general categories. First are warmup and stretch activities, conducted before other exercises. These exercises are low stress and intended to increase blood flow and range of motion, to help prevent injury. Second are aerobic activities such as

Table 19-2 Types of Breathing Techniques and Exercises for Pulmonary Rehabilitation

Breathing Exercise	Rationale
Pursed-lip breathing	To slow rate of breathing while creating back pressure to maintain airway patency, thereby preventing airway collapse and air trapping
Diaphragmatic breathing	Abdominal muscles promote diaphragmatic excursions, producing effective ventilation and reducing use of accessory muscles
Inspiratory resistance breathing	Flow-resistive devices use inspiratory load to strengthen ventilatory muscles
Threshold loading	Threshold-loading devices use inspiratory pressure as a prescribed load to strengthen ventilatory muscles
Incentive spirometry (sustained maximum inspiration)	Inspiratory capacity maneuver with breath hold at the end of inspiration promotes lung expansion in patients with restrictive lung diseases
Glossopharyngeal	Use of glossopharyngeal muscles promotes capture and swallowing of air

walking and cycling. These exercises build up participants' endurance to perform sustained ADLs. Last are strength-building exercises such as weight lifting and calisthenics, which can increase a participant's ability to hold a given position and lift objects.

Monitoring

During physical exercises, patients should be monitored using pulse oximetry (for oxygen saturation and heart rate), respiratory rate, and blood pressure. Their overall appearance should be considered as well. Most patients will exercise at up to 75% of their target heart rate in order to achieve the optimal cardiovascular benefit. You should terminate exercises if the patient experiences angina, muscle cramps, severe fatigue, excessive dyspnea, or other signs of distress. You should provide supplemental O_2 to those patients who have demonstrated oxygen desaturation during activity or the screening exercise test. If a patient experiences severe distress, you should stop the exercise routine, monitor vital signs, and contact the physician. In life-threatening emergencies, you may need to call a "code blue." All patient responses to exercises, favorable or adverse, should be documented.

Documenting Patient Progress

Records must be maintained by both program personnel and patients. These records should document all patient activities performed, responses to these activities, and overall progress. You should document patient progress made during each session in the *Progress Notes* section of the record. In addition, some institutions have a separate section in the patient record or chart entitled *Rehabilitation* or *Pulmonary Rehabilitation*, where such progress should be recorded. You should also encourage patients to maintain a log of all exercise activities performed at home, both for progress monitoring and as a motivational tool. All medical documentation should be kept on file for medical and legal reasons and for insurance reimbursement purposes.

Smoking Cessation and Nicotine Intervention

In addition to these components of pulmonary rehabilitation, many such programs either require patients who smoke to first enroll in a smoking cessation program or prohibit active smokers from participating. In any event, smoking cessation is essential to help control disease progression and obtain the full benefits of rehabilitation. Nicotine intervention should begin with in-depth counseling using the services of a counselor where possible and should be completed before program enrollment. One of the most important factors associated with success in smoking cessation is that smokers must be highly motivated to quit. The educational component should address tobacco dependence, which is a chronic, relapsing, and life-threatening condition with a neuropathological basis that requires treatment.

Education should review the difference between nicotine addiction and habit, as well as the myriad of symptoms related to nicotine withdrawal. The actual methods of nicotine intervention may include one or more of the following approaches:

- Individual counseling
- Group sessions
- Nicotine replacement therapy (nicotine gum, patches, lozenges, and/or sprays)
- Other pharmacologic intervention such as varenicline (Chantix)
- Hypnosis
- Follow-up and long-term support

Regarding pharmacologic therapy, a variety of medications are available, many of which are summarized in **Table 19-3**.

Combinations of these medications may be used in some patients. Note that some of these medications require a physician prescription.

Relapse from smoking cessation is a relatively common problem that may be detected via counseling sessions, interviews, or carbon monoxide breath analysis. In the case of a relapse, patients should be reminded not to be too discouraged. They should also be encouraged to continue trying and informed that smokers who are motivated to quit are often eventually successful after several attempts. This is especially true if they combine several approaches such as counseling and medication.

Table 19-3 Pharmacologic Treatment for Tobacco Dependence

Drug	Precautions	Side Effects	Dosage	Recommended Duration
Varenicline (**Chantix**—prescription)	Nausea	Constipation Insomnia Headache Dry mouth	Days 1–3: 0.5 mg OD Days 4–7: 0.5 mg BID Days 8–end of therapy: 1 mg BID	12 wk
Bupropion (**Zyban**—prescription)	Seizure Eating disorders	Insomnia Dry mouth	150 mg each morning for 3 days, then 150 mg BID (begin treatment 1–2 weeks pre-quit)	7–12 wk post-quit maintenance up to 6 mo
Nicotine gum (**Nicorette**—OTC)	Dependency	Mouth soreness Dyspepsia	1–24 cigs/day: 2-mg gum (up to 24/day) 25+ cigs/day: 4-mg gum (up to 24/day)	Up to 12 wk
Nicotine inhaler (**Nicotrol**—prescription)	Dependency	Local irritation of mouth and throat	6–16 cartridges/day	Up to 6 mo
Nicotine nasal spray (**Nicotrol** NS—prescription)	Dependency	Nasal irritation	8–40 doses/day	3–6 mo
Nicotine patch (**Nicoderm** CQ—OTC only)	Dependency	Local skin reaction	21 mg/24 h 14 mg/24 h 7 mg/24 h	4 wk then 2 wk then 2 wk

Abbreviations: BID, twice daily; cigs, cigarettes; mg, milligrams; OD, once daily; OTC, over the counter; h, hours; wk, weeks.

Respiratory Home Care

According to the AARC, respiratory home care includes prescribed respiratory care services provided in a patient's personal residence. As you prepare for the CRT exam, you should review the most common home care services and modalities, including safe operation, modification and troubleshooting of equipment, as well as related documentation.

Prescribed respiratory home care services include (but are not limited to):

- Patient assessment and monitoring
- Diagnostic and therapeutic modalities and services
- Disease management
- Patient and caregiver education
- Patient follow-up

All services require a physician's written or verbal order and must be practiced under appropriate law, regulation, and medical direction. Therapeutic modalities most commonly delivered in the home environment include:

- Supplemental oxygen therapy
- Invasive and noninvasive mechanical ventilation (positive and negative pressure)
- Continuous positive airway pressure (CPAP) and bi-level positive airway pressure (BiPAP™) therapy for the treatment of sleep apnea syndromes
- Apnea monitors
- Other modalities, including aerosol therapy and secretion clearance methods

Home Oxygen Therapy

Supplemental oxygen is the most common respiratory therapy used at home. General concepts related to oxygen therapy are discussed in Chapter 6 and elsewhere in this text. However, there are some unique aspects to providing O_2 therapy at home. First, in addition to a physician's order, the patient must first qualify for health insurance reimbursement of associated costs by meeting criteria related to accepted diagnosis and blood oxygen levels (either SpO_2 or PaO_2). For many patients with COPD or other chronic pulmonary disorders, this criteria includes an SpO_2 of 88% or less, or a PaO_2 of 55 mm Hg or less on room air. However, it is slightly easier for chronic lung patients with a secondary diagnosis such as pedal edema or cor pulmonale to qualify for home oxygen with either an SpO_2 of 89% or less, or a PaO_2 of 56 to 59 mm Hg. Home oxygen therapies also differ in the types of storage and delivery systems used. In general, the following types of oxygen systems can be found in home care:

- Oxygen concentrators: electrically powered devices that use sieve beds to physically separate nitrogen from oxygen.
- Liquid oxygen system (LOX): provides storage of liquid oxygen below its critical temperature. LOX offers the advantage of storing 860 times more oxygen per unit of volume.
- High pressure cylinders: gaseous oxygen that is compressed and stored in metal cylinders. Generally, "E" cylinders are used as a backup source for stationary systems such as concentrators and "D" cylinders, or are smaller for portability.

Oxygen Concentrators

An O_2 concentrator is an electrically powered device that physically separates the O_2 in room air from nitrogen. Most concentrators use sodium-aluminum silicate pellets to absorb nitrogen, CO_2, and water vapor and produce about 90–95% O_2 at up to 10 L/min. O_2 concentrators are the most cost-efficient supply method for patients in alternative settings who need continuous low-flow O_2. When used with patients receiving low-flow O_2, concentrators are just as effective in raising blood O_2 levels as more traditional supply systems (such as 100% cylinder gas with a cannula).

Liquid Oxygen Systems

Because 1 cubic foot of liquid O_2 equals 860 cubic feet of gas, liquid O_2 systems can store large quantities of O_2 in small spaces. These systems consist of a reservoir unit similar in design to a Thermos bottle. The inner container of liquid O_2 is suspended in an outer container, with a vacuum in between. The liquid O_2 is kept at approximately –300°F. When flow is turned on, O_2 passes through a vaporizing coil, where it is warmed and thus converted to a gaseous state. It then leaves the system through an outlet, where it is metered by a flow control valve.

Depending on manufacturer and model, small liquid O_2 cylinders hold between 45 and 100 pounds of liquid O_2. To calculate a liquid O_2 system's duration of flow, you should first convert the weight of liquid O_2 in pounds to the equivalent volume of gaseous O_2 in liters. At normal liquid cylinder operating pressures, 1 pound of liquid O_2 equals approximately 344 liters of gaseous O_2. Because of the extremely low temperature of liquid O_2, patients and caregivers must be extremely careful when refilling these portable systems.

Compressed Oxygen Cylinders

The primary use of compressed O_2 cylinders in home care and other alternative settings is either for ambulation (small cylinders) or as a backup to liquid or concentrator supply systems (H/K cylinders). In addition to the cylinder gas, a pressure-reducing valve with a metering device is needed to deliver O_2 at the prescribed flow. Standard clinical flow meters deliver flows up to 15 L/min; flows used in alternative settings are typically in the 0.25–4.0 L/min range.

Portable Oxygen Systems

Portable oxygen systems are generally used as a complement to a stationary O_2 system. They include smaller cylinders such as M-6/B, M-9/C, and D cylinders, refillable portable liquid units, and portable concentrators.

Flow durations for the M-6/B, M-9/C, and D cylinders are computed the same as for larger cylinders (refer to Chapter 6). **Table 19-4** provides the factors needed to compute the duration of flow for small cylinders filled to +10% of their service pressures, as well as example calculations for various flows.

Portable LOX units are filled at the in-home reservoir and can provide 5–8 hours of O_2 at 2 L/min. Portable concentrators typically can provide 90% O_2 for 2–3 hours on battery power, which can be recharged in about 3 hours. These units can also run continuously on either AC or 12-volt DC power.

Oxygen Appliances

The appliances of choice for home O_2 therapy are either simple low-flow devices or oxygen-conserving systems. Reservoir masks or other appliances designed to provide high O_2 concentrations are usually not used in the home care setting. High-flow systems may be used, but primarily for delivery of bland aerosols (covered subsequently).

Table 19-4 Duration of Flow in Hours for Full Portable O_2 Cylinders

L/min	Cylinder (Factor)			
	M-6/B (.07)	M-9/C (.11)	D (.16)	E (.28)
.5	5.5	8.2	13.8	22.7
.75	3.6	5.5	9.2	15.2
1.0	2.7	4.1	6.9	11.4
1.5	1.8	2.8	4.6	7.6
2.0	1.4	2.1	3.5	5.7
2.5	1.1	.7	2.8	4.5
3.0	0.9	1.4	2.3	3.8
3.5	0.8	1.2	2.0	3.2
4.0	0.7	1.0	1.7	2.8

The most common low-flow device used at home is the nasal cannula. In the home settings these devices generally are used at flows less than 4 L/min, so that the gas need not be humidified. Flows for infants being managed at home should be limited to no more than 2 L/min. The transtracheal catheter has been used as an alternative low-flow device. It offers the advantages of improved cosmetic appearance and lower flows to achieve the same therapeutic effect, while conserving O_2 and/or extending the available duration of flow. However, because insertion requires a surgical procedure, stoma complications such as pain, bleeding, or infection or abscess can occur. In addition, transtracheal catheters often become dislodged or obstructed. Due to the potential problems associated with this therapy, it is generally reserved for patients who meet one or more of the following criteria:

- Cannot be adequately oxygenated with standard therapy
- Do not comply when using other devices
- Experience complications from nasal cannula use
- Prefer the cosmetic appearance
- Need increased mobility

Other methods for conserving O_2 and extending its use time include pulse-dose and demand-flow delivery devices. As described in Chapter 6, these devices use either an electronic or pneumatic trigger mechanism to sense the user's breathing effort and deliver O_2 flow during inspiration. Some of these systems deliver a set bolus of O_2 early in inspiration only, while others deliver gas until the demand valve closes at the end of inspiration. These devices can be used with compressed gas cylinders, LOX systems, and O_2 concentrators. Indeed, most portable LOX systems and concentrators now include this conserving function as a built-in feature. Unfortunately, the performance of pulse-dose and demand-flow O_2 devices vary substantially, providing arterial oxygenation comparable to a nasal cannula at anywhere from a third to a sixth of the O_2 usage. Due to these performance variations, the only way to determine the appropriate flow setting is to adjust it under the conditions of use until the desired SpO_2 is achieved. In terms of troubleshooting these systems, you always should teach patients who suspect a problem to switch to a backup supply of continuous O_2 via nasal cannula at the equivalent liter flow (usually 2–4 L/min) until technical support can be provided.

Selecting and Recommending a Delivery System

Certain clinical scenarios regarding home oxygen systems commonly appear in some form on the CRT exam. For example, you should remember that a patient with restricted activity may be most suitable for an oxygen concentrator and a gaseous cylinder for backup. In contrast, it may be more appropriate to recommend a liquid system that is refillable and portable for an ambulatory patient. If such a patient is especially active or mobile, then the addition of a conserving device such as a demand-flow or pulse-dose unit should be considered.

Home Oxygen Troubleshooting and Modification

Another important aspect in home oxygen therapy involves equipment troubleshooting and modification. As such, related questions may appear in some form on the CRT exam. **Table 19-5** summarizes the most common problems encountered with home oxygen systems, as well as the recommended corrective actions or modifications.

Home Mechanical Ventilation

Whereas O_2 therapy is by far the most common respiratory modality used at home, mechanical ventilation is the most complex. While most patients are weaned from mechanical ventilation in either an acute care hospital or long-term facility, some ventilator-dependent patients are discharged to the home setting. Many of these patients have underlying cardiopulmonary conditions such as COPD or compromised cardiac status, while others may have been diagnosed with neuromuscular diseases or have sustained spinal cord trauma. In preparing for the CRT exam, you should keep in mind the following goals, patient characteristics, and contraindications.

Table 19-5 Basic Home Oxygen Troubleshooting

Type of O₂ System	Problem	Corrective Action/Modification
Concentrator	Machine won't turn on	Check electric power source including plug and circuit breaker. If power source is ok, place patient on backup gaseous system, as appropriate, and replace concentrator.
	Analyzed F$_{IO_2}$ is less than 85–90% or manufacturer's specifications	Sodium-aluminum silicate canisters are likely exhausted. Place patient on backup gaseous system, as appropriate, and replace concentrator.
	Patient on nasal cannula at 4 L/min or more complains of nasal dryness	Add a bubble humidifier.
Liquid	Liquid tank is making a slight intermittent hissing sound	Faint hissing can occasionally be heard from stationary liquid O₂ systems due to normal venting. It is likely that no action is needed, except to keep the tank upright.
	Liquid tank is making a very loud and constant hissing sound, and a steady stream of "mist" can be seen coming from the tank	Loud and constant hissing suggests a problem with liquid systems. Place the patient on backup oxygen and replace the liquid system.
Gaseous tanks	The oxygen regulator is turned on, but no oxygen is coming out	Either tank has not been turned on or it is empty. If no flow occurs with both tank and regulator turned on, replace tank.

Goals of home mechanical ventilation:
- Sustain and extend life
- Enhance the quality of life
- Reduce morbidity
- Improve or sustain physical and psychological function of all ventilator-dependent individuals and enhance growth and development in pediatric patients
- Provide cost-effective care

Prerequisites for patient discharge to the home:
- Patient and caregiver desire to go home.
- Patient is clinically stable for at least 2 weeks.
- Patient has been on continuous ventilation for at least 30 days with unsuccessful weaning.
- Patient is free of cardiac monitoring.
- Patient has a tracheostomy in place, unless using noninvasive ventilation.
- Patient demonstrates control of any seizure activity with medication protocol as prescribed.
- Patient is free of IV medications of an acute care nature such as vasodilators or beta-blockers.
- Family members and/or caregivers are willing and capable to accept home care responsibility.
- Patient has had a complete medical and financial assessment by the case manager (post acute).

As noted above, patients being considered for home mechanical ventilation must be clinically stable and have adequate caregiver support. In general, patients should *not* be considered for home ventilatory support if:

- They require more than 40% O₂ or more than 10 cm H₂O PEEP.
- They need continuous invasive monitoring.
- Their tracheostomy is still fresh (for invasive support only).
- The home physical environment is deemed unsafe by the discharge team.

Home environmental issues include fire, health, or safety hazards; unsanitary conditions; and inadequate heating, ventilation, or electrical service.

The choice of home care ventilator is based on a patient's clinical needs and available resources. The key patient factor is type of airway, i.e., tracheostomy or intact upper airway. For patients with trach tubes requiring continuous support, the common choice is an electrically powered, volume-cycled ventilator that uses a single-limb circuit. For patients with an intact upper airway who need only intermittent support (e.g., at night), electrically powered, pressure-limited ventilators with noninvasive interfaces are most common. Patients who would otherwise be suited for noninvasive positive pressure ventilation but object to mask or mouthpiece interfaces may be considered for negative pressure ventilation, usually via a chest cuirass or "pneumosuit."

Positive pressure ventilators for home use should:

- Be electrically powered with battery backup.
- Be simple, easy to use, and reliable.
- Provide a wide range of respiratory rates.
- Ensure accurate delivery of tidal volumes or pressures.
- Provide a range of modes, including assist/control, SIMV, PSV, and CPAP.
- Provide adequate humidification of inspired gas.
- Have variable flows.
- Allow variable F_{IO_2} (generally via an adjustable bleed-in port).
- Incorporate appropriate alarms:
  ○ Mandatory disconnect (low-pressure or low-volume) and high-pressure alarms
  ○ Remote and secondary (e.g., apnea monitor) disconnect alarms for high-risk patients

Additional considerations for home care ventilation include the following:

- A backup ventilator should be available for patients who:
  ○ Cannot maintain spontaneous ventilation for 4 or more consecutive hours
  ○ Live in an area where a replacement ventilator cannot be provided within 2 hours
- Caring for a ventilator-dependent patient in the home is a labor-intensive undertaking and involves extensive education and training for the family and/or caregivers, including infection control measures.
- Additional equipment needed may include hospital bed, supplemental oxygen, suction equipment, and related supplies.
- Arrangements must be in place for emergency situations, including power outages.

The NBRC will also expect you to be able to address common problems encountered during home care ventilatory support. While aspects of ventilator troubleshooting are covered elsewhere in this text, the most common problems and corrective actions or modifications specific to home ventilation are summarized in **Table 19-6**.

Nasal Continuous Positive Airway Pressure (CPAP)

Nasal CPAP is a relatively common form of respiratory therapy used in the home to treat sleep apnea–hypopnea syndrome (SAHS). With proper use, CPAP can dramatically lessen or resolve the many problems associated with SAHS, such as morning headaches, daytime hypersomnolence, and cognitive impairment. As a result, this therapy can enhance the patient's quality of life and may also lessen the incidence of more severe complications, such as systemic and pulmonary hypertension. For Medicare reimbursement, the sleep apnea diagnosis must be confirmed by polysomnography.

A CPAP setup consists of a flow generator, circuit, a patient interface (e.g., nasal mask, nasal pillows), and headgear. Most systems provide for pressures that may be adjusted to the 20–30 cm H_2O range. As discussed in Chapter 4, the optimal pressure is normally determined by a CPAP titration study. Many units now have a ramp feature that gradually raises the pressure to the prescribed level over a time interval. This helps some patients fall asleep and may increase therapy compliance.

A variation of nasal CPAP is BiPAP™. Whereas CPAP uses a single pressure level, BiPAP™ uses both an IPAP (inspiratory positive airway pressure) and an EPAP (expiratory positive airway pressure).

Table 19-6 Home Ventilator Troubleshooting

Problem	Corrective Action/Modification
Machine won't turn on	Ensure adequate ventilation and use backup ventilator or manual resuscitator bag, as appropriate; then check power source such as plug and circuit breaker
Ventilator-dependent patient lives in a rural area with frequent power outages	Ensure that utility company is notified in writing that a patient is on such equipment and that a backup power source such as a generator is in place
Caregiver can't immediately fix an alarm and patient appears to be in distress	Remove patient from ventilator, use backup ventilator or manual resuscitator bag as needed, and call 911; consider CPR as appropriate
Patient with tracheostomy is in distress; patient removed from the ventilator but extreme resistance is felt when manually ventilating	Call 911, attempt to pass suction catheter, and then resume manual ventilation with 100% FIO_2; consider CPR as appropriate
Patient on pressure-limited ventilation objects to the discomfort of the nasal mask	Consider different interface such as nasal pillows or recommend a negative-pressure ventilator

In other patients, the difference in IPAP and EPAP aids the patient's inspiratory effort, thus improving ventilation. BiPAP™ may also increase patient comfort and therefore improve patient compliance.

Although CPAP is an effective treatment for sleep apnea, there are several problems associated with this therapy that warrant corrective action or modification, as summarized in **Table 19-7**.

Other Respiratory Home Equipment and Modalities

In addition to home oxygen, mechanical ventilation, and CPAP therapy, there are other respiratory modalities that may be used in the home and therefore may appear on the CRT exam. They include apnea monitoring and aerosol therapy, as well as airway care and secretion clearance methods.

Apnea Monitoring

Apnea monitoring warns caregivers of certain cardiopulmonary life-threatening events; most notably cessation of breathing. The primary indication for home apnea monitoring is for neonates at risk of

Table 19-7 Problems Associated with CPAP and Corrective Action

Problem	Corrective Action/Modification
Patient complains of overall discomfort from excessive flow and noise	Use ramp feature to gradually build up to prescribed pressure
Skin irritation or excessive pressure from mask or other interface	Use different interface (mask or nasal pillows), adjust straps on headgear, and ensure proper cleaning of interface and headgear
Conjunctivitis	Adjust interface to eliminate leak around eyes
Epistaxis (nosebleed) or excessive nasal dryness	Add a humidifier or use room vaporizer
Inability to maintain adequate pressure	Check circuit connections for leak, use a chin strap to prevent pressure loss through mouth, use a different interface

recurrent apnea, bradycardia, and hypoxemia after hospital discharge. Other conditions that may require home apnea monitoring include:

- Infants receiving aminophylline or caffeine therapy for a history of apnea and bradycardia
- Infants with bronchopulmonary dysplasia requiring O_2 therapy, CPAP, or ventilatory support
- Infants with gastroesophageal reflux (GER) if symptomatic with color and tone change
- Infants of substance-abusing mothers if clinically symptomatic
- Infants with a tracheostomy or anatomic abnormalities at risk for airway compromise
- Infants with neurologic or metabolic disorders affecting respiratory control

Older children and adults may also require apnea monitoring, in particular those who are ventilator dependent, have conditions affecting regulation of breathing, or have symptomatic chronic lung disease. In addition, some patients are monitored for apnea at home because they are receiving patient-controlled analgesia agents that are respiratory suppressants.

Most apnea monitors detect both respirations and heart rate and activate audio and visual alarms when preset high or low limits are reached. In addition to the monitor, the equipment setup includes a patient cable, lead wires, and electrodes that are located on the infant's chest and abdomen. When setting up a baby on a monitor, pay particular attention to properly placing electrodes to avoid irritating the infant's skin. All connections should be checked to minimize false alarms.

The best home apnea monitoring programs and protocols involve a multidisciplinary team effort that integrates medical, educational, technical, psychosocial, and community support both before and after discharge. Key elements of this effort that should be considered prior to discharge include:

- A family conference to discuss ongoing management and 24-hour monitoring
- Emergency procedures, including CPR for parents and caregivers
- Notification and communication with primary caregiver
- Monitor setup, including electrode placement, cable and wire connections, and alarm settings
- Alarm evaluation and response
- Monitor troubleshooting
- Psychosocial support, including social services involvement, as appropriate
- Home care company contact information for questions and equipment ordering

You will need to confirm the monitoring competencies via return demonstration and reinforced, as necessary. These competencies and additional considerations are:

- Position the baby on the side or back, on a firm, flat surface when sleeping.
- Respond to all monitor alarms by:
    ○ Initially assessing the infant
    ○ Determining if real or false alarm
    ○ Responding to real alarm as appropriate (initially stimulate the baby)
    ○ Responding to false alarm by troubleshooting electrodes and wire connections
- Keep baby on the monitor at all times, except as instructed (e.g., during bathing).
- Keep the monitor plugged into a grounded outlet and use internal battery only for necessary travel (to physician's office) or during power outages.
- Do not use extension cords.
- Display CPR guidelines and emergency phone number near crib and telephone.
- Do not attempt to alter alarm settings or to reduce audible alarm.
- Ensure that there is an extra set of electrodes and lead wires.
- Disposable electrodes should be left in place no more than 2 days.
- The electrode belt, if in use, should be repositioned daily.
- Do not apply oils or lotions to electrode site.

In addition, you should anticipate and address the following post-discharge considerations:

- Family/caregivers' competency and confidence with all procedures
- Family/caregivers' stress level, coping mechanisms, and need for community resources
- Ongoing insurance/payer eligibility and related issues
- Active phone service and e-mail service
- Notification of utility company(s) and paramedics

Follow-up visits by a therapist are frequent at first, but become less needed as the family becomes skilled with the equipment and alarm responses. Some models record alarm events and can be useful to monitor the patient's progress. Event-storing monitors generally require periodic data downloading during follow-up visits. Apnea monitoring is usually discontinued after an infant demonstrates a negative pneumocardiogram or when apnea data logs reveal no events during a prescribed time frame. In general, most infants discharged with apnea monitors use them for 2–4 months.

Bland Aerosol Therapy

Bland aerosols may be used at home to help overcome a humidity deficit. This therapy may be provided continuously, for spontaneously breathing patients with a tracheostomy, or intermittently, as for patients with cystic fibrosis who may have difficulty clearing thick secretions. The aerosol can be produced by either an ultrasonic or a jet nebulizer. If using a jet nebulizer, a 50-psi air compressor is also required. Supplemental O_2 may be "bled in" from a concentrator or liquid supply system.

The major problem is infection from contaminated equipment. To reduce the incidence of infection, equipment and patient delivery systems must be cleaned and changed every 24 hours. Disinfection procedures are discussed in Chapter 7.

Aerosol Drug Administration

As in the acute care setting, the inhalation route can be used for drug administration to home care patients. Aerosol drugs commonly include adrenergic bronchodilators, anticholinergic agents, and anti-inflammatory drugs. Most inhaled drugs are available in either metered-dose inhaler (MDI) or dry powder inhaler (DPI) form. However, if these delivery methods are not feasible, the caregiver can use a small-volume nebulizer (SVN) powered by a low-output compressor. Note that Medicare limits reimbursement for home use of SVN/compressor systems by (1) requiring a certificate of medical necessity and (2) capping rental costs. Consequently, the reimbursable expenses for home aerosol drug administration are limited.

Airway Care and Secretion Clearance

Home care patients with tracheostomies require both daily stoma care and tracheobronchial suctioning. Tracheostomy care can be provided by most trained caregivers, but tube changes should only be performed by the patient's nurse, physician, or respiratory therapist.

As described in Chapters 6 and 11, tracheobronchial suctioning is accomplished using a portable electrically powered suction pump with collection bottle and suction tubing. In accordance with the AARC Clinical Practice Guideline for suctioning of the patient at home, some patients can be taught to suction themselves. However, it is more common to train caregivers on proper suctioning procedures. Daily maintenance and cleaning are a must. To help control home care supply costs, it is not uncommon for a single suction catheter to be used for 24 hours and then discarded. To prevent bacterial growth, catheters are placed in a disinfecting solution such as hydrogen peroxide or 2.5% acetic acid between suctioning attempts.

Secretion clearance methods available for patients with intact upper airways are also described in Chapter 11. These methods, which can be taught to home care patients and their caregivers, include directed coughing and postural drainage, percussion, and vibration. Additional assistance with secretion clearance, particularly useful for patients living alone, can be provided by mechanical adjuncts such as PEP devices, the flutter valve, and the high-frequency chest compression vest. Cough-assist devices such as the mechanical in-exsufflator also are gaining more widespread acceptance at home.

Infection Control

Chapter 7 covers the main infection control principles in respiratory therapy. In addition, you will need to consider these specific issues relating to infection control in the home setting, and you should cover them thoroughly when educating home care patients and their caregivers.

- Friends or relatives with respiratory infections should be discouraged from visiting the patient.
- Proper handwashing or disinfecting lotions should be applied to the hands before and after handling patients or home respiratory equipment.

- Disinfection of most home respiratory supplies such as nebulizers, humidifiers, and connectors may be achieved in the following manner:
  - First wash them with soap and warm water.
  - Soak them in a 50-50 solution of white vinegar and water for a minimum of 30 minutes.
  - Rinse them with water.
  - Leave them to air dry on a clean surface.
- Standard precautions, including gloves and eye/facial protection, should be used as appropriate.
- Sterile water should be used in large-volume nebulizers, although distilled water is acceptable for humidifiers.
- Wherever practical, disposable equipment (ventilator circuits) should be used.
- Nondisposable equipment should be scrubbed to remove organic material, then thoroughly washed, rinsed, and allowed to air-dry in a clean location.

Education of the Home Care Patient and Family/Caregivers

Regardless of type of equipment used, the family and caregivers must be educated on its safe application and maintenance, basic troubleshooting, and cleaning and disinfection. In providing this instruction, you should follow the general principles previously noted in the rehabilitation section of this chapter. In addition, the following education strategies apply in the home setting:

- Limit educational sessions to about one hour or less to avoid "information overload."
- Demonstrate the procedure(s) thoroughly.
- Ensure that the family and caregivers give a proper return demonstration for all procedures.
- Ensure that emergency procedures, such as power outages and patient emergencies, are adequately covered.
- Leave printed "EZ read" information about the procedures.
- Document all aspects of the education session(s) in the patient record.
- Follow up to reinforce material, as appropriate.

Beyond general educational strategies and principles, there are a variety of topics for which you should provide family and caregivers education. While some of these topics, such as infection control, are more general and apply to most respiratory modalities used in the home, others are more specific to the type of therapy. **Table 19-8** lists general home educational topics for which you should provide patient and caregiver instruction, as well as examples of specific topics for the most common home care modalities, including oxygen, mechanical ventilation, CPAP therapy, and apnea monitoring.

Interacting with the Case Manager

The intricacies of today's health care system and the complexities of patients and therapy often dictate that there be a case manager. The case manager is generally a clinician working for a health care facility or insurance provider, responsible for ensuring an appropriate care plan to optimize treatment outcomes and avoid unnecessary delays in discharge planning. In order to effectively interact with the case manager and other health care professionals such as physicians, you need to possess the following attributes:

- Professional appearance, vocabulary, and attitude
- Effective verbal and written communication skills
- Outstanding clinical and technical skills
- Strong team orientation
- Efficient use of time
- Effective organizational skills
- Outstanding follow-up abilities

In addition, there are common themes that are often the focus of the communication between you and the case manager. You can optimize your interaction with the case manager and contribution to achieving positive patient outcomes by being as knowledgeable as possible about the patient's

Table 19-8 Instructional Topics for Respiratory Home Care

Modality	Topic
General	Safe and effective use of equipment
	Basic equipment troubleshooting
	Equipment cleaning and disinfection
	Emergency procedures
	How to order supplies
	How to contact the home care company
Home oxygen	Posting "No Smoking" signs and ensuring that smoking is not allowed where O_2 is in use
	Avoiding trip/fall hazards from oxygen tubing
	Proper use of backup oxygen (gas cylinders)
	O_2 cylinders should be secured in carts/racks and never kept in closed spaces such as closets
Home mechanical ventilation	Basic response to ventilator alarms
	Basic airway clearance and maintenance (if trach in place)
	Use of backup ventilator and AMBU bag
CPAP and BiPAP™	Adjusting mask, nasal pillows, or other interface to ensure a proper fit and comfort
	Measures that may increase patient tolerance such as humidification and "ramp" feature
Apnea monitors	Infant CPR review and emergency procedures
	Responding to monitor alarms and troubleshooting

condition as well as by trying to anticipate specific topics that may arise during such encounters. These topics may include:

- Patient's diagnoses and chief complaints
- Initial therapy and clinical indications
- Modifications to therapy and justifications
- Ethical, cultural, and religious considerations
- Resuscitation status (full-code versus DNR)
- Patient's readiness for discharge
- Barriers to discharge, such as caregiver limitations
- Most suitable setting to which patient should be discharged
- Equipment and modalities the patient will need once discharged
- Reimbursement for equipment and procedures

Documentation

The documentation for home care is similar in some respects to that in other settings such as acute care in that a physician's order must be verified and a care plan should be devised (in conjunction with the case manager, as appropriate). In addition, all therapy and diagnostic procedures should be recorded along with the extent to which the patient tolerated such interventions. Furthermore, the extent to which the patient understood the education and tolerated the therapy should be noted in the *Progress Notes* or similar section of the patient record. However, the following are some unique aspects that apply to documentation for home care patients.

- Home care treatment plan: documents the assessment, outlines goals and therapies.
- Ongoing assessment form: provides a regular summary regarding the patient's clinical status, equipment functioning and cleanliness, as well as modifications to goals and therapies.
- A certificate of medical necessity: documents that a patient has met the qualifications for reimbursement of home oxygen, as previously mentioned in this chapter.
- Patient education checklists: may be used both as teaching tools and to document that the patient was properly instructed on all respiratory modalities.
- Assignment of benefits form: patient authorization for the home care company to receive direct reimbursement from third-party insurance payers for equipment and services.
- Discharge summary: describes the course of therapy and final status of goal attainment.

COMMON ERRORS TO AVOID

You can improve your score by avoiding these mistakes:

- Never explain planned goals and activities associated with pulmonary rehabilitation to the patient in highly technical or "textbook" terms. Instead, use understandable terms.
- Never inform a patient that pulmonary rehabilitation reverses the underlying disease process. Instead, communicate the essential aim of returning the patient to the highest functional capacity.
- Remember that pulmonary rehabilitation patients will never realize improvement in their pulmonary function but will tend to experience a greater level of activity.
- Participants in pulmonary rehabilitation should not just attend regularly scheduled classes. They also need to participate actively by exercising at home in accordance with their plan and maintaining a log or diary of activity.
- Avoid harsh criticism of patients who relapse from smoking cessation.
- Home oxygen instructions should never include how to change the flow. Such changes require a physician's order.
- Sterile water is not needed for most home care humidifiers. Distilled water is generally adequate.
- Sterilization is generally not needed for infection control in the home setting.
- To deliver an F_{IO_2} greater than 0.21, most home ventilators bleed in oxygen from a concentrator or liquid system.
- Never set up highly active oxygen-dependent patients on a concentrator, which is more suitable for those with restricted activity.

SURE BETS

In some situations you can be sure of the right approach to a clinical problem or scenario:

- Always use the cardiopulmonary exercise stress test to screen patients for pulmonary rehabilitation.
- Always have patients in pulmonary rehabilitation warm up before performing strengthening and aerobic activities to help avoid injury.
- The physical reconditioning component of pulmonary rehabilitation should always include aerobic and strength-training exercises.
- Always encourage patients in a smoking cessation program ("stay strong and don't get discouraged") and consider multiple approaches such as medication (buproprion SR, varenicline Chantix, nicotine replacement) and counseling.
- Patients enrolled in pulmonary rehabilitation will almost always experience a reduction in respiratory symptoms, increased exercise tolerance, and fewer hospitalizations.
- Patients with a pulse oximetry reading of less than 88% or a Pa_{O_2} of less than 55 mm Hg will generally always qualify for home oxygen therapy through Medicare and most other health payers.
- Always consider recommending oxygen conserving devices for highly active patients; however, those with limited mobility should generally be set up on a stationary system using an oxygen concentrator.
- Always supply a backup system for home oxygen and ventilator-dependent patients.

- Education of home oxygen patients should always focus on safe use, maintenance, cleaning, and fire precautions.
- During a home visit, always check the equipment's functioning and cleanliness, determine the patient's compliance with therapy, assess the patient, and modify goals as necessary.

PRE-TEST ANSWERS AND EXPLANATIONS

Below are this chapter's pre-test answers and explanations. Be sure to review each answer's explanation thoroughly to help you understand why it is correct. If the explanation is still unclear to you, review the chapter contents or the references and/or refer to this chapter's supplemental resources on the CD.

19-1. **Correct Answer: D.** Reverse lung damage. The goals of pulmonary rehabilitation include improving exercise tolerance, enhancing health-related quality of life, and reducing perceived dyspnea in participants. The goals do not include reversing lung damage.

19-2. **Correct Answer: C.** Mandatory participation for all COPD patients. The goals of pulmonary rehabilitation, which include returning the patient to the highest level of functional capacity, may be achieved by using a multidisciplinary approach, education and related counseling, as well as flexible approaches to meet varied patients' needs, but not through mandatory participation.

19-3. **Correct Answer: D.** I, II, III, and IV. Pulmonary rehabilitation programs will include patient education, breathing retraining, physical reconditioning, and smoking cessation and counseling. All of these areas are essential to the scope of practice as delineated for pulmonary rehabilitation.

19-4. **Correct Answer: B.** 75%. In order to achieve cardiovascular benefit and improvement during physical reconditioning, patients should safely exercise to 75% of their target heart rate. Working at levels less than this do not result in any significant improvement, and working at levels greater than this places the patient at risk for cardiovascular consequences.

19-5. **Correct Answer: A.** Demonstrate patient involvement and note outcomes. The other responses are valid but not the primary reason for documenting patient activity and response.

19-6. **Correct Answer: B.** Tension pneumothorax. Emergency situations that caregivers must be trained to recognize and properly deal with include ventilator or power failure, ventilator circuit problems, airway emergencies, and cardiac arrest.

19-7. **Correct Answer: A.** Put the patient on the selected device while still hospitalized. Ideally, the patient should be placed on the actual ventilator that will be used in the home setting before discharge.

19-8. **Correct Answer: C.** I and III only. The threshold for qualifying for oxygen therapy under Medicare is a resting PaO_2 of 55 torr or less or an SaO_2 of 88% or less for a single pulmonary diagnosis (COPD), or a PaO_2 between 56 and 59 torr or an SaO_2 of 89% with a secondary diagnosis (COPD and cor pulmonale).

19-9. **Correct Answer: A.** I and II only. Basic principles of infection control in the home care setting include: (1) proper handwashing technique by all caregivers; (2) discouraging visits to the patient from friends or relatives with respiratory infections; (3) proper cleaning and disinfection of all permanent equipment; and (4) NOT recycling disposable or single-patient use equipment on multiple patients.

19-10. **Correct Answer: C.** Inhaled steroids. Varenicline (Chantix), clonidine (Catapres), and buproprion SR are all medications that may be of help to those attempting to quit smoking. Inhaled steroids have no effect on smoking cessation efforts.

POST-TEST

A post-test for this chapter that includes automated scoring and feedback is available on the accompanying CD. Be sure to complete this additional assessment to confirm your mastery of this chapter's objectives.

REFERENCES

American Association for Respiratory Care. (2001). Clinical practice guideline. Exercise testing for evaluation of hypoxemia and/or desaturation. 2001 revision and update. *Respiratory Care, 46,* 514–522.

American Association for Respiratory Care. (2002). Clinical practice guideline. Pulmonary rehabilitation. *Respiratory Care, 47,* 617–625.

American Association for Respiratory Care. (2007). Long-term invasive mechanical ventilation in the home. 2007 revision and update. *Respiratory Care, 52,* 1056–1062.

American Association for Respiratory Care. (2007). Oxygen therapy in the home or alternate site health care facility. 2007 revision and update. *Respiratory Care, 52,* 1063–1068.

Butler, T. J. (2009). *Laboratory exercises for competency in respiratory care* (2nd ed.). Philadelphia: FA Davis.

Kasmarek, R. M., Dimas, S., & Mack, C. W. (2005). *The essentials of respiratory care* (4th ed.). St. Louis: Elsevier.

Ries, A. L., Bauldoff, G. S., Carlin, B. W., et al. (2007). Pulmonary rehabilitation: Joint ACCP/AACVPR evidence-based clinical practice guidelines. *Chest, 131* (5 Suppl), 4S–42S.

Wilkins, R. L., Stoller, J. K., & Kacmarek, R. M. (2009). *Fundamentals of respiratory care* (9th ed.). St. Louis: Mosby.

Wyka, K. A., Mathews, P. J., & Clark, W. F. (2002). *Foundations of respiratory care.* Albany: Delmar.

Perform Cardiopulmonary Calculations

Craig L. Scanlan

The CRT Exam does not have a separate major section on performing cardiopulmonary calculations. Instead, common calculations are embedded throughout the test, only being explicitly identified in subsections I-B-9-k (perform cardiopulmonary calculations) and III-A-1-b-2 (verify computations and note erroneous data). On average, you can expect 3–8 questions on the CRT Exam that require you to perform calculations.

Why then do we provide a whole chapter on this topic? The answer is simple. In our experience, too many candidates simply "write off" these questions, assuming that without access to a calculator they will get most of them wrong. As we have previously demonstrated, giving up on any CRT Exam questions simply lowers your probability of passing. Even if you lack confidence in your math skills, you simply cannot afford to concede any questions involving computations. The good news is that the computations you will likely encounter on the CRT Exam are predictable and relatively simple. With the preparation and practice we provide here, you should be able to score well on these items.

OBJECTIVES

After completion of this chapter, you should demonstrate the knowledge needed to:

- Perform cardiopulmonary calculations
- Verify computations

WHAT TO EXPECT ON THIS CATEGORY OF THE CRT EXAM

Number of questions: on average, you can expect 3–8 questions on the CRT Exam that require you to perform calculations or verify computations.

PRE-TEST

Carefully respond to each of the following questions. After completing the pre-test, compare your answers with those provided at the end of this chapter. Then thoroughly review each answer's explanation to help understand why it is correct.

20-1. A patient has a minute volume of 8.25 L/min and is breathing at a rate of 22/min. What is his average tidal volume?
  A. 182 mL
  B. 375 mL
  C. 275 mL
  D. 435 mL

20-2. A 5 foot 4 inch tall 110 lb woman with normal lungs has a tidal volume of 480 mL and is breathing at a rate of 14/min. What is her approximate alveolar ventilation?
  A. 6.72 L/min
  B. 3.42 L/min
  C. 5.18 L/min
  D. 15.4 L/min

20-3. A 150 lb patient has a tidal volume of 600 mL, an arterial P_{CO_2} (P_{aCO_2}) of 50 torr and a mixed expired P_{CO_2} (P_{ECO_2}) of 35 torr. What is the patient's physiologic deadspace?
  A. 200 mL
  B. 300 mL
  C. 180 mL
  D. 350 mL

20-4. A patient breathing 100% at sea level has a P_{aO_2} of 350 torr and a P_{aCO_2} of 40 torr. What is her A-a gradient or $P_{(A-a)O_2}$?
  A. 663 torr
  B. 363 torr
  C. 563 torr
  D. 313 torr

20-5. A patient receiving volume-limited ventilation with a tidal volume of 600 mL and 10 cm H_2O PEEP has a peak pressure of 45 cm H_2O and a plateau pressure of 30 cm H_2O. What is her static compliance?
  A. 13 mL/cm H_2O
  B. 15 mL/cm H_2O
  C. 20 mL/cm H_2O
  D. 30 mL/cm H_2O

20-6. A patient has a TLC of 5500 mL, a VC of 4000 mL, and an IC of 3000 mL. What is his functional residual capacity (FRC)?
  A. 2500 mL
  B. 1500 mL
  C. 1000 mL
  D. 7000 mL

20-7. A patient has a peak expiratory flow rate (PEFR) of 5.2 L/sec before bronchodilator treatment and 6.3 L/sec after treatment. What percent change in PEFR occurred?
  A. 8%
  B. 17%
  C. 21%
  D. 26%

20-8. A patient has a left ventricular stroke volume of 70 mL and a heart rate of 80/min. What is his cardiac output?
  A. 11.4 L/min
  B. 8.8 L/min
  C. 5.6 L/min
  D. 3.3 L/min

20-9. What inspiratory flow is needed for a patient receiving volume-limited ventilation at a rate of 20/min, I:E ratio of 1:2, and tidal volume of 500 mL?
  A. 60 L/min
  B. 50 L/min
  C. 40 L/min
  D. 30 L/min

20-10. A doctor orders 0.25 mL of 2.25% racemic epinephrine in 3 mL normal saline via small volume nebulizer for a child with croup. How many mg of racemic epinephrine are you delivering?
  A. 6.8 mg
  B. 5.6 mg
  C. 0.75 mg
  D. 12.0 mg

VENTILATION CALCULATIONS

Likely calculations regarding ventilation include the minute volume, tidal volume, physiologic dead-space, deadspace to tidal volume ratio and alveolar ventilation. Also possible are conversions between CO_2 percentages and partial pressures. **Table 20-1** provides the formulas for these parameters, example calculations, and "ballpark" rules to help you estimate or verify your computations.

Table 20-1 Computation Formulas and Example Problems for Ventilatory Parameters

Parameter/Formula	Example
Minute Volume	
$\dot{V}_E = f \times V_T$ *Ballpark rule*: at normal rates of breathing, the computed minute volume for adults will generally be in the 4–10 L/min range	*Problem 20.1* A patient has a tidal volume of 400 mL and is breathing at 14/minute. What is her minute volume? *Solution* $\dot{V}_E = f \times V_T$ $\dot{V}_E = 14$ breaths/min $\times 400$ mL/breath $\dot{V}_E = 5600$ mL/min or 5.6 L/min
Tidal Volume	
$V_T = \dot{V}_E \div f$ *Ballpark rule*: recheck your calculations if for an adult you obtain a $V_T < 100$ mL or > 1000 mL	*Problem 20.2* A patient has a minute volume of 8.25 L/min and is breathing at a rate of 22/min. What is his average tidal volume? *Solution* $V_T = \dot{V}_E \div f$ $V_T = 8.25$ L/min $\div 22$ breaths/min $V_T = 0.375$ L/breath $= 375$ mL
Physiologic Deadspace	
$V_D = V_T \times \dfrac{Pa_{CO_2} - PE_{CO_2}}{Pa_{CO_2}}$ *Ballpark rules*: (1) unless the patient has a trach (which lowers V_D), V_D will be ≥ 1 mL/lb PBW and usually less than 70% of the tidal volume; (2) large $Pa_{CO_2} - PE_{CO_2}$ differences (> 15–20 torr) indicate large deadspace volume	*Problem 20.4* A patient has a tidal volume of 450 mL, an arterial PCO_2 (Pa_{CO_2}) of 60 torr, and a mixed expired PCO_2 (PE_{CO_2}) of 30 torr. What is the patient's deadspace? *Solution* $V_D = V_T \times \dfrac{Pa_{CO_2} - PE_{CO_2}}{Pa_{CO_2}}$ $V_D = 450$ mL $\times [(60 - 30)/60]$ $V_D = 450$ mL $\times [30/60]$ $V_D = 225$ mL

(continues)

Table 20-1 Computation Formulas and Example Problems for Ventilatory Parameters (continued)

Parameter/Formula	Example
Deadspace to Tidal Volume Ratio	
$V_D/V_T = V_D \div V_T$ *Ballpark rule*: Unless the patient has a trach (which lowers V_D), V_D/V_T will range between 0.30 to 0.70	*Problem 20.5* A 6-foot-tall, 170-lb. patient with normal lungs has a tidal volume of 600 mL. What is his deadspace to tidal volume ratio? *Solution* With normal lungs, assume that V_D = 1 mL/lb. body weight V_D = 1 mL/lb × 170 lb. = 170 mL V_D/V_T = 170 ÷ 600 = 0.28
Deadspace (given V_D/V_T)	
$V_D = V_D/V_T \times V_T$ *Ballpark rule*: unless the patient has a trach (which lowers V_D), V_D will range between 30% and 70% of the tidal volume	*Problem 20.6* A 5-foot-tall, 105-lb. patient has a deadspace to tidal volume ratio of 0.40 and a tidal volume of 500 mL. What is her deadspace volume? *Solution* $V_D = V_D/V_T \times V_T$ V_D = 0.40 × 500 mL V_D = 200 mL
Alveolar Ventilation	
$V_A = f \times (V_T - V_D)$ *Ballpark rules*: (1) unless otherwise stated assume normal deadspace = 1 mL/lb; (2) $\dot{V}_A$ must always be less than the minute volume and in proportion to the V_D/V_T ratio—i.e., $\dot{V}_E - (V_D/V_T \times \dot{V}_E)$	*Problem 20.7* A 6-foot, 4-inch-tall 200-lb. man with normal lungs has a tidal volume of 680 mL and is breathing at a rate of 15 breaths/min. What is his approximate alveolar ventilation? *Solution* Assume normal deadspace 1 mL/lb × 200 lb = 200 mL $\dot{V}_A = f \times (V_T - V_D)$ $\dot{V}_A$ = 15 × (680 − 200) $\dot{V}_A$ = 15 × 480 $\dot{V}_A$ = 7200 mL/min or 7.2 L/min
Convert Expired CO_2% (Capnography) to P_{CO_2}	
$P_{ETCO_2} = F_{ETCO_2} \times (P_B - 47)$ *Ballpark rule*: normal F_{ETCO_2} range between 4% and 6%; a 5% F_{ETCO_2} is equivalent to a P_{ETCO_2} of 36 torr	*Problem 20.8* A patient at sea level has an end-expired CO_2 concentration (F_{ETCO_2}) of 0.043. What is her BTPS corrected end-tidal P_{CO_2} (P_{ETCO_2})? *Solution* Sea level P_B = 760 mm Hg Correction for BTPS = −47 mm Hg $P_{ETCO_2} = F_{ETCO_2} \times (P_B - 47)$ P_{ETCO_2} = 0.043 × (760 − 47) P_{ETCO_2} = 0.043 × 713 P_{ETCO_2} = 30.7 mm Hg (torr)

OXYGENATION CALCULATIONS

Likely calculations regarding oxygenation include the inspired and alveolar PO_2, the A-a gradient, percent shunt, P/F ratio, and arterial O_2 content. **Table 20-2** provides the formulas for these parameters, example calculations, and "ballpark" rules to help you estimate or verify your computations.

Table 20-2 Computation Formulas and Example Problems for Oxygenation Parameters

Parameter/Formula	Example
Inspired PO_2	
$P_{IO_2} = F_{IO_2} \times P_B$ *Ballpark rule*: at sea level with an F_{IO_2} of 1.0, the P_{IO_2} = 760 torr, therefore with an F_{IO_2} of 0.50, the $P_{IO_2} = \frac{1}{2} \times 760 = 370$ torr	*Problem 20.9* You are transporting a patient on 40% O_2 in a unpressurized airplane cabin at 8,000 ft altitude (P_B = 565 mm Hg). What is his P_{IO_2}? *Solution* $P_{IO_2} = F_{IO_2} \times P_B$ $P_{IO_2} = 0.40 \times 565$ mm Hg $P_{IO_2} = 226$ mm Hg (torr)
Alveolar PO_2	
$P_{AO_2} = F_{IO_2} (P_B - 47) - 1.25 \times P_{aCO_2}$ *Ballpark rules*: (1) maximum P_{AO_2} at sea level breathing room air $\approx$ 130 torr and breathing 100% $O_2 \approx$ 680 torr; (2) estimate as $(7 \times \%O_2) - P_{aCO_2}$	*Problem 20.10* A patient breathing 60% at sea level has a P_{aCO_2} of 28 torr. What is her alveolar PO_2 (P_{AO_2})? *Solution* Sea level P_B = 760 mm Hg $P_{AO_2} = F_{IO_2} (P_B - 47) - 1.25 \times P_{aCO_2}$ $P_{AO_2} = 0.60(760 - 47) - 1.25 \times 28$ $P_{AO_2} = 428 - 35$ $P_{AO_2} = 393$ mm Hg (torr)
A-a Gradient	
$P(A-a)_{O_2} = P_{AO_2} - P_{aO_2}$ *Ballpark rule*: (1) breathing 100% O_2, clinical range typically between 50 and 60 torr (normal) to 600 torr (severe shunting); (2) compare to %shunt (about 5% shunt per 100 torr $P_{AO_2} - P_{aO_2}$)	*Problem 20.11* A patient breathing 100% at sea level has a P_{aO_2} of 250 torr and a P_{aCO_2} of 60 torr. What is her A-a gradient or $P(A-a)_{O_2}$? *Solution* Sea level P_B = 760 mm Hg $P_{AO_2} = F_{IO_2} (P_B - 47) - 1.25 \times P_{aCO_2}$ $P_{AO_2} = 1.0(760 - 47) - 1.25 \times 60$ $P_{AO_2} = 713 - 75$ $P_{AO_2} = 638$ mm Hg (torr) $P(A-a)_{O_2} = P_{AO_2} - P_{aO_2}$ $P(A-a)_{O_2} = 638 - 250$ $P(A-a)_{O_2} = 388$ mm Hg (torr)

(continues)

Table 20-2 Computation Formulas and Example Problems for Oxygenation Parameters (continued)

Parameter/Formula	Example
Percent Shunt (estimate)	
$$\%shunt = \frac{P(A\text{-}a)o_2 \times 0.003}{[P(A\text{-}a)o_2 \times 0.003] + 5}$$ *Ballpark rule*: about 5% shunt per 100 torr $P(A\text{-}a)o_2$	*Problem 20.12* What is the estimated percent shunt of the patient in problem 20.11? *Solution* $$\%shunt = \frac{P(A\text{-}a)o_2 \times 0.003}{[P(A\text{-}a)o_2 \times 0.003] + 5}$$ $$\%shunt = \frac{388 \times 0.003}{[388 \times 0.003] + 5}$$ $$\%shunt = \frac{1.164}{1.164 + 5}$$ $$\%shunt = \frac{1.164}{6.164}$$ $\%shunt = .189 \times 100 = 19\%$
P/F Ratio	
$Pao_2/Fio_2 = Pao_2 \div Fio_2$ *Ballpark rule*: (1) expect P/F ratios of > 500 for patients with normal lung function; less than < 200 signifies acute lung injury; (2) estimate normal Pao_2 as $5 \times O_2\%$ (e.g., you would expect a patient breathing 50% O_2 oxygen to have a Pao_2 of about 250 torr)	*Problem 20.13* What is the P/F ratio of a patient breathing 50% O_2 with a Po_2 of 68 torr? *Solution* $Pao_2/Fio_2 = Pao_2 \div Fio_2$ $Pao_2/Fio_2 = 68 \div 0.50$ $Pao_2/Fio_2 = 136$
Arterial O_2 Content	
$Cao_2 = (O_2 \text{ bound to Hb}) + (\text{dissolved } O_2)$ $Cao_2 = (\text{total Hb} \times 1.36 \times Sao_2) + (0.003 \times Pao_2)$ *Ballpark rule*: if the Sao_2 is > 75% (most cases for arterial blood), the computed Cao_2 value in mL/dL will *always* be a bit larger than the total Hb present but never more than 40% larger—e.g., with a total Hb of 8 gm/dL and an Sao_2 of 90%, you would expect a Cao_2 between 8 and 11 mL/dL	*Problem 20.14* A patient has a hemoglobin concentration of 10 gm/dL, a Pao_2 of 50 torr and an Sao_2 of 80%. What is his total arterial O_2 content (Cao_2)? *Solution* O_2 bound to Hb = (total Hb $\times$ 1.36 $\times$ Sao_2) O_2 bound to Hb = (10 $\times$ 1.36 $\times$ 0.80) O_2 bound to Hb = 10.9 mL/dL Dissolved O_2 = 0.003 $\times$ Pao_2 Dissolved O_2 = 0.003 $\times$ 50 Dissolved O_2 = 0.15 mL/dL Cao_2 = (O_2 bound to Hb) + (dissolved O_2) Cao_2 = 10.9 + 0.15 = 11.05 mL/dL

PULMONARY MECHANICS

Likely calculations regarding pulmonary mechanics include static compliance and airway resistance of patients receiving ventilatory support. **Table 20-3** provides the formulas for these parameters, example calculations, and "ballpark" rules to help you verify your computations.

Table 20-3 Computation Formulas and Example Problems for Pulmonary Mechanics Parameters

Parameter/Formula	Example
Static Compliance	
$C_{LT} = \dfrac{V_T}{Pplat - PEEP}$ where C_{LT} = static compliance of the lungs and thorax; V_T = the corrected tidal volume; Pplat = the plateau pressure during a volume hold; and PEEP = the baseline airway pressure *Ballpark rule*: expect to see the C_{LT} range from 100 mL/cm H_2O (normal) to 10 mL/cm H_2O (severe reduction in compliance as might occur in ARDS)	*Problem 20.15* A patient receiving volume-limited ventilation with a tidal volume of 700 mL and 8 cm H_2O PEEP has a peak pressure of 42 cm H_2O and a plateau pressure of 35 cm H_2O. What is her static compliance? *Solution* $C_{LT} = \dfrac{V_T}{Pplat - PEEP}$ $C_{LT} = \dfrac{700}{35 - 8}$ $C_{LT} = 26$ mL/cm H_2O
Airway Resistance	
$R_{AW} = \dfrac{PIP - Pplat}{\dot{V}}$ Where R_{AW} = airway resistance (cm H_2O/L/sec); PIP = peak inspiratory pressure; Pplat = the plateau pressure during a volume hold; and $\dot{V}$ = inspiratory flow *in liters/sec* *Ballpark rule*: normal R_{AW} for orally intubated patients range from 10 to 15 cm H_2O/L/sec; expect higher computed values in patients with airway obstruction	*Problem 20.16* A patient receiving volume-limited ventilation with a tidal volume of 400 mL, inspiratory flow of 75 L/min, and 6 cm H_2O PEEP has a peak pressure of 45 cm H_2O and a plateau pressure of 30 cm H_2O. What is her airway resistance? *Solution* Convert 75 L/min to L/sec: 75 L ÷ 60 = 1.25 L/sec $R_{AW} = \dfrac{PIP - Pplat}{\dot{V}}$ $R_{AW} = \dfrac{45 - 30}{1.25}$ $R_{AW} = 12$ cm H_2O/L/sec

PULMONARY FUNCTION CALCULATIONS

Likely calculations related to pulmonary function testing include lung volumes and capacities, forced expiratory volume(time) as a percent of FVC, the percent change in a value, and the percent predicted compared to normal. **Table 20-4** provides the formulas for these parameters, example calculations and "ballpark" rules to help you estimate or verify your computations.

Table 20-4 Computation Formulas and Example Problems for Selected Pulmonary Function Parameters

Parameter/Formula	Example
Volumes/Capacities	
Most common formulas: $$VC = TLC - RV$$ $$VC = IRV + TV + ERV$$ $$TLC = FRC + IC$$ $$TLC = IRV + TV + ERV + RV$$ $$RV = FRC - ERV$$ $$RV = TLC - VC$$ $$FRC = RV + ERV$$ $$FRC = TLC - IC$$ *Ballpark rule*: verify the selected formula by drawing and labeling a graph of lung volumes and capacities before computation	*Problem 20.17* A patient has a FRC of 3800 mL, a tidal volume of 400 mL, and an expiratory reserve volume of 1300 mL. What is her residual volume? *Solution* $$RV = FRC - ERV$$ $$RV = 3800 - 1300$$ $$RV = 2500 \text{ mL}$$
Forced Expiratory Volume (time) Percent	
$$FEV_t\% = [FEV_t \div FVC] \times 100$$	*Problem 20.18* A patient has a forced vital capacity of 4.5 L and a FEV_3 of 4.0 L. What is his $FEV_3\%$? *Solution* $$FEV_3\% = [FEV_3 \div FVC] \times 100$$ $$FEV_3\% = [4.0 \div 4.5] \times 100$$ $$FEV_3\% = 89\%$$
Percent Change Value	
$$\% \text{ change} = \frac{post - pre}{pre} \times 100$$ where *pre* is the pretreatment value and *post* is the post-treatment for the parameter being measured *Ballpark rule*: if post > pre, then computed % change must be positive	*Problem 20.19* A patient has a FEV_1 of 2.4 L before bronchodilator treatment and an FEV_1 of 2.7 L after treatment. What percent change in FEV_1 occurred? *Solution* $$\% \text{ change} = \frac{2.7 - 2.4}{2.7} \times 100$$ $$\% \text{ predicted} = \frac{actual}{predicted} \times 100$$ $$\% \text{ change} = 11\%$$
Percent Predicted Value	
$$\% \text{ predicted} = \frac{actual}{predicted} \times 100$$ where actual is the patient's measured value and predicted is the patient's predicted normal value for that parameter. *Note:* when monitoring for changes over time for some measures like peak flow, we substitute the patient's personal best value for the predicted value *Ballpark rule*: if actual < predicted, then computed % predicted must be < 100%	*Problem 20.20* In the pulmonary lab, you measure a patient's forced vital capacity as 3.25 L. Her predicted normal FVC is 3.82 L. What percent of predicted normal is her FVC? *Solution* $$\% \text{ predicted} = \frac{actual}{predicted} \times 100$$ $$\% \text{ predicted} = \frac{3.25}{3.82} \times 100$$ $$\% \text{ predicted} = 85\% \text{ of normal}$$

CARDIOVASCULAR CALCULATIONS

Likely calculations regarding cardiovascular parameters include heart rate (from a ECG), pulse pressure, mean pressure, stroke volume, cardiac output, and cardiac index. **Table 20-5** provides the formulas for these parameters, example calculations and "ballpark" rules to help you estimate or verify your computations.

Table 20-5 Computation Formulas and Example Problems for Cardiovascular Parameters

Parameter/Formula	Example
Heart Rate (ECG)	
For regular rhythms: HR = 60 ÷ R-R (sec) where HR = heart rate; R-R is the R to R interval *Ballpark rule*: approximate HR = 300 ÷ R-R span in large (5-mm) boxes	*Problem 20.21* On an ECG strip run at standard recording speed of 25 mm/second, a patient has a regular rhythm with an R-R of 10 mm (two large boxes). What is the heart rate? *Solution* 10 mm × 0.04 = 0.40 sec 60 ÷ 0.40 = 150/min
Pulse Pressure	
pulse pressure = systolic – diastolic *Ballpark rules*: (1) compare to normal resting value of about 40 mm Hg (up to 100 mm Hg is normal during exercise); (2) expect high values with atherosclerosis, hyperthyroidism, aortic regurgitation; expect low values with CHF or shock	*Problem 20.22* A patient's arterial blood pressure is 165/90. What is her pulse pressure? *Solution* pulse pressure = systolic – diastolic pulse pressure = 165 – 90 pulse pressure = 75 mm Hg
Mean Blood Pressure (estimate)	
mean pressure = [systolic + (2 × diastolic)] ÷ 3 *Ballpark rule*: the mean pressure will be a bit *less* than halfway between the systolic and diastolic pressures	*Problem 20.23* A patient's arterial blood pressure is 100/70. What is his mean arterial pressure? *Solution* mean pressure = [systolic + (2 × diastolic)] ÷ 3 mean pressure = [100 + (2 × 70)] ÷ 3 mean pressure = [100 + 140] ÷ 3 mean pressure = 80 mm Hg
Cardiac Output	
CO = HR × SV where CO = cardiac output in L/min; HR = heart rate; and SV = average left ventricular stroke volume in L *Ballpark rules*: (1) compare to a "normal" output of 70 × 70 = 4900 or 4.9 L/min (HR = 70/min and SV = 70 mL); (2) for adult patients, expect to see the computed CO range between 3 to 10 L/min (normal 4–8 L/min)	*Problem 20.24* A patient has a left ventricular stroke volume of 60 mL and a heart rate of 105 beats/min. What is her cardiac output? *Solution* Convert SV in mL to L 60/1000 = 0.06 L CO = HR × SV CO = 105 × 0.06 CO = 6.3 L/min

(continues)

Table 20-5 Computation Formulas and Example Problems for Cardiovascular Parameters (continued)

Parameter/Formula	Example
Cardiac Output (Fick Method)	
$CO = \dfrac{\dot{V}O_2}{C(a\text{-}v)O_2 \times 10}$ where CO = cardiac output in L/min; $\dot{V}O_2$ = whole body oxygen consumption in mL/min; and $C(a\text{-}v)O_2$ = the arterial-mixed venous O_2 content difference *Ballpark rule*: (1) a normal $C(a\text{-}v)O_2$ is about 5 mL/dL; (2) all else being equal, the larger the $C(a\text{-}v)O_2$, the lower the cardiac output (inverse relationship!)	*Problem 20.25* A patient has an oxygen consumption of 300 mL/min, an arterial O_2 content of 18 mL/dL, and a mixed venous O_2 content of 12 mL/dL. What is his cardiac output? *Solution* $CO = \dfrac{\dot{V}O_2}{C(a\text{-}v)O_2 \times 10}$ $CO = \dfrac{300}{(18-12) \times 10}$ $CO = \dfrac{300}{60} = 5$ L/min
Cardiac Index	
$CI\ (L/min/m^2) = CO \div BSA$ where CI = cardiac index in L/min/m²; CO = cardiac output in L/min; and BSA = body surface area in m² (usually provided to you and based on the DuBois formula/nomogram) *Ballpark rules*: (1) for adults, the normal cardiac index will always be *less than* the cardiac output—about ½ as much for the average-size adult; (2) compare computed value to normal of 2.5–5.0 L/min/m²	*Problem 20.26* A patient has a cardiac output of 6.1 L/min and a body surface area of 2.3 m². What is his cardiac index? *Solution* CI = CO ÷ BSA CI = 6.1 ÷ 2.3 CI = 2.65 L/min/m²
Stroke Volume	
SV = CO ÷ HR where SV = average left ventricular stroke volume in mL; CO = cardiac output in mL/min; and HR = heart rate *Ballpark rule*: compare to normal of 60–130 mL	*Problem 20.27* A patient has a cardiac output of 4 L/min and heart rate of 80. What is her stroke volume? *Solution* Convert CO in L to mL 4 × 1000 = 4000 ml/min SV = CO ÷HR SV = 4000 ÷ 80 SV = 50 mL

EQUIPMENT CALCULATIONS

Likely calculations regarding equipment include cylinder duration of flow, air entrainment ratios, total output flows for air entrainment devices, mechanical ventilation time and flow parameters, suction catheter sizes and pressure conversions. **Table 20-6** provides the formulas for these parameters, example calculations and "ballpark" rules to help you estimate or verify your computations.

Table 20-6 Formulas and Example Problems for Equipment-Related Computations

Parameter/Formula	Example
Cylinder Duration of Flow	
time to empty (min) $= \dfrac{\text{psig} \times \text{factor}}{\text{flow}}$ where psig is the cylinder pressure in pounds per square inch gauge, factor is the cylinder factor, and flow is the flow in L/min. *Note:* See Tables 6-24 and 19-4 for cylinder factors. *Ballpark rule:* a full E cylinder at 10 L/min will last about 1 hour; a full H cylinder at 10 L/min will last about 10 times longer (10 hours)	*Problem 20.28* How long will an E cylinder of oxygen with a gauge pressure of 800 psi set to deliver 5 L/min last until empty? *Solution* time to empty (min) $= \dfrac{\text{psig} \times \text{factor}}{\text{flow}}$ time to empty (min) $= \dfrac{800 \times .28}{5}$ time to empty = 45 min
Air-Entrainment Ratio	
$\dfrac{\text{air}}{O_2} = \dfrac{100 - O_2\%}{O_2\% - 21}$ *Note:* the above formula is the same as the "magic box" that appears in many textbooks *Ballpark rule:* 60% O_2 is achieved with an air to O_2 ratio of about 1:1; lower $O_2\%$ mean higher ratios, and higher $O_2\%$ mean lower ratios	*Problem 20.29* What is the air-to-oxygen ratio for a 35% air-entrainment mask? *Solution* $\dfrac{\text{air}}{O_2} = \dfrac{100 - O_2\%}{O_2\% - 21}$ $\dfrac{\text{air}}{O_2} = \dfrac{100 - 35}{35 - 21}$ $\dfrac{\text{air}}{O_2} = \dfrac{65}{14} = 4.6:1 \approx 5:1$
Total Flow Air-Entrainment Device	
total flow = input flow $\times$ (air + O_2 ratio parts)	*Problem 20.30* Assuming an input O_2 flow of 8 L/min for the air-entrainment mask in problem 20.29, what would be the total flow delivered to the patient? *Solution* total flow = input flow $\times$ (air + O_2 ratio parts) total flow = $8 \times (5+1)$ total flow = 48 L/min

(continues)

Table 20-6 Formulas and Example Problems for Equipment-Related Computations (continued)

Parameter/Formula	Example
Time Parameters	
Note: Several mechanical ventilation time parameter computations may appear on the NBRC CRT exam. See Table 13-19 in Chapter 13 for a complete listing of the various parameters and their computations. *Here we provide an example only.* $$\text{total cycle time} = \frac{60}{f}$$ $$\text{inspiratory time} = \frac{\text{total cycle time}}{\text{sum of I:E ratio parts}}$$	*Problem 20.31* A patient receiving pressure control ventilation at a rate of 10 breaths/min has an I:E ratio of 1:3. What is her inspiratory time? *Solution* $$\text{total cycle time} = \frac{60}{10}$$ $\text{total cycle time} = 6$ seconds $$\text{inspiratory time} = \frac{\text{total cycle time}}{\text{sum of I:E ratio parts}}$$ $$\text{inspiratory time} = \frac{6}{(3+1)}$$ $\text{inspiratory time} = 1.5$ sec
Ventilator Inspiratory Flow (VCV)	
$$\dot{V}\text{insp} = \frac{\dot{V}_E}{\%\text{I-time}}$$ where $\dot{V}\text{insp}$ is the inspiratory flow in L/min, $\dot{V}_E$ is the minute volume in L/min, and %I-time is the percent inspiratory time (decimal) *Ballpark rule:* multiply the sum of the I:E parts by the minute volume	*Problem 20.32* What inspiratory flow is needed for a patient receiving volume-limited ventilation at a rate of 15 breaths/min, an I:E ratio of 1:3, and a tidal volume of 600 mL? *Solution* $\dot{V}_E = 15 \times 600$ mL $= 9000$ mL/min $= 9.0$ L/min %I-time (decimal) = [I-time÷(I-time + E-time)] = .25 $$\dot{V}\text{insp} = \frac{\dot{V}_E}{\%\text{I-time}}$$ $$\dot{V}\text{insp} = \frac{9.0}{.25}$$ $\dot{V}\text{insp} = 36$ L/min
Suction Catheter Size	
catheter size (Fr) = (3 × ET tube ID) ÷ 2 *Ballpark rule:* multiply the ET tube ID by 2 and use the next smallest size Fr catheter	*Problem 20.33* A patient has a 7-mm ID trach tube. What size suction catheter should you use? *Solution* catheter size (Fr) = (3 × ET tube ID) ÷ 2 catheter size (Fr) = (3 × 8) ÷ 2 catheter size (Fr) = 24 ÷ 2 = 12 Fr
Pressure Conversions	
See Table 6-28 for common pressure conversion factors. *Here we provide a common example only.* cm H_2O = 1.36 × mm Hg	*Problem 20.34* You record a patient's cuff pressure as 30 cm H_2O. What pressure is this in mm Hg? *Solution* cm H_2O = 1.36 × mm Hg mm Hg = cm H_2O ÷ 1.36 mm Hg = 30 ÷ 1.36 = 22 mm Hg

DRUG CALCULATIONS

Likely pharmacology-related calculations include dilution and dosage problems. **Table 20-7** provides the generic formulas for these problems, example calculations and "ballpark" rules to help you estimate or verify your computations.

Table 20-7 Formulas and Example Problems for Drug Dilution and Dosage Computations

Formula	Example
Dilution	
$V_1C_1 = V_2C_2$ (solve for unknown) *Ballpark rule*: doubling the volume halves the concentration of the solute	*Problem 20.35* A doctor orders 0.31 mg Xopenex (levalbuterol HCl) in 3 mL NS for a patient TID. All the pharmacy has on hand is the 1.25-mg 3-mL unit dose. How many mL of this unit dose would you administer to the patent for each treatment? *Solution* $V_1C_1 = V_2C_2$ $V_2 = \dfrac{V_1C_1}{C_2}$ $V_2 = \dfrac{3 \times 0.31}{1.25}$ $V_2 = 0.74$ mL
Dosage Computations	
mg/mL = 10 × % concentration % concentration = $\dfrac{\text{mg/mL}}{10}$ mL = $\dfrac{\text{dosage (mg)}}{\text{concentration (mg/mL)}}$ *Ballpark rule*: a 1% solution contains 10 mg/mL of solute with a 0.5% solution half as much and a 2% solution twice as much	*Problem 20.36* A doctor orders 2 mL of a 0.5% solution of a bronchodilator via SVN. How many mg of the drug are you administering? *Solution* mg/mL = 10 × % concentration mg/mL = 10 × 0.5 mg/mL = 5 mg/mL 5 mg/mL × 2 mL = 10 mg *Problem 20.37* A doctor orders 40 mg of a 0.25% solution of a bronchodilator for continuous nebulization, to be diluted with 200 mL normal saline. How many mL of the solution would you mix with the diluent? *Solution* mg/mL = 10 × % concentration mg/mL = 10 × 0.25 mg/mL = 2.5 mg/mL mL = $\dfrac{\text{dosage (mg)}}{\text{concentration (mg/mL)}}$ mL = $\dfrac{40}{2.5}$ mL = 16 mL

PRE-TEST ANSWERS AND EXPLANATIONS

Below are this chapter's pre-test answers and explanations. Be sure to review each answer's explanation thoroughly to help you understand why it is correct. If the explanation is still unclear to you, review the chapter contents or the references and/or refer to this chapter's supplemental resources on the CD.

20-1. **Correct Answer: B.** 375 mL. $V_T = 8.25 \div 22 = 0.375$ L or 375 mL

20-2. **Correct Answer: C.** 5.18 L/min. Assume normal deadspace 1 mL/lb × 110 lb = 110 mL. $V_A = 14 \times (480 - 110) = 5180$ mL/min or 5.18 L/min.

20-3. **Correct Answer: C.** 180 mL. $V_D = 600 \times [(50 - 35)/50] = 180$ mL.

20-4. **Correct Answer: D.** Sea level $P_B = 760$ mm Hg. $P_{AO_2} = 1.0 (760 - 47) - 1.25 \times 40 = 663$ mm Hg (torr). $P(A\text{-}a)O_2 = 663 - 350 = 313$ mm Hg (torr).

20-5. **Correct Answer: D.** 30 mL/cm H_2O. $C_{LT} = 600 \div (30 - 10) = 30$ mL/cm H_2O.

20-6. **Correct Answer: A.** 2500 mL. FRC = TLC − IC = 5500 − 3000 = 2500 mL.

20-7. **Correct Answer: C.** 21%. % change = $[(6.3 - 5.2) \div 5.2] \times 100 = 21\%$.

20-8. **Correct Answer: C.** 5.6 L/min. CO = HR × SV (L) = 80 × 0.07 = 5.6 L/min.

20-9. **Correct Answer: D.** 30 L/min. $\dot{V}_E = 10$ L/min; %I-time = 33%. $\dot{V}_{insp} = \dot{V}_E \div \%I\text{-time} = 10 \div .33 = 30$ L/min.

20-10. **Correct Answer: B.** 5.6 mg. mg/mL = 10 × 2.25 = 22.5 mg/mL. 22.5 mg/mL × 0.25 mL = 5.6 mg.

POST-TEST

A post-test for this chapter that includes automated scoring and feedback is available on the accompanying CD. Be sure to complete this additional assessment to confirm your mastery of this chapter's objectives.

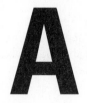
Entry Level CRT Examination Detailed Content Outline

National Board for Respiratory Care Entry Level CRT Examination Detailed Content Outline Effective Date: 7/10/2009 Open cells show an examination could include items from indicated cognitive levels. Shaded cells prevent appearance of items on examinations.	Recall	Application	Analysis	Totals
I. PATIENT DATA EVALUATION AND RECOMMENDATIONS	*11*	*14*	*1*	*26*
A. Review Data in the Patient Record	*4*	*0*	*0*	*4*
1. Patient history, e.g., • Present illness • Progress notes • Admission notes • Diagnoses • Respiratory care orders • DNR status • Medication history • Patient education (previous)				
2. Physical examination relative to the cardiopulmonary system, e.g., • Vital signs • Physical findings				
3. Laboratory data, e.g., • CBC • Culture and sensitivities • Electrolytes • Sputum Gram stain • Coagulation studies				
4. Pulmonary function results				
5. Blood gas results				
6. Imaging studies, e.g., • Radiograph • MRI • CT				

(continues)

National Board for Respiratory Care Entry Level CRT Examination Detailed Content Outline Effective Date: 7/10/2009 Open cells show an examination could include items from indicated cognitive levels. Shaded cells prevent appearance of items on examinations.	Recall	Application	Analysis	Totals
7. Monitoring data:				
a. Fluid balance				
b. Pulmonary mechanics, e.g., • Maximum inspiratory pressure • Vital capacity				
c. Respiratory, e.g., • Rate • I:E • Tidal and minute volume				
d. Pulmonary compliance, airways resistance, and work of breathing				
e. Noninvasive, e.g., • Pulse oximetry • Capnography • V_D/V_T • Transcutaneous O_2/CO_2				
8. Cardiac monitoring:				
a. ECG data results, e.g., • Heart rate • Rhythm				
b. Hemodynamic monitoring results, e.g., • Blood pressure • PA pressure • CVP • Cardiac output/index				
9. Maternal and perinatal/neonatal history and data, e.g., • Apgar scores • L/S ratio • Gestational age				
B. Collect and Evaluate Additional Pertinent Clinical Information	*6*	*11*	*1*	*18*
1. Assess a patient's overall cardiopulmonary status by **inspection** to determine:				
a. General appearance, e.g., • Venous distention • Diaphoresis • Edema • Clubbing • Accessory muscle activity • Cyanosis • Chest wall movement • Breathing pattern				
b. Airway assessment, e.g., • Macroglossia • Neck range of motion				
c. Cough, sputum amount, and character				
d. Apgar score, gestational age, and transillumination of chest				
2. Assess a patient's overall cardiopulmonary status by palpation to determine:				
a. Pulse, rhythm, and force				

(continues)

National Board for Respiratory Care Entry Level CRT Examination Detailed Content Outline Effective Date: 7/10/2009 Open cells show an examination could include items from indicated cognitive levels. Shaded cells prevent appearance of items on examinations.	Recall	Application	Analysis	Totals
b. Asymmetrical chest movements, tactile fremitus, crepitus, tenderness, secretions in the airway, and tracheal deviation			▒	▒
3. Assess a patient's overall cardiopulmonary status by **percussion**			▒	▒
4. Assess a patient's overall cardiopulmonary status by **auscultation** to determine presence of:	▒		▒	▒
a. Breath sounds				
b. Heart sounds and rhythm				
c. Blood pressure				
5. Interview a patient to determine:	▒		▒	▒
a. Level of consciousness and orientation, emotional state, and ability to cooperate				
b. Level of pain			▒	▒
c. Presence of dyspnea, sputum production, and exercise tolerance				
d. Nutritional status		▒	▒	▒
e. Social history, e.g., • Smoking • Substance abuse		▒	▒	▒
f. Advance directives, e.g., • DNR status		▒	▒	▒
6. Assess a patient's learning needs			▒	▒
7. Review a chest radiograph to determine:	▒		▒	▒
a. Position of endotracheal or tracheostomy tube				
b. Presence of, or change in, cardiopulmonary abnormalities e.g., • Pneumothorax • Pleural fluid • Consolidation • Pulmonary edema				▒
c. Position of indwelling tubes and catheters				
d. Presence of foreign bodies			▒	▒
e. Position of or change in hemidiaphragms or mediastinum			▒	▒
8. Review lateral neck radiographs, e.g., • Epiglottitis • Foreign body			▒	▒

(continues)

National Board for Respiratory Care Entry Level CRT Examination Detailed Content Outline Effective Date: 7/10/2009 Open cells show an examination could include items from indicated cognitive levels. Shaded cells prevent appearance of items on examinations.	Recall	Application	Analysis	Totals
9. Perform procedures:				
a. 12-lead ECG				
b. Transcutaneous monitoring				
c. Pulse oximetry and capnography				
d. Tidal volume, minute volume, vital capacity, and peak flow measurements				
e. Bedside spirometry, e.g., • FVC • FEV$_1$				
f. Arterial sampling—percutaneous or line				
g. Arterialized capillary blood sampling				
h. Timed walk test, e.g., • 6-minute				
i. Oxygen titration with exercise				
j. Blood gas/hemoximetry analysis				
k. Cardiopulmonary calculations e.g., • P(A-a)O$_2$ • V$_D$/V$_T$				
l. Hemodynamic monitoring, e.g., • Blood pressure • CVP				
m. Lung mechanics, e.g., • Plateau pressure • Airways resistance • MIP • Compliance • MEP				
n. Apnea monitoring				
o. Overnight pulse oximetry				
p. Tracheal tube cuff pressure and / or volume				
q. Arterial line insertion				
r. Stress testing, e.g., • ECG • Pulse oximetry				
s. Pulmonary function laboratory studies				
t. CPAP/BiPAP™ titration during sleep				

(continues)

National Board for Respiratory Care Entry Level CRT Examination Detailed Content Outline Effective Date: 7/10/2009 Open cells show an examination could include items from indicated cognitive levels. Shaded cells prevent appearance of items on examinations.	Recall	Application	Analysis	Totals
10. Interpret procedure results including:				
a. 12-lead ECG, e.g., • Rate • Artifacts • Irregular rhythm				
b. Transcutaneous monitoring				
c. Pulse oximetry and capnography				
d. Tidal volume, minute volume, vital capacity, and peak flow measurements				
e. Bedside spirometry, e.g., • FVC • FEV_1				
f. Arterial sampling—percutaneous or line				
g. Arterialized capillary blood sampling				
h. Timed walk test e.g., • 6-minute				
i. Oxygen titration with exercise				
j. Blood gas / hemoximetry analysis				
k. Cardiopulmonary calculations, e.g., • $P(A-a)O_2$ • V_D/V_T				
l. Hemodynamic monitoring, e.g., • Blood pressure • CVP				
m. Lung mechanics, e.g., • Plateau pressure • MEP • MIP				
n. Apnea monitoring				
o. Overnight pulse oximetry				
p. Tracheal tube cuff pressure and/or volume				
q. Arterial line insertion				
r. Stress testing, e.g., • ECG • Pulse oximetry				
s. Pulmonary function laboratory studies				
t. CPAP/BiPAP™ titration during sleep				

(continues)

National Board for Respiratory Care Entry Level CRT Examination Detailed Content Outline Effective Date: 7/10/2009 Open cells show an examination could include items from indicated cognitive levels. Shaded cells prevent appearance of items on examinations.	Recall	Application	Analysis	Totals
C. Recommend Procedures to Obtain Additional Data	*1*	*3*	*0*	*4*
1. Radiographic and other imaging studies				
2. Diagnostic bronchoscopy, e.g., • Evaluate hemoptysis • Atelectasis				
3. Sputum Gram stain, culture and sensitivities, e.g., • Pneumonia				
4. Bronchoalveolar lavage (BAL)				
5. Pulmonary function testing				
6. Lung mechanics, e.g., • Compliance • Airways resistance				
7. Blood gas analysis, pulse oximetry, and transcutaneous monitoring				
8. ECG				
9. Capnography				
10. Hemodynamic monitoring, e.g., • Blood pressure • CVP				
11. Sleep studies				
II. EQUIPMENT MANIPULATION, INFECTION CONTROL, AND QUALITY CONTROL	*5*	*15*	*9*	*29*
A. Manipulate Equipment by Order or Protocol	*4*	*10*	*8*	*22*
1. Oxygen administration devices:				
a. Low-flow devices, e.g., • Nasal cannula				
b. High-flow devices, e.g., • Air entrainment mask				
c. High-flow nasal cannula				
2. CPAP devices—mask, nasal, or bilevel				
3. Humidifiers				
4. Nebulizers				
5. Resuscitation devices, e.g., • Manual resuscitator (bag-valve) • Mouth-to-valve mask resuscitator				

(continues)

National Board for Respiratory Care Entry Level CRT Examination Detailed Content Outline Effective Date: 7/10/2009 Open cells show an examination could include items from indicated cognitive levels. Shaded cells prevent appearance of items on examinations.	Recall	Application	Analysis	Totals
6. Ventilators:				
a. Pneumatic, electric, fluidic, and microprocessor				
b. Noninvasive positive pressure				
7. Artificial airways:				
a. Oro- and nasopharyngeal airways				
b. Endotracheal tubes				
c. Tracheostomy tubes and devices				
d. Speaking tubes and valves				
e. Intubation equipment				
f. Laryngeal mask airway (LMA)				
g. Esophageal-tracheal Combitube®				
8. Suctioning devices				
9. Gas delivery, metering, and clinical analyzing devices:				
a. Gas cylinders, regulators, reducing valves, connectors and flowmeters, and air/oxygen blenders				
b. oxygen conserving devices, e.g., • Reservoir cannula • Pulse-dose				
c. Oxygen concentrators				
d. Air compressors				
10. Point-of-care analyzers, e.g., • Blood gas • Electrolytes				
11. Patient breathing circuits:				
a. Continuous mechanical ventilation				
b. IPPB				
c. CPAP and PEEP valve assemblies				
d. Noninvasive ventilation				
12. Environmental devices:				
a. Aerosol (mist) tents				
b. Oxygen hoods				
13. Incentive breathing devices				

(continues)

National Board for Respiratory Care Entry Level CRT Examination Detailed Content Outline Effective Date: 7/10/2009 Open cells show an examination could include items from indicated cognitive levels. Shaded cells prevent appearance of items on examinations.	Recall	Application	Analysis	Totals
14. Airway clearance devices:				
a. Percussors and vibrators				
b. Positive expiratory pressure (PEP) devices				
c. Vibratory PEP devices				
15. Manometers, e.g., • Aneroid • Digital • Water				
16. Respirometers, e.g., • Flow-sensing devices				
17. ECG monitors				
18. ECG machines (12-lead)				
19. Vacuum systems, e.g., • Pumps • Collection bottles • Regulators • Pleural drainage devices				
20. Oximetry monitoring devices, e.g., • Pulse oximeter • Transcutaneous				
21. Metered dose inhalers (MDI) and MDI spacers				
22. Dry powder inhalers				
23. Bedside screening spirometers				
24. CO, He, O_2, and specialty gas analyzers				
25. Bronchoscopes				
B. Ensure Infection Control	*0*	*2*	*1*	*3*
1. Ensure cleanliness of equipment by: • Selecting or determining appropriate agent and technique for disinfection and/or sterilization • Performing procedures for disinfection and/or sterilization • Monitoring effectiveness of sterilization procedures				
2. Assure proper handling of biohazardous materials				
3. Incorporate ventilator-associated pneumonia protocol				
4. Implement infectious disease protocols, e.g., • Avian flu • Transmission prevention • SARS				

(continues)

National Board for Respiratory Care Entry Level CRT Examination Detailed Content Outline Effective Date: 7/10/2009 Open cells show an examination could include items from indicated cognitive levels. Shaded cells prevent appearance of items on examinations.	Recall	Application	Analysis	Totals
5. Adhere to infection control policies and procedures, e.g., • Standard Precautions				
C. Perform Quality Control Procedures For	*1*	*3*	*0*	*4*
1. Blood gas analyzers, co-oximeters				
2. Gas analyzers				
3. Point-of-care analyzers				
4. Pulmonary function equipment				
5. Mechanical ventilators				
6. Gas metering devices, e.g., • Flowmeter				
7. Noninvasive monitors, e.g., • Transcutaneous				
8. Record and monitor QC data using accepted statistical methods				
III. INITIATION AND MODIFICATION OF THERAPEUTIC PROCEDURES	*19*	*45*	*21*	*85*
A. Maintain Records and Communicate Information	*2*	*3*	*0*	*5*
1. Record therapy and results using conventional terminology as required in the health care setting and/or by regulatory agencies:				
a. Specify therapy administered, date, time, frequency of therapy, medication, and ventilatory data				
b. Note and interpret patient's response to therapy				
1) Effects of therapy, adverse reactions, and patient's subjective and objective response to therapy				
2) Verify computations and note erroneous data				
3) Auscultatory findings, cough and sputum production, and characteristics				
4) Vital signs				
5) Pulse oximetry, heart rhythm, and capnography				
2. Communicate information:				
a. Regarding patient's clinical status to appropriate members of the health care team				

(continues)

National Board for Respiratory Care Entry Level CRT Examination Detailed Content Outline Effective Date: 7/10/2009 Open cells show an examination could include items from indicated cognitive levels. Shaded cells prevent appearance of items on examinations.	Recall	Application	Analysis	Totals
b. Relevant to coordinating patient care and discharge planning				
3. Accept and verify patient care orders				
4. Apply computer technology to:				
a. Document patient management				
b. Monitor workload assignments				
c. Patient safety initiatives, e.g., • Drug dispensing • Order entry				
5. Communicate results of therapy and alter therapy by protocol(s)				
6. Explain planned therapy and goals to a patient in understandable terms to achieve optimal therapeutic outcome				
7. Educate a patient and family concerning smoking cessation and health management				
B. Maintain a Patent Airway Including the Care of Artificial Airways	*2*	*2*	*3*	*7*
1. Properly position a patient				
2. Insert oro- and nasopharyngeal airways				
3. Perform endotracheal intubation				
4. Maintain position in the airway and appropriate cuff inflation of:				
a. LMA				
b. Esophageal-tracheal Combitube®				
c. Endotracheal tube				
d. Tracheostomy tube				
5. Assess tube placement				
6. Perform tracheostomy care				
7. Change tracheostomy tubes				
8. Maintain adequate humidification				
9. Perform extubation				

(continues)

National Board for Respiratory Care Entry Level CRT Examination Detailed Content Outline Effective Date: 7/10/2009 Open cells show an examination could include items from indicated cognitive levels. Shaded cells prevent appearance of items on examinations.	Recall	Application	Analysis	Totals
C. Remove Bronchopulmonary Secretions	*1*	*3*	*0*	*4*
1. Perform:				
a. Postural drainage, percussion, or vibration				
b. Nasotracheal suctioning				
c. Oropharyngeal suctioning				
d. Airway clearance using mechanical devices, e.g., • High frequency chest wall oscillation • Vibratory PEP				
2. Suction artificial airways				
3. Administer aerosol therapy with prescribed drugs				
4. Instruct and encourage bronchopulmonary hygiene techniques				
D. Achieve Adequate Respiratory Support	*2*	*5*	*1*	*8*
1. Instruct a patient in:				
a. Deep breathing and incentive spirometry techniques				
b. Inspiratory muscle training techniques				
2. Initiate and adjust:				
a. IPPB therapy				
b. Continuous mechanical ventilation settings				
c. Noninvasive ventilation				
d. Elevated baseline pressure, e.g., • CPAP • PEEP				
3. Select ventilator graphics, e.g., • Waveforms • Scales				
4. Initiate and select appropriate settings for high frequency ventilation				
5. Administer medications:				
a. Aerosolized				
b. Dry powder preparations				
c. Endotracheal instillation				

(continues)

National Board for Respiratory Care Entry Level CRT Examination Detailed Content Outline Effective Date: 7/10/2009 Open cells show an examination could include items from indicated cognitive levels. Shaded cells prevent appearance of items on examinations.	Recall	Application	Analysis	Totals
6. Administer oxygen				
7. Initiate and modify weaning procedures				
8. Position patient to minimize hypoxemia				
9. Prevent procedure-associated hypoxemia, e.g., • Oxygenate before and after suctioning and equipment changes				
10. Apply disease-specific ventilator protocols, e.g., • ARDS-Net protocol				
E. Evaluate and Monitor Patient's Objective and Subjective Responses to Respiratory Care	*3*	*7*	*5*	*15*
1. Recommend and review a chest radiograph				
2. Obtain a blood gas sample:				
a. By puncture				
b. From an arterial or pulmonary artery catheter				
c. From arterialized capillary blood				
3. Perform:				
a. Transcutaneous monitoring				
b. Pulse oximetry				
c. Blood gas and hemoximetry analyses				
d. Capnography				
e. Hemodynamic assessment				
4. Interpret results of:				
a. Blood gases				
b. Hemoximetry, e.g., • Carboxyhemoglobin				
c. Hemodynamics				
d. Pulse oximetry				
e. Capnography				
5. Observe for:				
a. Changes in sputum characteristics				
b. Signs of patient–ventilator dysynchrony				

(continues)

National Board for Respiratory Care Entry Level CRT Examination Detailed Content Outline Effective Date: 7/10/2009 Open cells show an examination could include items from indicated cognitive levels. Shaded cells prevent appearance of items on examinations.	Recall	Application	Analysis	Totals
6. Measure and record vital signs, monitor cardiac rhythm, and evaluate fluid balance (intake and output)				
7. Perform and interpret results of pulmonary function testing:				
a. Spirometry				
b. Compliance and airways resistance				
c. Lung volumes				
d. DLCO				
e. Exercise				
f. Bronchoprovocation studies				
8. Recommend blood tests, e.g., • Hemoglobin • Potassium				
9. Monitor airway pressures, and adjust and check alarm systems.				
10. Measure F_{IO_2} and/or oxygen flow				
11. Auscultate the chest and interpret changes in breath sounds				
F. Independently Modify Therapeutic Procedures Based on the Patient's Response	2	9	7	18
1. Terminate treatment based on patient's response to therapy.				
2. Modify treatment techniques:				
a. IPPB				
b. Incentive breathing devices				
c. Aerosol therapy				
1) Modify patient breathing patterns				
2) Change type of equipment and change aerosol output				
3) Change dilution of medication				
4) Adjust temperature of the aerosol				
d. Oxygen therapy				
1) Change mode of administration, flow, and F_{IO_2}				
2) Set up or change an O_2 blender				
3) Set up an O_2 concentrator or liquid O_2 system				

(continues)

2008 National Board for Respiratory Care, Olathe, KS. Provided by permission.

National Board for Respiratory Care Entry Level CRT Examination Detailed Content Outline Effective Date: 7/10/2009 Open cells show an examination could include items from indicated cognitive levels. Shaded cells prevent appearance of items on examinations.	Recall	Application	Analysis	Totals
e. Specialty gas therapy e.g., He/O₂, NO				
1) Change mode of administration				
2) Adjust flow or gas concentration				
f. Bronchial hygiene therapy				
1) Alter patient position and duration of treatment and techniques				
2) Coordinate sequence of therapies e.g., • Chest percussion • PEP • Postural drainage				
g. Maanagement of artificial airways				
1) Reposition or change endotracheal or tracheostomy tube				
2) Change type of humidification equipment				
3) Initiate suctioning				
4) Inflate and/or deflate the cuff				
5) Perform tracheostomy care				
h. Suctioning				
1) Alter frequency and duration of suctioning				
2) Change size and type of catheter				
3) Alter negative pressure				
4) Instill irrigating solutions				
i. Mechanical ventilation				
1) Improve patient synchrony				
2) Enhance oxygenation				
3) Improve alveolar ventilation				
4) Adjust I:E settings				
5) Modify ventilator techniques				
6) Adjust noninvasive positive pressure ventilation				
7) Monitor and adjust alarm settings				
8) Adjust ventilator settings based on ventilator graphics				
9) Change type of ventilator				

(continues)

2008 National Board for Respiratory Care, Olathe, KS. Provided by permission.

National Board for Respiratory Care Entry Level CRT Examination Detailed Content Outline Effective Date: 7/10/2009 Open cells show an examination could include items from indicated cognitive levels. Shaded cells prevent appearance of items on examinations.	Recall	Application	Analysis	Totals
10) Change patient breathing circuitry				
11) Alter mechanical dead space				
12) Initiate procedures for weaning				
G. Recommend Modifications in the Respiratory Care Plan Based on the Patient's Response	3	10	4	17
1. Recommend:				
a. Institution of bronchopulmonary hygiene procedures				
b. Treatment of pneumothorax				
c. Sedation and/or use of muscle relaxant(s)				
d. Adjustment of fluid balance				
e. Adjustment of electrolyte therapy				
f. Insertion or change of artificial airway				
g. Weaning from mechanical ventilation				
h. Extubation				
i. Discontinuing treatment based on patient response				
2. Recommend changes in:				
a. Patient position				
b. Inhaled drug dosage or concentration				
c. F_{IO_2} and oxygen flow				
3. Recommend changes in mechanical ventilation to:				
a. Improve patient synchrony				
b. Enhance oxygenation				
c. Improve alveolar ventilation				
d. Adjust I:E settings				
e. Modify ventilator techniques				
f. Adjust noninvasive positive pressure ventilation				
g. Monitor and adjust alarm settings				
h. Adjust ventilator settings based on ventilator graphics				
i. Change type of ventilator				

(continues)

National Board for Respiratory Care Entry Level CRT Examination Detailed Content Outline Effective Date: 7/10/2009 Open cells show an examination could include items from indicated cognitive levels. Shaded cells prevent appearance of items on examinations.	Recall	Application	Analysis	Totals
j. Change patient breathing circuitry				
k. Reduce auto-PEEP				
l. Reduce plateau pressure				
4. Recommend pharmacologic interventions including use of:				
a. Bronchodilators				
b. Antiinflammatory drugs e.g., • Leukotriene modifiers • Cromolyn sodium • Corticosteroids				
c. Mucolytics and Proteolytics e.g., • Acetylcysteine • Hypertonic saline • RhDNAse				
d. Cardiovascular drugs e.g., • ACLS protocol agents				
e. Antimicrobials e.g., • Antibiotics				
f. Sedatives				
g. Analgesics				
h. Paralytic agents				
i. Diuretics				
j. Surfactants				
k. Vaccines e.g., • Pneumovax • Influenza				
H. Determine the Appropriateness of the Prescribed Respiratory Care Plan and Recommend Modifications When Indicated by Data	1	3	0	4
1. Analyze available information to determine the pathophysiological state				
2. Review:				
a. Planned therapy to establish therapeutic plan				
b. Interdisciplinary patient and family plan				
3. Determine appropriateness of prescribed therapy and goals for identified pathophysiological state				
4. Recommend changes in therapeutic plan when indicated				

(continues)

National Board for Respiratory Care Entry Level CRT Examination Detailed Content Outline Effective Date: 7/10/2009 Open cells show an examination could include items from indicated cognitive levels. Shaded cells prevent appearance of items on examinations.	Recall	Application	Analysis	Totals
5. Perform respiratory care quality assurance				
6. Develop:				
a. Quality improvement program				
b. Respiratory care protocols				
7. Monitor outcomes of:				
a. Quality improvement programs				
b. Respiratory care protocols				
8. Apply respiratory care protocols				
I. Initiate, Conduct, or Modify Respiratory Care Techniques in an Emergency Setting	*1*	*1*	*1*	*3*
1. Treat cardiopulmonary emergencies according to:				
a. BCLS				
b. ACLS				
c. Pediatric Advanced Life Support (PALS)				
d. Neonatal Resuscitation Program (NRP)				
2. Treat a tension pneumothorax				
3. Participate in:				
a. Land/air patient transport				
b. Intra-hospital patient transport				
c. Disaster management				
d. Medical emergency team (MET) e.g., • Rapid response team				
J. Act As an Assistant to the Physician Performing Special Procedures	*1*	*1*	*0*	*2*
1. Intubation				
2. Bronchoscopy				
3. Thoracentesis				
4. Tracheostomy				
5. Chest tube insertion				
6. Moderate (conscious) sedation				

(continues)

National Board for Respiratory Care Entry Level CRT Examination Detailed Content Outline Effective Date: 7/10/2009 Open cells show an examination could include items from indicated cognitive levels. Shaded cells prevent appearance of items on examinations.	Recall	Application	Analysis	Totals
7. Cardioversion				
8. Ultrasound				
K. Initiate and Conduct Pulmonary Rehabilitation and Home Care	1	1	0	2
1. Monitor and maintain home respiratory care equipment				
2. Explain planned therapy and goals to a patient in understandable terms to achieve optimal therapeutic outcome				
3. Educate a patient and family in health management				
4. Interact with a case manager				
5. Counsel a patient and family concerning smoking cessation				
6. Instruct patient and family to assure safety and infection control				
7. Modify respiratory care procedures for use in home				
Totals	35	74	31	140

What Is On the CD

The CD included with this text provides customizable testing software to create, take, and review the chapter post-tests and mock exam as well as supplies an extensive set of links to respiratory care resources on the Internet.

HARDWARE AND SOFTWARE REQUIREMENTS

To use the resources on the CD, you must have access to a personal computer (PC) running Windows® and Internet Explorer 6 or higher. You also will need a CD-ROM drive and an SVGA color monitor with a display resolution of at least 1024×768. More details on recommended system requirements are provided on CD itself in the "ReadMe.rtf" file.

TESTING SOFTWARE

The testing software must be installed on your computer. Once installed on your computer, you will use this software to create, take, and review the chapter post-tests and mock exam.

Installation

To install the testing software, insert the CD into your CD-ROM drive. If the installation screen does not appear automatically, run D:\Setup.exe, substituting the appropriate CD-ROM drive letter if necessary. Follow the instructions for installation.

Use

After installation, you can use the testing software to create, take, and review the chapter post-tests and mock exam. To do so, click the Start button and choose Programs. Go to the *Certified Respiratory Therapist Exam Review Guide* folder and select the *CRT Exam Review Guide* icon.

Creating and Taking a Test

Once the program starts, you can create a customized chapter post-test or mock exam by clicking on the "Customize a Quiz" button at the top left side of the screen. From here, follow these three steps to create and take a quiz/test.

Step 1: Selecting the Content Area

Select the content area of the test you want to take by choosing either the desired book chapter or the "Mock Exam" topic. The question pool for the Mock Exam includes all of the questions from all of the chapters in this text. Each new quiz/test you create from a selected content area will be slightly different, since the program randomly samples questions from a pool of items.

Step 2: Choose the Number of Questions on Your Test

Use the indicator at the bottom of the page to choose exactly how many questions you would like to include on the quiz/test. The default setting is 10 questions. For chapter post-tests, we suggest choosing the following number of questions per test:

Chapter Number	Chapter Title	Suggested Post-Test Size
3	Review Data in Record	10
4	Collect & Evaluate Information	20
5	Recommend Additional Data	10
6	Manipulate Equipment	20
7	Ensure Infection Control	10
8	Perform Quality Control	10
9	Maintain Records/Communicate	10
10	Maintain Patent Airway	10
11	Remove Secretions	10
12	Achieve Respiratory Support	20
13	Evaluate Patient Responses	20
14	Modify Therapeutic Procedures	20
15	Recommend Modifications to Care	20
16	Determine Appropriateness of Care	10
17	Initiate/Modify Emergency Care	10
18	Act As an Assistant to the MD	10
19	Conduct Rehabilitation/Home Care	10
20	Cardiopulmonary Calculations	10

If you select the Mock Exam and are *not* assessing your test timing or pacing, we recommend setting it to deliver 140 questions. To assess your pacing (see Chapter 2), we recommend that you set the number of questions to 160 (140 + an extra 20 "pre-test" items) and limit your test time to 180 minutes.

Step 3: Taking a Quiz/Test

Click the "Start the Quiz" button to begin your quiz/test. For each question, click the circle (or checkbox) next to your answer choice. After you have made your selection, click the "Go to Next Question" button to proceed to the next question.

If you want to skip a question and return to it later, click on the "Bookmark" button. Clicking this button will create a "Jump to Bookmark" drop-down from which you can select and return to any skipped item. You also can use the "Previous" and "Next" buttons to navigate among the test items one-by-one.

Grading a Quiz

When you finish answering the questions to your satisfaction, click the "Grade Quiz" button located in the top menu. A new window will report your results. The left hand side of this window will display a score percentage bar chart. On the right side, you can review the individual questions and your score for that question as well as the related feedback. A red "X" indicates a wrong answer, and a green checkmark indicates a correct one.

Based on our experience, a score less than 75% correct on any post-test indicates that you need to spend additional time on that chapter's content, and/or you need to review the supplementary resources on the CD applicable to that chapter.

Exiting the Program

To quit the testing program, click the "Exit" button or select File > Exit from the main menu.

INTERNET RESOURCES

Access

The Internet resources are stored in a folder on the CD named "web_links." You can access these resources directly from the CD by opening this folder and double clicking on the applicable Internet resources file (a Web page that will open in your browser). Alternatively, you can copy the entire the "web_links" folder to your computer, where it will provide faster and more direct access to this important information.

Use

The included Internet resources files correspond to the 17 NBRC CRT content areas and carry both the corresponding book chapter and NBRC outline numbers. For example, you can review the Internet resources for Chapter 3 in this book (NBRC content area I-A) by selecting the file named *Chapter 3 (NBRC I-A)*. Alternatively, select the filename "Index" in the "web_links" folder to select from a complete list of all 17 Chapters/NBRC content areas.

Once you open an Internet resources file corresponding to a CRT content area, simply click on any of the described links to open it in your browser. All links will open in the *same window* as the Internet resources file. For this reason, to return to your Internet resources page when you finish reviewing a link, always use the "Back" button or command.

Please note that all links on the CD were verified just prior to production. However, because the Internet is a dynamic and ever-changing resource, it is possible that some of these links are no longer active. For updates to these Internet resources, visit CRTREVIEW.com (Appendix C).

JONES AND BARTLETT TECHNICAL SUPPORT

If you are having technical issues related to the use of this CD-ROM, please visit our support web site at http://www.jbpub.com/support.

Online CRT Review Course

This text, *Certified Respiratory Therapist Exam Review Guide*, evolved from an online course developed at the University of Medicine and Dentistry of New Jersey. Over the last decade, the *Online CRT Review* has helped hundreds of learners prepare for and pass the CRT exam. Beginning in 2009, this course will be available commercially on the Web at **CRTREVIEW.com**.

Like this text, the updated version of the Online CRT Review has been completely revised to include the new content tested in the most recent revision of the NBRC CRT exam. Other unique features include:

- Self-paced modular unit design—start anytime and take up to 90 days to finish.
- Available 24 hours/7 days—prepare anywhere/anytime at your convenience.
- Hundreds of prep sheets on procedures, equipment, and troubleshooting.
- Over 3,000 practice questions complete with answers and explanations.
- Unlimited practice testing on a mock exam with immediate scoring and feedback.
- Regularly updated knowledge bank of previously asked and answered questions.
- Online access to a tutor to assist you with content questions.
- One-time fee guarantee—participate until you pass the CRT exam.

Below are a few of the many unsolicited testimonials received from those who previously completed this course and passed the CRT exam:

> *"I would like to thank you and your staff for offering such a professional and well thought-out CRT Review. I would definitely recommend it to anyone over Kettering."* — C. S., Arizona

> *"I wanted to tell you I really benefited from the course and felt it was worth the money, time, and effort. I will strongly recommend it to future students."* — N. S., New Jersey

> *"Just wanted to let you know how impressed I was with this review course. The material/questions were very comprehensive. I was most impressed with the quick response time in answering questions and the thoroughness with which our questions were answered. I will definitely recommend this course to others."* — L. I., California

> *"I personally want to thank you for sharing your knowledge. This program is incredibly good. In my humble opinion, I learned more on this review than I did attending the Respiratory Care program from which I graduated. Thank you, thank you. My score was 120/140! This program took me from 88–120!"* — E. W., Texas

Purchasers of this text qualify for a special discounted enrollment fee for the Online CRT Review. For more details on the Online CRT Review and how to enroll for the reduced fee, please go to the course home page at **CRTREVIEW.com**.

Index